# THE DSM-IV PERSONALITY DISORDERS

## DIAGNOSIS AND TREATMENT
## OF MENTAL DISORDERS
### Allen Francis, *Series Editor*

# THE DSM-IV PERSONALITY DISORDERS

Edited by

## W. John Livesley

**THE GUILFORD PRESS**
New York   London

©1995 The Guilford Press
A Division of Guilford Publications, Inc.
72 Spring Street, New York, NY 10012

Printed in the United States of America

This book is printed on acid-free paper.

Last digit is print number:  9  8  7  6  5  4  3  2

**Library of Congress Cataloging-in-Publication Data**
The DSM-IV personality disorders / edited by W. John Livesley
    p.  cm.
  ISBN 0-89862-257-3
   1. Personality disorders—Classification.  2. Personality
disorders—Diagnosis.  3. Diagnostic and statistical manual
of mental disorders.  I Livesley, W. John.  II. Journal of
personality disorders.
   [DNLM: 1. Personality Disorders—diagnosis.  2. Personality
Disorders—classification.  WM 141 D811 1995]
RC554.D78  1995
616.85′8′012—dc20
DNLM/DLC
for Library of Congress                       94-25319
                                            CIP

DSM-IV is a trademark of the American Psychiatric Association.

# Preface

Over the last 15 years or so, the academic and scientific status of the study of personality disorders has changed considerably. From being a comparatively neglected area of psychopathology, personality disorders have emerged as an active and fertile field of clinical research. Slowly, a scientific understanding of these disorders is beginning to supplement earlier insights. Much of the credit for these developments must go to DSM-III. By classifying personality disorders on a separate axis, DSM-III drew attention to their clinical significance. At the same time, the decision to develop explicit diagnostic criteria for each disorder, although these were flawed and based on minimal empirical evidence, made it possible for the study of personality disorders to progress from the intuitive domain to that of more rigorous empirical analysis. The impact of these innovations can be seen in the enormous increase in articles on personality disorders; the establishment of a specialized journal, the *Journal of Personality Disorders,* devoted to the field; and an increase in specialized conferences and workshops.

## ORIGINS AND PURPOSE OF THE BOOK

This volume helps to document the growing literature on personality disorders as it relates to the DSM-IV classification. The origins of the book lie in three special issues of the *Journal of Personality Disorders* published in 1991 and 1993 that were devoted to reports from the DSM-IV Personality Disorders Work Group. These reports contained the results of detailed literature searches on given diagnoses, as well as new analyses of data sets on the performance of DSM-III-R criteria sets that were intended to provide the basis for the work group's decisions about the changes to be introduced in DSM-IV. By publishing these reports in the *Journal of Personality Disorders,* the work group hoped to keep journal readers informed about the rationale behind any changes and to involve them in the process of revision.

Three authors actively involved with these issues, Theodore Millon, M. Tracie Shea, and Thomas A. Widiger, suggested that these articles and associated commentaries from other experts be published as a separate volume. At their suggestion, Seymour Weingarten of The Guilford Press kindly invited me to be the editor. The resulting volume is organized around updated versions of the original papers and commentaries on each diagnosis. Additional sections contain new contributions that place DSM-IV in a historical and contemporary context and consider alternative approaches to the classification of personality disorders.

This volume is not intended to be a comprehensive textbook on personality disorders or a manual to guide the clinical use of the DSM-IV classification. Instead, it is intended to provide clinicians and others interested in personality disorders with an understanding of the way the DSM system evolved and why the changes made to DSM-III-R and DSM-IV came about. It also seeks to inform readers about the limitations of the DSM system and about some of the central unresolved issues in the classification of this domain of psychopathology.

The hope is that this work will contribute to the dialogue about the way personality disorders should be described and classified. It is also hoped that this volume will contribute a little to reshaping the research agenda. In recent years the field has been dominated by the DSM system, and research has focused almost entirely on the evaluation of DSM criteria sets. Alternative approaches and, equally important, conceptual research have been almost entirely neglected. Yet if the field is to progress, basic conceptual problems need to be addressed. It will not be possible to develop a valid system until some resolution is achieved on such issues as the definition of "personality disorder," the basis for distinguishing between Axis I and Axis II, the most optimal ways to represent personality disorders, and the relationsip between normal and abnormal personality. Only when these issues are addressed will it be posssible to make real progress on the contents of the classification and actual criteria. If this volume can help to stimulate debate on these issues, it will have more than fulfilled its purpose.

## PLAN OF THE BOOK

The volume is divided into four parts. Part I deals with the broader aspects of the DSM-IV classification; the two chapters that make up this part seek to place DSM-IV in its historical and contemporary context. The chapters in Part II provide in-depth reviews of each DSM-IV personality disorder diagnosis. They document the issues that the DSM-IV Personality Disorders Work Group considered important, and set out the rationale for changes in criteria sets. Part III contains similar reviews of disorders that are listed in DSM-IV Appendix B as diagnoses warranting further study; chapters are also included on diagnoses that were deleted from the classification. The chapters in Part IV provide a critical appraisal of some of the basic issues in the classification of personality disorders, and consider alternative approaches to that adopted for DSM-IV.

## Part I: The DSM-IV Classification of Personality Disorders

In the first chapter, Theodore Millon and Roger Davis untangle some of the complex and intertwined roots of current diagnostic concepts. They show how the current approach to classification and the diagnostic concepts included in DSM-IV have emerged from the contributions of the alienists, from classical psychopathology and phenomenology, from psychoanalytic thought, and from social learning theory. These diverse origins have created a system that is rich in ideas and understanding, and at the same time somewhat unwieldy and lacking in theoretical coherence.

In the second chapter, Peter Tyrer examines DSM-IV from a contemporary European perspective, and reminds us that the relatively uncritical acceptance of the system by North American psychiatry is not universal. Together, these chapters set the stage for a critical consideration of individual diagnoses. They remind us not only of the complex theoretical perspectives that have influenced the contents of DSM-IV, but also of the compromises that were required to formulate a system likely to gain widespread acceptability, as well as of the basic problems still to be addressed.

## Part II: DSM-IV Personality Disorder Diagnoses

Again, the chapters in Part II describe the 10 specific diagnoses listed in DSM-IV. As described above, many of these chapters are based on articles that first appeared in the special issues of the *Journal of Personality Disorders* devoted to the work group's reports. It was decided early in the DSM-IV process that a conservative approach would be adopted and that any changes would be minimal. For this reason, the process of revision in DSM-IV was different from that employed for earlier editions: Greater emphasis was placed on basing changes on evidence compiled from several sources. Concern has often been expressed that there was little theoretical or empirical justification provided for the selection of diagnoses and criteria sets in DSM-III or for the changes made in DSM-III-R. It was decided that this limitation would be remedied in DSM IV and that substantial documentation would be required to justify any proposed revisions. It was hoped that this requirement would open the process of revision to public scrutiny, and would also safeguard against arbitrary changes based on idiosyncratic opinions and political considerations.

Three sources of information provided the basis for the work group's deliberations: (1) a systematic review of the literature, organized around specific questions that the work group identified for each diagnosis; (2) reanalyses of existing data sets to provide additional information on criteria performance; and (3) field trials to evaluate the effectiveness of proposed revisions. The chapters in this section document this information. Each is organized in a similar way: The issues that the work group considered significant are listed, and the literature relevant to these issues is then presented, followed by recommendations for DSM-IV. In each chapter, a table is also provided for the reader's convenience that lists DSM-III-R and DSM-IV diagnostic criteria.

The significant issues addressed by the literature review vary a little across diagnoses, because some issues are specific to a given diagnosis or cluster of diagnoses. There is also considerable commonality, however, because issues such as diagnostic overlap, criterion performance, and diagnostic validity are fundamental problems that have not yet been solved for any personality diagnosis. All literature reviews were based on computer searches of the post-DSM-III literature, and in most cases this search was supplemented by a review of earlier sources. In addition, unpublished data were examined, and other data sets were reanalyzed to answer specific questions about criteria performance. The third component of the review process was the use of field trials to evaluate the effects of proposed changes. In the case of personality disorders, the only field trial that was conducted concerned antisocial personality disorder, and the results are described in Chapter 6.

These review chapters indicate plainly that one of the strengths of the DSM-IV process has been the importance placed on providing empirical evidence to support proposed changes. In Part II we see very clearly the major changes that have occurred in the study of personality disorders over the last decade and a half. The clinical-intuitive approach to understanding personality disorder has gradually been supplemented by empirical analysis. As a result, diagnostic concepts are less dependent on the insights of highly perceptive individual clinicians and more dependent on the results of empirical inquiry.

The literature reviews and reanalyses of the data were intended to provide the work group with objective information on which to base their conclusions. Such an objective is of course unattainable; inevitably, individual opinions and points of view influence the way literature is reviewed and interpreted. At the same time, the work group's interpretation of this material was also open to influences and pressures of various kinds. For this reason, it was decided that it would be interesting to ask experts who were not part of the DSM-IV process for their opinions about the outcome. Part II therefore includes commentaries by one or more experts on the DSM-IV diagnostic concepts and criteria sets. For most diagnoses the opinion of a single expert was obtained, but for the more controversial diagnoses (i.e., antisocial and borderline personality disorders), opinions were obtained from several experts who hold very different views. The commentaries contain interesting and at times controversial opinions. Sometimes they endorse the work group's conclusions and recommendations, but on occasions very different conclusions are drawn. They provide a useful reminder that DSM-IV is not the last word on the classification of personality disorders and that much has yet to be accomplished before a valid system will be achieved.

## Part III: Appended and Deleted Diagnoses

The DSM-IV classification of personality disorders has introduced several substantial changes. First, a new diagnosis, depressive personality disorder, has been included in Appendix B of DSM-IV for further study. Phillips, Hirschfeld, Shea, and Gunderson (Chapter 13) argue in support of this inclusion, based in the historical literature and empirical evidence. But as the commentary by McLean and Woody makes clear, the proposal promises to be extremely controversial.

A second change in DSM-IV is that passive–aggressive personality disorder has been moved from the main text to Appendix B for further study; at the same time, the diagnosis has been redefined to include a wider range of behaviors. The concept of passive–aggressive personality disorder, as discussed by Millon and Radovanov in Chapter 14, has been problematic since it was formally recognized in DSM-III. A major problem has been the fact that the diagnostic criteria cover a rather circumscribed set of behaviors that are associated with most personality disorders, rather than specific to a given disorder. This was recognized at the time in the DSM-III text, which stated that the diagnosis should not be made if any other personality disorder was present. This restriction was deleted from DSM-III-R. Concerns about the diagnosis, however, continued, leading to the proposal for a new diagnosis—negativistic personality disorder. (In the end, the new name was added in parentheses to the old one.) As Millon and Radovanov show, a strong case can be made for the reconceptualized disorder, although the evidence was not considered strong enough to justify its inclusion in the main text.

The other three chapters in Part III deal with two diagnoses—sadistic and self-defeating personality disorders (Chapters 15 and 16)—that were listed in the appendix to DSM-III-R but deleted from DSM-IV. They are included in this volume so that readers can be informed of the reasons for these decisions. Chapter 17, by Thomas Widiger, clearly enunciates the factors that led to the work group's recommendations. The chapters on these diagnoses are also included because many clinicians find these concepts useful in their clinical practice and may wish to decide for themselves whether the work group's decisions were justified.

## Part IV: Basic Issues and Alternative Perspectives

The reader will note several themes running through the reviews of specific disorders and the associated commentaries in Parts II and III. These themes include the question of the distinctiveness of diagnostic concepts, the relationships between and among diagnoses, and the appropriateness of the categorical approach to the classification of personality disorders. At the heart of these concerns is the validity not only of individual diagnostic concepts, but of the DSM approach to the classification of personality disorder. It will be apparent to readers that although considerable progress has been made

in the study of this important form of psychopathology, we are still a long
way from formulating a convincing system, and that there are many conceptual and empirical problems to be solved. The chapters in Part IV examine
some of these basic problems and consider alternatives to the approach so
firmly espoused by successive DSM committees. In doing so, they begin to
ask the question of how the DSM-V classification will be structured. By emphasizing conceptual and theoretical issues, these chapters nicely complement the empirical emphasis seen in Parts II and III.

Chapter 18 by Davis and Millon, provides an important introduction
to Part IV by reminding us of the vital importance of theory. Their chapter
contains the important message that not only must a classification of personality disorders provide a description of psychopathology that predicts
important clinical outcomes; it must also contribute to a theoretical understanding of these behaviors and possess theoretical coherence. Tracie Shea
examines the problem of diagnostic overlap in Chapter 19, and in so doing
raises the important issue of the nature and definition of the constructs underlying each diagnosis. This brings to the fore the question of categorical
versus dimensional approaches to classification, which is raised by most of
the commentators in Parts II and III.

Blashfield and McElroy continue to examine this issue in Chapter 20,
and point out some of the confusions that exist about the nature of dimensional and categorical models. They make the important point that these
models are not necessary incompatible. In Chapter 21, Schwartz, Wiggins,
and Norko pursue the issue of classificatory models from a different perspective, arguing strongly for a return to classical psychopathology. Their
argument that many current approaches to classification result in diagnos-
t c concepts that are little more than lists of characteristics reminds us not
to lose sight of the fact that "personality" refers to the coherence and integration of behavior, and that our task is to develop concepts that allow us to
understand the individual.

Widiger and Sanderson discuss dimensional models in depth in Chapter 22, and advocate adoption of the increasingly popular five factor model
to classify personality disorder. In Chapter 23, Jackson and I continue the
discussion of dimensional approaches and suggest that future revisions make
greater use of the psychological assessment methodology, both to develop
and evaluate the system and to examine empirically the evidence for categorical and dimensional models. We also build on Blashfield and McElroy's
point that dimensional and categorical models are not incompatible by showing how a dimensional system can be used to identify clinically meaningful
types. In Chapter 24 Lee Anna Clark provides an overview of the chapters
in Part IV, and seeks to identify underlying theories and to reconcile differences and inconsistencies. Finally, the concluding chapter seeks to identify
the more important achievements in the classification of personality disorders and to highlight future directions for classification research.

W. JOHN LIVESLEY

# Contributors

**Elizabeth Baerg, MD,** Department of Psychiatry, University of British Columbia, Vancouver, British Columbia

**David P. Bernstein, PhD,** Department of Veterans Affairs Medical Center, Bronx, New York; Mount Sinai School of Medicine, New York, New York

**Roger K. Blashfield, PhD,** Department of Psychiatry, College of Medicine, University of Florida, Gainesville, Florida

**Nancy Blum, MSW,** Department of Psychiatry, College of Medicine, University of Iowa, Iowa City, Iowa

**Lee Anna Clark, PhD,** Department of Psychology, College of Medicine, University of Iowa, Iowa City, Iowa

**Elizabeth M. Corbitt, PhD,** Department of Psychiatry, Western Psychiatric Institute and Clinic, Pittsburgh, Pennsylvania

**Alv A. Dahl, MD,** Department of Psychiatry, University of Oslo, Norway

**Roger Davis, MSc,** Department of Psychology, University of Miami, Coral Gables, Florida

**Susan J. Fiester, MD,** Private practice, Chevy Chase, Maryland

**Martha Gay, MD,** Department of Psychiatry, University of Colorado Health Sciences Center, Denver, Colorado

**John G. Gunderson, MD,** Personality and Psychosocial Research Program, McLean Hospital, Belmont, Massachusetts

**Robert D. Hare, PhD,** Department of Psychology, University of British Columbia, Vancouver, British Columbia

**Stephen D. Hart, PhD,** Mental Health, Law, and Policy Institute, Simon Fraser University, Burnaby, British Columbia

**Robert M. A. Hirschfeld, MD,** Department of Psychiatry and Behavioral Sciences, University of Texas Medical Branch, Galveston, Texas

**Douglas N. Jackson, PhD,** Department of Psychology, University of Western Ontario, London, Ontario

**Oren Kalus, MD,** Department of Veterans Affairs Medical Center, Bronx, New York; Mount Sinai School of Medicine, New York, New York

**Cassandra L. Kisiel, BA,** Personality and Psychosocial Research Program, McLean Hospital, Belmont, Massachusetts

**W. John Livesley, MD, PhD,** Department of Psychiatry, University of British Columbia, Vancouver, British Columbia

**Alexandra Martinez, MA,** Department of Psychology, University of Miami, Coral Gables, Florida

**Ross A. McElroy, PhD,** Department of Psychiatry, University of Florida, Gainesville, Florida

**Peter McLean, PhD,** Department of Psychiatry, University of British Columbia, Vancouver, British Columbia

**Harold Merskey, MD,** Department of Psychiatry, Robarts Research Institute, University of Western Ontario, London, Ontario; London Psychiatric Hospital, London, Ontario

**Theodore Millon, PhD,** Departments of Psychology and Psychiatry, University of Miami, Coral Gables, Florida; Harvard Medical School, Boston, Massachusetts

**Michael A. Norko, MD,** Department of Psychiatry, Yale University School of Medicine, New Haven, Connecticut

**Joel Paris, MD,** Department of Psychiatry, McGill University, Montreal, Quebec

**Bruce Pfohl, MD,** Department of Psychiatry, University of Iowa, Iowa City, Iowa

**Katharine A. Phillips, MD,** Personality and Psychosocial Research Program, McLean Hospital, Belmont, Massachusetts; Harvard Medical School, Boston, Massachusetts

**Paul A. Pilkonis, PhD,** Department of Psychiatry, Western Psychiatric Institute and Clinic, University of Pittsburgh School of Medicine, Pittsburgh, Pennsylvania

**Jerrold M. Pollak, PhD,** Department of Psychiatry, Rhode Island Hospital; Department of Psychiatry and Human Behavior, Brown University School of Medicine, Providence, Rhode Island

**Jelena Radovanov, MSc,** Department of Psychology, University of Miami, Coral Gables, Florida

**Lee Robins, PhD,** Department of Psychiatry, Washington University School of Medicine, St. Louis, Missouri

**Elsa Ronningstam, MD,** Personality and Psychosocial Research Program, McLean Hospital, Belmont, Massachusetts

**Cynthia J. Sanderson, PhD,** Division of Psychology, Cornell University Medical College, New York, New York

**Michael A. Schwartz, MD,** Department of Psychiatry, Case Western Reserve; University Hospitals of Cleveland, Cleveland, Ohio

**M. Tracie Shea, PhD,** Department of Psychiatry and Human Behavior, Brown University; Veterans Administration Medical Center, Providence, Rhode Island

**Larry J. Siever, MD,** Department of Veterans Affairs Medical Center, Bronx, New York; Mount Sinai School of Medicine, New York, New York

**Jeremy M. Silverman, PhD,** Department of Veterans Affairs Medical Center, Bronx, New York; Mount Sinai School of Medicine, New York, New York

**Lauren E. Smith, BA,** Personality and Psychosocial Research Program, McLean Hospital, Belmont, Massachusetts

**Steven Taylor, PhD,** Department of Psychiatry, University of British Columbia, Vancouver, British Columbia

**Svenn Torgersen, MD,** Center for Research in Clinical and Applied Psychology, Department of Psychology, University of Oslo, Norway

**Peter Tyrer, MD,** Academic Unit of Psychiatry, St. Mary's Hospital Medical School, London, England

**David Useda, BA,** Department of Psychology, University of Missouri, Columbia, Missouri

**Richard Weise, MEd,** Mood, Anxiety, and Personality Disorders Branch, National Institute of Mental Health, Bethesda, Maryland

**Thomas A. Widiger, PhD,** Department of Psychology, University of Kentucky, Lexington, Kentucky

**Osborne P. Wiggins, PhD,** Department of Philosophy, University of Louisville, Louisville, Kentucky

**Sheila Woody, PhD,** Department of Psychiatry, University of British Columbia, Vancouver, British Columbia

**Mary C. Zanarini, EdD,** Personality and Psychosocial Research Program, McLean Hospital, Belmont, Massachusetts

# Contents

## III. Appended and Deleted Diagnoses

## Part IV. Basic Issues and Alternative Perspectives

# THE DSM-IV PERSONALITY DISORDERS

# PART I

# THE DSM-IV CLASSIFICATION OF PERSONALITY DISORDERS

# CHAPTER 1

# Conceptions of Personality Disorders: Historical Perspectives, the DSMs, and Future Directions

THEODORE MILLON
ROGER DAVIS

Current conceptions of personality disorders are the result of a long and continuing history. Despite the desultory nature of our path to knowledge, there appear to be certain themes and concepts to which clinicians, researchers, and theorists return time and again; these are noted as the discussion proceeds in this chapter. Commonalities notwithstanding, the classification schemas to be summarized here represent different notions concerning which data are important to observe and how they should best be organized to represent personality.

It is not the intent of this chapter to enable the reader to master the details of personality disorder classification. The purpose is simply that of outlining the diverse formulations into which personality pathology has been cast through history. Much is to be gained by reading original or primary sources, but the aim of this synopsis is to distill the essentials of what clinicians have written and to present them as an orientation to the personality syndromes described in later chapters.

## HISTORICAL PERSPECTIVES

The history of formal personality characterization can be traced to the early Greeks. A survey of these notions can be found in the detailed reviews published by Roback (1927), Allport (1937), and Millon (1981). Given these fine secondary sources, there is no reason to record here any but the most central concepts of these early characterologists. Also worthy of brief mention are those who may be considered the forerunners of contemporary systems of classification.

"Character writing," a minor literary style originating in Athens, probably invented by Aristotle, was brought to its finest and most brilliant form through the pen of Theophrastus. Presented as "verbal" portraits, these depictions of character were brief sketches that captured certain common types so aptly as to be identified and appreciated by readers in all walks of life. In these crisp delineations, a dominant trait was brought to the forefront, and accentuated and embellished to highlight the major flaws or foibles of the individual. In essence, they were stylized simplifications that often bordered on the precious or burlesque.

For all its graphic and compelling qualities, literary characterology was a limited and often misleading form of personality description. In the hands of an astute observer, sensitive to the subtleties and contradictions of behavior, such portrayals provided a pithy analysis of both the humor and anguish of personal functioning. However, the very unique and picturesque quality of the presentations drew attention to the fascinating, and away from the mundane behaviors that typify everyday human conduct. The first explanatory system to specify personality dimensions is likely to have been the doctrine of bodily humors posited by the early Greeks some 25 centuries ago. Interestingly, history appears to have come full circle. The humoral doctrine sought to explain personality with reference to alleged body fluids, whereas much of contemporary psychiatry seeks answers with biochemical and endocrinological hypotheses.

In the 4th century B.C., Hippocrates described all disease as stemming from an excess of or imbalance among four bodily humors: yellow bile, black bile, blood, and phlegm. The humors were believed to be the embodiments of earth, water, fire, and air—the basic components of the universe, according to the philosopher Empedocles. Hippocrates identified four basic temperaments, the choleric, melancholic, sanguine, and phlegmatic; he saw these as corresponding, respectively, to excesses in yellow bile, black bile, blood, and phlegm. The Hippocratic system was modified by Galen centuries later. Galen associated the choleric temperament with a tendency toward irascibility, the sanguine temperament with a leaning toward optimism, the melancholic temperament with an inclination toward sadness, and the phlegmatic temperament with an apathetic disposition. Although the doctrine of humors has long since been abandoned, giving way to scientific studies on topics such as neurohormone chemistry, its terminology and connotations still persist in such contemporary expressions as being "sanguine" or "good-humored."

The ancients speculated also that body structure is associated with the character of personality. Whereas the humoral doctrine may be seen as the forerunner of contemporary psychiatric endocrinology, phrenology and physiognomy may be conceived as the forerunners of modern psychiatric morphology. Physiognomy, first recorded in the writings of Aristotle, sought to identify personality characteristics by outward appearances, particularly facial configurations and expressions. People have sought to appraise others throughout history by observing their countenances, the play in their faces, and the cast of their eyes, as well as their postural attitudes and the style of their movements. It was not until the late 18th century, however, that the first systematic effort was made to analyze external morphology and its relation to psychological functions. Despite the uses that some unscrupulous practitioners made of it, phrenology, as practiced by Franz Josef Gall, was an honest and serious attempt to construct a science of personology. Although Gall referred to his studies of "brain physiology" as "organology" and "cranioscopy," the term "phrenology," coined by a younger associate, came to be its popular designation. The rationale that Gall presented for measuring contour variations of the skull was not at all illogical, given the limited knowledge of 18th-century anatomy. In fact, his work signified an important advance over the naive and subjective studies of physiognomy of his time, in that he sought to employ objective and quantitative methods to deduce the inner structure of the brain. Seeking to decipher personality characteristics by their ostensible correlations with the nervous system, he was among the first to claim that a direct relationship exists between mind and body. Contending that the brain is the central organ of thought and emotion, Gall concluded, quite reasonably, that both the intensity and character of thoughts and emotions should correlate with variations in the size and shape of the brain or its encasement, the cranium. That these assertions proved invalid should not be surprising when we recognize, as we do today, the exceedingly complex structure of neuroanatomy and its tangential status as a substrate for personality functions. Despite the now transparent weaknesses of Gall's system, he was the first to attempt a reasoned thesis for the view that personality characteristics may correlate with body structure.

The first clear presentation of the clinical features of personality arose when psychiatrists at the end of the 18th century were drawn into age-old arguments concerning free will and whether certain moral transgressors are capable of "understanding" the consequences of their acts. It was Philippe Pinel (1801, 1806), referring to a form of madness known at the time as *la folie raisonnante*, who observed that certain of his patients engaged in impulsive and self-damaging acts, despite the fact that their reasoning abilities were unimpaired and they fully grasped the irrationality of what they were doing. Describing these cases under the name *mania sans délire* ("insanity without delirium"), Pinel was among the first to recognize that madness need not signify the presence of a deficit in reasoning powers. As he described it in 1801,

> I was not a little surprised to find many maniacs who at no period gave evidence of any lesion of understanding, but who were under the dominion of instinctive and abstract fury, as if the faculties of affect alone had sustained injury.

Until Pinel forcefully argued the legitimacy of this psychopathological entity, it was universally held that all mental disorders were disorders of the mind;

since mind was equated with reason, only a disintegration in the faculties of reason and intellect would be judged as insanity. However, beginning with Pinel there arose the belief that one could be insane (*mania*) without a confusion of mind (*sans délire*).

Benjamin Rush, the well-known American physician, wrote in the early 1800s of similar perplexing cases characterized by lucidity of thought combined with socially deranged behaviors. He spoke of these individuals as possessing an "innate, preternatural moral depravity" in which "there is probably an original defective organization in those parts of the body which are preoccupied by the moral faculties of the mind" (1812, p. 112). Rush appears to have been the first theorist to have taken Pinel's morally neutral clinical observation of defects in "passion and affect" and turned it into a social condemnation. He claimed that such individuals display a lifelong pattern of irresponsibility without a corresponding feeling of shame or hesitation over the personally destructive consequences of their actions. Describing the features characterizing this type, Rush wrote:

> The will might be deranged even in many instances of persons of sound understandings . . . the will becoming the involuntary vehicle of vicious actions through the instrumentality of the passions. Persons thus diseased cannot speak the truth upon any subject. . . . Their falsehoods are seldom calculated to injure anybody but themselves. (1812, p. 124)

As evident from the dates mentioned in the preceding paragraphs, the British alienist J. C. Prichard (1835) — credited by many as having been the first to formulate the concept of "moral insanity" — was in fact preceded in this realization by several theorists; nevertheless, he was the first to label it as such and to give it wide readership in English-speaking nations. Although he accepted Pinel's notion of *mania sans délire,* he dissented from Pinel's morally neutral attitude toward these disorders, and became the major exponent of the view that these behaviors signify a reprehensible defect in character that deserves social condemnation. He also broadened the scope of the original syndrome by including under the label "moral insanity" a wide range of previously diverse mental and emotional conditions. According to Prichard, all such individuals share a common defect in the power to guide themselves in accord with "natural feelings" — that is, a spontaneous and intrinsic sense of rightness, goodness, and responsibility. Those afflicted by this disease are swayed, despite their ability to intellectually understand the choices before them, by overpowering "affections" that compelled them to engage in socially repugnant behaviors.

Whereas "moral insanity" appeared to address defects of the male gender primarily, Ernst von Feuchtersleben (1847) depicted the female gender as disposed to hysterical symptoms as being sexually heightened, selfish, and "overprivileged with satiety and boredom." Attributing these traits to the unfortunate nature of female education, he wrote: "It combines everything that can heighten sensibility, weaken spontaneity, give a preponderance to the sexual sphere, and sanction the feelings and impulse that relate to it." Less oriented to matters of sexuality, Wilhem Griesinger (1845), the major psychiatric nosologist of mid-19th-century Germany, wrote that his hysterical women patients displayed an "immoderate sensitiveness, especially to the slightest reproach in which there is a tendency to refer everything to themselves, great irritability, great change of disposition on the least, or even from no, external motive." Among other distinguishing characteristics, according to Griesinger, were their volatile humor; their senseless caprices; and their inclination to deception, prevarication, jealousy, and malice.

　　Two major strands of thinking concerning personality types emerged in the early 20th century. On the one hand, there were the classical descriptive psychiatrists, such as Kraepelin, Bleuler, Kretschmer, and Schneider; on the other, there were those of a psychoanalytic persuasion, notably Freud, Abraham, and Reich. Despite their chronological overlap, they are separated here for purposes of considering their views of personality.

　　The prime psychiatric nosologist at the turn of the century, Emil Kraepelin, did not systematize his thinking on personality disorders until the third volume of the eighth edition of his major text, published in 1913. Until then, Kraepelin paid only scant attention to personality disturbances, concentrating his organizing efforts on the two major syndromes of "dementia praecox" and "maniacal–depressive insanity." In his efforts to trace the early course of these syndromes, Kraepelin "uncovered" two premorbid types: the "cyclothymic disposition," exhibited in four variants, each inclined to maniacal–depressive insanity; and the "autistic temperament," notably disposed to dementia praecox. In addition, Kraepelin wrote on a number of so-called "morbid personalities," those whom he judged as tending toward criminality and other dissolute activities. Kraepelin's autistic temperament serves as the constitutional soil for the development of dementia praecox. The most fundamental trait of this type is a narrowing or reduction of external interests and an increasing preoccupation with inner ruminations. Of particular note was Kraepelin's (1919) observation that children of this temperament frequently "exhibited a quiet, shy, retiring disposition, made no friendships, and lived only for themselves" (p. 109). They were disinclined to be open and become involved with others, were seclusive, and had difficulty adapting to new situations. They showed little interest in what went on about them; often refrained from participating in games and other pleasures; seemed resistant to influence (but in a passive rather than active way); and were inclined to withdraw increasingly in a world of their own fantasies.

　　In his eighth edition of the monumental *Lehrbuch* (1909–1915), Kraepelin began to formulate a number of subaffective personality conditions that are quite comparable to current borderline criteria. The "irritable temperament," elsewhere described by Kraepelin as the "excitable personality," was conceived as a "mixture of the fundamental states." It parallels the borderline features closely, as illustrated in the following excerpts from Kraepelin (1921):

The patients display from youth up extraordinarily great fluctuations in emotional equilibrium and are greatly moved by all experiences, frequently in an unpleasant way. . . . They flare up, and on the most trivial occasions fall into outbursts of boundless fury.

The colouring of mood is subject to frequent change . . . periods are interpolated in which they are irritable and ill-humoured, also perhaps sad, spiritless, anxious, they shed tears without cause, give expression to thoughts of suicide, bring forward hypochondriacal complaints, go to bed. . . .

They are mostly very distractible and unsteady in their endeavours.

In consequence· of their irritability and their changing moods their conduct of life is subject to the most multifarious incidents, they make sudden resolves, and carry them out on the spot, run off abruptly, go abruptly, enter a cloister. (pp. 130–131)

Of special note is the extent to which Kraepelin's description encompasses the central diagnostic criteria of borderline personality disorder as conceived today, especially the impulsivity, unstable relationships, inappropriate and intense anger, affective instability, and physically self-damaging acts.

Eugen Bleuler coined the term *schizoidie* (1922, 1929) to represent a pattern of traits closely allied to Hoch's "shut-in" type and Kraepelin's "autistic personality." The tendency to "schizoidness" was seen by Bleuler as present in everyone, differing among individuals only in the quantity of its potential biological penetrance. In its clinical or schizophrenic form, this tendency achieves its full level of morbid intensity, whereas in moderate form it may assume the character of only a mild schizoid personality, described by Bleuler as "people who are shut in, suspicious, incapable of discussion, people who are comfortably dull" (1924, p. 441). Bleuler believed the "fundamental symptoms" that he spelled out as pathognomonic for schizophrenia to be found in reduced magnitude among schizoids.

Despite Bleuler's seminal contributions to the schizophrenic concept, it was Ernst Kretschmer (1925) who introduced the most subtle refinements of the schizoid character portrayal. The distinctions first posited by Kretschmer closely parallel the DSM-III differentiation between the schizoid and avoidant types. Kretschmer considered psychotic disorders to be accentuations of essentially normal personality types—a position not commonly held by the majority of his psychiatric colleagues. Thus, he saw the schizophrenic, the schizoid, and the schizothymic as possessing different quantities of the same disposition or temperament: a distinctly pathological level among schizophrenics, a moderate degree among schizoids, and a minimal amount among relatively well-adjusted schizothymics. Similarly, cycloids were viewed as moderately affected variants of those with manic–depressive psychosis, and cyclothymic personalities were seen as normal types possessing minor portions of the disposition. As for the relationship between bodily structure and temperament, Kretschmer contended that normal "asthenic" (physically thin) individuals are inclined toward introversion, timidity, and a lack of personal warmth—that is, lesser intensities of the more withdrawn and unresponsive schizophrenics to whom they are akin. Normal "pyknics" (heavy-set) are gregarious, friendly, and interpersonally dependent—that is, as less extreme variants of the moody and socially excitable manic–depressive. Although Kretschmer noted that schizoids may exhibit certain "peculiari-ties of character" and display contrasting temperaments in "different rela-tive proportions," he wrote at length about two subgroups, which he termed the "hyperaesthetic" and the "anaesthetic" schizoid types. Those in the form-er group, the hyperaesthetics, were described quite similarly to what the re-cent DSMs have labeled the avoidant personality. A few phrases are quoted below from Kretschmer to convey how this type contrasts with the anaesthetic, akin to the DSM schizoid personality. Kretschmer portrayed the hyperaesthet-ic as follows:

> Timid, shy, with fine feelings, sensitive, nervous, excitable. . . .
> Abnormally tender, constantly wounded . . . "all nerves." . . .
> [Hyperaesthetics] feel all the harsh, strong colours and tones of everyday life . . . as shrill, ugly . . . even to the extent of being psychically painful. Their autism is a painful cramping of the self into itself. They seek as far as possible to avoid and deaden all stimulation from the outside. (1925, pp. 155–161)

Descriptively, and in contrast to the hyperaesthetic/avoidant, Kretschmer por-trayed the anaesthetic/schizoid personality as follows:

> We feel that we are in contact with something flavourless, boring . . . What is there in the deep under all these masks? Perhaps there is a nothing, a dark, hollow-eyed nothing—affective anaemia. Behind an ever-silent facade, which twitches uncertainly with every expiring whim—nothing but broken pieces, black rubbish heaps, yawning emotional emptiness, or the cold breath of an arctic soullessness. (1925, p. 150)

Kurt Schneider (1923) differed from many of his contemporaries, most notably Kretschmer, in that he did not view personality pathology as a precur-sor to other mental disorders, but conceived it as a separate entity that covaried with them. In the last edition of his text on "psychopathologic per-sonalities," Schneider described the following 10 variants seen often in psy-chiatric work. "Hyperthymic" personalities reflect a mix of high activity, optimism, and shallowness; they tend to be uncritical, cocksure, impulsive, and undependable. Many seem unable to concentrate, and those who achieve occasional insights fail to retain them as lasting impressions. Those in the second category, the "depressive" personalities, have a skeptical view of life, tend to take things seriously, and display little capacity for enjoyment. They are often excessively critical and deprecatory of others; at the same time, they are full of self-reproach and exhibit hypochondriacal anxieties. "Inse-cure" personalities were grouped by Schneider into two subvarieties, the "sen-sitives" and the "anankasts" (compulsives). These individuals ruminate excessively over everyday experience, but have little capacity for expressing

or discharging the feelings these thoughts stir up. Chronically unsure of themselves, they are apt to see life as a series of unfortunate events. They tend
to behave in a strict and disciplined manner, holding closely to what is judged
as socially correct. "Fanatic" personalities are expansive individuals inclined
to be uninhibited, combative, and aggressive in promoting their views; they
are often querulous and litigious. Among the "attention-seeking" personalities are those with heightened emotional responses, who delight in novelty
and give evidence of excess enthusiasms, vivid imaginations, and a striving
to be in the limelight; showy and capricious, many are boastful and inclined
to lie and distort. "Labile" personalities do not evidence a simple chronic
emotionality, but are characterized by abrupt and volatile mood changes,
impulsive urges, sudden dislikes, and a "shiftless" immaturity. The "explosive" personality is characterized by being impulsively violent, disposed to
be fractious, and likely to become combative without warning or provoca-
tion. "Affectionless" personalities lack compassion and are often considered
callous and cold; they appear distant or indifferent to friends and strangers
alike. Historically, these patients correspond to those identified in the literature as exhibiting "moral insanity." The so-called "weak-willed" personalities are not only docile and unassuming but are easily subjected to seduction
by others and readily exploited "to no good end"; they are inevitably fated
to trouble and disillusionment. The last of Schneider's types, the "asthenic"
personality, subjects himself or herself to intense hypochondriacal scrutiny,
and is so preoccupied with bodily functions that external events fade into
the background and appear strange or unreal.

Sigmund Freud (1908, 1932), Karl Abraham (1921, 1925), and Wilhelm
Reich (1933) laid the foundation of the psychoanalytic character typology.
These categories were conceived initially as a product of frustrations or in-
dulgences of instinctual or libidinous drives especially in conjunction with
specific psychosexual stages of maturation. Freud's (1908) paper set the seeds
for psychoanalytic character types. His primary interest at that time was not
in tracing the formation of character structure, but rather in discovering
the derivatives of instincts as they evolve during particular psychosexual
stages. Although Freud noted that developmental conflicts give rise to broadly
generalized defensive tendencies, these were noted only incidentally, written largely as minor digressions from the main point of his early papers;
unlike Karl Abraham, he did not focus on character structure derivatives,
but attempted to identify the psychosexual roots of specific and narrowly
circumscribed symptoms (such as compulsions or conversions).

It was not until the writings of Wilhelm Reich in 1933 that the concept
of character appeared in its fullest psychoanalytic form. Reich asserted that
the neurotic solution of psychosexual conflicts is accomplished by a pervasive restructuring of the individual's defensive style—a set of changes that
ultimately crystallizes into what he spoke of as a "total formation" of character. In contrast to his forerunners, Reich claimed that the emergence of specific pathological symptoms is of secondary importance when compared to the

total character structuring that evolves as a consequence of these experiences. As Reich put it, "Our problem is not the content or the nature of this or that character trait" (1949, p. 46). To him, the particular defensive modes acquired in dealing with early experience become stable, even ossified, or as he put it, "a character armour." As the consolidation process hardens, the response to earlier conflicts becomes "transformed into chronic attitudes, into chronic automatic modes of reaction" (p. 46).

It may be useful at this point to briefly summarize the major character types. Organizing the various formulations that have been proposed in the psychoanalytic literature is no simple task. The most common practice (and the one followed here) differentiates types into the psychosexual stage associated with their development.

The "oral" period is usually differentiated into two phases: the "oral-sucking" phase, in which food is accepted indiscriminately, followed by the "oral-biting" phase, in which food is accepted selectively, occasionally rejected, and aggressively chewed. An overly indulgent sucking stage leads to what is frequently referred to as the "oral-dependent" type. Characteristic of these individuals is an imperturbable optimism and naive self-assurance; such persons are inclined to be happy-go-lucky and emotionally immature, in that serious matters do not seem to affect them. An ungratified sucking period is associated with excessive dependency and gullibility. For example, deprived children may learn to "swallow" anything in order to ensure that they get something; here, external supplies are all-important, but the children yearn for them passively. Frustrations experienced at the oral-biting stage typically lead to the development of aggressive oral tendencies such as sarcasm and verbal hostility in adulthood. Sometimes referred to as the "oral-sadistic" character, this person is in many ways the characterological opposite of the oral-sucking or dependent character. The basic pattern is one of pessimistic distrust, an inclination to blame the world for unpleasant matters, and a tendency to be cantankerous and petulant.

Difficulties associated with the "anal" period likewise lead to distinctive modes of adult personality. During this time, children can both control their sphincter muscles and comprehend the expectancies of their parents; for the first time in their lives, children have the power to thwart their parents' demands actively and knowingly, and they now have the option of either pleasing them or frustrating their desires. Depending on the outcome, children will adopt attitudes toward authority that will have far-reaching effects. So-called "anal" characters are quite different from each other, depending on whether their conflict resolutions occur during the "anal-expulsive" or the "anal-retentive" period. Characteristics emerging from the anal-expulsive period are primarily those of suspiciousness and megalomania; a tendency toward extreme conceit and ambitiousness; and a pattern of self-assertion, disorderliness, and negativism. Difficulties that emerge in the late anal, or anal-retentive, phase are usually associated with frugality, obstinacy, and orderliness. There is a predominance of parsimony and pedantry, a hair-splitting meticulousness, and a rigid devotion to societal rules and regula-tions. As Fenichel (1945) put it, these individuals are in constant conflict between "I want to be naughty" and "I must be good."

Although writers such as Fenichel (1945) have proposed what may be called a "urethral" character, there is little consensus that a distinct pattern exists. The most outstanding personality features attributed here are those of ambition and competitiveness, both of which are presumed to be reac-tions against feelings of shame and inadequacy.

The next major psychosexual phase in which a distinct set of character types are associated is the so-called "phallic stage." This period of psychosexual development is one that Reich (1933) conceived as troubled by narcissistic sexuality. Although libidinal impulses are normally directed toward the op-posite sex, they may become excessively self-oriented. Either intense frus-tration or overindulgence during this period of need for genital contact may produce conflict and defensive armouring. As a result, according to Reich, there will be a striving for leadership, a need to stand out in a group, and poor reactions to even minor "defeats." This phallic narcissistic character was depicted by Reich as vain, brash, arrogant, self-confident, vigorous, cold, reserved, and defensively aggressive. If these persons succeed in gaining the attentions of others, they often become delightful and spontaneous high achievers; conversely, if they are not greatly appreciated or sought after, they are inclined to downgrade themselves or to become exhibitionistic and provocative.

In early analytic theory, the "genital" stage was viewed as the pinnacle of maturity, the attainment of a fully socialized and adjusted adult. However, Reich, in disagreement with other analysts, saw two pathological complica-tions associated with this final period: the "hysterical" and the "masochistic" characters. Among the hysterical characters are people fixated at the geni-tal level, who have little inclination to sublimate their impulses and are preoc-cupied with sexual excitations and discharge. They are noted by a characteristic fearfulness and skittishness, a pseudoseductiveness, interper-sonal superficiality and flightiness, and an inability to sustain endeavors. In what he referred to as the masochistic character, Reich described a pattern resulting from the repression of exhibitionistic tendencies during the geni-tal stage. The masochist is characterized by self-criticism, a querulous dis-position, and a habit of tormenting both self and others. The masochist, however, is in a terrible bind. Love and affection are sought but result in pain; by making themselves unlovable, masochists avoid pain, but as a con-sequence prevent themselves from achieving the love they desire.

Karen Horney's descriptive eloquence is perhaps without peer; neverthe-less, difficulties arise in attempting to summarize what she refers to as the major "solutions" to life's basic conflicts. Although her primary publications were written over a short period, she utilized different terms to represent similar conceptions (Horney, 1937, 1939, 1942, 1945, 1950). An attempt is made here to synthesize these diverse formulations, albeit briefly. When a person is faced with the insecurities and inevitable frustrations of life, Horney identified three broad modes of relating that will emerge: "moving toward" people, "moving against" people, or "moving away" from them. In her 1945 book, Horney formulated three character types to reflect these solutions: Moving toward is found in a "compliant" type; moving against, in an "aggressive" type; and moving away, in a "detached" type. In 1950, Horney reconceptualized her typology in line with the manner in which individuals solve intrapsychic conflicts. Corresponding roughly to the prior trichotomies, they were termed the "self-effacement" solution, the "expansive" solution, and the solution of "neurotic resignation." Although these sets of three do not match perfectly, they do correspond to the essential themes of Horney's characterology.

Although central to the development of the interpersonal orientation in psychiatry, the personality typology presented by Harry Stack Sullivan (1947) may best be grouped with that of Schneider, in that both are atheoretical, comprise 10 varieties, and attempt to identify syndromes seen in everyday clinical practice. The first type, labeled the "nonintegrative" personality, is characterized by fleeting involvements with people, a failure to profit from experience, and a disregard for the consequences of one's behavior; these individuals constantly disappoint others by their superficiality and wandering inclinations, but this does not dispose them to experience discontent or to wonder why others react as they do. The second of Sullivan's syndromes, termed the "self-absorbed" or "fantastic" personality, is characterized by autistic and wish-fulfilling thinking. Conflicted as to whether the world is essentially "good" or "bad," these persons see relationships as either marvelous or despicable; they engage in a series of intimacies that inevitably terminate in profound disillusionment, only to be sought after and repeated again. The "incorrigible" personality is identified by hostility toward others and a pattern of unfriendly, morose, and forbidding behaviors. Authority is viewed as especially hostile, and there is a tendency to complain bitterly about those in superior positions. The fourth syndrome is termed the "negativistic" personality; these individuals cope with their considerable insecurity by refusing to subscribe to the views of others, by passively or subtly resisting social norms, or by engaging in a cynical form of conciliation. The fifth type, which Sullivan conceives as a supernegativistic variety, is termed the "stammerer"; stammering is perceived as a symptom disorder by most theorists, and Sullivan offers little reason for categorizing stammerers as a personality type. "Ambition-ridden" personalities are noted by their exploitation of others, their competitiveness, and their unscrupulous manipulations. Those with the seventh syndrome, "asocial" personalities, are typically detached and lonely, unable to establish and maintain warm and gratifying personal relationships. They seem unable to appreciate the possibility that others may value them; though some asocials are sensitive, others seem obtuse and drift through life without intimate relationships. The "inadequate" personality is distinguished by a need for guidance from a strong person who will take responsibility for everyday decisions; these persons appear to have learned that a clinging helplessness is an adequate adaptation to life. The ninth syndrome is labeled by Sullivan the "homosexual" personality; its distinguishing feature is that love appears to extend only to persons of the same sex. Here, again, Sullivan has identified a specific symptom with the totality of a personality. The final syndrome is labeled the "chronically adolescent" personality. These individuals are perennially seeking to achieve ideals, but rarely are able to fulfill their aspirations in either love objects or mature vocations; some will ultimately resolve their frustrations, whereas some will become cynical, others will turn lustful or celibate, and so on.

## THE DSMs

Classificatory confusion reigned in the late 1940s as clinicians found it necessary to employ different systems for different purposes — one nomenclature for hospitalized patients, another taxonomy for statistical reporting, a third for disability coverage, and so on. Compounding this polyglot were the idiosyncratic modifications and syntheses proposed by clinicians who had returned from their diverse military experiences, each seeking to persuade their equally enthusiastic colleagues of the validity of some new syndromal entity or the applicability of some innovative classification system.

So great a diversity as this necessitated action on the part of the American Psychiatric Association (APA). Accordingly, the APA Board of Trustees requested that its Committee on Nomenclature and Statistics review the utility of the major taxonomies then in use. Disorders of personality, transient stress reactions, and organic brain disease were the realms in which primary deficits were noted. Further recommendations were obtained from leading university and hospital training centers as well as from those who had been engaged in developing the armed forces and Veterans Administrations nomenclatures. The committee was further charged with the task of preparing a separate and new *Diagnostic and Statistical Manual of Mental Disorders*. First published in 1952, this manual has retrospectively been referred to as DSM-I (American Psychiatric Association, 1952).

### DSM-I

In the first official DSM, the broad category of "personality disorders" subsumed five subclasses — namely, personality pattern disturbances, personality trait disturbances, sociopathic personality disturbance, special symptom reactions, and transient situational personality disorders. Each of these encompassed several subvarieties. All of these disorders ostensibly reflected developmental defects with minimal subjective anxiety and little or no personal distress. Most characteristic was a lifelong pattern of action or behavior rather than emotional symptomatology. The personality pattern disturbances were considered deep-seated and rarely alterable by therapy; they included the inadequate, schizoid, cyclothymic, and paranoid personalities. The second broad category, personality trait disturbances, typified individuals who were unable to maintain their emotional equilibrium under conditions of minor or major stress. It included what were termed the emotionally unstable, the passive–aggressive (with subvariants), and the compulsive. Sociopathic disturbances signified characteristics conflicting with the prevailing cultural milieu and its conventions; subsumed here were not only overt antisocial behaviors, but acts of a socially unacceptable nature, such as homosexuality and alcoholism.

Although listed under the personality disorder grouping, both the special symptom reactions and transient disorders were not personality pathologies in the sense we currently view them; they included disturbances such as enuresis, learning deficiencies, and posttraumatic stress disorders.

## DSM-II

The formal and intimate involvement of the APA in the construction of the eighth revision of the *International Classification of Diseases* (ICD-8) was a potent factor in motivating the organization to refashion its DSM-I in a manner fully compatible with the new international nosology. Hence, shortly following approval of what was to be the ICD-8 at the World Health Organization's International Revision Conference in 1965, the APA reactivated its Committee on Nomenclature and Statistics. With its tasks clearly defined, the committee was able to submit, as early as 1967, an initial draft of the new DSM-II for review and comment to a select group of 120 psychiatrists. Suggestions for revision were received, collated, and incorporated in a mid-1967 final draft manuscript. This proposal was submitted to the APA Executive Committee, where it was approved in late 1967 and subsequently published in 1968 as DSM-II.

A paragraph or two comparing the DSM-I and the DSM-II may be useful as a précis for later discussions on both the character of, and the extensive changes introduced in, DSM-III. Notable among the conceptual innovations was the DSM-II committee's decision to avoid terms that implied acceptance of a particular theoretical viewpoint, especially with regard to syndromes, where matters of causality were notably controversial. Among other DSM-II modifications was the judgment to disband the functionally irrelevant distinction that had been drawn in DSM-I between personality trait and personality pattern disturbances; both were now to be grouped under the heading of "personality disorders." New personality syndromes were added to the list, while others were eliminated. Furthermore, the transient situational disorders and the special symptom reactions were retitled and transferred elsewhere in the classification schema. Only the antisocial personality designation of the DSM-I sociopathic group remained in the personality disorder section; both sexual deviations and alcoholism headed up their own categorical groups. An important shift in the characterization of personality disorders was made when the assumption of emotional indifference was no longer a defining attribute of the personality disturbances. In contrast to DSM-I, DSM-II clearly stipulated that these disorders must involve both impaired functioning and personally experienced distress. Also stipulated was the expectancy that these diagnoses had to be qualitatively different and essentially nonoverlapping with either neurotic or psychotic disorders. Added to the personality list were two new disorders, the asthenic and explosive personalities.

## DSM-III

In addition to the framework they constructed to give it shape and structure, the DSM-III Task Force's members shared a number of implicit values as well as explicit goals that guided their review of the text and criteria drafts. They recognized that no ideal classification was possible in clinical psychopathology; that all nosological systems would be imperfect; and that, regardless of what advances were made in knowledge and theory, the substantive and professional character of mental health would be simply too multidimensional in structure and too multivariate in function ever to lend itself to a single, fully satisfactory system. It was acknowledged also that no consensus was likely ever to be found among either psychiatrists or psychologists as to how a classification might be best organized (e.g., dimensions, categories, observable qualities), much less what it should contain (etiology, prognosis, structure, severity).

In the light of the foregoing, the DSM-III Task Force agreed to take an explicitly nondoctrinaire approach—not only by avoiding the introduction of particular theoretical biases concerning the nature and etiology of mental disorders, but by actively expunging them wherever they were found in DSM-II. The task force was equally committed to the goal of syndromal inclusiveness. The intent here was to embrace as many conditions as are commonly seen by practicing clinicians, thereby maximizing the opportunity of further investigators to evaluate the character of each condition as a valid syndromal entity. The initial requirement for a potentially new category was that its diagnostic criteria be outlined with specificity and relative distinctness from other syndromes. The ultimate inclusion test was whether the conditions had been utilized with reasonable frequency by, as well as drawing positive comments concerning its clarity from, a significant number of clinicians participating in the field trials.

In addition to the principles enunciated above, the task force was guided by the following considerations in its DSM-III plans: to expand the classification to maximize its utility for outpatient populations; to differentiate levels of severity and course within syndromes; to maintain compatibility, where feasible, with the forthcoming ICD-9; to rely on empirical data to establish the diagnostic criteria; and to be receptive to the concerns and critiques submitted by interested professional and patient representatives. DSM-III was published in 1980.

The most important facts concerning the DSM-III personality disorders were their partition from the main body of clinical syndromes and their placement in a separate axis. Clinicians in the past were often faced with the task of deciding whether a patient was best diagnosed as possessing a personality or a symptom syndrome; that choice was no longer necessary. Henceforth, clinicians were able to record not only the current clinical picture, but also those characteristics that typified the individual's behaviors over extended periods, both prior to and concurrent with the present complaint. The new multiaxial format enabled practitioners to place the clinical syndromes of Axis I within the context of the individual's lifelong and pervasive style of functioning, recorded on Axis II.

The formal adoption of the multiaxial schema in DSM-III signified a reformulation of the task of psychodiagnoses that approached the magnitude described by Kuhn (1962) as a paradigm shift. It represented a distinct divergence from the traditional medical disease model, in which the clinician's job is to disentangle and clear away "distracting" symptoms and signs so as to pinpoint the underlying or "true" psychopathological state. As far as personality disorders are concerned, this bifurcation assured that the more enduring and often more prosaic styles of personality functioning would not be overlooked when attention was given to the frequently more urgent and behaviorally dramatic clinical syndromes. It also took cognizance of the fact that the lifelong coping styles and emotional vulnerabilities comprising personality can provide a context within which the more salient and usually transient clinical states are likely to arise and be understood. Although the DSM-III text noted that an individual could have disorders on both axes, the task force was more purposeful in recommending that both axes be routinely recorded whenever this was justified. Toward that end, it encouraged the formal notation of all relevant personality "traits" on Axis II, even when a distinctive personality "disorder" was not in evidence.

Brief note should be made of a number of DSM-II personality disorders that were no longer part of the DSM-III group. Among them were the asthenic and inadequate personalities, both of which were discarded because of the infrequency with which they were utilized. The cyclothymic personality was transferred to the affective disorders classification—a decision that raised some controversy among task force members. Similarly, the explosive personality disorder was transferred from the personality classification to that of the impulsive disorders, in light of its highly circumscribed and intermittent nature.

The personality disorders of DSM-III were grouped, somewhat arbitrarily, into three clusters: the first characterized by odd or eccentric behaviors; the second by dramatic, emotional, or erratic behaviors; and the third by the notable presence of anxiety or fear. Among the new DSM-III categories were the avoidant, dependent, and narcissistic personalities. Considerable attention was given to the contrast between the avoidant and the schizoid disorders. The avoidant's detachment was seen as based upon a strong desire for social acceptance combined with a fear of rejection; the schizoid's was viewed as a passively detached style of interpersonal behavior stemming from a presumed intrinsic deficit in the capacity for affective and social gratification. The dependent personality disorder paralleled an earlier (DSM-I) description, in that it was thought to represent a diminished self-confidence combined with a search for security-providing relationships. The description of the narcissistic personality was written within the framework of currently popular psychoanalytic theories, notably those of Kohut (1971) and Kernberg (1975), as well as that of a social learning developmental model (Millon, 1969). The schizotypal was conceived largely as an advanced or more severely dysfunctional variant of the schizoid and avoidant personalities, and was believed to be characterized by intense social detachment and eccentric behaviors. The borderline personality was thought to signify that an individual's personality cohesion and interpersonal competence had insidiously deteriorated. Among the more controversial discussions at task force meetings were those pertaining to the concept of an antisocial personality disorder. The diagnostic criteria selected for this syndrome appeared to many to be more properly suited for what might be termed the "criminal personality"; despite serious objections from many quarters, the criteria were retained with only modest alterations.

## DSM-III-R

Two major elements comprised the revisions introduced in the 1987 DSM-III-R. First, appreciable changes were made in several of the criteria sets for extant disorders, most notably for the avoidant and dependent types; criteria for the former were designed to highlight features of the analytically conceived phobic character. The second revision was the introduction of two ultimately controversial disorders that were assigned provisional status by virtue of having been placed in the manual's Appendix A; these disorders were entitled the self-defeating (*née* masochistic) and the sadistic personality disorders.

## DSM-IV

A major intent of DSM-III-R was to refine the criteria of all disorders, not only those of personality disorders. Progress toward that end was minimal, owing to the modest body of systematic research that had been carried out subsequent to the publication of DSM-III. However, by the late 1980s numerous researchers had developed well-designed structured interviews and self-report inventories, which provided the basis for systematic studies that could evaluate the reliability and validity of the DSM-III-R personality disorders and their criteria. DSM-IV has just been published (American Psychiatric

Association, 1994). As illustrated and discussed in later chapters of this book, innumerable changes were introduced into the DSM-IV criteria sets for the personality disorders—changes informed largely by scientifically grounded data.

Beyond the refinements of diagnostic criteria and the reduction of problematic overlaps between Axis II categories, a number of modifications were made in the status of several disorders. Most notably, the two disorders placed in DSM-III-R Appendix A—the self-defeating and sadistic personalities—were dropped on the grounds of their failure to obtain adequate empirical support, as well as their continued controversial character. The narrow scope of attributes comprising the passive–aggressive personality was broadened to encompass the diverse ways in which oppositional attitudes and behaviors express themselves; given an alternative designation, that of negativistic personality disorder, this category was placed in DSM-IV Appendix B for further study. Another addition to Appendix B was the depressive personality disorder; despite its similarity to and possible overlap with certain of the Axis I mood disorders, there was strong support for its inclusion as a means of assuring continued empirical evaluation of its validity and prevalence.

## FUTURE DIRECTIONS

Where does current thinking appear to be headed? Historically, most conceptions of personality pathology have been rooted in clinical observation and speculation. In recent years, growth has moved the field toward an increasing dependence on empirical studies of broad-based and representative populations who are administered standardized instruments, the results of which are analyzed statistically. Despite this empiricist drift, the growth of theorizing continues unabated; increasingly sophisticated models and stronger scientific bases are employed. The following paragraphs touch briefly on a number of these empirical and theoretical developments. They are presented to alert the reader to the diverse concepts and methods that are likely to guide our future understanding of the personality disorders.

### Dimensional Models

A major issue confronting the DSM-IV Personality Disorders Work Group was whether or not a dimensional schema should replace the categorical format that has been employed for the personality disorders' taxonomy (see Widiger, 1991; Widiger & Sanderson, Chapter 22, this volume). The dimensional model has its roots in early psychological studies of normal personality, and has been most clearly illuminated in research employing factor analytic statistical methods. Factor analysis is a statistical method that calculates intercorrelations among a large group of variables (traits, behaviors, symptoms, etc.). Patterns or clusters among these correlations are referred to as "first-order," or "primary," factors; the elements making up these factors are interpreted to provide them with relevant psychological meaning. "Second-order," or "higher-order," factors may be derived from the original factors by clustering them into larger units; these second-order factors are usually the ones possessing the scope necessary to correspond to the breadth of a concept such as personality.

Among the earliest and most productive of those utilizing a factorial approach to the construction of personality dimensions has been Raymond Cattell (1957, 1965). His research has led him to identify 16 primary factors, or source traits, which he has arranged in sets of bipolar dimensions. Cattell's second-order factor dimensions may be described as follows: creativity versus conventionality, independence versus dependence, toughness versus sensitivity, neuroticism versus stability, leadership versus followership, high anxiety versus low anxiety, and introversion versus extraversion. Cattell gives primacy to the latter two second-order factors in constructing four personality types. The first type, "high anxiety–introversion," is noted as being tense, excitable, suspicious, insecure, jealous, unstable, silent, timid, and shy. The second type, "low anxiety–introversion," tends to be phlegmatic, unshakable, trustful, adaptable, mature, calm, self-sufficient, cold, timid, unconcerned, and resourceful. In the third personality type, the "high anxiety–extraversion" group, is found someone who is tense, excitable, insecure, suspicious, jealous, and unstable, but at the same time sociable, enthusiastic, talkative, practical, and dependent. The last of the types, "low anxiety–extraversion," is identified by being phlegmatic, confident, unshakable, adaptable, mature, calm, warm, sociable, enthusiastic, practical, and conventional.

Hans Eysenck (1952, 1960) has selected three dimensions of personality that are fundamental to psychopathology: "neuroticism," "introversion–extraversion," and "psychoticism." Stimulated by the ideas of Jung, Kretschmer, and Pavlov, Eysenck has constructed an explanatory schema in terms of autonomic nervous system reactivity and ease of conditionability. Those who are highly autonomically reactive are prone to neurotic disorders, whereas those who readily form conditioned responses are inclined to introverted behavior. People at the high end of both conditionability and autonomic reactivity are disposed to develop fears and compulsions, whereas those who are subject to minimal conditioning are likely to become extraverted and potentially antisocial. As in the case of Cattell, Eysenck's formulations provide us with a rather skimpy range of clinically diverse personality types.

A more recent and promising development may be found in what has come to be known as the "five-factor model," a schema that has had numerous critics-turned-followers (Goldberg, 1993), as well as a substantial degree of generalizability and empirical support (Costa & Widiger, 1994). Despite its proponents' effective arguments regarding the model's utility as a foundation for understanding and explicating the personality disorders (Costa & McCrae, 1990), a number of otherwise sympathetic investigators have raised serious questions concerning both its logic and applicability (Clark, 1993; Davis & Millon, 1993; Tellegen, 1993).

An especially promising use of factorial models has been developed by Livesley and his associates (Livesley, Jackson, & Schroeder, 1989; Schroeder, Wormworth, & Livesley, 1992). Selecting diagnostic features from clinical rather than normal personality sources, they sought to examine the correspondence of these features with the DSM's personality disorders. Modest consonance was evident. More significant was the data resolution, which produced 18 factors ostensibly representing a comprehensive schema for personality pathology. Although Livesley and colleagues have recently been drawn to the five-factor solution as a framework for a higher-order personality model, their first-order factorial dimensions may prove a more apt basis for detailing and differentiating many varieties of personality pathology.

Problematic among all factorial methods is the bias incumbent in the original selection of descriptive items; as is well known, what is put into the analysis has a powerful effect on what will emerge. Similarly troublesome is the failure of these methods to provide a rationale for how and why certain factors interrelate and develop as they do. This failure leaves open to speculation both the dynamics and the pathogenesis of personality disorders.

## Interpersonal Models

Akin to trait-oriented dimensional models that depend on factor-analytic solutions are trait-oriented approaches that center their attention on variations in one trait domain, that of interpersonal behavior (McLemore & Brokaw, 1987). Drawing inspiration from the work of Horney and Sullivan, Timothy Leary (1957), along with associates at the Kaiser Permanente Foundation, constructed an interpersonal typology based on two dimensions: dominance–submission and hate love. Utilizing gradations and permutations, Leary separated 16 behavioral segments, which he then grouped into eight distinct interpersonal types. Each is identified by two variants, a mild and an extreme form. Two labels are used to designate each of the eight types—the first to signify the mild or more adaptive variant; the second, the more extreme or pathological variant. For example, the "rebellious distrustful" personality is characterized by an attitude of resentment and by feelings of deprivation. These persons handle anxiety and frustration by actively distancing themselves from others and by displaying bitterness, cynicism, and passively resistant behaviors. Although they do not wish to be distant (they desire both closeness and tenderness as alternatives), experience has taught them that it is best not to trust others, to be skeptical of the so-called goodwill of others, and to be alert to and rebel against signs of phoniness and deceit in others. In several regards, this interpersonal type foreshadowed major features of the DSM's avoidant personality disorder.

Employing a circumplex model to represent the interrelationships and commonalities, as well as the differences among the types they have generated, several contemporary theorists—notably Benjamin (1974, 1993), Kiesler (1986), and Wiggins (1982)—have articulated correspondences between these types and the various DSM personality disorders. Especially promising is the rich diversity of descriptive features each of these thinkers has formulated to characterize these disorders. In the case of Benjamin (1986), she has, along with Millon (1969, 1984), attempted to create circumplex models that include affective, intrapsychic, and cognitive traits, as well as those of an interpersonal nature. From this theoretical base, Benjamin (1993) has constructed a schema that portrays for the reader many of the dimensions comprising the complexity of personality functions. Thus, she rephrases the standard criteria of the DSM-III-R and DSM-IV to highlight each personality's diverse attributes. The following excerpts of criteria for the histrionic type illustrate this approach: "Commandeers the role of 'the life of the party' "; "Characteristically emphasizes sexual attractiveness"; "Seems . . . compelled to project an image of being attractive"; "Goes to great lengths . . . to elicit praise"; "Is . . . interested in creating an image that is pleasantly dependent"; "Has a sense of self as colorful"; "Sees others as . . . able to provide whatever is needed" (Benjamin, 1993, pp. 175–177).

## Cognitive Models

The emergence of a broad-ranging cognitive science in psychological thought in the past two decades is evident most notably in clinical areas through the growth of the cognitive–behavioral approach to therapy—a movement led by several thinkers, most recently in the realm of personality disorders by Beck and his associates (Beck, Freeman, & Associates, 1990). Although the focus of Beck and colleagues' attention is on cognitive dysfunctions, these are seen as part of a nexus of motivational aims, affective styles, and interpersonal strategies. What is most promising is the insight provided readers into the beliefs, assumptions, and expectancies that characterize each of the personality disorders. Also elaborated is how the idiosyncratic pattern of an individual's cognitive schema contributes to both the formation and the perpetuation of the various disorders. Especially illuminating are the pattern of beliefs and strategies predominating in each of the personalities. Together with the enlightening characterizations by interpersonal theorists such as Benjamin, the cognitive approach begins to "fill out" the full scope of attributes comprising what is meant by personality. Thus, to Beck et al., (1990) the cognitive profile of dependent personalities consists of the following elements: They have a picture of themselves as helpless, needy, weak, and incompetent. Dependents see the strong "caretaker" in an idealized way, as nurturant and supportive. They believe that they need others (specifically, a strong person) to "survive," and that their happiness rests on having such a figure to lean upon. Their main fear is that they will be abandoned, and their protective strategy is to cultivate a dependent relationship, to subordinate themselves, to placate and please, and never to offend.

## Analytic Models

The "character" types briefly noted earlier in this chapter remain a foundation for much of personality disorder thought, having played an important role in guiding the Axis II sections of the DSM. With the advent and central role of self and object relations theorizing in recent decades, analytic models have taken a new turn, contributing ideas that have resulted in several of the newer personality disorders in recent DSMs (notably the borderline and narcissistic personalities).

Although numerous analytic theorists have contributed in recent years to the study of character, the work of Otto Kernberg (1975, 1984) deserves special note. Offering a new characterology, Kernberg has also constructed a useful framework for organizing types in terms of their level of severity. Breaking away from a rigid adherence to the psychosexual model, Kernberg proposes another dimension as primary—that of structural organization. Coordinating character types in accord with severity and structural organization leads Kernberg to speak of "higher," "intermediate," and "lower" levels of character pathology; both the intermediate and lower levels are referred to as "borderline personality organizations." To illustrate his ordering of types, Kernberg assigns most hysterical, obsessive–compulsive, and depressive personalities to the higher level. At the intermediate level of organization, Kernberg locates the "infantile" and most narcissistic personalities. Last, clear-cut antisocial personalities are classified as distinctly of a lower-level borderline organization.

Because the basis for generating their ideas is largely inferential rather than quantitative and replicable, analytic theorists continue to be judged by many contemporary researchers as unscientific. Despite their less than optimal methodologies, their observations are often the most astute among those of current clinicians, and their deductions concerning development and pathogenesis are often the most fertile and synthesizing.

## Biological Models

Clinicians since the days of Hippocrates have posited that biological and chemical elements undergird temperament and psychic pathology. The proliferation in recent years of sophisticated neurobiological knowledge and methodologies, as well as the upsurge of the biological orientation in psychiatric practice, has led to a renaissance in the conviction that the long-sought discovery of biogenetic substrates for all disorders (including those of personality) is close at hand. Beyond genetic studies seeking to uncover familial patterns of heritability, a number of researchers and theorists have sought to construct personality classification systems based on biological dispositions. Notable here is the ongoing work of Siever and associates (Siever & Davis, 1991; Weston & Siever, 1993) and of Cloninger (1986, 1987).

Siever's group's hypotheses take the form of a dimensional model anchored to the Axis I disorders. Building on findings with the schizophrenic, affective, impulse control, and anxiety disorders, Siever and colleagues propose that they represent severe variants on continua that have as their grounding four defects, respectively termed "cognitive/perceptual organization," "affective regulation," "impulse control," and "anxiety modulation." At one end are the extreme and discrete symptoms manifest in Axis I disorders. At the milder end of the continua are styles of personality functioning that may crystallize into pervasive difficulties taking the form of Axis II disorders. Thus, milder cognitive/perceptual disorganization may result in schizotypal personalities; impulse control difficulties may underlie the development of antisocial patterns; and so on.

Another recent neurobiological schema has been presented by Cloninger (1986, 1987). Drawing on family and developmental studies, personality psychometrics, and (most significantly) neuropharmacological and neuroanatomical correlates of behavioral conditions, Cloninger has generated a theoretical model composed of three dimensions, which he terms "reward dependence," "harm avoidance," and "novelty seeking." Proposing that each is a heritable personality disposition, he relates them explicitly to specific monoaminergic pathways. For example, high reward dependence is thought to be connected to low noradrenergic activity; harm avoidance is associated with high serotonergic activity; and high novelty seeking is relateed to low dopaminergic activity. Cloninger portrays those high on reward dependence as sociable, sympathetic, and pleasant; in contrast, those low on this polarity are characterized as detached, cool, and practical. Those high on harm avoidance are characterized as cautious, apprehensive, and inhibited; those low on this valence are likely to be confident, optimistic, and carefree.

Not only are there sound reasons to approach neurobiological speculations with a measure of skepticism, given the tenuous nature of our knowledge concerning the complexities of neurochemical interaction; hesitation must also be expressed concerning hypotheses that propose direct parallels between neurobiological and behavior–emotion systems. Nonetheless, it is encouraging when promising areas of convergence among diverse fields of inquiry are encountered.

## Evolutionary Models

Convergence among diverse fields of inquiry provides the framework for Millon's own model of personality classification (Millon, 1990). Convinced that there exist "deeper" principles of adaptation that are common to all aspects of evolution, Millon has set forth the elements comprising those commonalities. Developed as a model for personality classifications over the past 30 years or so, this model currently serves as a deductive framework for both

deriving and explicating both the DSM personality disorders and other normal and abnormal personality patterns (Millon, 1991).

The evolutionary model, as well as its "biosocial learning" forerunner (Millon, 1969, 1981), has generated several new personality categories, several
of which have found their way into DSM-III, DSM-III-R, and DSM-IV (Kernberg, 1984). Drawing on a threefold polarity framework (pleasure–pain, active–passive, and self–other), Millon deduced a series of IO personality
"prototypes" and three severe variants, of which a few have proved to be "original" derivations in the sense that they were never formulated as categories
in prior psychiatric nosologies. For example, the avoidant personality was
first described (and the term "avoidant" was coined) by Millon (1969); this
disorder had its origins in biosocial learning theory and was described as
the personality pattern representing an active–detached coping style. Progressive research will determine whether the network of concepts comprising
this theory provides an optimal structure for a comprehensive nosology of
personality pathology. At the very least, it contributes to the view that formal theory can lead to the deduction of new categories worthy of consensual and empirical verification.


## CONCLUDING COMMENTS

Heterogeneous requirements are especially problematic in classically structured syndromes—that is, those requiring singly necessary or jointly sufficient diagnostic criteria. Personality categories, by contrast, are composed
intentionally in a heterogeneous manner; that is, they accept the legitimacy
of syndromic diversity and overlap. Nevertheless, there is still a need to
reduce the "fuzziness" between boundaries, so as to eliminate excessive numbers of unclassifiable and on-the-boundary cases. One step toward the goal
of sharpening diagnostic discriminations is to spell out a distinctive criterion for every diagnostically relevant clinical attribute aligned with every personality category. For example, if the attribute "interpersonal conduct" is
deemed to be of clinical value in assessing personality disorders, then singular diagnostic criteria should be specified to represent the characteristic
or distinctive manner in which each personality "conducts its interpersonal
life."

A taxonomic schema that includes all relevant clinical attributes (e.g.,
behavior, affect, cognition), and specifies a defining feature on every attribute for each of the personality disorders, would be fully comprehensive in
its clinical scope and would possess parallel and directly comparable criteria among all Axis II categories. A format of this nature will not only furnish
logic and symmetry to the DSM taxonomy, but will enable investigators to
be systematic in determining the relative diagnostic efficacy of characterological covariates. Moreover, clinicians would be able to appraise both typical and unusual syndromal patterns, as well as to establish the coherence

(if not the "validity") of both dimensionally generated and classically established categorical entities.

## REFERENCES

Abraham, K. (1921). Contributions to the theory of the anal character. In K. Abraham, *Selected papers on psychoanalysis.* London: Hogarth Press, 1927.

Abraham, K. (1925). Character formation on the genital level of the libido. In K. Abraham, *Selected papers on psychoanalysis.* London: Hogarth Press, 1927.

Allport, G. W. (1937). *Personality: A psychological interpretation.* New York: Holt.

American Psychiatric Association. (1952). *Diagnostic and statistical manual of mental disorders* (1st ed.). Washington, DC: Mental Hospitals Service.

American Psychiatric Association. (1968). *Diagnostic and statistical manual of mental disorders* (2nd ed.). Washington, DC: Author.

American Psychiatric Association. (1980). *Diagnostic and statistical manual of mental disorders* (3rd ed.). Washington, DC: Author.

American Psychiatric Association. (1987). *Diagnostic and statistical manual of mental disorders* (3rd ed., rev.). Washington, DC: Author.

American Psychiatric Association. (1994). *Diagnostic and statistical manual of mental disorders* (4th ed.). Washington, DC: Author.

Beck, A. T., Freeman, A., & Associates. (1990). *Cognitive therapy of personality disorders.* New York, Guilford Press.

Benjamin, L. S. (1974). Structural Analysis of Social Behavior. *Psychological Review, 81,* 392–425.

Benjamin, L. S. (1986). Adding social and intrapsychic descriptors to Axis I of DSM-III. In T. Millon & G. L. Klerman (Eds.), *Contemporary directions in psychopathology.* New York: Guilford Press.

Benjamin, L. S. (1993). *Interpersonal diagnosis and treatment of personality disorders.* New York: Guilford Press.

Bleuler, E. (1922). Die probleme der schizoidie und der syntonie. *Zeitschrift fuer die Gesamte Neurologie und Psychiatrie, 78,* 373–388.

Bleuler, E. (1924). *Textbook of psychiatry* (A. A. Brill, Trans.). New York: Macmillan.

Bleuler, E. (1929). Syntonie-schizoidie, schizophrenie. *Neurologie und Psychopathologie, 38,* 47–64.

Cattell, R. B. (1957). *Personality and motivation: Structure and measurement.* New York: World.

Cattell, R. B. (1965). *The scientific analysis of personality.* Chicago: Aldine.

Clark, L. A. (1993). Personality disorder diagnosis: Limitations of the five-factor model. *Psychological Inquiry, 4,* 100–104.

Cloninger, C. R. (1986). A unified biosocial theory of personality and its role in the development of anxiety states. *Psychiatric Developments, 3,* 167–220.

Cloninger, C. R. (1987). A systematic method for clinical description and classification of personality variants. *Archives of General Psychiatry, 44,* 573–588.

Costa, P., & McCrae, R. (1990). Personality disorders and the five-factor model of personality. *Journal of Personality Disorders, 4,* 62–371.

Costa, P., & Widiger, T. (Eds.). (1994). *Personality disorders and the five-factor model of personality.* Washington, DC: American Psychological Association.

Davis, R. D., & Millon, T. (1993). The five-factor model for personality disorders: Apt or misguided. *Psychological Inquiry, 4,* 104–109.

Eysenck, H. J. (1952). *The scientific study of personality.* London: Routledge & Kegan Paul.

Eysenck, H. J. (1960). *The structure of human personality.* London: Routledge & Kegan Paul.

Fenichel, O. (1945). *The psychoanalytic theory of neurosis.* New York: Norton.

Feuchtersleben, E. von. (1847). *Lehrbuch der arzlichen seelenkunde.* Vienna: Gerold.

Freud, S. (1908). Character and anal eroticism. In E. Jones (Ed.), *Sigmund Freud: Collected papers* (Vol. 2). London: Hogarth Press, 1925.

Freud, S. (1932). Libidinal types. In E. Jones (Ed.), *Sigmund Freud: Collected papers* (Vol. 5). London: Hogarth Press, 1925.

Goldberg, L. (1993). The structure of phenotypic personality traits. *American Psychologist, 48,* 26–34.

Griesinger, W. (1845). *Mental pathology and therapeutics.* London: New Sydenham Society, 1867.

Horney, K. (1937). *The neurotic personality of our time.* New York: Norton.

Horney, K. (1939). *New ways in psychoanalysis.* New York: Norton.

Horney, K. (1942). *Self analysis.* New York: Norton.

Horney, K. (1945). *Our inner conflicts.* New York: Norton.

Horney, K. (1950). *Neurosis and human growth.* New York: Norton.

Kernberg, O. (1975). *Borderline conditions and pathological narcissism.* New York: Jason Aronson.

Kernberg, O. (1984). *Severe personality disorders.* New Haven, CT: Yale University Press.

Kiesler, D. J. (1986). The 1982 interpersonal circle: An analysis of DSM-III personality disorders. In T. Millon & G. L. Klerman (Eds.), *Contemporary directions in psychopathology.* New York: Guilford Press.

Kohut, H. (1971). *The analysis of the self.* New York: International Universities Press.

Kraepelin, E. (1909–1915). *Psychiatrie: Ein Lehrbuch* (8th ed.). Leipzig: Barth.

Kraepelin, E. (1913). *Psychiatrie: Ein Lehrbuch* (8th ed., Vol. 3). Leipzig: Barth.

Kraepelin, E. (1919). *Dementia praecox and paraphrenia.* Edinburgh: Livingstone.

Kraepelin, E. (1921). *Manic-depressive insanity and paranoia.* Edinburgh: Livingstone.

Kretschmer, E. (1925). *Physique and character.* London: Kegan Paul, 1926.

Kuhn, T. (1962). *The structure of scientific revolutions.* Chicago: University of Chicago Press.

Leary, T. (1957). *Interpersonal diagnosis of personality.* New York: Ronald Press.

Livesley, W. J., Jackson, D. N., & Schroeder, M. L. (1989). A study of the factorial structure of personality pathology. *Journal of Personality Disorders, 3,* 292–306.

McLemore, C., & Brokaw, D. (1987). Personality disorders as dysfunctional interpersonal behavior. *Journal of Personality Disorders, 1,* 270–285.

Millon, T. (1969). *Modern psychopathology.* Philadelphia: W. B. Saunders.

Millon, T. (1981). *Disorders of personality: DSM-III, Axis II.* New York: Wiley–Interscience.

Millon, T. (1984). On the renaissance of personality assessment and personality theory. *Journal of Personality Assessment, 48,* 450–456.

Millon, T. (1990). *Toward a new personology: An evolutionary model.* New York: Wiley–Interscience.

Millon, T. (1991). Normality: What may we learn from evolutionary theory. In D. Offer & M. Sabshin (Eds.), *The diversity of normal behavior.* New York: Basic Books.

Pinel, P. (1801). *Traité medico-philosophique sur l'alienation mentale.* Paris: Richard, Caille & Ravier.

Pinel, P. (1806). *A treatise on insanity* (D. Davis, Trans.). New York: Hafner.

Prichard, J. C. (1835). *A treatise on insanity.* London: Sherwood, Gilbert & Piper.

Reich, W. (1933). *Charakter Analyse.* Leipzig: Sexpol Verlag.

Reich, W. (1949). *Character analysis* (3rd ed.) (V. R. Carafagno, Trans.). New York: Farrar, Straus.

Roback, A. A. (1927). *The psychology of character.* New York: Harcourt, Brace.

Rush, B. (1812). *Medical inquiries and observations on the diseases of the mind.* Philadelphia: Kimber & Richardson.

Schneider, K. (1923). *Psychpathic personalities.* London: Cassell, 1950.

Schroeder, M. L., Wormworth, J. A., & Livesley, W. J. (1992). Dimensions of personality disorder and their relationships to the big five dimensions of personality. *Psychological Assessment, 4,* 47–53.

Siever, L., & Davis, K. (1991). A psychobiological perspective on the personality disorders. *American Journal of Psychiatry, 148,* 1647–1658.

Sullivan, H. S. (1947). *Conceptions of modern psychiatry.* New York: Norton.

Tellegen, A. (1993). Folk concepts and psychological concepts of personality and personality disorder. *Psychological Inquiry, 4,* 122–130.

Weston, S., & Siever, L. (1993). Biologic correlates of personality disorders. *Journal of Personality Disorders, 7,* 129–148.

Widiger, T. (1991). Personality disorder dimensional models proposed for DSM-IV. *Journal of Personality Disorders, 5,* 386–398.

Wiggins, J. S. (1982). Circumplex models of interpersonal behavior in clinical psychology. In P. C. Kendall & J. N. Butcher (Eds.), *Handbook of research methods in clinical psychology.* New York: Wiley.

CHAPTER 2

# Are Personality Disorders Well Classified in DSM-IV?

PETER TYRER

Although the personality disorders described in DSM-III, DSM-III-R, and DSM-IV (American Psychiatric Association [APA], 1980, 1987, 1994) represent a major advance on earlier classifications, including those of historical interest described so well by Theodore Millon and Roger Davis in Chapter 1, they are still far from adequate in describing the phenomena that constitute the clinical core of personality disturbance. They are useful in indicating the areas in which personality disturbance is manifested, so that these can be separated from mental state (Axis I) disorders, and the introduction of better operational criteria has improved the reliability of their description. However, the degree of overlap between and among the different personality disorders is far too great, and the specious use of the term "comorbidity" hides diagnostic confusion. Moreover, there is insufficient emphasis on the concept that "personality disorder" refers to long-term functioning, and too much reliance is placed on self-report. The continuing reliance on a categorical system of diagnosis fails to recognize the wide variation of personality abnormality, which has only been acknowledged partly in changes introduced to DSM-IV. The personality disorders described in the classification can be described with greater reliability and confidence in cross-sectional research studies, but still lack validity in clinical practice.

The separation of personality disorder by the APA (1980) in DSM-III as a discrete axis of classification was a major advance in psychiatric nosology. It has forced attention on a group of disorders that has been long neglected, although it lies at the heart of psychiatric practice. This separation has led to an apparently improved classification and better definition, and it has stimulated a degree of research endeavor that would have been unthinkable 15 years ago. However, a great proportion of this endeavor is still preoccupied with the definition and measurement of DSM personality disorders, and this suggests that all is far from well in the classification. Although the introduction of a classificatory system based on operational criteria has been an excellent stimulus to research work, the fact that much of the research engendered has been concerned with this same classification is an indictment of academia. An addition to the famous laws of C. Northcote Parkinson could be "Research creates unproductive research," and this is exemplified by much of the activity in psychiatric classification since the introduction of DSM-III.

We now have two main classifications of personality disorder: DSM-IV and the 10th revision of the *International Classification of Diseases* (ICD-10; World Health Organization [WHO], 1992). As ICD-10 has replicated many of the features of DSM-III-R, the DSM and ICD classification schemes can often be discussed together.

In reviewing DSM-IV personality disorders, I am aware of the many excellent reviews and commentaries that have already been published in recent years (Frances, 1980; Frances & Widiger, 1986; Widiger & Frances, 1985; Livesley & Jackson, 1992). However, there may be some advantages in looking at the disorders from an external perspective and inserting them in a broader context. The European literature on personality disorders can be criticized on many grounds, not least on those of methodology; as Chapter 1 has indicated, however, it is a rich source and can teach us a great deal. This can be divided usefully into four headings: those of classification, definition, separation of Axis I and Axis II disorders, and the merits of categorical and dimensional approaches to personality disorders.

## CLASSIFICATION

Classification depends on consensus, which is best achieved through the structure of a committee. Committees concerned with classification usually include many members with special (and sometimes vested) interests in one or more categories, and sometimes with an aversion to others amounting to prejudice. If a committee meets for the purpose of revising a classification, it will make changes whether or not there are data to support them, because otherwise it will seem to be failing in its task. In the absence of satisfactory data, there may be a tendency for committees to make even more changes than if good data are available, because they are more likely to be swayed by arguments and opinion. The introduction of the sadistic and self-defeating personality disorder categories in an appendix of DSM-III-R is a prime example of the risks of classification without adequate data being available, and readers will be aware of the furor of criticism that these new categories created (Shainess, 1987; Walker, 1987).

Although the classification of personality disorders in DSM-III-R and DSM-IV has in some cases been successful, a broader approach, taking into account a historical perspective, needs to be incorporated. The busy activity of classifying personality disorders in the United States in the 1980s and

1990s should be set against two millennia of recording abnormal personalities. Some of our clinical forefathers were very wise, and their descriptions of personality disorders have an uncanny accuracy in hitting the target. True, none of them approach the methodological sophistication of recent DSM classifications. However, when one reads classical descriptions of, for example, paranoid personality disorder through a cultural and temporal range extending from Theophrastus (1925) over 2,000 years ago to Kraepelin (1904) and Schneider (1923) and through to the classifications of DSM-III and the ICD (World Health Organization & Alcohol, Drug Abuse and Mental Health Administration [ADAMHA], 1983), the descriptions have a stability and underlying validity denied to other categories such as schizotypal personality disorder and other recent newcomers. It would be unwise to dismiss past work on personality disorders on the grounds that it is largely anecdotal and impressionistic, and that it cannot be replicated. The unreliability of psychiatric measurement in the distant past detracts little from the fundamental validity of many observations. If one relies entirely on recent U.S. data, a type of personality disorder could be derived that is so culturally bound to, for example, the eastern seaboard of the United States that it may be a disorder known only to that specific cultural setting. It is only those personality disorders that are robust enough to persist across cultures and generations that are worthy of an international classification.

In the absence of good data, as is common in personality disorders, the committee is subject to pressures that are more political than scientific. Thus, if any group represented on the committee wants a new diagnosis, it will tend to get its way. It seems to be commoner in these situations for new diagnoses to be included than for old ones to be removed (Kendell, 1975).

Even if one accepts the validity of the 10 personality disorders in DSM-IV, there is no satisfactory way of classifying patients who have more than one personality disorder. There are now many studies suggesting that mixed personality disorders as defined by DSM-III are the rule rather than the exception (Frances, Clarkin, Gilmore, Hurt, & Brown, 1984; Stangl, Pfohl, Zimmerman, Bowers, & Corenthal, 1985; Pfohl, Coryell, Zimmerman, & Stangl, 1986; Fyer, Frances, Sullivan, Hurt, & Clarkin, 1988). Some combined disorders are so frequent that it is difficult to decide whether they are measuring separate entities. Borderline personality disorder, for example, is rarely found alone and is difficult to distinguish from others in the "flamboyant cluster" of histrionic, antisocial, and narcissistic personality disorders (Barasch, Kroll, & Carey, 1983; Kroll, Carey, Simes, & Roth, 1982). Also, the avoidant may overlap with the dependent category (Reich, Noyes, & Troughton, 1987). Although it is possible to argue — as Widiger and Frances (1985) have done — that a prototypal model of categorization is more appropriate for these disorders, in which boundaries overlap and membership is heterogeneous, a classification of personality disorders consisting of multiple categories is unwieldy and unlikely to achieve widespread use in clinical practice.

Rutter (1987) has suggested that because the characteristic that defines all personality disorders "is a pervasive persistent abnormality in maintaining social relationships" (p. 453), the classification should be into "one overall category defined in terms of relationship abnormalities" (p. 454). Although this proposal has merits, it may extend diagnostic "lumping" too far and it does not take account of some important qualitative differences among personality disorders. Factor- and cluster-analytic studies support the notion of four main personality disorder groupings, rather than the three corresponding with those of Cloninger (1987) and the DSM-III flamboyant, withdrawn, and anxious–fearful clusters. These four have been called the sociopathic, dependent, withdrawn, and compulsive personality disorders (Kass, Skodol, Charles, Spitzer, & Williams, 1985; Tyrer & Alexander, 1979, Tyrer , Alexander, & Ferguson, 1988; Livesley & Jackson, 1992; Schroeder & Livesley, 1991). It is possible that these could be extended to five disorders, subserving the dimensions identified by Costa and McCrea (1990), but it is doubtful whether more conditions deserve description.

If several personality disorders are identified in a single individual, which should take precedence? DSM-III made only a half-hearted attempt to decide this issue by relegating passive–aggressive personality disorder to a lower position on the hierarchy, only for this procedure to be abolished in DSM-III-R. All other personality disorders (except for those included in an appendix for further study) have equivalent status. One can appreciate the dilemma in which the committee members have been placed. On the one hand, they would like to have a set of "clean," separated personality disorders; on the other, they wish to reflect the diversity and rich variation in personality that makes each person unique.

One way of overcoming this difficulty is to rate the degree of social maladjustment created by each personality disorder subtype or trait. In one schedule, the Personality Assessment Schedule (PAS; Tyrer & Alexander, 1979), the severity of personality abnormality depends on the amount of social impairment produced by the characteristic in question. The results are subjected to a cluster analysis procedure that reveals four major groupings of abnormal personality—sociopathic, passive–dependent, anankastic (obsessional), and schizoid—with nine further subcategories. Analysis has shown that sociopathic personality disorders (which would cover the antisocial, borderline, and histrionic personality disorders in DSM-III) produce consistently greater social malfunction than anankastic and schizoid personality disorders (which would include the schizoid [but probably not schizotypal], avoidant, obsessive–compulsive, and passive–aggressive personality disorders in DSM-III) (Ferguson & Tyrer, 1988). As personality disorder manifests itself through social maladjustment (and personal distress arising from such maladjustment), then it is reasonable to postulate that the disorders causing greater social impairment should take precedence over those causing less when several disorders coexist. It is therefore an advantage to have a separate assessment procedure for social maladjustment when assessing patients with personality disorders. In a recent modification of the PAS, in which ICD-10 personality disorder criteria are scored using the criterion of social dysfunction, successful separation of severe and less severe personality disorders is achieved with an overall interrater reliability of .86 ($R_I$ statistic) (Merson, Tyrer, Duke, & Henderson, 1994).

## DEFINITION

The precise definition of terms has been one of the assets of the DSM classification and has generated lists of operational criteria for personality disorders, where concepts have been generally vague and precise description conspicuously lacking, might appear self-evident. There are two distinct levels of definition, general and specific. The general definition is necessary to separate personality disorders from normal personality variations. This has tended to follow Schneider's (1923) concepts that those with personality disorders suffer because of their disorders and also cause society to suffer.

This is a common feature in both DSM and ICD descriptions of personality disorders. DSM-IV states: "Only when personality traits are inflexible and maladaptive and cause significant functional impairment or subjective distress do they constitute Personality Disorders" (American Psychiatric Association, 1994, p. 630). The meanings of these terms are not defined elsewhere, which is perhaps surprising, given the attention to detail that characterizes the specific criteria for each personality disorder. However, this rather loose description needs to be kept in mind by the clinician when deciding whether a patient satisfies the criteria necessary for a specific disorder.

At present there are no links between the specific operational criteria for each disorder and the general description quoted above. This leads to problems. For example, how does one classify a patient who "lacks close friends or confidants other than first-degree relatives" (American Psychiatric Association, 1994, p. 641) if he or she is not suffering as a consequence of this apparent isolation or causing others to suffer? One of the operational criteria for schizoid personality disorder has been satisfied, and yet the severity of disturbance is not sufficient to permit us to regard this attribute as disordered.

There are many other examples throughout the operational criteria in DSM-IV that can be satisfied without any obvious distress or suffering to the subject, although they may have an adverse effect on others. These include the following (all quoted from APA, 1994): "appears indifferent to the praise or criticism of others" (schizoid personality disorder, p. 641); "behavior or appearance that is odd, eccentric, or peculiar" (schizotypal personality disorder, p. 645); "consistently uses physical appearance to draw attention to self" (histrionic personality disorder, p. 658); "is interpersonally exploitative, i.e., takes advantage of others to achieve his or her own ends" (narcissistic personality disorder, p. 661); and "passively resists fulfilling routine social and occupational tasks" (passive–aggressive [negativistic] personality disorder, p. 735).

Even the better operational criteria can be criticized. Nowhere in these criteria is there any indication of the persistence or level of subjective distress or social dysfunction that needs to be created by the attribute in question in order to qualify for the label of personality disorder. As Widiger and Frances (1985) point out, "personality disorders are defined as chronic and pervasive (maladaptive) personality traits, but most of the criteria for their diagnosis fail to indicate how the central features of chronicity and pervasiveness are to be established" (p. 619).

Hope springs eternal that each criterion will be so comprehensive that the exact description of a behavioral characteristic will somehow make it pathognomonic of a personality disorder in the absence of any other external criteria. This is unrealistic. Some external criteria are essential because personality disorders, unlike Axis I disorders, are defined on a broad canvas that involves the position of patients in their relationships with society over a long period. Societies change and vary from culture to culture, so it is likely that diagnoses of personality disorders will also vary similarly. This is unsatisfactory for those who would like to see operational criteria for diagnosis that are independent of the whims of society, but it does not accord with clinical reality.

Some abnormal personality characteristics may be considered adaptive because they fit into the cultural setting. Antisocial personality characteristics were an advantage during the 12 years of the Third Reich; obsessional ones, in Victorian England; and Type A features, in the United States at (or at least just before) the present time. This may appear to be a problem in cross-national studies of personality disorders, but if the abnormality is defined in terms of social maladjustment, then good reliability can be achieved (Tyrer et al., 1984). Even with the variation of diagnosis introduced by cultural setting, it seems likely that the more severe personality disorders will be maladaptive in all situations, and these are the ones that need to be identified and separated from the rest.

For those who are unhappy about the use of social dysfunction as a major criterion of personality diagnosis, the hypothesis put forward by Cloninger (1987) has attractions. Cloninger suggests that personality variations and disorders can be explained by malfunction in the three main heritable biological systems governing behavior: novelty seeking, primarily mediated through dopaminergic pathways; harm avoidance, primarily mediated through serotonergic pathways; and reward dependence, primarily mediated through noradrenergic pathways. This tridimensional structure allows up to nine major disorders of personality to be identified; those predicted by the model match eight of the personality disorders in DSM-III and resurrect another, cyclothymic, from DSM-II. Cloninger's work deserves further testing. Even if only part of it is verified, it would be an important anchor for the untethered empiricism that is rife in current research on personality disorder.

## SEPARATION OF AXIS I AND AXIS II DISORDERS

Personality disorders owe their diagnostic renaissance primarily to the separation of personality and mental state diagnoses. It is very important for this difference to be maintained, but there is an increasing tendency in revisions of DSM to blur this distinction. This will lead to problems of classification. An important distinction between ICD-10 and DSM-IV is that the presence of subjective distress and presence of social malfunctioning are combined in ICD but separated in DSM. Thus a patient who has apparent personality features leading to subjective distress but no evidence of social dysfunction can still qualify for a diagnosis of personality disorder in DSM-IV; in ICD-10, however, the behavior has to be inflexible, maladaptive, or otherwise dysfunctional across a broad range of personal and social situations to qualify for personality disorder (World Health Organization, 1992). Because Axis I disorders are characterized mainly by symptoms (i.e., forms of subjective distress) and abnormal patterns of behavior, it is not clear how Axis I and Axis II disorders should be distinguished. In particular, there is likely to be major difficulty in separating chronic Axis I disorders from Axis II ones.

The relative persistence of abnormal personality is important, but this is difficult to measure using the operational criteria of DSM. Therefore, assessments of personality status are placing increasing reliance on present personality and functioning. This leads to increased reliability, but that reliability may be achieved at the cost of poor validity. There is also considerable inconsistency in DSM's decisions about categorizing disorders as either Axis I or Axis II. For example, explosive personality disorder was excluded from Axis II in DSM-III because it is an episodic rather than a persistent abnormality (Lion, 1981). However, borderline personality disorder, which overlaps considerably with explosive personality disorder (it is also characterized by episodic mood disturbance, impulsivity, and lack of control), is classified in Axis II. The justifications for removing explosive personality disorder and classifying it elsewhere are poor until better evidence is available. In ICD-10, explosive personality disorder (renamed impulsive personality disorder) is included and shares many of the features of borderline personality disorder.

It is more important to make clear distinctions between Axis I and Axis II disorders and to classify conditions accordingly. Thus the removal from ICD and DSM of cyclothymic (or affective) personality disorder on the basis that this probably represents *formes frustes* of manic–depressive psychosis is supported by empirical research. When cluster analysis is used to identify premorbid personality characteristics independent of mental state disorders, a cyclothymic personality cannot be identified (Tyrer & Alexander, 1979), and the temporal reliability of cyclothymia as a personality characteristic is sufficiently poor (Mann, Jenkins, Cutting, & Cowan, 1981) that the condition is more likely to be a mental state abnormality than a personality diagnosis.

Longitudinal studies that record the temporal reliability of Axis II disorders have been extremely useful in identifying those DSM-III personality disorders that assess temporal reliability (McGlashan, 1986; Pope, Jonas, Hudson, Cohen, & Gunderson, 1983), but they are relatively small in number compared with the large numbers of cross-sectional studies of DSM-III personality diagnoses. These studies have shown that personality diagnoses do not remain consistent and have thrown into doubt some of the criteria for defining them. Similar studies in Europe have shown a reasonable degree of temporal reliability over a 6-month to 3-year period, although the kappa values achieved (.6, .65) could still be regarded as unsatisfactory (Mann, Jenkins, Cuttings, & Cowan, 1981; Tyrer, Strauss, & Cicchetti, 1983).

In order to separate long-standing personality characteristics from the more ephemeral mental state disorders, investigators in the United Kingdom have tended to rely more on information derived from close informants than on information from the patients themselves (Mann et al., 1981; Tyrer & Alexander, 1979; Tyrer, Alexander, Cicchetti, Cohen, & Remington, 1979). This also accords with the emphasis that the Schneiderian definition of personality disorders places on their impact on society. There is good evidence that personality characteristics can be affected by the presence of Axis I disorders, particularly depression and anxiety (Coppen & Metcalfe, 1965; Hirschfeld & Klerman, 1979; Hirschfeld et al., 1983; Reich, Noyes, Coryell, & O'Gorman, 1986). When informants are interviewed, the contaminating effect of present mental state is at least partly removed, and clinical observations of personality that may affect assessments are also discounted. It is perhaps no coincidence that of the eight structured interview schedules currently in use for the assessment of abnormal personality, two—the PAS (Tyrer & Alexander, 1979) and the Standardized Assessment of Personality (Mann et al., 1981)—have been introduced by the skeptical British and obtain information primarily from an informant interview. The other six—the Schedule for Interviewing Borderlines (Baron, 1982); the Borderline Personality Disorder Scale (Perry, 1982); the Structured Clinical Interview for DSM-III, Axis II (Spitzer, Williams, & Gibbs, 1987); the Structured Interview for the DSM-III Personality Disorders (Stangl et al., 1985); the Diagnostic Interview for Borderlines (Gunderson, 1982); and the Personality Disorder Examination (Loranger, Susman, Oldham, & Russakoff, 1985)—have all been introduced by the more trusting North American investigators and rely mainly on an interview with the patient. Perhaps this is a true cross-national difference in personality assessment.

There are some advantages in assessing the personality status of patients by interviewing them directly when they do not have another mental disorder or have a relatively mild degree of abnormal personality. If these conditions do not apply (as is frequently the case in clinical practice), then the merits of using informants are strong and sometimes overwhelming. Informants can also be used for those major psychiatric disorders in which interviewing patients is clearly not appropriate because the patient's testimony is so obviously impaired by their mental condition (e.g., functional and organic psychoses). Neither DSM-III-R nor DSM-IV can be used to assess personality disorders in the presence of a major psychosis, and this is an important handicap of the classification. Finally, informants can also assess the degree of personality change produced by an Axis I disorder. This is particularly important in the case of schizophrenia, and the category of "personality change" is recognized in ICD-10 (World Health Organization, 1992).

In North America there is reluctance to use informants in assessing personality disorders. Part of this may be cultural; there is perhaps greater concern over the privacy and confidentiality of personal information in the United States and Canada than in many countries, and agreement from patients to involve informants may be more difficult to obtain. There appears to be another reason that is less praiseworthy: Put simply, informants spoil things. Their testimony often conflicts with those of patients (e.g., Tyrer et al., 1979; Zimmerman, Pfohl, Coryell, Stangl, & Corenthal, 1988), and because so much worship takes place at the altar of reliability in personality disorder research, these findings are somewhat embarrassing. It is therefore much easier to forget about informants and concentrate on patients alone. This is head-in-the-sand mentality, as every clinician involved in the care of the severely personality-disordered can point to the importance of getting corroborating information from other sources before accepting the versions presented by patients.

The trouble is that the operational criteria of DSM are moving closer and closer to the subjective version, and will have to be drastically altered to include equivalent criteria for informants. Much more needs to be done to identify the criteria determining good and bad informants. For example, are spouses and cohabiters better informants than friends, as some research has suggested (Brothwell, Casey, & Tyrer, 1992)? If so, the tendency in North American studies to rely on information predominantly from friends rather than closer informants may be defective.

If an informant interview were to be regarded as an essential component of the assessment of personality disorder in DSM, many of the operational criteria currently in use would have to be revised greatly. At present, far too many of the criteria used can be examined only with patients themselves and are influenced heavily by current mental state. In particular, schizotypal personality disorder is extremely difficult to distinguish from schizophrenia, as the criteria include ideas of reference, odd beliefs and magical thinking, abnormal perception, and eccentric behavior. It is questionable whether this type of malfunctioning is a long-term personality characteristic independent of Axis I disorders, and this can only be evaluated adequately with the help of an informant. It would also be extremely difficult to evaluate borderline personality disorder using the current operational criteria if an informant interview were to take place. How can an informant assess "frantic efforts to avoid real or imagined abandonment" or "chronic feelings of emptiness" (American Psychiatric Association, 1994, p. 654) as a personality dimension? The overlapping dynamic and descriptive aspects of borderline personality disorder are difficult to separate even with interviews with the patients, but are impossible to separate when informants are providing the information. There is no doubt that a syndrome of impulsivity, recurrent mood disturbance, and identity difficulties exists, but it may not be a personality disorder, and this is supported by its relative lack of stability in longitudinal studies (Pope et al., 1983; Trull, Widiger, & Frances, 1987). Further studies including interviews with informants may help to clarify the position of this unfortunately named hybrid.

Much more research is necessary on the relative advantages of using patients or informants in the assessment of personality disorders. There are often ethical difficulties in getting adequate informants (and this may be a particular problem in the United States), but access to independent information is really essential before personality status can be determined satisfactorily.

## CATEGORICAL VERSUS DIMENSIONAL CLASSIFICATION OF PERSONALITY DISORDERS

DSM-III and its successors have enjoyed considerable popularity because they have improved the delineation of categories of Axis I disorders. The same procedure has been adopted with Axis II disorders, but has been conspicuously less successful. This is because most of the disorders described in Axis I, despite argument about their distinct identity, have in most cases been accepted by the psychiatric community as useful diagnoses. The DSM classification has improved their definition and thereby helped categorization. Personality disorders cannot be treated in the same way. The idea of qualitatively distinct (preferably single) personality disorders, which is the aim of the classification, is not borne out by experimental work. The results of almost all the structured interview schedules based on DSM-III suggest that a single personality disorder is much less common than multiple ones (Reich, 1987), and in severe personality disorders most areas of personality functioning become disorganized and maladaptive (Tyrer et al., 1983). The aim of identifying mutually exclusive personality disorder categories therefore seems to be a mirage; it can be achieved only by distortion of natural data.

The dimensional approach has many advantages. If, as many argue, personality disorders are regarded as the extremes of a continuum in which various degrees of personality difficulty grade toward normal personality variation, then it is obviously more appropriate to record the abnormality in dimensional terms (Cloninger, 1987; Bronisch, 1992; Livesley & Jackson, 1992). By doing this, one avoids the Procrustean distinction of a cutoff point between normal (and allegedly healthy) personality functioning and the extreme categories of personality disorders. It also allows examination of the relative importance of different types of personality disorders.

The concept of personality accentuation — initially introduced in ICD-10 implicitly, but subsequently dropped—recognizes the advantages of the dimensional approach. This concept acknowledges degrees of personality abnormality that are not universally maladaptive but that can affect the course of Axis I disorders and make individuals more vulnerable to distress when environmental conditions are adverse (Leonhard, 1968). Indeed, there may be important psychiatric syndromes that include a combination of personality abnormality and Axis I disorders, but these will be missed unless Axis I and Axis II are recorded separately (Tyrer, 1985; Tyrer Seivewright, Ferguson, & Tyrer, 1992).

## SUGGESTED IMPROVEMENTS

It would be wrong to abandon the well-tried and tested methods that have led to the development of consecutive revisions of DSM. Nevertheless, these could be modified to (1) give less weight in personality disorders to operational criteria of description, with omission of those that do not rely on experimental evidence; (2) introduce external criteria of social dysfunction into definitions of the DSM personality disorders; (3) improve the descriptions of personality disorders and separation of Axis II from Axis I disorders by systematic use of information derived from informants; and (4) allow both categorical and dimensional systems of classification to coexist. A start has already been made on the first of these suggestions by Livesley (1987) and Schroeder and Livesley (1991), who have shown that many of the behavioral items covering the range of DSM personality disorders are duplicated; this suggests that several items of the present system are redundant.

My prediction is that making these modifications will open up the classification to improve research methodology, so that it will be more common for investigators to ask "Is this a valid description of abnormal personality?" than to ask the restricted and ultimately sterile question "Is this a reliable index of the DSM criteria of personality disorder?" To speculate further, I suspect that such research will also reveal that the number of personality disorders in DSM could be reduced substantially without any loss to clinical or research practice. There is far too great a degree of overlap among existing categories to justify the retention of all of them (Tyrer, Casey, & Ferguson, 1991). These are exciting times in the development of our knowledge of abnormal personality, and it would be a shame if too much time and effort were directed into shoring up those structures in the DSM-IV classification that have no external validity and maintain their position through political rather than scientific arguments.

## REFERENCES

American Psychiatric Association. (1980). *Diagnostic and statistical manual of mental disorders* (3rd ed.). Washington DC: Author.

American Psychiatric Association. (1987). *Diagnostic and statistical manual of mental disorders* (3rd ed., rev.). Washington, DC: Author.

American Psychiatric Association. (1994). *Diagnostic and statistical manual of mental disorders* (4th ed.). Washington, DC: Author.

Barasch, J., Kroll, J., & Careym K. (1983). Discriminating borderline from other personality disorders. *Archives of General Psychiatry, 40,* 1297–1302.

Baron, M. (1982). *Schedule for Interviewing Borderlines (SIB).* New York: New York State Psychiatric Institute.

Bronisch, T. (1992). Diagnostic procedures of personality disorders according to the criteria of present classification systems. *Verhaltenstherapie, 2,* 140–150.

Brothwell, J., Casey, P. R., & Tyrer, P. (1992). Who gives the most reliable account of a psychiatric patient's personality? *Irish Journal of Psychological Medicine, 9,* 90–93.

Cloninger, C. R. (1987). A systematic method of clinical description and classification of personality variants. *Archives of General Psychiatry, 44,* 573–588.

Coppen, A., & Metcalfe, M. (1965). Effects of a depressive illness on MPI scores. *British Journal of Psychiatry, 111,* 236–239.

Costa, P. T., & McCrea, R. R. (1990). Personality disorders and the five-factor model of personality. *Journal of Personality Disorders, 4,* 362–371.

Ferguson, B. G., & Tyrer, P. (1988). Classifying personality disorder. In P. Tyrer (Ed.), *Personality disorders: Diagnosis, management and course* (pp. 12–32). London: Wright.

Frances, A. J. (1980). The DSM-III personality disorders: A commentary. *American Journal of Psychiatry, 137,* 1050–1054.

Frances, A. J., Clarkin, J., Gilmore, M., Hurt, S. W., & Brown, R. (1984). Reliability of criteria for borderline personality disorder: A comparison of DSM-III and DIB. *American Journal of Psychiatry, 141,* 1080–1084.

Frances, A. J., & Widiger, T. (1986). The classification of personality disorders: An overview of problems and solutions. In A. J. Frances & R. E. Hales (Eds.), *Psychiatry update: American Psychiatric Association annual review* (Vol. 5, pp. 240–257). Washington, DC: American Psychiatric Press.

Fyer, M. R., Frances, A. J., Sullivan, T., Hurt, S. W., & Clarkin, J. (1988). Co-morbidity of borderline personality disorder. *Archives of General Psychiatry, 45,* 348–352.

Gunderson, J. (1982). *Diagnostic Interview for Borderline Patients* (2nd ed.). Belmont, MA: Harvard Medical School.

Hirschfeld, R. M. A., & Klerman, G. L. (1979). Personality attributes and affective disorder. *American Journal of Psychiatry, 136,* 67–70.

Hirschfeld, R. M. A., Klerman, G. L., Clayton, P. J., Keller, M. B., McDonald-Scott, P., & Larkin, B. H. (1983). Assessing personality: Effects of the depressive state on trait measurement. *American Journal of Psychiatry, 140,* 695–699.

Kass, F., Skodol, A. E., Charles, E., Spitzer, R. L., & Williams, J. B. W. (1985). Scaled ratings of DSM-III personality disorders. *American Journal of Psychiatry, 142,* 627–630.

Kendell, R. E. (1975). *The role of diagnosis in psychiatry.* Oxford: Blackwell.

Kraepelin, E. (1904). *Lectures on clinical psychiatry.* (T. Johnstone, Ed. and Trans.). London: Balliere, Tindall & Cox.

Kroll, J., Carey K., Simes, L., & Roth, M. (1982). Are there borderlines in Britain? A cross validation of U.S. findings. *Archives of General Psychiatry, 39,* 60–63.

Leonhard, K. (1968). *Akzentuierte Personlichkeiten.* East Berlin: Verlag Volk und Gesundheit.

Lion, J. R. (1981). A comparison between DSM-III and DSM-II personality disorder.

In J. R. Lion (Ed.), *Personality disorders: Diagnosis and management* (pp. 1–31). Baltimore: Williams & Wilkins.

Livesley, W. J. (1987). A systematic approach to the delineation of personality disorders. *American Journal of Psychiatry, 144,* 772–777.

Livesley, W. J., & Jackson, D. N. (1992). Guidelines for developing, evaluating and revising the classification of personality disorders. *Journal of Nervous and Mental Disease, 180,* 609–618.

Loranger, A. W., Susman, V. L., Oldham, J. M., & Russakoff, H. (1985). *Personality Disorder Examination (PDE): A structured interview for DSM-III-R personality disorders.* White Plains, NY: New York Hospital–Cornell University Medical Center, Westchester Division.

Mann, A. H., Jenkins, R., Cuttings, J. C., & Cowan, P. J. (1981). The development and use of a standardized assessment of abnormal personality. *Psychological Medicine, 11,* 839–847.

McGlashan, T. H. (1986). Schizotypal personality disorder: Chestnut Lodge Follow-Up Study. VI. Long-term follow-up perspectives. *Archives of General Psychiatry, 43,* 329–334.

Merson, J., Tyrer, P., Duke, P., & Henderson, F. (1994). Interrates reliability of ICD-10 guidelines for the diagnosis of personality disorders. *Journal of Personality Disorders, 8,* 89–95.

Perry, J. (1982). *The Borderline Personality Disorder Scale (BPD Scale).* Cambridge, MA: Cambridge Hospital.

Pfohl, B., Coryell, W., Zimmerman, M., & Stangl, D. (1986). DSM-III personality disorders: Diagnostic overlap and internal consistency of individual DSM-III criteria. *Comprehensive Psychiatry., 27,* 21–34.

Pope, H. G., Jonas, J. M., Hudson J. I., Cohen, B. M., & Gunderson, J. G. (1983). The validity of DSM-III borderline personality disorder: A phenomenologic family history, treatment response and long term follow up study. *Archives of General Psychiatry, 40,* 23–30.

Reich, J. (1987). Instruments measuring DSM-III and DSM-III-R personality disorders. *Journal of Personality Disorders, 1,* 220–240.

Reich, J., Noyes, R. Jr., Coryell, W., & O'Gorman, T. W. (1986). The effects of state anxiety on personality measurement. *American Journal of Psychiatry, 143,* 760–763.

Reich, J., Noyes, R. Jr., & Troughton, E. (1987). Dependent personality disorders associated with phobic avoidance in patients with panic disorder. *American Journal of Psychiatry, 144,* 329–326.

Rutter, M. (1987). Temperament, personality and personality disorder. *British Journal of Psychiatry, 150,* 443–458.

Schneider, K. (1923). *Die psychopathischen Personlichkeiten.* Berlin: Springer-Verlag.

Schroeder, M. L., & Livesley, W. J. (1991). An evaluation of DSM-III-R personality disorders. *Acta Psychiatrica Scandinavica, 84,* 512–519.

Shainess, N. (1987). Masochism or self-defeating personality. *Journal of Personality Disorders, 1,* 174–177.

Spitzer, R. L., Williams, J. B., & Gibbs. (1987). *Structured Clinical Interview for DSM-III Personality Disorders (SCID-II).* New York: New York State Psychiatric Institute.

Stangl, D., Pfohl, B., Zimmerman, M., Bowers, W., & Corenthal, C. (1985). A structured interview for the DSM-III personality disorders: A preliminary report. *Archives of General Psychiatry, 42,* 591–596.

Theophrastus. (1925). *A book of characters.* (R. Adlington, Ed. and Trans.) London: Dutton.

Trull, T. J., Widiger, T. A., & Frances, A. (1987). Co-variation of criteria sets for avoidant, schizoid and dependent personality disorders. *American Journal of Psychiatry, 144,* 767–771.

Tyrer, P. (1985). Neurosis divisible? *Lancet, i,* 685–688.

Tyrer, P., & Alexander, J. (1979). The classification of personality disorder. *British Journal of Psychiatry, 135,* 163–167.

Tyrer, P., Alexander, J., & Ferguson, B. (1988). Personality Assessment Schedule. In P. Tyrer (Ed.), *Personality disorders: Diagnosis, management and course* (pp. 140–167). London: Butterworth/Wright.

Tyrer, P., Alexander, M. S., & Cicchetti, D., Cohen, M. S., & Remington, M. (1979). Reliability of a schedule for rating personality disorders. *British Journal of Psychiatry, 135,* 168–174.

Tyrer, P., Casey, P. R., & Ferguson, B. (1991). Personality disorder in perspective. *British Journal of Psychiatry, 159,* 463–471.

Tyrer, P., Cicchetti, D. V., Casey, P. R., Fitzpatrick, K., Oliver, R., Balker, A., Giller, E., & Harkness, L. (1984). Cross-national reliability study of a schedule for assessing personality disorders. *Journal of Nervous and Mental Disease, 172,* 718–721.

Tyrer, P., Seivewright, N., Ferguson, B., & Tyrer, J. (1992). The general neurotic syndrome: A coaxial diagnosis of anxiety, depression and personality disorder. *Acta Psychiatrica Scandinavica, 85,* 201–206.

Tyrer, P., Strauss, J., & Cicchetti, D. (1983). Temporal reliability of personality in psychiatric patients. *Psychological Medicine, 13,* 393–398.

Walker, L. E. A. (1987). The inadequacy of the masochistic personality disorder diagnosis for women. *Journal of Personality Disorders, 1,* 183–189.

Widiger, T. A., & Frances, A. (1985). The DSM-III personality disorders. *Archives of General Psychiatry, 42,* 615–623.

World Health Organization. (1992). *The ICD-10 classification of mental and behavioural disorders: Diagnostic criteria for research.* Geneva: Author.

World Health Organization (WHO), & Alcohol, Drug Abuse and Mental Health Administration (ADAMHA). (1983). Diagnosis and classification of mental disorders and alcohol and drug-related problems: A research agenda for the 1980's. *Psychological Medicine, 13,* 907–921.

Zimmerman, M., Pfohl, B., Coryell, W., Stangl, D., & Corenthal, C. (1988). Diagnosing personality disorder in depressed patients: A comparison of patient and informant interviews. *Archives of General Psychiatry, 45,* 733–737.

# PART II

# DSM-IV PERSONALITY DISORDER DIAGNOSES

CHAPTER 3

# Paranoid Personality Disorder

DAVID P. BERNSTEIN
DAVID USEDA
LARRY J. SIEVER

Since the time of Kraepelin (1921), a pervasive and unwarranted mistrust of others has been considered the defining feature of paranoid personality disorder. Other clinical characteristics that have figured prominently in the descriptive literature on this disorder are the paranoid individual's hypersensitivity to criticism (Kretschmer, 1925; Cameron, 1943, 1963), antagonism and aggressiveness (Schneider, 1923; Sheldon, 1940; Sheldon & Stevens, 1942), rigidity (Shapiro, 1965), hypervigilance (Cameron, 1963; Shapiro, 1965), and excessive need for autonomy (Millon, 1969, 1981). This body of clinical literature formed the basis of the diagnostic criteria for paranoid personality disorder that were incorporated in to DSM-III (American Psychiatric Association [APA], 1980). DSM-III required that patients meet three criteria for suspiciousness, two for hypersensitivity, and two for restricted affectivity in order to receive a diagnosis of paranoid personality disorder. In DSM-III-R (American Psychiatric Association, 1987), the grouping of diagnostic criteria into sets was replaced by a truly polythetic system, in which no single feature (or group of features) was required and any combination of four of seven criteria was sufficient for a paranoid personality disorder diagnosis.

In this chapter, some of the major nosological issues concerning paranoid personality disorder are raised and addressed in light of current research findings. Particular emphasis is placed on research pertaining to the development of diagnostic criteria for paranoid personality disorder in DSM-IV (American Psychiatric Association, 1994).

An earlier version of this chapter was published in the *Journal of Personality Disorders*, 1993, 7, 53–62. Copyright 1993 by The Guilford Press. Adapted by permission.

## SIGNIFICANT ISSUES

A central issue regarding paranoid personality disorder is its status as a possible "schizophrenia spectrum" disorder. Kraepelin (1921) observed that premorbid "paranoid personalities" were often present in individuals who later developed paranoid psychoses, including dementia praecox. Subsequent writers also considered premorbid traits such as suspiciousness and hostility to be predisposing factors in the emergence of later delusional illness, particularly in the "late paraphrenias" of old age (Herbert & Jacobson, 1967). Historically, then, some authors have considered paranoid personality disorder a possible precursor of other, more severe paranoid conditions. More recent speculations have concerned the position of paranoid personality disorder on a hypothetical "schizophrenia spectrum" (Siever & Davis, 1991) that includes DSM-III-R Axis I schizophrenia and Axis II schizoid and schizotypal personality disorders.

The conceptualization of paranoid personality disorder as a possible "schizophrenia spectrum" disorder raises issues concerning syndromal boundaries. First, what is the relationship between paranoid personality disorder and schizotypal personality disorder, an Axis II disorder with which paranoid personality disorder shares certain diagnostic features (e.g., suspiciousness)? The high rate of diagnostic overlap between these disorders raises questions about their discriminant validity and suggests the possibility of subsuming paranoid personality disorder within a broadly redefined schizotypal category.

Second, what is the relationship between paranoid personality disorder and Axis I delusional disorder? The differential diagnosis between paranoid personality disorder and delusional disorder rests on the absence of systematized delusions in the former; yet "true" delusions are sometimes difficult to distinguish from the cognitive distortions of patients with paranoid personality disorder, and delusional beliefs may appear in individuals with long-standing paranoid personality traits. These findings raise the possibility of a spectrum that encompasses both paranoid personality disorder and delusional disorder, and that is distinct from (or only partially overlapping with) the schizophrenia-related disorders.

An additional set of issues concerns the formulation of the diagnostic criteria for paranoid personality disorder in DSM-IV: Namely, which of the DSM-III-R paranoid personality disorder criteria were candidates for modification or eliminated in DSM-IV, on the basis of their diagnostic efficiency (e.g., sensitivity and specificity)? Also, to what extent could North American approaches to the definition of the disorder (i.e., DSM-III-R and DSM-IV) have been made compatible with other diagnostic systems, particularly the World Health Organization's 10th revision of the *International Classification of Diseases* (ICD-10)? Increasing compatibility between the two systems would have the desirable effect of facilitating international communication and collaboration regarding both research and clinical practice.

The resolution of these nosological issues will require studies employing diagnostic validators, such as phenomenology, family history, laboratory findings, and treatment response; however, research on the validation of paranoid personality disorder has been limited. This chapter has therefore attempted to reach some preliminary conclusions, based on the empirical studies that have been conducted to date. This review process was not intended to be exhaustive, but rather to focus on issues germane to the refinement of the diagnostic criteria for paranoid personality disorder.

## LITERATURE REVIEW

### Epidemiology

Paranoid ideation has long been reported to be especially prevalent among groups such as prisoners (Faergeman, 1963; Slater & Roth, 1969), refugees and immigrants (Eitinger, 1959; Mezey, 1960), the elderly (Christenson & Blazer, 1984; Fish, 1960; Post, 1966), and the hearing-impaired (Kay & Roth, 1961). The extent to which these groups are truly "at risk" for paranoid personality disorder, however, is uncertain, because the different methodologies and diagnostic criteria used in these studies (most of which were conducted prior to the publication of DSM-III) make it difficult to evaluate the findings. Furthermore, many studies failed to distinguish paranoid personality traits, which may accompany a variety of psychiatric or physical conditions, from paranoid personality disorder, and to determine whether paranoid personality disorder was primary or secondary to organic causes (e.g., as in hearing impairment).

Most clinically based studies using DSM-III or DSM-III-R criteria have reported a preponderance of paranoid personality disorder in males (Alnaes & Torgersen, 1988a; Reich, 1987), although the sex distribution of paranoid personality disorder in the general population has not been established. Though overall prevalences of paranoid personality disorder in clinically based studies have varied widely (Table 3.1), it appears that the extensive revision of the diagnostic criteria for this disorder in DSM-III-R has resulted in an increased diagnostic prevalence of the disorder. Prevalences of paranoid personality disorder in 11 clinical studies employing DSM-III criteria ranged from less than 1% to 20%, with a median prevalence of 5.5% (Mellsop, Varghese, Joshua, & Hicks, 1982; Clarkin, Widiger, Frances, Hurt, & Gilmore, 1983; Kass, Skodol, Charles, Spitzer, & Williams, 1985; Khantzian & Treece, 1985; Koenigsberg, Kaplan, Gilmore, & Cooper, 1985; Dahl, 1986; Pfohl, Coryell, Zimmerman, & Stangl, 1986; Widiger, Frances, Warner, & Bluhm, 1986; Reich, 1987; Alnaes & Torgersen, 1988a; Zanarini, 1989), whereas prevalences of paranoid personality disorder in the four studies using DSM-III-R criteria ranged from 15% to 30%, with a median prevalence of 18% (Morey & Heumann, 1988; Skodol, Rosnick, Kellman, Oldham, &

TABLE 3.1. Prevalence of DSM-III and DSM-III-R Paranoid Personality Disorder in 15 Clinical Studies

| Study | Sample size | Diagnostic nomenclature | Type of sample | Prevalence | |
|---|---|---|---|---|---|
| | | | | $n$ | % |
| Mellsop et al. (1982) | 77 | DSM-III | Inpatient | 8 | 10 |
| Clarkin et al. (1983) | 76 | DSM-III | Outpatient | 6 | 8 |
| Kass et al. (1985) | 609 | DSM-III | Outpatient | 30 | 5 |
| Khantzian & Treece (1985) | 87 | DSM-III | Outpatient | 2 | 2 |
| Koenigsberg et al. (1985) | 2,462 | DSM-III | Mixed | 11 | 0 |
| Dahl (1986) | 103 | DSM-III | Inpatient | 1 | 1 |
| Pfohl et al. (1986) | 131 | DSM-III | Outpatient | 17 | 20 |
| Widiger et al. (1986) | 84 | DSM-III | Inpatient | 17 | 20 |
| Reich (1987) | 170 | DSM-III | Outpatient | 11 | 6 |
| Morey & Heumann (1988) | 291 | DSM-III-R | Mixed | 64 | 22 |
| Skodol et al. (1988) | 97 | DSM-III-R | Inpatient | 14 | 14 |
| Alnaes & Torgersen (1988) | 298 | DSM-III | Outpatient | 15 | 5 |
| Zanarini (1989) | 253 | DSM-III | Mixed | 16 | 6 |
| Millon & Tringone (1989) | 809 | DSM-III-R | Mixed | 12 | 1 |
| Freiman & Widiger (1989) | 50 | DSM-III-R | Inpatient | 15 | 30 |

Hyler, 1988; Millon & Tringone, 1989; Freiman & Widiger, 1989). The prevalence of paranoid personality disorder in the general population is unknown, although one epidemiological study has estimated it as 3.3% in young adults aged 18 to 21 (Bernstein, Cohen, Velez, Schwab-Stone, & Siever, 1993) — an estimate slightly higher than those obtained in four published studies of adult nonpsychiatric control subjects (range = 0.5% to 2.3%, median prevalence = 1.4%) (Baron et al., 1985; Coryell & Zimmerman, 1989; Drake & Vaillant, 1985; Kendler & Gruenberg, 1982).

## Criterion Performance

Only a handful of studies have systematically examined the diagnostic efficiency of the clinical features of paranoid personality disorder, using DSM-III or DSM-III-R diagnostic criteria. Two studies (Livesley, 1986; Zanarini, 1989) have called into question the diagnostic efficiency of the DSM-III paranoid personality disorder features grouped under the heading "restricted affectivity" ("appears cold and unemotional," "presents himself as objective and rational," "lacks a sense of humor," and "absence of tender feelings towards others"; American Psychiatric Association; 1980, p. 309). These criteria were eliminated in DSM-III-R.

Most of the DSM-III-R paranoid personality disorder diagnostic criteria have exhibited satisfactory sensitivity and specificity in the few clinical studies that have examined their diagnostic efficiency (Millon & Tringone, 1989; Morey & Heumann, 1988; Freiman & Widiger, 1989). However, paranoid personality disorder criterion 6 ("is easily slighted ...") was found to

TABLE 3.2. DSM-III-R and DSM-IV Diagnostic Criteria for Paranoid Personality Disorder

| DSM-III-R criteria | DSM-IV criteria |
|---|---|
| A. A pervasive and unwarranted tendency, beginning by early adulthood and present in a variety of contexts, to interpret the actions of people as deliberately demeaning or threatening, as indicated by at least *four* of the following: | A. A pervasive distrust and suspiciousness of others such that their motives are interpreted as malevolent, beginning by early adulthood and present in a variety of contexts, as indicated by four (or more) of the following: |
| (1) expects, without sufficient basis, to be exploited or harmed by others | (1) suspects, without sufficient basis, that others are exploiting, harming, or deceiving him or her |
| (2) questions, without justification, the loyalty or trustworthiness of friends or associates | (2) is preoccupied with unjustified doubts about the loyalty or trustworthiness of friends or associates |
| (3) reads hidden demeaning or threatening meanings into benign remarks or events, e.g., suspects that a neighbor put out trash early to annoy him | (3) is reluctant to confide in others because of unwarranted fear that the information will be used maliciously against him or her |
| (4) bears grudges or is unforgiving of insults or slights | (4) reads hidden demeaning or threatening meanings into benign remarks or events |
| (5) is reluctant to confide in others because of unwarranted fear that the information will be used against him or her | (5) persistently bears grudges, i.e., is unforgiving of insults, injuries, or slights |
| (6) is easily slighted and quick to react with anger or to counterattack | (6) perceives attacks on his or her character or reputation that are not apparent to others and is quick to react angrily or to counterattack |
| (7) questions, without justification, fidelity of spouse or sexual partner | (7) has recurrent suspicions, without justification, regarding fidelity of spouse or sexual partner |
| B. Occurrence not exclusively during the course of Schizophrenia or a Delusional Disorder. | B. Does not occur exclusively during the course of Schizophrenia, a Mood Disorder With Psychotic Features, or another Psychotic Disorder and is not due to the direct physiological effects of a general medical condition. **Note:** If criteria are met prior to the onset of Schizophrenia, add "Premorbid," e.g., "Paranoid Personality Disorder (Premorbid)." |

*Note.* From APA (1987, p. 339) and APA (1994, pp. 537–638). Copyright 1987 and 1994 by the American Psychiatric Association. Reprinted by permission.

be the least specific of any in the paranoid criteria set (range = .62 to .64, median = .63), and criterion 7 ("questions, without justification, fidelity of spouse or sexual partner") exhibited poor sensitivity in two of the three studies surveyed (range = .17 to .60, median = .38). Although the diagnostic efficiency of criteria 6 and 7 was sufficient to warrant their continued inclusion in the paranoid personality disorder criteria set, there were thus reasons to consider modifying them in DSM-IV. These modifications are discussed later in this chapter. Table 3.2 lists the DSM-III-R and DSM-IV criteria for paranoid personality disorder.

## Comparison of DSM and ICD-10 Diagnostic Criteria

The DSM-III-R criteria set for paranoid personality disorder was found to overlap only partially with the proposed paranoid personality disorder items in the ICD-10, based on a meeting between APA and World Health Organization representatives (Dr. Michael First, personal communication, November 1991). Corresponding ICD-10 items were found for DSM-III-R criterion 4 ("bears grudges . . . ") (ICD-10 criterion 3), DSM-III-R criterion 5 ("is reluctant to confide in others . . . ") (ICD-10 criterion 2), DSM-III-R criterion 6 ("is easily slighted . . . ") (ICD-10 criterion 3), and DSM-III-R criterion 7 ("questions . . . fidelity of spouse or sexual partner") (ICD-10 criterion 5). Corresponding items were not found for DSM-III-R criteria 1 ("expects . . . to be exploited or harmed"), 2 ("questions . . . trustworthiness of friends or associates"), and 3 ("reads hidden demeaning or threatening meanings into benign remarks or events . . . "). Four additional items were included in ICD-10: items 1 ("excessive sensitiveness to setbacks and rebuffs"), 4 ("a combative and tenacious sense of personal rights out of keeping with the actual situation"), 6 ("a tendency to experience excessive self-importance, manifest in a persistent self-referential attitude"), and 7 ("preoccupation with unsubstantiated 'conspiratorial' explanations of events around the subject or in the world at large"). At this time, there are no empirical data that might help resolve these discrepancies. Nor do the revised criteria in DSM-IV bridge these gaps (see below).

## Comorbidity

Fewer than one-fourth of patients with paranoid personality disorder in clinically based samples are free of other personality disorder diagnoses (Zanarini, 1989; Millon & Tringone, 1989). Table 3.3 presents rates of overlap between paranoid personality disorder and other Axis II disorders as reported in six clinically based studies. Rates of overlap with specific Axis II disorders varied considerably across the studies. For example, the percentage of patients with paranoid personality disorder receiving comorbid diagnoses of schizotypal personality disorder ranged from 17% (Millon & Tringone, 1989) to 71% (Widiger et al., 1986). Such high overlap is possibly attibut-

TABLE 3.3. Comorbidity among Axis II Disorders in Six Clinical Studies

| | SZD | SZT | HST | NAR | BDL | ATS | AVD | DEP | OCP | PAG | SDF | SAD |
|---|---|---|---|---|---|---|---|---|---|---|---|---|
| Percentage of patients with paranoid personality disorder receiving indicated diagnosis | | | | | | | | | | | | |
| Widiger et al. (1986) | 18 | 71 | 23 | 2 | 41 | 29 | 18 | 12 | 0 | 53 | — | — |
| Morey & Heumann (1988) | 23 | 25 | 28 | 36 | 48 | 8 | 48 | 30 | 8 | 17 | — | — |
| Skodol et al. (1988)[a] | 0 | 43 | 14 | 57 | 93 | 14 | 86 | 57 | 50 | 29 | 43 | — |
| Zanarini (1989) | 0 | 50 | 56 | 38 | 100 | 13 | 56 | 31 | 19 | 50 | — | — |
| Millon & Tringone (1989)[b] | 8 | 17 | 8 | 75 | 0 | 25 | 8 | 0 | 33 | 17 | 0 | 0 |
| Freiman & Widiger (1989) | 3 | 33 | 27 | 47 | 53 | 33 | 60 | 27 | 0 | 40 | 13 | 27 |
| Percentage of patients with indicated diagnosis receiving a diagnosis of paranoid personality disorder | | | | | | | | | | | | |
| Widiger et al. (1986) | 43 | 25 | 10 | 22 | 13 | 16 | 11 | 5 | 0 | 20 | — | — |
| Morey & Heumann (1988) | 47 | 59 | 29 | 36 | 32 | 28 | 39 | 29 | 22 | 31 | — | — |
| Skodol et al. (1988)[a] | 0 | 38 | 12 | 38 | 21 | 25 | 31 | 24 | 33 | 67 | 30 | — |
| Zanarini (1989) | 0 | 10 | 8 | 13 | 9 | 2 | 17 | 7 | 17 | 14 | — | — |
| Millon & Tringone (1989)[b] | 0 | 12 | 1 | 4 | 3 | 0 | 0 | 0 | 0 | 1 | 0 | 6 |
| Freiman & Widiger (1989) | 62 | 46 | 44 | 64 | 47 | 36 | 47 | 33 | 0 | 75 | 50 | 44 |

Note. Key to personality disorder abbreviations: SZD, schizoid; SZT, schizotypal; HST, histrionic; NAR, narcissistic; BDL, borderline; ATS, antisocial; AVD, avoidant; DEP, dependent; OCP, obsessive–compulsive; PAG, passive–aggressive; SDF, self-defeating; SAD, sadistic.
[a]Prevalence of SZT in this table based on the Personality Disorder Examination. (Skodol et al., 1988, also reported prevalences based on other diagnostic instruments.)
[b]Prevalence of SZT in this table based on the Millon Clinical Multiaxial Inventory. (Millon & Tringone, 1989, also reported prevalences based on other diagnostic instruments.)

able to shared diagnostic criteria (e.g., paranoid ideation). High rates of overlap were also reported with narcissistic, borderline, avoidant, and passive–aggressive personality disorders.

Few studies employing DSM-III or DSM-III-R criteria have reported rates of diagnostic overlap between paranoid personality disorder and Axis I disorders. In a study of 298 psychiatric outpatients, Alnaes and Torgersen (1988b) found that patients with paranoid personality disorder were 3.5 times more likely to receive a DSM-III Axis I diagnosis of agoraphobia without panic than would be expected on the basis of the prevalence of this disorder in the total sample. No other Axis I diagnosis was significantly associated with paranoid personality disorder. Coryell and Zimmerman (1989) examined the relationship between DSM-III Axis I and Axis II disorders in a combined sample of 797 relatives of psychiatric and nonpsychiatric control probands. When compared to relatives without personality disorder diagnoses, relatives with paranoid personality disorder were at significantly increased lifetime risk for Axis I diagnoses of alcohol and drug abuse/dependence, schizophrenia, obsessive–compulsive disorder, phobic disorder, and bulimia, as well as for a history of attempted suicide. However, when compared to relatives with other personality disorders, relatives with paranoid personality disorder were at greater risk only for Axis I diagnosis of bulimia.

## Family/Genetic Studies

Studies reporting on the familial aggregation of paranoid personality disorder in the relatives of schizophrenic probands have produced mixed results. Although paranoid personality disorder appears to be slightly more prevalent in the relatives of schizophrenics than in the family members of control subjects, statistically significant findings have been reported in only two (Baron et al., 1985; Kendler & Gruenberg, 1982) of five published studies (Baron et al., 1985; Coryell & Zimmerman, 1989; Kendler & Gruenberg, 1982; Kendler, Masterson, & Davis, 1985; Stephens, Atkinson, Kay, Roth, & Garside, 1975).

There is some evidence that paranoid personality disorder may have a stronger familial relationship with Axis I delusional disorder than with schizophrenia. Kendler et al. (1985) reported that the morbid risk of paranoid personality disorder was significantly greater in the first degree relatives of probands with delusional disorder (4.8%) than in the relatives of schizophrenics (0.8%) and medical controls (0%). There is some evidence, however, that schizophrenia and delusional disorder do not share a similar genetic basis. For example, Kendler and Hays (1981) found that cases of schizophrenia were significantly less common in the first- and second-degree relatives of probands with delusional disorder (0.6%) than in the relatives of schizophrenic probands (3.8%). Thus, paranoid personality disorder and delusional disorder may share a genetic basis that is stronger than, and distinct from, the basis they share with schizophrenia. In contrast, schizophrenia may share a genetic basis with Axis II schizotypal personality disorder because an excess of relatives with schizotypal personality disorder has been found in many (Baron et al., 1985; Siever et al., 1991) but not all (Coryell & Zimmerman, 1989), studies in which schizophrenic patients have served as probands.

## Treatment Response

Although case reports have appeared on the successful treatment of paranoid personality disorder with cognitive therapy (Turkat, 1985; Turkat &

Maisto, 1985; Williams, 1988), no controlled studies have examined the response of paranoid personality disorder to either psychotherapy or pharmacotherapy. Paranoid individuals are often considered difficult to engage in a psychotherapeutic relationship because of their mistrust of the therapist's motives, denial of difficulties, and reluctance to disclose personal information (Bullard, 1960). Siever and Kendler (1985) have reported that in their clinical experience, patients with paranoid personality disorder can sometimes benefit from low doses of neuroleptic medication, but this claim has not been evaluated in a controlled trial.

## DISCUSSION

Evidence from phenomenological studies offers some tentative support for the diagnostic validity of paranoid personality disorder, and does not appear to justify subsuming paranoid personality disorder within a broadly redefined schizotypal diagnostic category. Although paranoid and schoizotypal personality disorders exhibit a high rate of overlap in clinically based studies, a substantial proportion of paranoid patients do not meet the diagnostic criteria for schizotypal personality disorder. Furthermore, patients with paranoid personality disorder frequently share the clinical characteristics of several other Axis II disorders, particularly narcissistic, borderline, avoidant, and passive–aggressive personality disorders. Phenomenologically, paranoid personality disorder appears to be a heterogeneous diagnostic category whose members may share none, some, or many schizotypal diagnostic features.

Family/genetic studies also support the discriminant validity of paranoid personality personality. Although research findings largely support the hypothesis of schoizotypal personality disorder as a "schizophrenia spectrum" disorder, findings regarding the relationship of paranoid personality disorder to schizophrenia have been less consistent. There is also evidence that paranoid personality disorder and Axis I delusional disorder may share a genetic basis that is more substantial than the basis they share with schizophrenia. However, at this early stage of family/genetic research, it would be premature to characterize paranoid personality disorder as either a "schizophrenia spectrum" or a "delusional spectrum" disorder.

Although only a few studies have assessed the diagnostic efficiency of the DSM-III and DSM-III-R criteria for paranoid personality disorder, it was decided that criterion 6 ("is easily slighted and quick to react with anger or to counterattack") should be modified to increase diagnostic specificity, and that criterion 7 ("questions, without justification, fidelity of spouse or sexual partner") should be altered to increase its sensitivity.

It appears that there are substantial differences between the paranoid personality disorder criteria included in DSM-III-R and DSM-IV and those proposed for ICD-10. However, empirical studies comparing these criteria sets are needed before these discrepancies can be resolved.

## CHANGES MADE IN DSM-IV

The following changes have been made to the diagnostic criteria for para-noid personality disorder in DSM-IV. These changes are minor because of the nascent state of research in the area. Slight changes have been made in criteria 6 and 7. Criterion 6 has been modified to read, "perceives attacks on his or her character or reputation that are not apparent to others and is quick to react with anger or to counterattack" (see Table 3.2). This modifi-cation indicates that the defensive outbursts of paranoid individuals are responses to perceived attacks; it provides greater differentiation from similar reactions based on wounded self-esteem (e.g., as in dependent and avoidant personality disorders) or impulsivity and/or affective liability (e.g., as in bor-derline and histrionic personality disorders). Criterion 7 has been modified as follows: "has recurrent suspicions, without justification, regarding fidel-ity of spouse or sexual partner." This modification emphasizes the intensity and pervasiveness of the paranoid individual's pathological jealousy, with the aim of increasing the item's sensitivity.

In addition, the "stem" for the seven paranoid personality disorder in-clusion criteria has been changed as follows: "A pervasive distrust and sus-piciousness of others such that their motives are interpreted as malevolent, beginning by early adulthood and present in a variety of contexts, as indi-cated by four (or more) of the following." This modification emphasizes the fact that suspiciousness and mistrust of others are the central defining fea-tures of the disorder.

Although it was considered premature to propose substantial changes to the DSM-IV and ICD-10 criteria sets in order to increase the compatibili-ty between the two sets, DSM-III-R criterion 4 ("bears grudges or is unforgiv-ing of insults or slights") has been revised slightly in becoming criterion 5 ("persistently bears grudges, i.e., is unforgiving of insults, injuries, or slights"), in order to increase compatibility with ICD-10 item 2 ("tendency to bear grudges persistently, i.e., to be unforgiving of insults, injuries, or slights").

## REFERENCES

Alnaes, R., & Torgersen, S. (1988a). DSM-III symptom disorders (Axis I) and perso-nality disorders (Axis II) in an outpatient population. *Acta Psychiatrica Scandinavica, 78,* 348–355.

Alnaes, R., & Torgersen, S. (1988b). The relationship between DSM-III symptom dis-orders (Axis I) and personality disorders (Axis II) in an outpatient population. *Acta Psychiatrica Scandinavica, 78,* 485–492.

American Psychiatric Association. (1980). *Diagnostic and statistical manual of mental dis-orders* (3rd ed.). Washington, DC: Author.

American Psychiatric Association, (1987). *Diagnostic and statistical manual of mental dis-orders* (3rd ed., rev.). Washington, DC: Author.

American Psychiatric Association. (1994). *Diagnostic and statistical manual of mental dis-orders* (4th. ed.). Washington, DC: Author.

Baron, M., Gruen, R., Rainer, J. D., Kane, J., Asnis, L., & Lord, S. (1985). A family study of schizophrenic and normal control probands: Implications for the spectrum concept of schizophrenia. *American Journal of Psychiatry, 142*, 447–454.

Bernstein, D. P., Cohen, P., Velez, C. N., Schwab-Stone, M., & Siever, L. (1993). The prevalence and stability of the DSM-III-R personality disorders in a community-based survey of adolescents. *American Journal of Psychiatry, 150*(8), 1237–1243.

Bullard, D. (1960). Psychotherapy of paranoid patients. *Archives of General Psychiatry, 2,* 137–141.

Cameron, N. (1943). The paranoid pseudo-community. *American Journal of Sociology, 49,* 32–38.

Cameron, N. (1963). *Personality development and psychopathology.* Boston: Houghton Mifflin.

Christenson, R., & Blazer, D. (1984). Epidemiology of persecutory ideation in an elderly population in the community. *American Journal of Psychiatry, 141,* 1088–1091.

Clarkin, J. F., Widiger, T. A., Frances, A., Hurt, S. W., & Gilmore, M. (1983). Prototypic typology and the borderline personality disorder. *Journal of Abnormal Psychology, 92,* 263–273.

Coryell, W. H., & Zimmerman, M. (1989). Personality disorder in the families of depressed, schizophrenic, and never-ill probands. *American Journal of Psychiatry, 146,* 496–502.

Dahl, A. (1986). Some aspects of the DSM-III personality disorders illustrated by a consecutive sample of hospitalized patients. *Acta Psychiatrica Scandinavica, 73*(Suppl. 328), 61–67.

Drake, R., & Vaillant, G. (1985). A validity study of Axis II of DSM-III. *American Journal of Psychiatry, 142*, 533–558.

Eitinger, L. (1959). The incidence of mental disease among refugees in Norway. *Journal of Mental Science, 105,* 326–338.

Faergeman, P. (1963). *Psychogenic psychoses.* London: Butterworths.

Fish, F. (1960). Senile schizophrenia. *Journal of Mental Science, 106,* 938–946.

Freiman, K., & Widiger, T. (1989). [Co-occurrence and diagnostic efficiency statistics]. Unpublished raw data.

Herbert, M.E., & Jacobson, S. (1967). Late paraphrenia. *British Journal of Psychiatry, 113,* 461–469.

Kass, F., Skodol, A. E., Charles, E., Spitzer, R. L., & Williams, J. B. W. (1985). Scaled ratings of DSM-III personality disorders. *American Journal of Psychiatry, 142,* 627–630.

Kay, D. W. K, & Roth, M. (1961). Environmental and hereditary factors in the schizophrenias of old age ("late paraphrenia") and their bearing on the general problem of causation in schizophrenia. *Journal of Mental Sciences, 107,* 649–686.

Kendler, K. S., & Hays, P. (1981). Paranoid psychosis (delusional disorder) and schizophrenia: A family history study. *Archives of General Psychiatry, 38,* 547–987.

Kendler, K. S., & Gruenberg, A. M. (1982). Genetic relationship between paranoid personality disorder and the "schizophrenic spectrum" disorders. *American Journal of Psychiatry, 139,* 1185–1186.

Kendler, K. S., Masterson, C. C., & Davis, K. L. (1985). Psychiatric illness in first-degree relatives of patients with paranoid psychosis, schizophrenia and medical illness. *British Journal of Psychiatry, 147,* 524–531.

Khantzian, E. J., & Treece, C. (1985). DSM-III psychiatric diagnosis of narcotic addicts: Recent findings. *Archives of General Psychiatry, 42,* 1067–1071.

Koenigsberg, H. W., Kaplan, R. D., Gilmore, M. M., & Cooper, A. M. (1985). The relationship between syndrome and personality disorder in DSM-III: Experience with 2,462 patients. *American Journal of Psychiatry, 142,* 207–212.

Kraepelin, E. (1921). *Manic–depressive insanity and paranoia.* Edinburgh: Livingstone.

Kretschmer, E. (1925). *Physique and character.* London: Kegan Paul, 1926.

Livesley, W. J. (1986). Trait and behavioral prototypes of personality disorder. *American Journal of Psychiatry, 143,* 728–732.

Mellsop, G., Varghese, F., Joshua, S., & Hicks, A. (1982). The reliability of Axis II of DSM-III. *American Journal of Psychiatry, 139,* 360–361.

Mezey, A. (1960). Personal background, emigration and mental disorder in Hungarian refugees. *Journal of Mental Science, 106,* 618–627.

Millon, T. (1969). *Modern psychopathology: A biosocial approach to maladaptive learning and functioning.* Philadelphia: W. B. Saunders.

Millon, T. (1981). *Disorders of personality: DSM-III, Axis II.* New York: Wiley–Interscience.

Millon, T., & Tringone, R. (1989). [Co-occurrence and diagnostic efficiency statistics]. Unpublished raw data.

Morey, L., & Heumann, K. (1988). [Co-occurrence and diagnostic efficiency statistics]. Unpublished raw data.

Pfohl, B., Coryell, W., Zimmerman, M., & Stangl, D. (1986). DSM-III personality disorders: Diagnostic overlap and internal consistency of individual DSM-III criteria. *Comprehensive Psychiatry, 27,* 21–34.

Post, F. (1966). *Persistent persecutory states of the elderly.* Oxford: Pergamon Press.

Reich, J. (1987). Sex distribution of DSM-III personality disorders in psychiatric outpatients. *American Journal of Psychiatry, 144,* 485–488.

Roth, M. (1955). The natural history of mental disorder in old age. *Journal of Mental Science, 101,* 281–301.

Schneider, K. (1923). *Die psychopathischen—ersonlichkeiten.* Berlin: Springer-Verlag.

Shapiro, D. (1965). *Neurotic styles.* New York: Basic Books.

Sheldon, W. H. (1940). *The varieties of human physique: An introduction to constitutional psychology.* New York: Harper.

Sheldon, W. H., & Steven, S. S. (1942). *The varieties of temperament: A psychology of constitutional differences.* New York: Harper.

Siever, L. J., & Davis, K. (1991). A psychobiologic perspective on the personality disorders. *American Journal of Psychiatry, 148,* 1647–1658.

Siever, L. J., & Kendler, K. S. (1985). Paranoid personality disorder. In R. Michels, J. Cavenar, & H. Bradley (Eds.), *Psychiatry: Vol. 1. The personality disorders and neuroses* (pp. 1–11). New York: Basic Books.

Siever, L. J., Silverman, J. Horvath, T., Klur, H., Collaro, E., Keet, R., Pinkham, L., Rinaldi, P., Mohs, R., & Davis, K. (1991). Increased morbid risk for schizophrenic related disorders in relatives of schizotypal personality disordered patients. *Archives of General Psychiatry, 47,* 634–640.

Skodol, A. E., Rosnicle, L., Kellman, D., Oldham, J. M., & Hylar, S. E. (1988). Validating structured DSM-III-R personality disorder assessments with longitudinal data. American *Journal of Psychiatry, 145,* 1297–1299.

Slater, E., & Roth, M. (1969). *Clinical psychiatry.* Baltimore: Williams & Wilkins.

Stephens, D. A., Atkinson, M. W., Kay, D. W. K., Roth, M., & Garside, R. F. (1975). Psychiatric morbidity in parents and sibs of schizophrenics and non-schizophrenics. *British Journal of Psychiatry, 127,* 97–108.

Turkat, I. D. (1985). Paranoid personality disorder. In I. D. Turkat (Ed.), *Behavioral case formulation* (pp. 155–198). New York: Plenum.

Turkat, I. D., & Maisto, S. A. (1985). Application of the experimental method to the formulation and modification of the personality disorders. In D. H. Barlow (Ed.), *Clinical handbook of psychological disorders* (pp. 503–570). New York: Guilford Press.

Widiger, T., Frances, A., Warner, L., & Bluhm, C. (1986). Diagnostic criteria for the borderline and schizotypal personality disorders. *Journal of Abnormal Psychology, 95*, 43–51.

Williams, J. (1988). Cognitive intervention for a paranoid personality disorder. *Psychotherapy, 25*, 570–575.

World Health Organization. (1992). *The ICD-10 classification of mental and behavioural disorders: Diagnostic criteria for research.* Geneva: Author.

Zanarini, M. (1989). [Co-occurrence and diagnostic efficiency statistics]. Unpublished raw data.

CHAPTER 4

# Schizoid Personality Disorder

OREN KALUS
DAVID P. BERNSTEIN
LARRY J. SIEVER

Schizoid personality disorder is one of the three DSM "odd cluster" personality disorders (schizotypal and paranoid personality disroders are the
others), characterized by phenomenological similarities to schizophrenia.
Schizoid personality disorder is distinguished from the other two personality disorders in this cluster by the prominence of social, interpersonal, and
affective deficits (i.e., "negative symptoms") in the absence of psychotic-like
cognitive/perceptual distortions.

Despite a rich and extensive clinical and theoretical tradition regarding the schizoid character, its pre-DSM-III status was handicapped by considerable heterogeneity and lack of clearly operationalized diagnostic criteria.
The architects of DSM-III (American Psychiatric Association [APA], 1980)
attempted to subdivide and sharpen the boundaries of this heterogeneous
area by adding schizotypal and paranoid personality disorders to the "odd
cluster" and avoidant personality disorder to the "anxious cluster." The narrowing of the schizoid personality disorder diagnosis that resulted from these
changes raised further questions, however, about the location of its diagnostic
boundaries and about whether the diagnosis is a valid and separate entity.
Evidence of extensive criteria overlap, as well as comorbidity with other personality disorders, has been of particular concern in this regard. The low
prevalence rates of DSM-III schizoid personality disorder have further complicated attempts to address these issues empirically. Although modifications
of the diagnostic criteria in DSM-III-R (American Psychiatric Association,
1987) appear to have increased the sensitivity and prevalence of the diagnosis, the scarcity of empirical data on either DSM-III or DSM-III-R schizoid

An earlier version of this chapter was published in the *Journal of Personality Disorders,* 1993, 7(1),
43–52. Copyright 1993 by The Guilford Press. Adapted by permission.

personality disorder has remained a significantly limiting factor in resolving these concerns in DSM-IV (American Psychiatric Association, 1994).

## SIGNIFICANT ISSUES

Some of the key issues in resolving the nosological status of schizoid personality disorder include the following:

1. As noted above, one matter of concern is the extent to which schizoid personality disorder overlaps with and is difficult to separate from other personality disorders, particularly schizotypal and avoidant personality disorders. This concern arises from evidence that a number of the key features of schizoid personality disorder, such as social isolation, pursuit of solitary activities, absence of intimate relationships, and restricted expression of affect, may be shared with schizotypal and paranoid personality disorders. Extensive comorbidity among schizoid, schizotypal, paranoid, and avoidant personality disorders raises the possibility that schizoid personality disorder may have been annexed by these other disorders.

The distinction between schizoid and avoidant personality disorders is also problematic, given the extensive overlap between these presumably mutually exclusive diagnoses. Although they share prominent social isolation, they are theoretically distinguishable by the avoidant individual's intimacy needs and sensitivity to rejection. This distinction may not be as clear-cut in the clinical setting, however, as prominent concerns centering around intimacy (such as ambivalence and fear of engulfment) (Akhtar, 1987) and social anxiety (Overholser, 1989) may also be involved in the social isolation seen in schizoid personality disorder.

Lastly, schizoid personality disorder was rarely diagnosed when DSM-III criteria were used. Although the prevalence of the diagnosis appears to have increased with the use of DSM-III-R criteria, its low prevalence still casts doubt on whether it is a valid diagnosis. Taken together, these concerns raised the question of whether schizoid personality disorder should be retained or deleted as a separate diagnosis in DSM-IV.

2. The similarities of schizoid personality disorder to the residual and prodromal phases of schizophrenia suggest that some schizophrenia patients may have been misdiagnosed as having schizoid personality disorder. A related issue is the extent to which schizoid personality disorder is genetically and familially part of the schizophrenia continuum. Although schizotypal personality disorder has specifically been singled out as having a genetic/familial relationship to schizophrenia, this issue has not been adequately addressed in schizoid personality disorder. The evidence supporting genetic transmission of "negative" rather than "positive" symptoms in schizophrenia, and the prominence of "negative symptoms" in schizoid personality disorder, would suggest a possible link between schizophrenia and schizoid personality disorder (Gunderson, Siever, & Spaulding, 1983).

A number of features reported by Akiskal (1987) as describing chronically dysthymic individuals (i.e., introversion, anhedonia, and psychomotor inertia) bear a resemblance to schizoid personality disorder, raising the issue of possible overlap and/or comorbidity with affective disorders. Alternatively, chronic low-grade depressive symptoms may be characterological—a possibility that inspired consideration of a "depressive personality disorder" in DSM-IV (see Chapter 13).

3. A number of the revisions to the schizoid personality disorder criteria in DSM-IV were motivated in part by a desire to increase compatibility with the World Health Organization's 10th revision of the *International Classification of Diseases* (ICD-10; World Health Organization, 1990). This was considered important because increased compatibility will facilitate international clinical and research efforts.

## LITERATURE REVIEW

The pre-DSM-III clinical literature and the post-DSM-III/III-R empirical and clinical literature were reviewed to address the issue of clinical overlap and possible annexation of schizoid personality disorder by avoidant and schizotypal personality disorders. Recent, unpublished data sets based on the DSM-III and DSM-III-R schizoid personality disorder criteria sets were also examined for their implications for criteria modification in DSM-IV.

### Historical and Clinical Literature

The term "schizoid" was originated by Bleuler (1924) to describe a tendency to turn inwardly and away from the external world, the absence of emotional expressiveness, simultaneous contradictory dullness and sensitivity, and pursuit of vague interests. Although most historical clinical descriptions of schizoid personality disorder appear consistent with DSM-III and DSM-III-R criteria, there also appear to be some discrepancies. In addition to describing the familiar "negative" symptoms of schizoid personality disorder outlined in the DSM criteria, many clinicians also described the presence of contradictory affective and cognitive states in schizoid personality disorder that were not recognized in DSM-III (some of these features may have been absorbed into other personality disorders, such as schizotypal and avoidant). Kretschmer (1925), for example, differentiated between two types of schizoid characteristics—the "hyperaesthetic" and "anaesthetic"—that contrasted overt insensitivity with inner sensitivity. Rather than separating these contrasting behavioral tendencies into two distinct diagnostic groups, as DSM-III did with the schizoid and avoidant categories, Kretschmer suggested that these characteristics may in fact coexist in the same person. Several clinicians have observed that the schizoid's apparent outward insensitivity and indifference often belies marked inner sensitivity. Heston (1970) and Wolff and Chick (1980), for example, pointed to a contradictory emotional detachment and appearance associated with inner sensitivity in the schizoid. This association highlights a problem in the DSM-III-R schizoid personality disorder criterion that is based on an inferred intrapsychic state — subjective indifference to rejection or criticism — rather than a more purely "objective" descriptive manifestation.

Another area in which the traditional literature differs from DSM-III and DSM-III-R concerns the schizoid's sexuality. Observations by Terry and Rennie (1938) and others of deviant sexuality (compulsive masturbation and perverse sexuality) are consistent with the DSM criterion of absent heterosexual relationships, but not with the absence of sexual desire. Other clinical features either not reported or de-emphasized in DSM-III and its revision include autistic thinking, fragmented self-identity, and symptoms of derealization/depersonalization. Numerous clinicians (particularly psychodynamically oriented ones) have stressed the fragmented personality structure and the use of primitive defensive mechanisms such as splitting. Others have described the false sense of self and the artificial quality of the schizoid, as in Winnicott's (1965) "false self." Guntrip (1969) and other clinicians have reported the frequent presence of depersonalization, derealization, absence of feeling, and disembodiment. The psychoanalytic literature also makes extensive references to the "primitive character structure" of the schizoid, and in particular to an identity disturbance that may contrast with the more dramatic and affectively charged identity disturbance reported in borderline personality disorder patients. Bleuler (1954) and other clinicians also emphasized the phenomenological similarities between the schizoid personality and schizophrenia, which anticipated current questions on the relationship of all three Cluster A diagnoses to schizophrenia.

The DSM-III criteria for schizoid personality disorder were somewhat limited in scope and variety of symptomatology, and appeared to reflect minimally much of the preceding descriptive literature. The changes incorporated in DSM-III-R provided a richer and potentially more sensitive description, and reduced the risk of oversimplification (Akhtar, 1987). The use of a polythetic system that does not require any single feature added further flexibility and may have increased sensitivity of the diagnosis.

## Prevalence

Estimates of the prevalence of schizoid personality disorder in the general population based on community survey (Reich, Yates, & Nduaguba, 1989), nonpsychiatric controls (Drake & Vaillant, 1985), and relatives of psychiatric patients (Zimmerman & Coryell, 1990) have ranged from 0.5% to 7%. In a longitudinal epidemiological study of adolescents and children using DSM-III-R criteria, Bernstein (1990) reported a prevalence rate of 1.7% for schizoid personality disorder, 1.2% for schizotypal personality disorder, and 4.1% for paranoid personality disorder.

Considerable variation in the prevalence rates in clinical settings is apparent. Studies using DSM-III-R criteria generally report higher prevalence rates than those using DSM-III criteria (see Table 4.1). Morey (1988), for example, comparing DSM-III with DSM-III-R schizoid personality disorder diagnoses in the same group of 291 personality-disordered patients, reported a substantially higher prevalence using DSM-III-R criteria (1.4% vs. 11.0%). For those studies using DSM-III criteria, prevalence rates ranged from 0% to 5%, with a median of 1%; for those using DSM-III-R criteria, the rates ranged from 1% to 16%, with a median of 8.5%.

## Criterion Performance

The criteria for DSM-III-R and DSM-IV schizoid personality disorder are shown in Table 4.2. The results of three studies examining the performance of the DSM-III-R criteria (Millon & Tringone, 1989 [$n = 26$]; Morey & Heumann, 1988 [$n = 32$]; Freiman & Widiger, 1989 [$n = 8$] were divergent, although some trends were apparent (Table 4.3). Of the three criteria reflecting impaired capacity for interpersonal relationships, only criterion 1 ("neither desires nor enjoys close relationships . . . ") demonstrated high sensitivity and specificity and was considered prototypical by clinicians. Criterion 2 ("almost always chooses solitary activities") had high sensitivity and was judged prototypical but had moderate specificity. Criterion 6 ("has no close friends or confidants . . . ") also demonstrated high sensitivity, but it had the

TABLE 4.1. Prevalence of DSM-III and DSM-III-R Schizoid Personality Disorder in 15 Clinical Studies

| Study | Sample size | Diagnostic nomenclature | Type of sample | Prevalence $n$ | % |
|---|---|---|---|---|---|
| Mellsop et al. (1982) | 77 | DSM-III | Inpatient | 3 | 4 |
| Clarkin et al. (1983) | 76 | DSM-III | Outpatient | 1 | 1 |
| Kass et al. (1985) | 609 | DSM-III | Outpatient | 6 | 1 |
| Khantzian & Treece (1985) | 87 | DSM-III | Outpatient | 3 | 2 |
| Koenigsberg (1985) | 2,462 | DSM-III | Mixed | 0 | 0 |
| Dahl (1986) | 103 | DSM-III | Inpatient | 5 | 5 |
| Pfohl et al. (1986) | 131 | DSM-III | Outpatient | 1 | 1 |
| Widiger et al. (1986) | 84 | DSM-III | Inpatient | 7 | 8 |
| Reich (1987) | 170 | DSM-III | Outpatient | 0 | 0 |
| Morey (1988) | 291 | DSM-III-R | Mixed | 32 | 11 |
| Skodol et al. (1988) | 97 | DSM-III-R | Inpatient | 1 | 1 |
| Alnaes & Torgerson (1988a) | 298 | DSM-III | Outpatient | 5 | 2 |
| Zanarini (1989) | 253 | DSM-III | Mixed | 1 | 1 |
| Millon & Tringone (1989) | 809 | DSM-III-R | Mixed | 46 | 6 |
| Freiman & Widiger (1989) | 50 | DSM-III-R | Inpatient | 8 | 16 |

TABLE 4.2. DSM-III-R and DSM-IV Diagnostic Criteria for Schizoid Personality Disorder

| DSM-III-R criteria | DSM-IV criteria |
|---|---|
| A. A pervasive pattern of indifference to social relationships and a restricted range of emotional experience and expression, beginning by early adulthood and present in a variety of contexts, as indicated by at least *four* of the following: | A. A pervasive pattern of detachment from social relationships and a restricted range of expression of emotions in interpersonal settings, beginning by early adulthood and present in a variety of contexts, as indicated by four (or more) of the following: |
| (1) neither desires nor enjoys close relationships, including being part of a family | (1) neither desires nor enjoys close relationships, including being part of a family |
| (2) almost always chooses solitary activities | (2) almost always chooses solitary activities |
| (3) rarely, if ever, claims or appears to experience strong emotions, such as anger and joy | (3) has little, if any, interest in having sexual experiences with another person |
| (4) indicates little if any desire to have sexual experiences with another person (age being taken into account) | (4) takes pleasure in few, if any, activities |
| (5) is indifferent to the praise and criticism of others | (5) lacks close friends or confidants other than first-degree relatives |
| (6) has no close friends or confidants (or only one) other than first-degree relatives | (6) appears indifferent to the praise or criticism of others |
| (7) displays constricted affect, e.g., is aloof, cold, rarely reciprocates gestures or facial expressions, such as smiles or nods | (7) shows emotional coldness, detachment, or flattened affectivity |
| B. Occurrence not exclusively during the course of Schizophrenia or a Delusional Disorder | B. Does not occur exclusively during the course of Schizophrenia, a Mood Disorder With Psychotic Features, another Psychotic Disorder, or a Pervasive Developmental Disorder and is not due to the direct physiological effects of a general medical condition. |
| | **Note:** If criteria are met prior to the onset of Schizophrenia, add "Premorbid," e.g., "Schizoid Personality Disorder (Premorbid)." |

*Note.* From APA (1987, p. 340) and APA (1994, p. 641). Copyright 1987 and 1994 by the American Psychiatric Association. Reprinted by permission.

TABLE 4.3. Criterion Performance of Schizoid Personality Disorder

| DSM-III-R diagnostic criterion | Sensitivity | | Specificity | | Proto typicality |
|---|---|---|---|---|---|
| | Range | Median | Range | Median | |
| 1 | .62–.87 | .69 | .86–.93 | .99 | 78 |
| 2 | .73–.88 | .75 | .78–.88 | .88 | 76 |
| 3 | .35–.63 | .38 | .92–.94 | .93 | 55 |
| 4 | .62–.75 | .63 | .78–1.00 | .86 | 71 |
| 5 | .00–.34 | .13 | .93–.95 | .95 | 55 |
| 6 | .69–.91 | .87 | .55–.68 | .67 | 50 |
| 7 | .50–.72 | .69 | .71–.90 | .86 | 66 |

lowest specificity (median = .67) of all the schizoid criteria. The low specificity of criteria 2 and 6 indicates that these features are shared with other personality disorders.

In contrast to the high sensitivity and low to moderate specificity of the criteria referring to interpersonal relationships, criterion 3 ("rarely if ever, claims or appears to experience strong emotions . . . "), criterion 4 ("indicates little if any desire to have sexual experiences . . . "), and criterion 5 ("is indifferent to the praise and criticism of others") demonstrated low sensitivity and low prototypicality but high specificity. These criteria may define a subgroup of schizoid personality disorder patients dominated by deficits in affective responsivity and capacity for pleasure. It was concluded that retaining them in DSM-IV despite their low sensitivity might be justified by their possible ability to identify atypical cases. Criterion 5 had the lowest sensitivity of all the schizoid criteria (range = .00–.34; median = .13); thus, modifying this item was thought to be justified on the basis of its low frequency. Criterion 7 ("displays constricted affect . . . ") demonstrated intermediate sensitivity, specificity, and prototypicality.

## Compatibility of DSM and ICD-10 Diagnostic Criteria

The revisions to schizoid personality disorder criteria introduced in DSM-III-R appear to have significantly increased compatibility with ICD-10, and the revisions introduced in DSM-IV should further enhance their correspondence (see below). DSM-III-R criteria 1, 2, 3, 5, 6, and 7 are closely matched with the ICD-10 criteria 6, 5, 4, 6, 3, and 2, respectively. DSM-III-R criterion 3 ("rarely, if ever, claims or appears to experience strong emotions, such as anger or joy") diverges from the corresponding ICD-10 criterion 1, which emphasizes lack of pleasure ("incapacity to experience pleasure"). ICD-10 criterion 7 ("marked difficulty in recognizing and adhering to social convention, resulting in eccentricity of behaviour") does not have a corresponding DSM-III-R item.

## Comorbidity

Rates of comorbidity of schizoid personality disorder with other personality disorders are listed in Table 4.4. The highest co-occurrence was with schizotypal personality disorder, perhaps because of the high overlap between the two criteria sets (e.g., social isolation, restricted affect). Avoidant personality disorder also demonstrated high comorbidity with schizoid personality disorder. Lesser degrees of comorbidity were demonstrated with paranoid, antisocial, borderline, and passive–aggressive personality disorders.

In a study examining Axis I and Axis II comorbidity, Alnaes and Torgersen (1988b) reported that the Cluster A personality disorders as a group showed high comorbidity with dysthymic disorder, social phobia, and agoraphobia. Of seven relatives of psychiatric patients diagnosed with schizoid personality disorder, Zimmerman and Coryell (1989) reported a 14.3% rate of mania, a 28.6% rate of alcohol abuse/dependence, and a 14.3% rate of drug abuse/dependence.

## Genetic/Family Studies

Some family/genetic studies suggest that the boundaries of schizophrenia-related disorders may extend beyond schizotypal personality disorder to include schizoid and paranoid personality disorders (Gunderson et al., 1983; Baron et al., 1985), whereas other studies suggest that the relationship ex-

TABLE 4.4. Comorbidity of Schizoid Personality Disorder with Other Axis II Disorders

|  | PRN | SZT | ATS | BDL | HST | NAR | AVD | DPD | OCP | PAG |
|---|---|---|---|---|---|---|---|---|---|---|
|  | Percentage of criterion group receiving schizoid diagnosis | | | | | | | | | |
| Dahl (1986) | 0 | 80 | 40 | 20 | 20 | 0 | 60 | 0 | 0 | 0 |
| Morey (1988) | 47 | 38 | 3 | 19 | 9 | 98 | 53 | 19 | 16 | 19 |
| Freiman & Widiger (1989) | 62 | 62 | 25 | 38 | 0 | 38 | 88 | 0 | 0 | 50 |
| Skodol et al. (1988) | 40 | 60 | 0 | 60 | 0 | 20 | 80 | 20 | 20 | 0 |
| Millon & Tringone (1989)[a] | 4 | 27 | 0 | 0 | 0 | 8 | 23 | 15 | 8 | 0 |
| Millon & Tringone (1989)[b] | 0 | 32 | 0 | 0 | 0 | 4 | 46 | 7 | 7 | 4 |
| Millon & Tringone (1989)[c] | 0 | 2 | 0 | 0 | 0 | 7 | 39 | 20 | 17 | 11 |

Note. Key to personality disorder abbreviations: PRN, paranoid; SZT, schizotypal, ATS, antisocial; BDL, borderline; HST, histrionic; NAR, narcissistic; AVD, avoidant; DEP, dependent; OCP, obsessive–compulsive; PAG, passive–aggressive.
[a]Clinical interview.
[b]Diagnostic checklist.
[c]Millon Clinical Multiaxial Inventory.

tends to schizotypal but not to schizoid personality disorder (Baron et al., 1985). Some studies examining the genetic characteristics of the schizophrenic spectrum may also have been confounded by a failure to distinguish clearly between schizoid and schizotypal personality disorders. Evidence that "negative" rather than "positive" symptoms are associated with increased heritability in schizophrenia (Dworkin & Lenzenweger, 1984) would theoretically support a familial/genetic link between schizophrenia and schizoid personality disorder, because the latter is also largely exposed through "negative" symptoms.

## Treatment Response

Few data exist in the form of systematic treatment studies on patients with schizoid personality disorder, partly because such patients are unlikely to request treatment. When they do present for treatment, it is usually in the context of an acute stress or shift in life circumstances (Siever & Kendler, 1987). Major changes and modifications of character structure are unlikely, probably because of constitutionally determined limitations in affective response and expression (Millon, 1981). Therapy should probably be aimed at achieving modest reductions in social isolation and in promoting more effective adjustment to new circumstances. Cognitive interventions, social skills training, and group therapy may be of some benefit, whereas intensive psychoanalytically oriented therapies are less likely to succeed. The role of drug therapy remains an open question.

# DISCUSSION

Distinguishing schizoid personality disorder from other phenomenologically similar personality disorders in the odd cluster and from avoidant personality disorder remains a key concern. Whether the issue is one of more refined differential diagnosis or diagnostic validity will require additional research. However, the high comorbidity of schizoid personality disorder, particularly with schizotypal personality disorder, suggests that more discriminating diagnostic features are needed. Most DSM-III-R criteria with high specificity demonstrated unsatisfactory sensitivity, and those with high sensitivity generally had low specificity. Although schizoid personality disorder shares several social deficit symptoms with schizotypal personality disorder, the two disorders can be distinguished by the absence of positive psychotic-like symptoms in schizoid personality disorder. Schizotypal personality disorder also appears to have clearer familial and genetic links to schizophrenia than does schizoid personality disorder.

Some studies suggest that schizoid personality disorder can be distinguished from avoidant personality disorder (Trull, Widiger, & Frances, 1987) on the basis of intimacy needs and sensitivity to rejection. However, contrasting historical descriptions suggesting that sensitivity and insensitivity coexist in schizoid personality disorder, and more recent empirical studies suggesting that anxiety and other clinical symptoms occur in both disorders (Overholser, 1989), call for additional investigation. The poor performance of indifference to criticism as a schizoid personality disorder criterion is consistent with this concern. The discrepancy between the appearance and experience of sensitivity also highlights the need for more reliable and sensitive behavioral measures beyond mere clinical observation.

These concerns, along with the low prevalence of schizoid personality disorder when DSM-III criteria have been used, raised the question of whether schizoid personality disorder should be retained as an independent diagnosis in DSM-IV. However, the increased prevalence of schizoid personality disorder observed when DSM-III-R criteria have been used, as well as historical and recent clinical evidence, were thought to support a separate schizoid personality distinct from both avoidant and schizotypal personality disorders.

Although the DSM-III-R schizoid personality disorder criterion set has demonstrated increased compatibility with that of ICD-10, some discrepancies remained prior to DSM-IV. It was decided that revising DSM-III-R criterion 3, which refers to experience and expression of strong emotion, to emphasize lack of pleasure (anhedonia) as adopted in ICD-10 criterion 1, would increase compatibility. In contrast, ICD-10 criterion 7 (". . . eccentricity of behaviour") was not adopted in DSM-IV because of its close correspondence to the DSM-III-R schizotypal personality disorder criteria.

The question of whether schizoid personality disorder is part of the schizophrenic spectrum disorders will require additional investigation. Future research should incorporate biological markers (e.g., deviant eye tracking and attentional deficits) that have been observed in schizotypal personality disorder and schizophrenia.

## CHANGES MADE IN DSM-IV

A few modifications in the schizoid personality disorder diagnostic criteria have been made in DSM-IV to increase the clarity of the criterion set and increase compatibility with ICD-10. The introductory description to the A criteria replaces "indifference to" social relationships with "detachment from" social relationships, and "restricted range of emotional experience and expression" with "restricted range of expression of emotions in interpersonal settings" (see Table 4.2). The first modification emphasizes a more objective behavioral description (rather than an inferred subjective state); the second modification provides increased specificity for the context in which the relative lack of emotional expression takes place. Criterion 4 in DSM-IV has been modified from criterion 3 in DSM-III-R to emphasize the individual's difficulty in taking pleasure in everyday activities (i.e., emphasizing anhedonia, rather than difficulty in experience and expression of strong emotions). Criterion 6 in DSM-IV has been modified from criterion 5 in DSM-III-R to include individuals who *appear* indifferent to praise or criticism, but who do indeed have an underlying insensitivity. The modifications in DSM-IV items 3, 4, 5, and 7 should increase compatibility with ICD-10.

## REFERENCES

Alnaes, R., & Torgerson, S. (1988a). DSM-III symptom disorders (Axis I) and personality disorders (Axis II) in an outpatient population. *Acta Psychiatrica Scandinavica,
78,* 348–355.

Alnaes, R., & Torgersen, S. (1988b). The relationship between DSM-III symptom disorders (Axis I) and personality disorders (Axis II) in an outpatient population.
*Acta Psychiatrica Scandinavica, 78,* 485–492.

Akhtar, S. (1987). Schizoid personality disorder: A synthesis of developmental, dynamic, and descriptive features. *American Journal of Psychotherapy, 41,* 499–518.

Akiskal, H. (1987). The clinical management of affective fisorders. In R. Michels et
al. (Eds.), *Psychiatry.* New York: Basic Books.

American Psychiatric Association. (1980). *Diagnostic and statistical manual of mental disorders* (3rd ed.). Washington, DC: Author.

American Psychiatric Association. (1987). *Diagnostic and statistical manual of mental disorders* (3rd ed., rev.). Washington, DC: Author.

American Psychiatric Association. (1994). *Diagnostic and statistical manual of mental disorders* (4th ed.). Washington, DC: Author.

Baron, M., Gruen, R., Rainer, J. D., Kane, J., Asnis, L., & Lord, S. (1985). A family
study of schizophrenic and normal control probands: Implications for the spectrum concept of schizophrenia. *American Journal of Psychiatry, 142,* 447–454.

Bernstein, D. P. (1990). *The prevalence and stability of the DSM-III-R personality disorders
in adolescence.* Unpublished doctoral dissertation, New York University.

Bleuler, E. (1924). *Textbook of psychiatry* (A. A. Brill, Trans.). New York: Macmillan.

Bleuler, M., (1954). The concept of schizophrenia [Letter to the editor]. *American Journal
of Psychiatry, 11,* 382–383.

Clarkin, J. F., Widiger, T.A., & Frances, A., Hurt, S. W. & Gilmore, M. (1983). Prototypic typology and the borderline personality disorder. *Journal of Abnormal Psychology, 92,* 263–273.

Dahl, A. (1986). Some aspects of the DSM-III personality disorders illustrated by a
consecutive sample of hospitalized patients. *Acta Psychiatrica Scandinavica,
73*(Suppl. 228), 61–66.

Drake, R., & Vaillant, G. (1985). A validity study of Axis II of DSM-III. *American Journal of Psychiatry, 142,* 553–558.

Dworkin, R., & Lenzenweger, M. (1984). Symptoms and the genetics of schizophrenia: Implications for diagnosis. *American Journal of Psychiatry, 141,* 1541–1546.

Freiman, K., & Widiger, T. (1989). [Co-occurrence and diagnostic efficiency statis-
tics]. Unpublished raw data.

Gunderson, J. G., Siever, L. J., & Spaulding, E. (1983). The search for a schizotype:
Crossing the border again. *Archives of General Psychiatry, 40,* 15–22.

Guntrip, H. (1969). *Schizoid phenomena, object relations and the self.* New York: International Universities Press.

Heston, L. L. (1970). The genetics of schizophrenia and schizoid disease. *Science, 167,* 249–256.

Kass, F., Skodol, A. E., Charles, E., Spitzer, R. L., & Williams, J. B. W. (1985). Scaled ratings of DSM-III personality disorders. *American Journal of Psychiatry, 142.* 627–630.

Khantzian, E. J., & Treece, C. (1985). DSM-III psychiatric diagnosis of narcotic addicts: Recent findings. *Archives of General Psychiatry, 42.* 1067–1071.

Koenigsberg, H. W., Kaplan, R. D., Gilmore, M. W., & Cooper, A. M. (1985). The relationship between syndrome and personality disorder in DSM-III: Experience with 2,462 patients. *American Journal of Psychiatry, 142*(2), 207–212.

Kretschmer, E. (1925). *Physique and character.* London: Kegan Paul, 1926.

Mellsop, G., Varghese, F., Joshua, S., & Hicks, A. (1982). The reliability of Axis II of DSM-III. *American Journal of Psychiatry, 139,* 360–361.

Millon, T. (1981). *Disorders of personality: DSM-III, Axis II.* New York: Wiley–Interscience.

Millon, T., & Tringone, R. (1989). [Co-occurrence and diagnostic efficiency statistics]. Unpublished raw data.

Morey, L. (1988). Personality disorders in DSM-III and DSM-III-R: Convergence, coverage, and internal consistency. *American Journal of Psychiatry, 145,* 573–577.

Morey, L., & Heumann, K. (1988). [Co-occurrence and diagnostic efficiency statistics]. Unpublished raw data.

Overholser, J. C. (1989). Differentiation between schizoid and avoidant personalities: An empirical test. *Canadian Journal of Psychiatry, 34*(8), 785–790.

Pfohl, B., Coryell, W., Zimmerman, M., & Stangl, D. (1986). DSM-III personality disorders: Diagnostic overlap and internal consistency of individual DSM-III criteria. *Comprehensive Psychiatry, 27,* 21–34.

Reich, J. (1987). Sex distribution of DSM-III personality disorders in psychiatric outpatients. *American Journal of Psychiatry, 144,* 485–488.

Reich, J., Yates, W., & Nduaguba, M. (1989). Prevalence of DSM-III personality disorders in the community. *Social Psychiatry and Psychiatric Epidemiology, 24,* 12–16.

Siever, L. J., & Kendler, K.S. (1987). Schizoid/schizotypal/paranoid personality disorders. In J. O. Cavenar (Ed.), *Psychiatry.* New York: Basic Books.

Skodol, A. E., Rosnick, L., Kellman, D., Oldham, J., & Hyler, S. (1988). Validating structured DSM-III-R personality disorder assessments with longitudinal data. *American Journal of Psychiatry, 145,* 1297–1299.

Terry, G. C., & Rennie, T. (1938). Analysis of paraergesia. *American Journal of Orthopsychiatry, 9,* 817–918.

Trull, T. J., Widiger, T. A., & Frances, A. (1987). Covariation of criteria sets for avoidant, schizoid and dependent personality disorders. *American Journal of Psychiatry, 144*(6), 767–771.

Widiger, T., Frances, A., Warner, L., & Blum, C. (1986). Diagnostic criteria for the borderline and schizotypal personality disorders. *Journal of Abnormal Psychology, 95,* 43–51.

Winnicott, D. W. (1965). *The maturational process and the facilitating environment.* New York: International Universities Press.

Wolff, S., & Chick, J. (1980). Schizoid personality in childhood. *Psychological Medicine, 10,* 85–101.

World Health Organization. (1992) *International classification of diseases* (10th revision). Geneva: Author.

Zanarini, M. (1989). [Co-occurrence and diagnostic efficiency statistics]. Unpublished raw data.

Zimmerman, M., & Coryell, W. (1989). DSM-III personality disorder diagnoses in a nonpatient sample. *Archives of General Psychiatry, 46,* 682–689.

Zimmerman, M., & Coryell, W. H. (1990). Diagnosing personality disorders in the community: A comparison of self-report and interview measures. *Archives of General Psychiatry, 47,* 527–531.

# CHAPTER 5

# Schizotypal Personality Disorder

LARRY J. SIEVER
DAVID P. BERNSTEIN
JEREMY M. SILVERMAN

Schizotypal, paranoid, and schizoid personality disorders constitute the "odd cluster" of the DSM personality disorders. All are characterized by a degree of social detachment and "odd" or idiosyncratic behavior that can be observed in much more extreme form in the schizophrenic disorders. Schizotypal personality disorder is distinguished from the others by eccentricity and cognitive/perceptual distortions; paranoid personality disorder, by suspiciousness and mistrust of others; and schizoid personality disorder, by a preference for solitary activities that does not necessarily involve distortions in perceptions of reality.

Schizotypal personality disorder is the most recently adopted disorder of this cluster. It also represents the first personality disorder defined in part by its genetic relationship to chronic schizophrenia. For these reasons, the establishment of schizotypal personality disorder in DSM-III (American Psychiatric Association [APA], 1980) provided the stimulus for investigation of this disorder and its relationship both to other personality disorders and to the schizophrenic disorders. Increasingly compelling evidence suggests that schizotypal personality disorder is related to schizophrenia in terms of common phenomenological (Kendler, 1985; Siever & Gunderson, 1983), genetic (Kendler, 1985; Kendler, Gruenberg, & Straus, 1981; Torgersen, 1985), biological (Siever, 1985), outcome (McGlashan, 1986), and treatment response (Goldberg et al., 1986; Serban & Siegel, 1984) characteristics.

A statement of the issues for the DSM-IV revision process is first presented, followed by a review of epidemiological, phenomenological (including reliability, comorbidity, and diagnostic efficiency studies), genetic, biological,

An earlier version of this chapter was published in the *Journal of Personality Disorders*, 1991, 5, 178–193. Copyright 1991 by The Guilford Press. Adapted by permission.

outcome, and treatment response studies. Finally, these results are discussed with regard to the specific issues; changes proposed for and actually made in DSM-IV (American Psychiatric Association, 1994) are described; and recommendations regarding future investigation are made.

## SIGNIFICANT ISSUES

The major issues regarding schizotypal personality disorder in particular and the Cluster A disorders in general center around the extent to which they overlap with one another, the other personality disorders, and the Axis I psychotic disorders, specifically the schizophrenic and paranoid disorders. The issues for the DSM-IV revision process can be summarized as follows:

1. Should schizotypal personality disorder and possibly the other "odd cluster" diagnoses be included with other schizophrenia-related disorders on Axis I? The schizophrenia-related disorders appear to represent a continuum from severe, chronic, "Kraepelinian" schizophrenia to the milder schizophrenia-related personality disorders, of which schizotypal personality disorder is the prototype. Investigations suggesting that schizotypal personality disorder is closely related to schizophrenia have sharpened questions regarding the relationship of the Axis I to the Axis II disorders, and prompted questions as to whether schizotypal personality disorder would not more properly be placed with the Axis I disorders. On the other hand, the Axis II disorders are defined in DSM-III-R in terms of "enduring patterns of perceiving, relating to, and thinking about the environment and oneself" (American Psychiatric Association, 1987, p. 335). The DSM-III-R criteria for schizotypal personality disorder reflect persistent disturbances in perception/cognition of, and relatedness between, self and others, so that schizotypal personality disorder would appear to meet fully the definition for an Axis II disorder.

2. Could the substantial overlap between borderline and schizotypal personality disorder be reduced by refining the criteria for schizotypal personality disorder, particularly the psychotic-like criteria? The well-documented overlap between schizotypal and borderline personality disorder could be a function of random overlap, an artifact of the inclusion of psychotic-like symptoms solely in schizotypal personality disorder criteria, or a result of genuine synergism in pathophysiological antecedents to these disorders. To the extent that overlap might be reduced by sharpening criteria, how could the criteria for schizotypal personality disorder be revised to be more specific?

3. Could the specificity of the relationship of schizotypal personality disorder to schizophrenia as opposed to the affective disorders be enhanced by modifying the schizotypal personality disorder criteria? The offspring and relatives of affective disorder and schizophrenic disorder patients show an

increased prevalence of schizotypal personality disorder (Ingraham, 1989; Squires-Wheeler, Skodol, Friedman, & Erlenmeyer-Kimling, 1988), prompting questions as to whether some of the DSM-III-R criteria for schizotypal personality disorder encompass affective-related characteristics and whether criteria changes would increase the specificity of the relationship between schizotypal personality disorder and schizophrenia. In order to clarify these issues and potential paradoxes, the relationship of schizotypal personality disorder to schizophrenia and to other personality disorders was reviewed from phenomenological, genetic, biological, outcome, and treatment response vantage points.

## LITERATURE REVIEW

The issues described above were approached by reviewing published studies and unpublished data sets. Particular attention was given to studies of reliability and diagnostic efficiency of criteria; overlap with other disorders; comorbidity with the Axis I disorders; and studies using external validators, such as family history, biological indices, outcome, and response to treatment.

### Phenomenological Studies

The impetus for the designation of schizotypal personality disorder as a new diagnostic category in DSM-III emerged from concerns on the part of Spitzer and other architects of DSM-III that the definition of borderline conditions had become too diffuse by including both affectively unstable and schizophrenia-related personality disorders, and that the criteria for schizoid personality disorder were too broadly defined to specifically characterize individuals with enduring psychotic-like traits (Spitzer, Endicott, & Gibbon, 1979). In order to define a prototypical personality disorder based on the chronic psychotic-like characteristics observed in the relatives of chronic schizophrenic patients, the case histories of individuals diagnosed as having "borderline" or "latent" and uncertain schizophrenia in the Danish adoptive studies (Kety, Rosenthal, Wender, Schulsinger, & Jacobsen, 1975) were reviewed. The features identified provided the basis for the DSM-III criteria for schizotypal personality disorder. As the diagnoses made by Kety et al. (1975) had a demonstrable genetic relationship to chronic schizophrenia, schizotypal personality disorder is the only Axis II disorder defined empirically on the basis of a genetic relationship to an Axis I disorder.

However, through the individual latent or uncertain schizophrenic case histories selected from the Danish adoptive studies included biological relatives of chronic schizophrenic patients, they also included relatives and probands with no demonstrated genetic relationship to chronic schizophrenia (Gunderson, Siever, & Spaulding, 1983). The criteria selected for DSM-III may not, therefore, have defined precisely the personality characteristics reflective of a genetic relationship to schizophrenia. Furthermore, it was not the intention of Spitzer and colleagues to restrict the definition to a personality disorder that was necessarily specifically related to schizophrenia; rather, it was to use the adoptive studies as a starting point to define a personality disorder having chronic psychotic-like characteristics associated with social withdrawal rather than with affective instability, as in contemporary definitions of borderline personality (Spitzer et al., 1979). To further this aim, they then refined the defining characteristics on the basis of a questionnaire sent to members of the APA in order to differentiate schizotypal personality disorder from "unstable personality disorder," which included impulsive and effectively unstable but not psychotic-like characteristics (since changed to borderline personality disorder). Thus, although schizotypal personality disorder was defined in part on the basis of a genetic relationship to chronic schizophrenia, it was conceived by its architects as a clinical personality disorder characterized by chronic psychotic-like characteristics, rather than specifically as a milder schizophrenia-related disorder.

In fact, relatives of schizophrenics from the Danish adoptive studies (Gunderson et al., 1983) and the Iowa non-500 study (Kendler, Gruenberg, & Tsuang, 1985) appear to have been more likely to manifest the "negative" symptoms of schizotypal personality disorder (e.g., social isolation, poor rapport, and eccentricity) than the "positive," psychotic-like symptoms (e.g., magical thinking, referential ideation, and perceptual distortion). In contrast, clinically defined schizotypal personality disorder patients may be specifically defined by their psychotic-like characteristics (Jacobsberg, Hymowitz, Barasch, Frances, 1986; Widiger, Frances, Warner, & Bluhm, 1986). Therefore, according to Frances (1985), schizotypal personality disorder should be defined as a clinical personality disorder that may not necessarily be the same as the schizophrenia-related personality disorders observed in the relatives of chronic schizophrenic patients.

## Sensitivity and Specificity of Criteria

Attempts to identify symptoms that are sensitive and specific for schizotypal personality disorder have utilized comparisons between schizotypal and other personality disorder patients, particularly patients with borderline personality disorder. In a review of the studies of schizotypal criteria, McGlashan (1987) suggested that odd communication, suspiciousness/paranoid ideation, and social isolation represent the most characteristic or "core" criteria for schizotypal personality disorder, whereas illusions, depersonalization, and derealization were not characteristic in his sample. Undue social anxiety, although nearly universal among schizotypal patients (Pfohl, Coryell, Zimmerman, & Stangl, 1986), is not particularly specific for this disorder. The discriminating power of "positive" symptoms, such as odd communication, ideas of reference, magical thinking, and illusions, was emphasized by Jacobsberg et al. (1986) in a study comparing schizotypal and borderline patients.

In a similarly designed study, Widiger et al. (1986) found ideas of reference, odd speech, and paranoid ideation to be most closely correlated with the total number of schizotypal symptoms. Although these studies have not been entirely consistent and have employed different clinical populations and analytic tools, most tend to support social withdrawal, odd/eccentric speech and behavior, and suspicious/paranoid ideation as central disturbances in the schizotypal patient.

Although studies specifically comparing borderline and schizotypal patients have tended to identify "positive" symptoms as discriminators of the schizotypal diagnosis, these results may reflect the fact that the schizotypal–borderline overlap patients may be characterized by prominent psychotic symptoms, whereas borderline patients without a schizotypal diagnosis are unlikely to have "positive" symptoms or they would have met the schizotypal criteria. Recent phenomenological, familial, and biological data suggest that the overlap group may represent variants of borderline personality disorder characterized by psychotic-like symptoms, but not necessarily related to schizophrenia per se (Siever, Klar, et al., 1987). Alternatively, they may represent synergistic effects of biogenetic and psychosocial precursors to each disorder.

## Comorbidity

The overlap between schizotypal personality disorder and Axis I disorders has not been extensively studied, but a substantial overlap with major depressive disorder has been found in several studies. McGlashan (1983) retrospectively assigned DSM-III Axis II diagnoses to former patients at the Chestnut Lodge, and found that at time of hospital admission, 9% of the 75 patients diagnosed with schizotypal personality disorder were also given a diagnosis of mania, and that 29% received a diagnosis of depression. Pfohl, Stangl, and Zimmerman (1984) reported that of 78 patients with major depressive disorder, 9% also met DSM-III criteria for schizotypal personality disorder. Siever (1988) found that 49% of patients with schizotypal personality disorder also met criteria for major depressive disorder at the time of the study, and 63% had a history of at least one major depressive episode. Conversely, 51% of the patients presenting with major depressive disorder also received a schizotypal diagnosis.

Because personality disorders are rarely diagnosed in the presence of more florid schizophrenic symptomatology, few studies have examined the comorbidity of schizophrenia and Axis II disorders. McGlashan (1983) found that 44% of the 75 Chestnut Lodge patients retrospectively diagnosed as having schizotypal personal disorder also qualified for a diagnosis of schizophrenia. At follow-up 15 years later, 55% of the schizotypal patients received a schizophrenic diagnosis. No other personality disorder showed such a high rate of overlap with schizophrenia. Schizotypal personality disorder often coexists with other personality disorders, as do all of the Axis II personality disorders (Table 5.1). These associations do not appear to be random, but may occur in two patterns. On the one hand, schizotypal personality disorder co-occurs with the other "odd cluster" diagnoses and with personality disorders from other clusters reflecting social isolation and detachment, such as compulsive and avoidant personality disorder (Kass, Skodol, Charles, Spitzer, & Williams, 1985; Siever, 1985). On the other hand, many patients meeting DSM-III criteria for schizotypal personality disorder also carry a concurrent borderline personality disorder diagnosis (Jacobsberg et al., 1986, McGlashan, 1987). In seven clinical studies reporting rates of diagnostic overlap among all DSM-III or DSM-III-R Axis II disorders (Table 5.1), the percentage of patients with schizotypal personality disorder receiving comorbid borderline diagnoses ranged from 33% (Skodol, 1989) to 91% (Zanarini, 1989) (median = 50%), and the percentage of borderline patients given comorbid schizotypal diagnoses ranged from 0% (Millon & Tringone, 1989) to 53% (Freiman & Widiger, 1989) (median = 23%).

TABLE 5.1. Cormorbidity among Axis II Disorders in Seven Clinical Studies

| | SZD | PRN | HST | NAR | BDL | ATS | AVD | DEP | OCP | PAG | SDF | SAD |
|---|---|---|---|---|---|---|---|---|---|---|---|---|
| Percentage with schizotypal personality disorder receiving indicated diagnosis | | | | | | | | | | | | |
| Dahl (1986) | 10 | 2 | 15 | 2 | 41 | 32 | 15 | 0 | 0 | 0 | — | — |
| Pfohl et al. (1986) | 0 | 0 | 33 | 8 | 50 | 8 | 58 | 0 | 17 | 50 | — | — |
| Morey (1988) | 44 | 59 | 18 | 33 | 33 | 4 | 59 | 30 | 11 | 15 | — | — |
| Skodol (1989)[a] | 0 | 38 | 12 | 44 | 88 | 19 | 88 | 62 | 31 | 12 | 50 | 0 |
| Zanarini (1989) | 0 | 10 | 71 | 29 | 91 | 38 | 29 | 39 | 8 | 32 | — | — |
| Millon & Tringone (1989)[b] | 12 | 12 | 0 | 3 | 47 | 3 | 68 | 15 | 0 | 9 | 26 | 3 |
| Freiman & Widiger (1989) | 46 | 46 | 0 | 45 | 54 | 46 | 54 | 46 | 0 | 50 | 18 | 27 |
| Percentage with indicated diagnosis receiving a diagnosis of schizotypal personality disorder | | | | | | | | | | | | |
| Dahl (1986) | 80 | 100 | 17 | 33 | 45 | 38 | 35 | 0 | 0 | 0 | — | — |
| Pfohl et al. (1986) | 0 | 0 | 13 | 20 | 21 | 20 | 47 | 0 | 29 | 33 | — | — |
| Morey (1988) | 38 | 25 | 8 | 14 | 9 | 6 | 20 | 12 | 13 | 11 | — | — |
| Skodol (1989)[a] | 0 | 43 | 12 | 33 | 23 | 38 | 36 | 30 | 24 | 33 | 40 | 0 |
| Zanarini (1989) | 0 | 50 | 48 | 51 | 40 | 29 | 43 | 45 | 33 | 45 | — | — |
| Millon & Tringone (1989)[b] | 8 | 17 | 8 | 75 | 0 | 25 | 8 | 0 | 33 | 17 | 0 | 0 |
| Freiman & Widiger | 33 | 33 | 27 | 47 | 53 | 33 | 60 | 27 | 0 | 40 | 13 | 27 |

Note. Key to personality disorder abbreviations: SZD, schizoid; PRN, paranoid; HST, histrionic; NAR, narcissistic; BDL, borderline; ATS, antisocial; AVD, avoidant; DEP, dependent; OCP, obsessive–compulsive; PAG, passive–aggressive; SDF, self-defeating; SAD, sadistic.
[a]Prevalence of schizotypal personality disorder in this table based on the Personality Disorder Examination. (Skodol, 1989, also reported prevalences based on other diagnostic instruments.)
[b]Prevalence of schizotypal personality disorder in this table based on the Millon Clinical Multiaxial Inventory. (Millon & Tringone, 1989, also reported prevalences based on other diagnostic instruments.)

## Genetic/Family Studies

Adoptive (Gunderson et al., 1983; Kendler, 1985; Kendler et al., 1981; Torgersen, 1985) and familial (Baron et al., 1985: Schulz et al., 1986; Soloff & Millward, 1983; Stone, 1977) studies are consistent with a common genetic diathesis to schizophrenia and schizotypal personality disorder. Although phenomenologically oriented psychiatrists since the time of Bleuler have observed that the family members of schizophrenic patients are often eccentric and socially isolated, the first definitive evidence for a genetic relationship between chronic schizophrenia and schizotypal personality disorder derives from the adoptive studies of Kety et al. (1975) and subsequent reanalyses of the case histories in these studies using DSM-III criteria. Schizotypal personality disorder was found to be more common among the biological relatives of schizophrenic patients than among their adoptive relatives or among the biological or adoptive relatives of controls (Gunderson et al., 1983; Kendler, 1985). In fact, schizotypal personality disorder has been diagnosed more frequently than chronic schizophrenia itself in the relatives of schizophrenic probands, raising the possibility that schizotypal symptoms may represent a more common phenotypic expression than chronic schizophrenia of an underlying diathesis to the schizophrenia-related disorders.

Further support for a relationship between schizotypal personality disorder and chronic schizophrenia is provided by studies of the first-degree relatives, siblings, and cotwins of chronic schizophrenic probands (Torgersen, 1985). Preliminary results of a more recent direct-interview family study suggests that schizotypal personality disorder is more prevalent in the relatives of schizophrenic probands than in those of controls, and that schizotypal signs are more discriminating than schizotypal symptoms (Kendler et al., 1989). Studies identifying schizotypal patients as probands, and psychiatrically evaluating their relatives (Baron et al., 1985; Schulz et al., 1986; Soloff & Millward, 1983; Stone, 1977) or cotwins (Torgersen, 1985), suggest familial transmission of schizotypal personality disorder as part of a continuum of schizophrenia-related disorders. The cumulative risk for schizophrenia-related disorders is greater in the relatives of schizotypal personality disorder probands than in the relatives of probands with other non-schizophrenia-related personality disorders, whereas the cumulative risk for other psychiatric disorders (including major affective disorders, antisocial disorders, and other personality disorders) does not differ between groups (Silverman et al., 1986). Indications of a reciprocal familial/genetic relationship of schizotypal personality disorder to chronic schizophrenia have been reported (Schulz et al., 1986; Soloff & Millward, 1983), although sample sizes to date have been too small to establish or disconfirm this hypothesis. Thus, these studies support the relationship between schizotypal personality disorder and schizophrenia, and provide strong evidence for the familial/genetic transmission of schizotypal personality disorder itself.

The genetic specificity of current definitions of schizotypal personality disorder is less clearly established. Biological relatives of adopted individuals with major affective disorders may also demonstrate schizotypal characteristics (S. Kety, personal communication, December 1987), although it is not clear whether these represent the "core" or "positive" symptoms. Schizotypal patients in the clinical setting frequently present with depressive symptoms, and such patients have an increased familial cumulative risk for major affective disorders (Silverman, Siever, Pinkham, Mohs, & Davis, 1988). Relatives of schizotypal–borderline patients have an increased morbid risk for schizophrenia-related disorders (primarily schizophrenia-related personality disorders), and for those personality disorders with marked affective and impulsive features (Silverman, Siever, Mohs, & Davis, 1987). Could the psychotic-like symptoms and broad social dysfunction as represented in the DSM-III-R criteria for schizotypal personality disorder be, in some cases, related to affective and impulsive disorders? Would the symptoms of such individuals differ in character from the truly schizophrenia-related schizotypal personality?

## Biological Studies

Biological correlates of chronic schizophrenia may also be abnormal in at least some forms of schizotypal personality disorder. Impaired smooth-pursuit eye movements (SPEMs) have been reported in 60–80% of schizophrenic patients and approximately half of their relatives, in contrast to a much smaller proportion of the relatives of manic–depressive patients (Holzman, Solomon, Levin, & Waternaux, 1984; Lipton, Levin, Holzman, & Leven, 1983). SPEM impairment has been specifically associated with schizotypal personality disorder, but not with other types of psychopathology, in volunteer subjects (Siever, Coursey, Alterman, Buchsbaum, & Murphy, 1984; Siever et al., 1989), personality disorder patients (Siever et al., 1990), and the offspring of schizophrenic parents (P. S. Holzman, personal communication, November 1988), supporting a biological association between schizotypal personality disorder and schizophrenia. Performance on a backward masking task (an information-processing test) shows abnormalities in schizotypal personality disorder patients that are similar to, though milder than, those observed in schizophrenic patients (Braff, 1986). Decreased activity of platelet monoamine and/or plasma amine oxidase has been reported in schizotypal volunteers and schizotypal relatives of schizophrenic patients (Baron & Levitt, 1980; Baron, Levitt, & Perlman, 1980; Baron, Gruen, Asnis, & Kanc, 1983) although in other studies it seems to be more closely related to sensation seeking and affective symptomatology (Buchsbaum, Coursey, & Murphy, 1976). Abnormalities in galvanic skin orienting response and evoked potential responses similar to those observed in schizophrenic patients have been reported in studies of college volunteers selected on the basis of a psychological test profile similar to that of schizophrenic patients

(Siever, 1985; Simons, 1981, 1982), as well as in preliminary studies of schizotypal personality disorder patients. Computerized tomographic scan (CT scan) studies have shown increases in the ventricular–brain ratio (VBR) in schizophrenic patients (Shelton & Weinberger, 1986) and schizotypal patients (Siever, Coccaro, et al., 1987). These studies cumulatively suggest that schizotypal individuals and at least a subgroup of clinically defined patients with schizotypal personality disorder demonstrate biological/psychophysiological abnormalities characteristic of chronic schizophrenia. Thus, biological studies complement genetic studies in supporting a relationship between schizotypal personality disorder and schizophrenia that extends to include clinically defined schizotypal patients.

These biological correlates (e.g., SPEM impairment, increased VBR, abnormalities on backward masking) are often associated with chronic attentional/cognitive dysfunction, apparently reflecting structural alteration of the central nervous system. These biological factors tend to be correlated with the "negative" or deficit symptoms of schizophrenia, whereas neurochemical variables such as catecholamine metabolites, which may be more state-related, may be associated with the "positive" or psychotic-like symptoms of schizophrenia. Plasma homovanillic acid (HVA), the major metabolite of dopamine, has been found to be correlated with psychotic symptoms in drug-free schizophrenic patients (Davis et al., 1985) and to diminish in parallel with psychotic symptoms with neuroleptic treatment (Pickar et al., 1986). Preliminary studies of schizotypal patients suggest that cerebrospinal fluid and plasma HVA are increased in schizotypal patients compared to other personality-disordered controls, and that these increases may be partially associated with increased psychotic-like symptoms (Siever, 1987).

Some preliminary evidence suggests that patients with a more prototypical schizotypal profile emphasizing the core deficit features without concomitant borderline features may be more likely to evidence biological correlates related to schizophrenia than the schizotypal–borderline group may be (Siever, 1985; Siever, Coccaro, et al., 1987), although larger samples with measures that are relatively more specific for schizophrenic versus affective disorders are required to clarify this issue.

## Outcome

Schizotypal patients have been shown to have a long-term outcome more similar to that of chronic schizophrenia than to that of another severe personality disorder, borderline personality disorder (McGlashan, 1986). The premorbid and illness characteristics of schizotypal patients, however, were more similar to those of McGlashan's other personality-disordered groups than to those of schizophrenics, with the exception of their premorbid social adjustment and their frequency of social contacts. Most specific outcome measures fell between those of schizophrenic patients and of personality-disordered groups (McGlashan, 1986). The patients with schizotypal and borderline features were more socially related than the pure schizotypal patients and "functioned" more like borderline patients, although their capacity for more intimate relationships seemed poorer than did that of the pure borderline personality disorder patients (McGlashan, 1986).

The proportion of patients with schizotypal personality disorder who actually go on to develop chronic schizophrenia is not clear, although as high as 25% of one sample of schizotypal patients were reported to have satisfied criteria for schizophrenia upon follow-up 2 years later (Schulz & Soloff, 1987), and 17% of the Chestnut Lodge sample received a later schizophrenic diagnosis (Fenton & McGlashan, 1989). This proportion was substantially lower in a sample of male veterans (Siever, 1987), and in those patients diagnosed as having schizophrenia on follow-up, at least two may have had schizophrenic symptoms that they were concealing on initial evaluation. In the Chestnut Lodge outcome study, symptoms of paranoid ideation, social isolation, and magical thinking were good predictors of the later onset of schizophrenia in character disorder patients (Fenton & McGlashan, 1989). In summary, the course of schizotypal personality disorder is similar to, although not quite as severe as, that of chronic schizophrenia, particularly with respect to social relatedness. Paranoid symptomatology and social impairment may be associated with worse outcome.

## Treatment Response

Like schizophrenic patients, schizotypal personality disorder patients have been found to respond positively to neuroleptics such as thiothixene and haloperidol (Goldberg et al., 1986; Serban & Siegel, 1984). Psychotic-like and anxiety symptoms—that is, illusions, ideas of reference, psychoticism, obsessive–compulsive symptoms, and phobic anxiety—responded specifically to the neuroleptic treatment (Goldberg et al., 1986). Although antidepressants such as monoamine oxidase inhibitors, tricyclics, and lithium carbonate were reported to cause symptomatic improvement in diagnoses that were forerunners to the schizotypal diagnosis, such as "pseudoneurotic schizophrenia" (Klein, 1967; Rifkin, Quitkin, & Carrillo, 1972), they have not been proven to have benefit in rigorously diagnosed schizotypal patients. Thus, schizotypal patients resemble chronic schizophrenic patients in their response to neuroleptics, particularly with respect to reduction of psychotic-like symptoms. Patients with borderline personality disorder, however, have also been reported to respond to neuroleptic medications (Soloff, George, & Nathan, 1986).

Controlled studies of the treatment response of schizotypal personality disorder to psychotherapy are not available. However, Searles (1965), Knight (1954), Frosch (1983), and Hoch and Polatin (1949) discussed problems encountered in treating patients with characteristics similar to DSM-III-R criteria for schizotypal personality disorder. Such patients tend to decompensate in the setting of unmodified analytic treatment, but may respond to a psychotherapeutic approach that emphasizes reality testing, attention to interpersonal boundaries, and educative interventions (Stone, 1985), if the goals are not too ambitious. The psychotherapeutic approach to schizotypal patients thus incorporates techniques utilized in the treatment of both schizophrenic patients and patients with severe personality disorders.

## DISCUSSION

### Schizotypal Personality Disorder—Axis I or Axis II?

The commonalities between chronic schizophrenia and schizotypal personality disorder suggest that the boundaries of the schizophrenia spectrum extend beyond chronic schizophrenia to include at least a substantial subset of schizotypal individuals. Although the strength and specificity of this relationship for schizotypal patients identified in a clinical setting require further investigation, initial results of studies evaluating family history, biological characteristics, outcome, and treatment response of schizotypal patients support the existence of such a relationship. These considerations would seem to argue for the inclusion of schizotypal personality disorder as one of the schizophrenia-related disorders, which are currently placed among the Axis I disorders.

Genetic and epidemiological studies, however, suggest that schizophrenia-related personality disorders may be more common manifestations of genotypes predisposing individuals to the schizophrenia-related disorders than chronic schizophrenia itself may be. That is, that the schizophrenia spectrum may include more individuals with Axis II than with Axis I disorders. The multiaxial system introduced in DSM-III does not easily accommodate or acknowledge the existence of spectrum disorders that may include both the episodic, symptomatic disorders included on Axis I and the stable psychopathological characteristics of the Axis II disorders. However, as our knowledge of the genetics, biology, outcome, and treatment response of both the Axis I and Axis II disorders increases, it seems likely that there will be increasing evidence not only for a schizophrenia spectrum, but also for an affective spectrum, an anxiety spectrum, and an impulse disorder spectrum, with manifestations varying from exacerbating and remitting symptoms to more persistent character traits. Simply to remove schizotypal personality disorder from Axis II and include it in Axis I might set a problematic precedent. It would raise questions as to whether schizoid or paranoid personality disorder as defined in DSM-III-R should also be included with the Axis I schizophrenic disorders; whether avoidant personality disorder should be included with the Axis I phobic anxiety disorders; whether borderline personality disorder should be included with the Axis I impulse disorders; or whether depressive or self-defeating personality disorder should be included with the Axis I affective disorders. Although these relationships are less clearly established than that between schizotypal personality disorder and schizophrenia, these personality disorders have been less intensively investigated using the approaches applied to schizotypal personality disorder. Available evidence, however, suggests that the possibility that at least some of these personality disorders will be found to be related to the corresponding Axis I disorders is not a remote one.

One potential solution to this dilemma that would not involve restructuring the multiaxial format would be to acknowledge schizotypal personality disorder explicitly on both Axes I and II. The concept of spectrums could be introduced in the introduction to and explanation of the multiaxial system, to clarify why schizotypal personality disorder is noted in both Axis I and Axis II. This solution would orient the clinician to the fact that schizotypal personality disorder should be potentially considered as a schizophrenia-related disorder that also meets the criteria for an Axis II disorder (i.e., it involves an enduring constellation of traits that describes an individual's interpersonal, cognitive, and affective style), but that it may not invariably, at least according to current criteria, define a disorder related to chronic schizophrenia. Investigators would be encouraged to examine a larger range of characteristics than those included in DSM-III-R or even DSM-IV in order to identify which schizotypal characteristics are most specific for the personality disorder(s) related to schizophrenia, as opposed to those schizotypal criteria (e.g., possibly some variants of psychotic-like symptoms) with etiologies unrelated to schizophrenia. Such an endeavor not only would be important in furthering our understanding of the schizophrenia-related disorders, but could have important implications for the diagnosis, prognosis, and treatment of the severe personality disorders. Premature closure of the status of schizotypal personality disorder in a dichotomous Axis I–Axis II framework might impair further research in the areas of both schizophrenic and personality disorders, which has been quite productive with the present framework. The acknowledgment of a spectrum or dimensional model of schizophrenia-related disorders that includes both Axis I and Axis II disorders might enhance both clinicians' and investigators' appreciation of the relationship between these two axes.

## Overlap between Schizotypal and Borderline Personality Disorders

Available data raise the possibility that some of the overlap between schizotypal and borderline personality disorders may be an artifact of less specific psychotic-like features that may occur with both disorders. The resolution of this question will require larger empirical studies that attempt to define more discriminating criteria that might reduce the overlap between these two disorders. Ultimately, external validating studies will be required to determine whether patients with schizotypal personality disorder and concomitant borderline personality disorder differ from "pure" schizotypal patients on genetic, biological, outcome, and treatment response variables.

Preliminary studies suggest that patients with both schizotypal and border-line personality disorders have characteristics falling between those of "pure" schizotypal patients and "pure" borderline patients, suggesting that there is some genuine overlap as well as artifactual overlap.

## Specificity of Relationship between Schizotypal Personality Disorder and Schizophrenia

Affective characteristics, which may be observed in both borderline patients and relatives of affective disorder patients, may lead to cognitive/perceptual distortions, difficulty in maintaining relationships, suspiciousness and projection under stress, and social anxiety. However, these characteristics would be expected to be most prominent in altered affective states. Again, studies attempting to refine the criteria for schizotypal personality disorder, as well as studies of external validators, are needed to resolve this question conclusively.

# CHANGES PROPOSED FOR AND MADE IN DSM-IV

Modifications to the diagnostic criteria for schizotypal personality disorder initially proposed for DSM-IV were directed toward reducing the high degree of diagnostic overlap between schizotypal and other personality disorders that are considered to fall outside of the "schizophrenia spectrum," particularly borderline personality disorder. Phemenological studies have suggested that the occurrence of psychotic-like symptomatology in "non-schizophrenia-related" personality disorders may be an important source of this diagnostic overlap. The changes proposed in the schizotypal criteria set were directed toward improving specificity by taking into account the persistence of psychotic-like symptomatology outside of the context of discrete periods of affective symptoms (e.g., depression, anxiety, and anger). It was hypothesized that the appearance of psychotic-like symptomatology among borderline patients would be associated with these affective periods, whereas psychotic-like features in schizotypal patients would be persistent and relatively independent of affective symptoms. Therefore, the proposed DSM-IV schizotypal criteria set included the requirement that schizotypal "signs and symptoms must not be limited to discrete periods of affective symptomatology (c.g., depression, anxiety, anger)." These distinctions were similar to the assessments required for the full diagnosis of schizoaffective disorder, where schizophrenia-like psychotic symptoms are assessed for the context in which they occur—that is, whether or not they overlap entirely with affective symptoms.

An example may clarify this point. Suppose that a patient reports numerous instances over the course of his life in which he has had the distinct feeling that strangers were discussing him and deriding his character. Upon further evaluation, it becomes clear that this feeling consistently emerges only after some untoward event has occurred (e.g., when he was fired from his job; in the period immediately after his mother's death; after a loud, angry argument with his estranged wife), and that it is associated with a clearly depressed, angry, or anxious mood. Although the patient experiences several such episodes in a year, he reports extended periods of normal mood when he does not feel any acute affective distress and displays no referential symptoms.

This patient is reporting clear examples of "ideas of reference" (DSM-III-R criterion 1). Because this feature only emerges in the context of affective symptomatology, however, it would not be considered present under the originally proposed DSM-IV criteria. Each DSM-III-R schizotypal personality disorder criterion would seem to be amenable to such contextual assessment.

In cases where information regarding the context in which a particular schizotypal feature appears is unavailable, the proposed modification could be interpreted either less restrictively (i.e., the feature would be considered to be present) or more restrictively (i.e., the feature would be considered to be absent). The former alternative would be less restrictive, as it would preserve the schizotypal diagnosis unless exclusionary information can be obtained; in contrast, the latter approach would limit schizotypal diagnoses to cases where data are available regarding the affective context in which schizotypal symptomatology occurs. For clinical purposes, the less restrictive approach would be recommended, although researchers might wish to use the more restrictive approach in order to obtain more homogeneous samples of schizotypal patients.

Additional changes originally proposed to the criteria set concerned social isolation and social anxiety. The following addition was proposed to the social isolation criterion: "no close friends or confidants (or only one) other than first-degree relatives due primarily to lack of desire, persuasive discomfort with others, or eccentricities." Thus a patient who avoids or otherwise lacks close friendships because of past troubles associated with their intensity, instability, or emotional turmoil would not be considered to meet this criterion, whereas a patient who has never had any interest in establishing a close connection with others would be considered to meet the criterion.

The following addition was also proposed for social anxiety: "excessive social anxiety, e.g., extreme discomfort in social situations involving unfamiliar people that does not diminish with familiarity and tends to be associated with paranoid fears rather than fears of negative judgments about self." This revision would mean that this criterion would not be met by those socially anxious individuals who are generally able to "warm up" to novel social situations over time or who are primarily concerned that they will be judged negatively (e.g., being seen as "unattractive" or "a jerk").

It was hoped that all of the proposed changes would identify a more homogeneous group of schizotypal patients, with less overlap with borderline diagnoses. The degree to which this was the case was evaluated in a multicenter study. The DSM-III-R criteria and the proposed DSM-IV criteria, in which the features as defined must not be limited to periods of affective symptomatology, were assessed in 270 subjects from four study sites. Three of the participating study sites — the Mount Sinai/Bronx Department of Veterans Affairs outpatient departments, McLean Hospital, and the Eastern Pennsylvania Psychiatric Institute — assessed clinically identified subjects with prominent personality disorder traits, though not necessarily schizotypal personality disorder. The fourth group of subjects, obtained from the Mount Sinai Family Studies Program, were relatives of psychiatric probands (primarily schizophrenic, though some had a major affective disorder). Each site assessed subjects using a comprehensive structured personality disorder interview designed to assess all DSM-III-R personality disorder categories. A second questionnaire, Supplemental Questions for Assessing Schizophrenia Spectrum Disorders, was also employed. This interview was designed to work in conjunction with the more encompassing personality disorder assessment interviews to evaluate the presence or absence of the additional refinements associated with the proposed DSM-IV schizotypal personality disorder criteria.

As expected, the number of subjects diagnosed with schizotypal personality disorder by the proposed DSM-IV criteria was substantially reduced (DSM-III-R, $n$ = 43; proposed DSM-IV, $n$ = 25). In addition, compared to the DSM-III-R criteria, most of the individual items associated with the proposed set of criteria had comparable or slightly increased sensitivity and specificity for the overall schizotypal personality disorder diagnosis. The reduction in overlap between schizotypal and borderline personality disorders with the proposed criteria, however, was trivial. Thus, most of the criteria changes proposed for DSM-IV did not achieve the objective of increasing the discriminant validity of the diagnosis. As a result, it was decided that most of the DSM-III-R criteria, with only minor changes in wording and numbering, should be retained for DSM-IV (see Table 5.2; note in DSM-IV criterion 9 that a version of the proposed change for social anxiety *has* been made). Phenomenological, family/genetic, and biological studies suggest that schizotypal personality disorder is a valid diagnostic entity and one that is related to schizophrenia. Further research will be required to explicate the exact nature of this relationship and to refine diagnostic criteria.

TABLE 5.2. DSM-III-R and DSM-IV Diagnostic Criteria for Schizotypal Personality Disorder

| DSM-III-R criteria | DSM-IV criteria |
|---|---|
| A. A pervasive pattern of deficits in interpersonal relatedness and peculiarities of ideation, appearance, and behavior, beginning by early adulthood and present in a variety of contexts, as indicated by at least *five* of the following: | A. A pervasive pattern of social and interpersonal deficits marked by acute discomfort with, and reduced capacity for, close relationships as well as by cognitive or perceptual distortions and eccentricities of behavior, beginning by early adulthood and present in a variety of contexts, as indicated by five (or more) of the following: |
| (1) ideas of reference (excluding delusions of reference) | (1) ideas of reference (excluding delusions of reference) |
| (2) excessive social anxiety, e.g., extreme discomfort in social situations involving unfamiliar people | (2) odd beliefs or magical thinking that influences behavior and is inconsistent with subcultural norms (e.g., superstitiousness, belief in clairvoyance, telepathy, or "sixth sense"; in children and adolescents, bizarre fantasies or preoccupations) |
| (3) odd beliefs or magical thinking, influencing behavior and inconsistent with subcultural norms, e.g., superstitiousness, belief in clairvoyance, telepathy, or "sixth sense," "others can feel my feelings" (in children and adolescents, bizarre fantasies or preoccupations) | (3) unusual perceptual experiences, including bodily illusions |
| (4) unusual perceptual experiences, e.g., illusions, sensing the presence of a force or person not actually present (e.g., "I felt as if my dead mother were in the room with me") | (4) odd thinking and speech (e.g., vague, circumstantial, metaphorical, overelaborate, or stereotyped) |
| (5) odd or eccentric behavior or appearance, e.g., unkempt, unusual mannerisms, talks to self | (5) suspiciousness or paranoid ideation |
| (6) no close friends or confidants (or only one) other than first-degree relatives | (6) inappropriate or constricted affect |
| (7) odd speech (without loosening of associations or incoherence), e.g., speech that is impoverished, digressive, vague, or inappropriately abstract | (7) behavior or appearance that is odd, eccentric, or peculiar |
| (8) inappropriate or constricted affect, e.g., silly, aloof, rarely reciprocates gestures or facial expressions, such as smiles or nods | (8) lack of close friends or confidants other than first-degree relatives |

*(cont.)*

**TABLE 5.2.** (cont.)

| DSM-III-R criteria | DSM-IV criteria |
|---|---|
| (9) suspiciousness or paranoid ideation | (9) excessive social anxiety that does not diminish with familiarity and tends to be associated with paranoid fears rather than negative judgments about self |
| B. Occurrence not exclusively during the course of Schizophrenia or a Pervasive Developmental Disorder | B. Does not occur exclusively during the course of Schizophrenia, a Mood Disorder With Psychotic Features, another Psychotic Disorder, or a Pervasive Developmental Disorder. |
| | **Note:** If criteria are met prior to the onset of Schizophrenia, add "Premorbid," e.g., "Schizotypal Personality Disorder (Premorbid)." |

*Note.* From APA (1987, pp. 341–342) and APA (1994, p. 645). Copyright 1987 and 1994 by the American Psychiatric Association. Reprinted by permission.

## REFERENCES

American Psychiatric Association. (1980). *Diagnostic and statistical manual of mental disorders* (3rd ed.). Washington, DC: Author.

American Psychiatric Association. (1987). *Diagnostic and statistical manual of mental disorders* (3rd ed., rev.). Washington, DC: Author.

American Psychiatric Association. (1994). *Diagnostic and statistical manual of mental disorders* (4th ed.). Washington, DC: Author.

Baron, J. M., Gruen, R., Asnis, L., & Kane, J. (1983). Familial relatedness of schizophrenia and schizotypal states. *American Journal of Psychiatry, 140,* 1437–1442.

Baron, M., Gruen, R.. Rainer, J. D., Kane, J., Asnis, L., & Lord, S. (1985). A family study of schizophrenic and normal control probands: Implications for the spectrum concept of schizophrenia. *American Journal of Psychiatry, 142,* 447–454.

Baron, M., & Levitt, M. (1980). Platelet monoamine oxidase activity: Relation to genetic load of schizophrenia. *Psychiatry Research, 3,* 69–74.

Baron, M., Levitt, M., & Perlman, R. (1980). Low platelet monoamine oxidase activity: A possible biochemical correlate of borderline schizophrenia. *Psychiatry Research, 3,* 329–335.

Braff, D. L. (1986). Impaired speed of information processing in nonmedicated schizotypal patients. *Schizophrenia Bulletin, 7,* 499–508.

Buchsbaum, M. S., Coursey, R. D., & Murphy, D. L. (1976). The biochemical and high-risk paradigm: Behavioral and familial correlates of low platelet monoamine oxidase activity. *Science, 193,* 339–341.

Dahl, A. (1986). Some aspects of the DSM-III personality disorders illustrated by a consecutive sample of hospitalized patients. *Acta Psychiatrica Scandinavica, 73*(Suppl. 328), 61–66.

Davis K. L., Davidson, M., Mohs, R. C., Kendler, K., Davis, B., Johns, C., DeNigris, Y., & Horvath, T. (1985). Plasma HVA concentrations correlate with the severity of schizophrenic illness. *Science, 227,* 1601–1602.

Fenton, T. S., & McGlashan, T. H. (1989). Risk of schizophrenia in character disordered patients. *American Journal of Psychiatry, 146,* 1280–1284.

Frances, A. (1985). Validating schizotypal personality disorders: Problems with the schizophrenia connection. *Schizophrenia Bulletin, 11*(4), 595–597.

Freiman, K., & Widiger, T. (1989). [Co-occurrence and diagnostic efficiency statistics]. Unpublished raw data.

Frosch, J. (1983). *The psychotic process.* New York: International Universities Press.

Goldberg, S. C., Schulz, S. C., Schulz, P. M., Resnick, R. J., Hamer, R. M., & Friedel, R. O. (1986). Borderline and schizotypal personality disorders treated with low dose thiothixelle vs. placebo. *Archives of General Psychiatry, 43,* 680–686.

Gunderson, J. G., Siever, L. J., & Spaulding, E. (1983). The search for a schizotype: Crossing the border again. *Archives of General Psychiatry, 40,* 15–22.

Hoch, P., & Polatin, P. (1949). Pseudoneurotic forms of schizophrenia. *Psychiatric Quarterly, 23,* 248–276.

Holzman, P. S., Solomon, C. M., Levin, S., & Waternaux, C. S. (1984). Pursuit eye movement dysfunctions in schizophrenia. *Archives of General Psychiatry, 41,* 136–140.

Ingraham, L. J. (1989). Genetic factors in schizophrenia and schizophrenia-like illness from a national sample of adopted individuals and their families. *Abstracts of the 28th Annual Meeting of the American College of Neuropsychopharmacology.*

Jacobsberg, L., Hymowitz, P., Barasch, A., & Frances, A. (1986). Symptoms of schizotypal personality. *American Journal of Psychiatry, 143,* 1222–1227.

Kass, F., Skodol, A. E., Charles, E., Spitzer, R. L., & Williams, J. B. W. (1985). Scaled ratings of DSM-III personality disorders. *American Journal of Psychiatry, 142,* 627–630.

Kendler, K. (1985). Diagnostic approaches to schizotypal personality disorder: A historical perspective. *Schizophrenia Bulletin, 11,* 538–553.

Kendler, K. S., Gruenberg, A. M., & Strauss, J. S. (1981). An independent analysis of the Copenhagen sample of the Danish adoption study of schizophrenia. *Archives of General Psychiatry, 38,* 982–987.

Kendler, K. S., Gruenberg, A. M., & Tsuang, M. T. (1985). Psychiatric illness in first degree relatives of schizophrenic and surgical control patients: A family study using DSM-III criteria. *Archives of General Psychiatry, 42,* 770–779.

Kendler, K. S., Walsh, D., Su, Y., McGuire, M., Spellman, M., Lytle, C. H., McCormick, O., O'Neil, A. O., Shinkwin, R., Nuallain, M. N., O'Hare, A., Kidd, K. K., MacLean, C. J., & Diehl, S. R. (1989). The Roscommon family and linkage study of schizophrenia: Preliminary report. *Abstracts of the 28th Annual Meeting of the American College of Neuropsychopharmacology,* p. 56.

Kety, S. S., Rosenthal, D., Wender, P. H., Schulsinger, F., & Jacobsen, B. (1975). Mental illness in the biological and adoptive families of adopted individuals who have become schizophrenics: A preliminary report based on psychiatric interviews. In R. R. Fieve, D. Rosenthal, & H. Brill (Eds.), *Genetic research in psychiatry* (pp. 147–165). Baltimore: John Hopkins University Press.

Klein, D. F. (1967). Importance of psychiatric diagnosis in prediction of clinical drug effects. *Archives of General Psychiatry, 16,* 118–126.

Knight, R. P. (1954). Management and psychotherapy of the borderline schizophrenic patient. In R. P. Knight & C. R. Friedman (Eds.), *Psychoanalytic psychiatry and psychology* (pp. 110–122). New York: International Universities Press.

Lipton, R. B., Levin, S., Holzman, P. S., & Leven, S. (1983). Eye movement dysfunctions in psychiatric patients: A review. *Schizophrenia Bulletin, 9,* 13–32.

McGlashan, T. H. (1983). The borderline syndrome: II. Is it a variant of schizophrenia or affective disorder? *Archives of General Psychiatry, 40,* 1319–1323.

McGlashan, T. H. (1986). Schizotypal personality disorder: Chestnut Lodge Follow-Up Study. VI. Long-term follow-up perspective. *Archives of General Psychiatry, 43,* 329–334.

McGlashan, T. H. (1987). Testing DSM-III symptom criteria for schizotypal and borderline personality disorders. *Archives of General Psychiatry, 44,* 15–22.

Millon, T., & Tringone, R. (1989). [Co-occurrence and diagnostic efficiency statistics]. Unpublished raw data.

Morey, L. (1988). Personality disorders in DSM-III and DSM-III-R: Convergence, coverage, and internal consistency. *American Journal of Psychiatry, 145,* 573–577.

Pfohl, B., Coryell, W., Zimmerman, M., & Stangl, D. (1986). DSM-III personality disorders: Diagnostic overlap and internal consistency of individual DSM-III criteria. *Comprehensive Psychiatry, 27,* 21–34.

Pfohl, B., Stangl, D., & Zimmerman, H. (1984). The implications of DSM-III personality disorders for patients with major depression. *Journal of Affective Disorders, 7,* 299–315.

Pickar, D., Labarca, R., Doran, A., Wolkowitz, O., Roy, A., Brier, A., Linnoila, M., & Paul, S. (1986). Longitudinal measurement of plasma homovanillic acid levels in schizophrenic patients. *Archives of General Psychiatry, 43,* 669–676.

Rifkin, A., Quitkin, F., & Carrillo, C. (1972). Lithium carbonate in emotionally unstable character disorder. *Archives of General Psychiatry, 27,* 519–523.

Schulz, P. M., Schulz, S. C., Goldberg, S. C., Ettigi, P., Resnick, R. J., & Friedel, R. O. (1986). Diagnoses of the relatives of schizotypal outpatients. *Journal of Nervous and Mental Disorders, 174,* 457–463.

Schulz, P. M., & Soloff, P. H. (1987, May). *Still borderline after all these years.* Paper presented at the 140th Annual Meeting of the American Psychiatric Association.

Searles, H. F. (1965). *Collected papers on schizophrenia and related subjects.* New York: International Universities Press.

Serban, G., & Siegel, S. (1984). Response of borderline and schizotypal patients to small doses of thiothtxene and haloperidol. *American Journal of Psychiatry, 141,* 1455–1458.

Shelton, R. C., & Weinberger, D. R. (1986). X-ray computerized tomography studies of schizophrenia: A review and synthesis. In H. A. Nasrallah & D. R. Weinberger (Eds.), *The neurology of schizophrenia* (pp. 325–348). Amsterdam: Elsevier.

Siever, L. J. (1985). Biological markers in schizotypal personality disorder. *Schizophrenia Bulletin, 11,* 564–575.

Siever, L. J. (1987). [Unpublished data.]

Siever, L. J. (1988). [Unpublished data.]

Siever, L. J., Coursey, R. D., Alterman, I. S., Buchsbaum, M. S., & Murphy, D. L. (1984). Impaired smooth pursuit eye movement: Vulnerability markers for schizotypal personality disorder in a volunteer population. *American Journal of Psychiatry, 141,* 1560–1565.

Siever, L. J., Coursey, R. D., Alterman, I. S., Zahn, T., Brody, L., Bernad, P., Buchsbaum, M., Lake, C. R., & Murphy, D. L. (1989). Clinical, psychophysiological, and neurological characteristics of volunteers with impaired smooth pursuit eye movements. *Biological Psychiatry, 26,* 35–51.

Siever, L. J., Coccaro, E. F., Zemishlany, Z., Silverman, J., Klar, H., Losonczy, M. F., Davidson, M., Friedman, R., Mohs, R. C., & Davis, K. L. (1987). Psychobiology of personality disorder: Pharmacologic implications. *Psychopharmacology Bulletin,* *23,* 333–336.

Siever, L. J., & Gunderson, J. G. (1983). The search for a schizotypal personality: Historical origins and current status. *Comprehensive Psychiatry, 24,* 199–212.

Siever, L. J., Keefe, R., Bernstein, D. P., Coccaro, E. F., Klar, H. M., Zemishlany, Z., Peterson, A., Davidson, M., Mahon, T., Horvath, T., & Mohs, R. (1990). Eye tracking impairment in clinically identified schizotypal personality disorder patients. *American Journal of Psychiatry, 147,* 740–745.

Siever, L. J., Klar, H., Coccaro, E. F., Silverman, J., Sween, L., & Davis, K. L. (1987, May). Schizotypal and borderline personality overlap. *Abstracts of the 140th Annual Meeting of the American Psychiatric Association.*

Silverman, J. M., Siever, L. J., Mohs, R. C., & Davis, K. L. (1987). Risk for affective and personality disorders in relatives of personality disordered patients. *Abstracts of the Annual Meeting of the Society of Biological Psychiatry.*

Silverman, J. M., Mohs, R. C., Siever, L. J., Kendler, K. S., Breitner, J. C. S., & Davis, K. L. (1986). Heritability for schizophrenia-spectrum disorder in schizophrenia and schizophrenia-related personality disorder. *Clinical Neuropharmacology, 9*(4), 271–273.

Silverman, J. M., Siever, L. J., Pinkham, L., Mohs, R. C., & Davis, K. L. (1988). Risk for affective, schizophrenia-related and personality disorders in relatives of depressed personality disordered patients. *Abstracts of the Annual Meeting of the Society of Biological Psychiatry.*

Simons, R. F. (1981). Electrodermal and cardiac orienting in psychometrically high risk subjects. *Psychiatry Research, 4,* 347–256.

Simons, R. F. (1982). Physical anhedonia and future psychopathology: A possible electrocortical continuity. *Psychophysiology, 19,* 433–441.

Skodol, A. E. (1989). [Co-occurrence and diagnostic efficiency statistics]. Unpublished raw data.

Soloff, P. H., George, A.. & Nathan, R. S. (1986). Progress in pharmacotherapy of borderline disorders. *Archives of General Psychiatry, 43,* 698–700.

Soloff, P. H., & Millward, J. W. (1983). Psychiatric disorders in the families of borderline patients. *Archives of General Psychiatry, 40,* 37–44.

Spitzer, R. L., Endicott, J., & Gibbon, M. (1979). Crossing the border into borderline personality and borderline schizophrenia: The development of criteria. *Archives of General Psychiatry, 36,* 17–24.

Squires-Wheeler, E., Skodol, A. E., Friedman, D., & Erlenmeyer-Kimling, L. (1988). The specificity of DSM-III schizotypal personality traits. *Psychological Medicine, 18,* 757–765.

Stone, M. (1977). The borderline syndrome: Evolution of the term, genetic aspects and prognosis. *American Journal of Psychotherapy, 31,* 345–365.

Stone, M. (1985). Schizotypal personality: Psychotherapeutic aspects. *Schizophrenia Bulletin, 11,* 576–589.

Torgersen, S. (1985). Relationship of schizotypal personality disorder to schizophrenia: Genetics. *Schizophrenia Bulletin, 11,* 554–563.

Widiger, T. A., Frances, A., Warner, L., & Bluhm, C. (1986). Diagnostic criteria for the borderline and schizotypal personality disorders. *Journal of Abnormal Psychology, 95,* 43–51.

Zanarini, M. (1989). [Co-occurrence and diagnostic efficiency statistical]. Unpublished raw data.

# Commentary on Paranoid, Schizoid, and Schizotypal Personality Disorders

SVENN TORGERSEN

The aim of this chapter is not to discuss the fundamental problems of defining personality disorders; that is done by other authors in this volume. Instead, I present some dilemmas that arise when we follow the DSM system for classifying personality disorders, and then consider the implications of these dilemmas for the classification of paranoid, schizoid, and schizotypal personality disorders.

## DILEMMAS IN THE CLASSIFICATION OF PERSONALITY DISORDERS

### Definition of Disorder

First, we should ensure that the criteria selected to diagnose a personality disorder really describe dysfunction, distress, or limitations in self-realization and pleasure. Conventional studies of specificity and sensitivity in patient populations do not address this question. These studies only tell us what kind of criteria discriminate between disorders, not what kind of criteria discriminate between personality disorders and normality. This issue is important because many specific personality disorders are highly correlated with normal personality dimensions (Torgersen & Alnaes, 1989; Costa & McCrae, 1992). Criteria describing introverted traits may therefore have high sensitivity and specificity because they differentiate between the "odd, eccentric" Cluster A and "dramatic, erratic" Cluster B personality disorders, but they will not necessarily discriminate normal individuals from those with personality disorders. Even if such criteria appear helpful in diagnosis with patient samples, a high frequency of false positives may result if these criteria are used to detect cases of personality disorders in a sample with a large proportion of normal subjects. DSM-III-R states that "It is only when *person-ality traits* are inflexible and maladaptive and cause either significant func-tional impairment or subjective distress that they constitute *Personality Disorders*" (American Psychiatric Association, 1987, p. 335; italics in original). DSM-IV makes a similar statement (American Psychiatric Association, 1994, p. 630). In practice, however, diagnosis is usually determined by the num-ber of criteria present, not by the degree of distress and dysfunction.

## Delineation of Individual Diagnoses

Another problem is how the criteria for personality disorders should be grouped to constitute separate diagnostic entities. Basically, there are two methods of delineating personality disorders. Criteria may be grouped together as in factor analysis, on the basis of intercorrelations among criter-ia. Or, as with cluster analysis, criteria that co-occur within a group of personality-disordered individuals may define a diagnosis. According to this procedure, the same criteria can be used to define several disorders. Lives-ley, Jackson, and Schroeder (1989) have applied the former method; my col-leagues and I (Torgersen, Skre, Onstad, Edvardsen, & Kringlen, 1993) have used both; and DSM-III-R and DSM-IV are based on the latter. This means, for instance, that social isolation and paranoid ideation may occur in more than one disorder. Although such a procedure may be valid, it creates an artificial overlap among the disorders. This could be avoided, however, by establishing a hierarchy. For example, a group of affect-constricted disor-ders might be delineated using a few criteria, and then further subdivided using new sets of criteria. Possible ways of doing this based on cluster analy-sis are proposed elsewhere (Torgersen, Skre, et al., 1993).

## Level of Inference

A problem with DSM-III-R is the level of inference required to assess diag-nostic criteria. Generally, DSM-III (American Psychiatric Association, 1980) and DSM-III-R aimed to achieve satisfactory reliability by making diagnos-tic criteria overtly behavioral rather than covertly emotional or motivation-al. This probably increased reliability at the expense of validity. For example, in order to differentiate between schizoid and avoidant personality disor-ders, it is important to establish whether the social isolation is due to lack of desire or fear of rejection. The criteria adopted for DSM-IV require more inference than the criteria found in DSM-III-R—a development that involves a return to the situation before DSM-III. It remains to be seen whether or not reliability will decline as a result of this change. I will return to these dilemmas later. But, first, three issues are discussed in connection with the "odd, eccentric" personality disorders (Cluster A). The first issue relates to validity: For what reasons have these specific disorders been retained in DSM-IV? To answer this question, validation data must be discussed. Such data can come from family/genetic studies, studies of the relevance of the diagnosis for the outcome of treatment, and so on. The second issue is whether these disorders should be included among the personality disorders on Axis II or among the symptom disorders on Axis I. This issue pertains to the spectrum question—that is, whether the personality features are so closely related to a symptom disorder that some of these diagnoses may be better grouped with the symptom disorders. Family/genetic data can also help to resolve this question. The third issue concerns the choice of criteria in DSM-IV. Have the criteria that have been retained from DSM-III-R performed satisfactorily, and are the changes made to the criteria sets in DSM-IV really improvements? These questions are addressed using the information presented in Chapters 3–5 and as yet unpublished data from my own research. Finally, a new delineation within Cluster A, and between the Cluster A and other personality disorders, is discussed.

## PARANOID PERSONALITY DISORDER

### Validity

The concept of paranoid personality disorder has a long history in psychiatry. Kraepelin, as well as E. Bleuler, described the distrust of others and the rigidity in the belief systems of paranoid individuals. Schneider (1923) also proposed such a disorder, labeled the "fanatic type." DSM-II (American Psychiatric Association, 1968) included a paranoid personality, as did the eighth and ninth revisions of the *International Classification of Diseases* (ICD-8 and ICD-9; World Health Organization, 1974, 1978). Finally, paranoid personality disorder is also included in ICD-10 (World Health Organization, 1992). Thus, different diagnostic systems have recognized the necessity of incorporating a paranoid personality syndrome.

Is paranoid personality disorder validated through family/genetic studies? Two twin studies have investigated the heritability of paranoid traits. In a large Australian twin study of normal subjects, Kendler, Heath, and Martin (1987) found that suspiciousness as measured by a few questionnaire items seemed to be genetically influenced. Recently, in a population-based sample, Kendler and Hewitt (1992) found that paranoid traits, assessed with the Claridge Paranoid Ideation Questionnaire, were more than 40% heritable. Paranoid traits seem to be partly genetically anchored and thus have some validity.

What about clinical usefulness? Does the existence of a paranoid personality disorder or paranoid traits influence treatment outcome or affect the prognosis of Axis I disorders? Generally, the presence of personality disorder decreases the prognosis of symptom disorders. Pfohl, Stangl, and Zimmerman (1984) found that the number of personality disorder criteria present correlated with an unfavorable outcome in depression. But what about para-

noid personality disorder specifically? Joffe and Regan (1989) unexpectedly found that depressed patients who responded positively to antidepressants had higher scores on the Paranoid scale of the Millon Clinical Multiaxial Inventory. However, most patients had very low scores, and the authors
suggested that the differences were attributable to higher scores being more
autonomous and self-determined. Pilkonis and Frank (1988), on the other
hand, found that depressive subjects with Cluster A personality disorders
responded more slowly to antidepressants. To date, there is no clear evidence that the presence of paranoid personality disorder predicts the development of Axis I symptom disorders. This lack of evidence can be attributed more to the lack of studies than to negative results. Therefore, as evidence now stands, the validity of paranoid personality disorder can be accepted.

## Axis II or Axis I?

Bernstein, Useda, and Siever, in Chapter 3, thoroughly discuss the overlap
between paranoid personality disorder and Axis I disorders. They cite evidence from family/genetic studies suggesting that paranoid personality disorder is more frequent among relatives of schizophrenic probands than
among relatives of controls. My colleagues and I (Torgersen, Onstad, Skre,
Edvardsen, & Kringlen, 1993) have confirmed these findings to a certain extent: Paranoid personality disorder was slightly more frequent among cotwins and relatives of schizophrenic probands than among cotwins and
relatives of subjects with major depression, but the difference was not statistically significant. The same was true for the criterion of suspiciousness in
schizotypal personality disorder (see below).
    Bernstein et al. (Chapter 3) also cite a study showing that paranoid per-
sonality disorder and delusional disorder are familially related, as well as
a study showing a small familial relationship between schizophrenia and delusional disorder. Two twin studies (Farmer, McGuffin, & Gottesman, 1987;
Onstad, Skre, Torgersen, & Kringlen, 1991) suggest that this familial transmission may be genetic. Because a genetic relationship exists between
schizotypal personality disorder and schizophrenia (Torgersen, Onstad, et
al., 1993) and some overlap exists between schizotypal and paranoid personality disorders, we may see a pattern that Bernstein et al. suggest: A common genetic etiology exists for some overlapping cases of paranoid and
schizotypal personality disorders, perhaps because of overlapping criteria.
Some cases of schizophrenia and delusional disorder may also have a common etiology. This would create a weak relationship between paranoid personality disorder and schizophrenia, as the Kendler and Gruenberg (1984)
re-examination of the Danish adoption study showed, and possibly also between schizotypal personality disorder and delusional disorder. However,
the main etiological links are between schizotypal personality disorder and

schizophrenia and between paranoid personality disorder and delusional disorder, respectively, as Bernstein et al. conclude in Chapter 3.

Does such a family/genetic relationship between paranoid personality disorder and delusional disorder warrant the inclusion of paranoid personality disorder within the delusional disorders on Axis I? I agree with Bernstein et al. that such an inclusion would be premature, because the relationship is too weakly established. Furthermore, paranoid personality disorder is also related to other Axis I disorders. For example, we (Alnaes & Torgersen, 1988a) found a strong comorbidity between paranoid personality disorder and agoraphobia without panic. An explanation for this may be that paranoid fears may be just as good reasons for staying at home and avoiding public places as the fear of having panic attacks or experiencing dizziness.

## Criteria Changes

Generally, based on analysis of internal consistency and correlations between the criteria and the disorder, my colleagues and I found the DSM-III-R criteria for paranoid personality disorder to be among the best of those for the various personality disorders (Torgersen, Skre, et al., 1993). Nevertheless, we found reason to suggest modification of DSM-III-R criterion 4 ("bears grudges . . ."), criterion 6 ("is easily slighted . . ."), and criterion 7 ("questions . . . fidelity of spouse or sexual partner"), because these criteria correlated least well with the overall criteria set. In fact, criterion 7 did not correlate at all with the overall set. The modification of criterion 6 in DSM-IV as described in Chapter 3 appears to be successful, according to a recent, not yet published study (Torgersen & Alnaes, 1995) of nearly 300 outpatients in Norway. The sensitivity was .86 and the specificity was .80. These values are far higher than any reported for the original DSM-III-R criterion. The modification of criterion DSM-III-R item 4 (it is now criterion 5 in DSM-IV) was less successful: Sensitivity was only .43 although specificity was .95, and the correlation with the sum of the other criteria was only .28. The modified criterion 7, which concerns suspicions about fidelity, also appeared to have low sensitivity (.38), and high specificity (.97), and the correlation with the sum of the other criteria was only .19. It seems reasonable to conclude that DSM-IV criterion 7 is very weak. This item was first included in DSM-III-R and it has never discriminated well, probably because it is impossible to discern on the basis of the patient's report alone whether the suspicion in fact is or is not justified. Even if the clinical impression is that paranoid individuals are very jealous, this applies more to psychotic patients with apparent delusional ideas about infidelity. A conservative rating would imply that one would not score criterion 7 when assessing an individual with infidelity worries without independent information. This would create a very low base rate and consequently, the sensitivity would be too low.

## SCHIZOID PERSONALITY DISORDER

### Validity

As Kalus, Bernstein, and Siever note in Chapter 4, the term "schizoid" has been especially popular in traditional European psychiatry (E. Bleuler, Kretschmer) and early British object relations theory (Winnicott, Guntrip). Also, neo-Reichians such as Lowen (1967) have elaborated what they call "the schizoid split." DSM-II included a schizoid personality, as did ICD-8, ICD-9, and ICD-10. As Kalus and colleagues state, schizoid personality disorder was somewhat pushed aside by schizotypal and avoidant personality disorders in DSM-III, although the changes in DSM-III-R increased the prevalence of the disorder in clinical populations. This is also the case with the DSM-IV criteria: We (Alnaes & Torgersen, 1988b) observed a frequency of 2% for DSM-III schizoid personality disorder among 298 psychiatric outpatients. Six years later, a frequency of 15% was recorded for the same population when diagnosis was based on the criteria for the DSM-IV.

Family/genetic studies of schizoid personality disorder are almost completely lacking. Preliminary results from a Norwegian twin study show that schizoid personality disorder has negligible heritability and that approximately one-third of the variance could be attributed to family environmental factors. This represents some validation of the disorder—not on a genetic basis, as is usual, but on an environment-shared-in-families basis.

As far as I know, the usefulness of the diagnostic concept in clinical practice has not yet been studied.

### Axis I

As Kalus et al. state in Chapter 4, neither family studies nor studies of comorbidity suggest any specific relation between schizoid personality disorder and any Axis I disorder. It might be added that a twin/family study ruled out any genetic/familial relationship between schizoid personality disorder and schizophrenia (Torgersen, Onstad, et al., 1993).

### Criteria Changes

Kalus and colleagues present a review of data from studies of DSM-III-R criteria showing that, on the basis of sensitivity, criterion 3 ("rarely . . . claims or appears to experience strong emotions") and criterion 5 ("is indifferent to the praise and criticism of others") discriminated poorly. We have made similar observations (Torgersen, Skre, et al., 1993). Furthermore, these criteria correlated poorly with other schizoid criteria. In fact, along with criterion 7 ("displays constricted affect"), they seem to belong with the criteria for schizotypal personality disorder.

Our unpublished study of the DSM-IV criteria (Torgersen & Alnæs,

1995) showed that the new criteria set did not discriminate better than the DSM-III-R criteria set. The sensitivity and specificity of DSM-IV criterion 4 (modified from DSM-III-R criterion 3) were .57 and .96, respectively, and the correlation with the sum of the remaining criteria was .37. The sensitivity of DSM-IV criterion 6 (modified from DSM-III-R criterion 5) was .10, with a specificity of 1.00, and the correlation with the remaining criteria was only .16. Kalus and colleagues also question DSM-III-R criterion 4 ("indicates little if any desire to have sexual experiences . . . "). In our study, this criterion (modified as criterion 3 in DSM-IV) showed a sensitivity and specificity of .33 and .98, respectively; the correlation with the other criteria was .30.

It is surprising that Kalus and colleagues recommended keeping the criteria pertaining to emotions and indifference, in view of their poor discriminatory power. The modifications included in DSM-IV have not improved their performance. The consequence is that the current DSM-IV concept of schizoid personality disorder really consists of two disorders, one introverted and the other affect-constricted. This creates an overlap with schizotypal personality disorder — a problem to which I return later.

## SCHIZOTYPAL PERSONALITY DISORDER

### Validity

Schizotypal personality disorder has a long history in European psychiatry. Kraepelin, E. Bleuler, and Kretschmer described relatives of schizophrenics who were not overtly schizophrenic, although they were unsocial and displayed a strange mixture of hypersensitivity and indifference. Even though Rado, Meehl, and others used the term, it did not appear in any classification prior to the Spitzer, Endicott, and Gibbon (1979) study, which lead to its inclusion in DSM-III.

The results of family studies (Baron, Gruen, Asnis, & Lord, 1985; Dahl, 1987; Siever et al., 1990, Battaglia et al., 1992) are equivocal regarding the familial transmission of schizotypal personality disorder. A study of 59 pairs of schizotypal twins suggested a genetic transmission of the disorder (Torgersen, 1984). A recent twin study of a nonpatient population also showed some hereditary influence on most schizotypal scales (Kendler & Hewitt, 1992). However, as is the case with most genetic studies (Torgersen, 1985), the genetic influences is greater for the "negative" features than for the "positive," perceptual/cognitive features of the disorder. Twin and family studies suggest that schizotypal personality disorder has some construct validity, especially the negative, affect-constricted component of the disorder. As Siever, Bernstein, and Silverman point out in Chapter 5, studies of biological correlates and treatment responses reach the same conclusion: There is evidence of validity, although the disorder appears to be heterogeneous.

## Axis I

In Chapter 5, Siever and colleagues provide a detailed discussion of family, adoption, and twin studies that point to a relationship between schizotypal personality disorder and schizophrenia. We (Torgersen, Onstad, et al., 1993) have also shown that schizotypal personality disorder is the only personality disorder that is more frequent among the co-twins and relatives of schizophrenics than among the cotwins and relatives of major depressives. Furthermore, only the eccentric, affect-constricted criteria of schizotypal personality disorder — odd behavior, odd speech, inappropriate affect, and excessive social anxiety — are more frequent among the cotwins and relatives of schizophrenics. Other schizotypal features appear to fall outside the schizophrenic spectrum. This raises the question of whether the eccentric, affect-constricted component of schizotypal personality disorder should be classified as part of schizophrenia on Axis I, as in ICD-10, and the other component should be classified as a personality disorder on Axis II. This is a possibility that I discuss in more detail later.

## Criteria Changes

The studies of the sensitivity and specificity of schizotypal personality disorder criteria cited by Siever et al. in Chapter 5 show inconsistent results. Our own data on the criteria are more in accordance with the genetic and biological studies (Torgersen, Skre, et al., 1993): DSM-III-R criterion 8 ("inappropriate or constricted affect ... "), criterion 5 ("odd or eccentric behavior ... "), and criterion 4 ("odd speech ... ") constitute the core of schizotypal personality disorder. These criteria also correlate strongly with the affect-constricted criteria of schizoid personality disorder. The remaining DSM-III-R schizotypal criteria are closer to other personality disorders than to the core of schizotypal personality disorder. Criteria 1 ("ideas of reference ... "), 3 ("odd beliefs or magical thinking ... "), and 4 ("unusual perceptual experiences ... ") are associated with the criteria for borderline personality disorder. Criterion 9 ("suspiciousness or paranoid ideation") is, of course, closer to paranoid personality disorder, and criterion 6 ("no close friends ... ") is closer to the seclusive part of schizoid personality disorder. And finally, criterion 2 ("excessive social anxiety ... ") is closer to avoidant personality disorder.

This overwhelming multidimensionality of the schizotypal criteria set might explain the conflicting results of different studies. It also means that a study of the sensitivity and specificity of the various criteria is of questionable value. Nevertheless, we analyzed our data on the DSM-IV criteria set and found that the internal consistency assessed with Chronbach's alpha was only .62 — a result that is not surprising, given the heterogeneity of the criteria set (Tornersen & Alnaes, 1995). Most criteria differentiated poorly between diagnoses, with criterion 8 (constricted affect) being the best-discriminating criterion.

I think that a more fundamental revision of the criteria for schizotypal personality disorder would have been preferable to that adopted for DSM-IV. The odd, eccentric, affect-constricted part of the disorder should have been the point of departure for extensive changes. Adding the affect-constricted criteria of schizoid personality disorder would delineate a disorder related to schizophrenia. Whether this disorder should be located on Axis I or Axis II is a minor question. When a disorder develops relatively early in life and encompasses thoughts, feelings, motivational aspects, and behavior, it is usually described in terms of personality features. When the disorder is ego-syntonic rather than ego-dystonic, there is reason to locate it on Axis II even if it is etiologically related to an Axis I disorder. A prerequisite would be that the personality disorder develops before the related symptom disorder. In addition, it is of significance that it does not always develop into a symptom disorder, but may remain a personality disorder throughout life. Even with these rules, the conceptual delineation between the prodromal symptoms of schizophrenia and schizotypal personality disorder is not easy. For the time being, however, we have to contend with this ambiguity.

## CONCLUSION

What is to be done with the Cluster A disorders? An easy solution would have been to make minimal changes to DSM-III-R, and this was the course of action adopted for DSM-IV. But what would constitute the ideal revision?

First, paranoid personality disorder could be left as it is, with the exclusion of the criterion pertaining to suspicions of infidelity. Second, a seclusive disorder could be created, consisting of the seclusive criteria for schizoid personality disorder and the "lack of close friends" criterion for schizotypal personality disorder. Third, an eccentric, affect-constricted disorder might be constructed from the affect-constricted criteria for DSM-III-R schizoid and schizotypal personality. Most of the other schizotypal personality disorder criteria could be included in borderline personality disorder, along with the criterion "transient, stress-related paranoid ideation or severe dissociative symptoms." I see little reason for including a criterion for suspiciousness in schizotypal personality disorder, because it only creates overlap with paranoid personality disorder.

As currently conceptualized, schizoid personality disorder really consists of two disorders—an affect-constricted disorder that is similar to schizotypal personality disorder, and a seclusive disorder that is similar to avoidant personality disorder. It is not surprising, therefore, that schizotypal and avoidant personality disorders overlap most often with schizoid personality disorder, as Kalus and colleagues show in Chapter 4. The proposed changes would solve this comorbidity problem.

Freeing schizotypal personality disorder from the pseudopsychotic criteria would also reduce the comorbidity with borderline personality disorder. As Siever and colleagues point out in Chapter 5, borderline is the most frequently co-occurring personality disorder among individuals with schizotypal personality disorder.

Earlier in this commentary, I have mentioned three important dilemmas for consideration in the development of a diagnostic system for personality disorders: (1) identifying diagnostic criteria to describe the disordered features of personality; (2) establishing adequate delineation of the various disorders, using factor-analytic or cluster-analytic methods; and (3) deciding upon the level of inference required to assess criteria. The first issue confronts us with the continuing quest to find criteria that really define the disordered features of personality. This is an important issue for future research. As indicated earlier, I currently support a factor-analytic approach to the resolution of the second issue, although this may change as we learn more about the origins and nature of personality disorders. In the case of the third issue, Siever and colleagues have argued in Chapter 5 for the introduction of criteria that require greater inferential judgment. They note that the criterion originally proposed (though not finally adopted) for social isolation in DSM-IV schizotypal personality disorder was as follows: "no close friends or confidants (or only one) other than first-degree relatives *due primarily to lack of desire, pervasive discomfort with others, or eccentricities*" (emphasis added). Furthermore, they note that the following criterion was proposed for social anxiety (a version of this *was* adopted in DSM-IV): "excessive social anxiety, e.g. extreme discomfort in social situations involving unfamiliar people that does not diminish with familiarity *and tends to be associated with paranoid fears rather than fears of negative judgment about self*" (emphasis added). It remains to be seen what will happen to diagnostic reliability when more inference is required. As for validity, this may increase. The first-cited criterion, however, does not differentiate among seclusive lack of desire, affect-constricted eccentricities, and avoidant discomfort; only borderline troubles are left out. The second criterion excludes avoidant fears, but admits paranoid fears. Thus, we see that when we start to elaborate criteria, problems arise. Even so, I think that Siever et al. have made an important start. In the future, we cannot avoid paying more attention to the conceptual content of the criteria. Currently, however, the overall structure of the realm of the odd, eccentric, Cluster A personality disorders is still unresolved.

## REFERENCES

Alnaes, R., & Torgersen, S. (1988a). The relationship between DSM-III symptom disorders (Axis I) and personality disorders (Axis II) in an outpatient population. *Acta Psychiatrica Scandinavica, 78,* 485–492.

Alnaes, R., & Torgersen, S. (1988b). DSM-III symptom disorders (Axis II) in an outpatient population. *Acta Psychiatrica Scandinavica, 78,* 348–355.

American Psychiatric Association. (1968). *Diagnostic and statistical manual of mental disorders* (2nd ed.). Washington, DC: Author.

American Psychiatric Association. (1080). *Diagnostic and statistical manual of mental disorders* (3rd ed.). Washington, DC: Author.

American Psychiatric Association. (1987). *Diagnostic and statistical manual of mental disorders* (3rd ed., rev.). Washington, DC: Author.

American Psychiatric Association. (1994). *Diagnostic and statistical manual of mental disorders* (4th ed.). Washington, DC: Author.

Baron, M., Gruen, R., Asnis, L., & Lord, S. (1985). Familial transmission of schizotypal and borderline personality disorders. *American Journal of Psychiatry, 142,* 927–934.

Battaglia, M., Gasperini, M., Sciuto, G., Scherillo, P., Diaferia, G., & Bellodi, L. (1991). Psychiatric disorders in the families of schizotypal subjects. *Schizophrenia Bulletin, 17,* 659–668.

Costa, P.T. Jr., & McCrae, R.R. (1992). The five-factor model of personality and its relevance to personality disorders. *Journal of Personality Disorders, 6,* 343–359.

Dahl, A. A. (1987). *Borderline disorders: A comparative study of hospitalized patients.* Oslo: University of Oslo Faculty of Medicine.

Farmer, A. E., McGuffin, P., & Gottesman, I. I. (1987). Twin concordance for DSM-III schizophrenia: Scrutinizing the validity of the definition. *Archives of General Psychiatry, 44,* 634–641.

Joffe, R. T., & Regan, J. J. (1989). Personality and response to tricyclic antidepressants in depressed patients. *Journal of Nervous and Mental Disease, 177,* 745–749.

Kendler, K. S., & Gruenberg, A. M. (1984). An independent analysis of the Danish study of schizophrenia: VI. The relationship between psychiatric disorders as defined by DSM-III in the relatives and adoptees. *Archives of General Psychiatry, 41,* 555–564.

Kendler, K. S., Heath, A., & Martin, N.G. (1987). A genetic epidemiologic study of self-report suspiciousness. *Comprehensive Psychiatry, 28, 187*–196.

Kendler, K. S., & Hewitt, J. (1992). The structure of self-report schizotypy in twins. *Journal of Personality Disorders, 6,* 1–17.

Livesley, W. J., Jackson, D. N., & Schroeder, M. L. (1989). A study of the factorial structure of personality pathology. *Journal of Personality Disorders, 3,* 292–306.

Lowen, A. (1967). *The betrayal of the body.* London: Collier Macmillan.

Onstad, S., Skre, I., Torgersen, S., & Kringlen, E. (1991). Twin concordance for DSM III-R schizophrenia. *Acta Psychiatrica Scandinavica, 83,* 395–401.

Pfohl, B., Stangl, D., & Zimmerman, M. (1984). The implications of DSM-III personality disorders for patients with major depression. *Journal of Affective Disorders, 7,* 309–318.

Pilkonis, P. A., & Frank, E. (1988). Personality pathology in recurrent depression: Nature, prevalence, and relationship to treatment response. *American Journal of Psychiatry, 145,* 435–441.

Schneider, K. (1923). *Psychopathic personalities.* London: Cassell, 1958.

Siever, L. J., Silverman, J. M., Horvath, T., Klar, H., Coccaro, E., Keefe, R. S. E., Pinkham, L., Rinaldi, P., Mohs, R. C., & Davis, K. L. (1990). Increased morbid risk for schizophrenia related disorders in relatives of schizotypal personality disorder patients. *Archives of General Psychiatry, 47,* 634–640.

Spitzer, R. L., Endicott, J., & Gibbon, M. (1979). Crossing the border into borderline personality and borderline schizophrenia: The development of criteria. *Archives of General Psychiatry, 36,* 17–24.

Torgersen, S. (1984). Genetic and nosological status of schizotypal and borderline personality disorders: A twin study. *Archives of General Psychiatry, 41,* 546–554.

Torgersen, S. (1985). Relationship of schizotypal personality disorder to schizophrenia: Genetics. *Schizophrenia Bulletin, 11,* 554–563.

Torgersen, S., & Alnaes, R. (1989). Localizing DSM-III personality disorders in a three-dimensional structural space. *Journal of Personality Disorders, 3,* 274–281.

Torgersen, S. & Alnaes, R. (1995). *A psychometric investigation of the DSM-IV options/91 criteria for personality disorders.* Unpublished manuscript.

Torgersen, S., Onstad, S., Skre, I., Edvardsen, J., & Kringlen, E. (1993). "True" schizotypal personality disorder: A study of co-twins and relatives of schizophrenic probands. *American Journal of Psychiatry, 150,* 1662–1667.

Torgersen, S., Skre, I., Onstad, S., Edvardsen, J., & Kringlen, E. (1993). The psychometric genetic structure of DSM-III-R personality disorder criteria. *Journal of Personality Disorders, 7,* 196–213.

World Health Organization. (1974). *Glossary of mental health disorders and guide to their classification for use in conjunction with the International Classification of Diseases* (8th rev. ed.). Geneva: Author.

World Health Organization. (1978). *Mental health disorders: Glossary and guide to their classification in accordance with the ninth revision of the International Classification of Diseases.* Geneva: Author.

World Health Organization. (1992). *The ICD-10 classification of mental and behavioural disoders: Diagnostic criteria for research.* Geneva: Author.

CHAPTER 6

# Antisocial Personality Disorder

THOMAS A. WIDIGER
ELIZABETH M. CORBITT

Frances (1980), in his early and often-cited review of the DSM-III (American Psychiatric Association [APA], 1980) personality disorders, suggested that antisocial "was the most controversial of all the personality disorders" (p. 1053). Millon (1983) also suggested that "among the more controversial topics at task force meetings (which covered all of the mental disorder diagnoses) were discussions pertaining to the concept of an Antisocial Personality Disorder" (p. 812). Antisocial personality disorder may not, in fact, be the most controversial personality disorder diagnosis in DSM-III or DSM-III-R (American Psychiatric Association, 1987), but it has received substantial criticism (e.g., Frances, 1980; Gunderson, 1983; Hare, Hart, & Harpur, 1991; Kernberg, 1989; Millon, 1981, 1983; Perry, 1990; Reid, 1987; Rogers & Dion, 1991; Skodol, 1989; Vaillant, 1984; Wulach, 1983). Much of this criticism has suggested that there is an overemphasis on overt criminal acts and related behaviors, to the neglect of more general personality traits of psychopathy. It is felt that this has contributed to (1) a failure to represent traditional concepts of psychopathy adequately; (2) an overdiagnosis of antisocial personality disorder in criminal and forensic settings; (3) an underdiagnosis of antisocial personality disorder in various noncriminal settings; (4) difficulties in the differentiation of antisocial personality disorder from substance use disorders; and (5) an overly complex and cumbersome criteria set. Each of these issues is discussed here in turn.

An earlier version of this chapter was published in the *Journal of Personality Disorders*, 1993, 7, 63–77. Copyright 1993 by The Guilford Press. Reprinted by permission.

## REPRESENTATION OF CLINICAL TRADITION

Hare et al. (1991), Kernberg (1989), Millon (1981, 1983), and others have suggested that the DSM-III and DSM-III-R criteria for antisocial personality disorder are discrepant with historical and clinical tradition. "Despite the history of alternative models and theories available for consideration, the DSM-III Task Force voted to base its diagnostic guidelines in accord with [(Robins, 1966)a] single, albeit well-designed, follow-up study of delinquency cases referred to one child guidance clinic in a large midwestern city" (Millon, 1981, p. 197). The DSM-III criteria set was not based solely on Lee Robins's (1966) study, but the description of antisocial personality disorder presented in DSM-II was closer to the original formulations of psychopathy developed by Cleckley (1941), McCord and McCord (1964), and others than were the DSM-III diagnostic criteria. The DSM-III criteria were based primarily on the criteria sets developed by Feighner et al. (1972), L. Robins (1966), and Spitzer, Endicott, and E. Robins (1978). Table 6.1 presents a summary of the DSM-III-R antisocial personality disorder criteria.

There is some empirical support for the hypothesis that the DSM-III and DSM-III-R criteria for antisocial personality disorder fail to match closely clinicians' concepts of antisocial personality disorder/psychopathy (hereafter, "DSM-III(-R)" is used to refer to both DSM-III and DSM-III-R). DSM-III(-R) antisocial personality disorder has obtained at least adequate agreement of clinicians' diagnoses with semistructured and/or self-report inventory assessments (e.g., Hyler et al., 1989; Skodol, Oldham, Rosnick, Kellman, & Hyler, 1991), suggesting perhaps a congruency between the diagnoses of clinicians and the DSM-III(-R), but this agreement could simply reflect the clinicians' adherence to the official nomenclature rather than their preferred formulations. Blashfield and Breen (1989) suggested on the basis of their face validity study that clinicians do not believe such criteria as unemployment for 6 months, traveling from place to place without a prearranged job, and a child's illness resulting from minimal hygiene to reflect antisocial personality traits adequately. These behaviors and events may be diagnostic of antisocial personality disorder within particular clinical settings, but they may not adequately describe for clinicians the personality traits of someone with antisocial personality disorder (Widiger & Trull, 1987). Livesley, Reiffer, Sheldon, and West (1987) reported higher prototypicality ratings by the clinicians they surveyed for such traits as unstable interpersonal relationships, failure to learn from experience, disregard for consequences, egocentricity, manipulativeness, and disregard for the feelings of others than for many of the DSM-III antisocial personality disorder criteria. Tennent, Tennent, Prins, and Bedford (1990) obtained ratings from British psychiatrists, psychologists, and probation officers. The items that were consistently rated as the most important and/or essential were an onset no later than the early 20s, impulsivity, pathological egocentricity, little response to special consideration or kindness, callous unconcern for others, behavior unaffected by

TABLE 6.1. DSM-III-R Diagnostic Criteria for Antisocial Personality Disorder

A. Current age at least 18.

B. Conduct disorder with onset before age 15 [12 subcriteria].

C. A pattern of irresponsible and antisocial behavior since the age of 15, as indicated by at least *four* of the following:

  (1) is unable to sustain consistent work behavior, as indicated by any of the following (including similar behavior in academic settings if the person is a student):
    (a) significant unemployment for six months or more within five years when expected to work and work was available
    (b) repeated absences from work unexplained by illness in self or family
    (c) abandonment of several jobs without realistic plans for others
  (2) fails to conform to social norms with respect to lawful behavior, as indicated by repeatedly performing antisocial acts that are grounds for arrest (whether arrested or not), e.g., destroying property, harassing others, stealing, pursuing an illegal occupation
  (3) is irritable and aggressive, as indicated by repeated physical fights or assaults (not required by one's job or to defend someone or oneself), including spouse- or child-beating
  (4) repeatedly fails to honor financial obligations, as indicated by defaulting on debts or failing to provide child support or support for other dependents on a regular basis
  (5) fails to plan ahead, or is impulsive, as indicated by one or both of the following:
    (a) traveling from place to place without a prearranged job or clear goal or clear idea about when the travel will terminate
    (b) lack of a fixed address for a month or more
  (6) has no regard for the truth, as indicated by repeated lying, use of aliases, or conning others for personal profit or pleasure
  (7) is reckless regarding own or others' personal safety, as indicated by driving while intoxicated, or recurrent speeding
  (8) if a parent or guardian, lacks ability to function as a responsible parent, as indicated by one or more of the following:
    (a) malnutrition of child
    (b) child's illness resulting from lack of minimal hygiene
    (c) failure to obtain medical care for a seriously ill child
    (d) child's dependence on neighbors or nonresident relatives for food or shelter
    (e) failure to arrange for a caretaker for young child when parent is away from home
    (f) repeated squandering, on personal items, of money required for household necessities
  (9) has never sustained a totally monogamous relationship for more than one year
  (10) lacks remorse (feels justified in having hurt, mistreated, or stolen from another)

D. Occurrence of antisocial behavior not exclusively during the course of Schizophrenia or Manic Episodes.

punishment, lack of a sense of responsibility, being chronically or currently antisocial, inability to experience guilt, and inability to form meaningful relationships.

## OVERDIAGNOSIS WITHIN PRISON AND FORENSIC SETTINGS

Many critiques of DSM-III(-R) antisocial personality disorder have suggested that the criteria set results in an overdiagnosis of antisocial personality disorder within criminal and forensic settings. Frances (1980) and Wulach (1983) cited Guze, Goodwin, and Crane (1969) as indicating that 80% of criminals would be diagnosed with antisocial personality disorder. Guze et al. followed 223 convicted male felons from 1959 through 1968. Seventy-nine percent met their research criteria for "sociopathy" at intake (although on follow-up only 52% of the remaining 176 subjects continued to meet these same criteria). Generalizing from the Guze et al. study to DSM-III(-R), however, may not be appropriate: The criteria for sociopathy used by Guze et al. do have a historical relationship to DSM-III(-R) antisocial personality disorder, but they appear to be more inclusive. The Guze et al. criteria consisted of a history of police trouble (other than traffic arrests), plus any two of five items (history of excessive fighting, school delinquency, poor job record, period of wanderlust, or running away from home; prostitution could substitute for any of these five for female subjects).

Hare (1980) reported that 76% of 146 prison inmates satisfied (initial draft) DSM-III criteria for antisocial personality disorder, compared to only 33% who met research criteria for psychopathy. Hare (1983) subsequently compared the DSM-III antisocial personality disorder criteria to an early version of the Psychopathy Checklist (PCL) in 159 federal inmates. Half of the inmates received a DSM-III antisocial personality disorder diagnosis from at least one of two clinicians, whereas only 35% received a diagnosis of psychopathy by the PCL when the recommended cutoff score of 33 was used (total score = 44). The kappa coefficient for agreement between the DSM-III antisocial personality disorder and PCL diagnoses was .51. In a further study, Hare (1985) found that 49% of 274 inmates received a DSM-III diagnosis of antisocial personality disorder by at least one of two raters, in comparison to only 33% who received a score of 34 on the PCL. Hart and Hare (1989) reported that 50% of 80 men remanded by the courts to a forensic unit met the DSM-III criteria for antisocial personality disorder, whereas only 12.5% were given a diagnosis of psychopathy by an initial version of the revision of the PCL.

Hare (1991) summarized the association of the PCL and the PCL—Revised (PCL-R) with the DSM-III and DSM-III-R across 10 data sets (all prison or forensic settings). The point-biserial correlation of the antisocial personality disorder diagnoses with total PCL(-R) scores varied between .54 and .63 for seven of the data sets. The two lowest findings were point-biserial correlations of only .13 and .08, and in both cases the base rate for antisocial personality disorder was about 80%. Cote and Hodgins (1990) administered the National Institute of Mental Health (NIMH) Diagnostic Interview Schedule (DIS; Robins, Helzer, Croughan, & Ratcliff, 1981) to a random sample of 495 male inmates of Quebec penitentiaries. Antisocial personality disorder was diagnosed in 61.5% of these subjects. Similar findings were reported by Bland, Newman, Dyck, and Orn (1990).

Robins, Tipp, and Przybeck (1991), however, have argued that if the criticism were warranted that antisocial personality disorder "medicalizes" criminality, then most persons with an antisocial personality disorder diagnosis would have a criminal history. On the basis of the NIMH Epidemiologic Catchment Area (ECA) data, they reported that only 47% of those who met the DSM-III antisocial personality disorder criteria had a significant arrest record (total $n$ = 628). "Rather than criminality, the adult symptoms that typify the antisocial personality are job troubles (found in 94%), violence (found in 85%), multiple moving traffic offenses (found in 72%), and severe marital difficulties (desertion, multiple separations or divorces, multiple infidelities, found in 67%)" (Robins et al. 1991, p. 260). In addition, the occurrence of a significant arrest record was not predictive of an antisocial personality disorder diagnosis. Only 37% of those with multiple nontraffic arrests (40% for males) met the DSM-III antisocial personality disorder criteria. The ECA sample also included prisoners, and on the basis of these data, Robins et al. (1991) suggested that "only about half of all prison residents meet criteria for the disorder" (p. 289). This prevalence is comparable to the results reported by Hare (1983, 1985), but Robins et al. (1991) suggest that a 50% base rate for antisocial personality disorder within a prison is within theoretical and clinical expectations.

## UNDERDIAGNOSIS WITHIN OTHER NONCLINICAL SETTINGS

Critical reviews of the DSM-III(-R) antisocial personality disorder criteria have also suggested that the behaviorally specific criteria may contribute to an underdiagnosis of antisocial personality disorder/psychopathy within nonclinical settings other than prison and forensic institutions. To the extent that the DSM-III(-R) criteria emphasize criminal and delinquent activity, psychopathic persons who operate within the letter of the law would not be diagnosed as having antisocial personality disorder. However, there are few empirical data that pertain directly to this concern. Loranger (1988) compared the prevalence of personality disorders diagnosed by DSM-II and DSM-III within the same psychiatric hospital. Antisocial personality disorder was diagnosed in 9.3% of the cases with DSM-II, and in only 4.6% using DSM-III (p < .001), despite the fact that there was a twofold increase in the overall rate of personality disorder diagnoses (from 19% to 49%). Loranger (1988) suggested that "the focus on criminal behavior in the DSM-III antisocial criteria may have excluded some cases identified in DSM-II by clinicians using the more traditional Cleckley concept" (p. 674).

Robins et al. (1984) reported antisocial personality disorder lifetime prevalences of 2.1%, 2.6%, and 3.3% in three of the NIMH ECA sites (New Haven, Connecticut; Baltimore, Maryland; and St. Louis, Missouri, respectively). Bland, Orn, and Newman (1988) reported a lifetime rate of 3.7%, based on a sample of 3,258 Edmonton, Alberta urban community residents. Regier et al. (1988) reported 1-month prevalence rates from five NIMH ECA sites of 0.3% (New Haven, Connecticut), 0.5% (Baltimore, Maryland), 0.8% (St. Louis, Missouri), 0.4% (Durham, North Carolina), and 0.4% (Los Angeles, California). Zimmerman and Coryell (1989) reported that 3.3% of 797 relatives of patients and normals met the DSM-III criteria for antisocial personality disorder, the highest rate for any personality disorder. Interpretation of these findings, however, is somewhat complicated by the absence of any theoretical or clinical consensus for what the rate of psychopathy/antisocial personality disorder should be within a community, and none of these studies have focused on populations or professions in which "successful" or "adaptive" psychopaths would most likely be found (e.g., law, politics, or business).

Widom (1977) lamented some time ago that "we have no knowledge of the extent to which psychopathy remains undetected in the general population or even whether the concept is a meaningful one outside the prison or psychiatric hospital" (p. 675). She therefore placed advertisements in a Boston counterculture newspaper seeking (for example) "adventurous carefree people who've led exciting impulsive lives" (p. 675). Seventy-three persons responded, and 28–30 subjects participated in a series of tests and interviews. The psychopaths she identified, however, were not appreciably different from those who would be sampled from a clinical setting. Sixty-one percent reported some form of psychiatric experience, 46% had been in outpatient treatment, 21% had been inpatients, and 29% had a history of suicide attempts. They were somewhat distinct from a prison/forensic sample. Seventy-four percent had been arrested, but only 18% of those arrested had ever been convicted (50% had been incarcerated, but only 25% for longer than 2 weeks). In any case, 79% met Robins's (1966) criteria for the diagnosis of sociopathy (e.g., 79% had a poor work history, 68% used excessive drugs, and 43% had school problems or truancy). Similar results were provided in a subsequent report by Widom and Newman (1985).

Sutker and Allain (1983) used the Minnesota Multiphasic Personality Inventory (MMPI) to identify "adaptive sociopaths" within a medical student population. Only 2.4% of the 450 students met the MMPI criteria for sociopathy; eight of the male sociopaths were studied in more detail. None met the DSM-III criteria for antisocial personality disorder, although five met the antisocial personality disorder conduct disorder criterion. Prior to the age of 15, 50% had had repeated sexual intercourse in casual relationships (vs. none of eight comparison males), 63% acknowledged vandalism (vs. 25%), 63% acknowledged chronic violations of rules at home and/or at school (vs. 13%), and 50% acknowledged the initiation of fights (vs. 0%). By adulthood, at least half admitted to difficulties in maintaining an enduring sexual relationship, honoring financial obligations, and refraining from recklessness, and 88% admitted to being arrested (vs. 25% of the comparison males), but none of the subjects met a sufficient number of criteria to receive a DSM-III antisocial personality disorder diagnosis. Sutker and Allain suggested that these were indeed psychopathic persons who exhibited (in laboratory testing) impulsive errors, disregard for details of instruction, and exaggerated needs for excitement seeking, but that "strong desires for the rewards often associated with respectable professional status motivated and sustained adaptiveness" (p. 77).

Additional research would be necessary to determine whether the DSM-III-R antisocial personality disorder criteria could or should identify the successful and/or adaptive psychopath. Widom (1977) suggested that her approach was useful in identifying "the more 'successful' psychopath who may be arrested frequently but convicted infrequently" (p. 682), but one might question whether these persons were really successful, given their history of inpatient and/or outpatient treatment, arrests, school difficulties, suicide attempts, and poor employment. A psychopathic lawyer, politician, or businessperson without a significant history of unemployment, arrests, marital instability, and defaults on debts would probably fail to meet the DSM-III-R antisocial personality disorder criteria, but it may then be questionable whether such persons should receive a mental disorder diagnosis. If these persons are indeed successful and/or adaptive, then they may not be displaying sufficient maladaptivity to warrant a mental disorder diagnosis, unless the threshold for a diagnosis is lowered to include more subtle indicators of impairment (e.g., marital difficulties, superficial relationships, and exploitation of others).

## DIFFERENTIATION OF ANTISOCIAL PERSONALITY DISORDER FROM SUBSTANCE USE DISORDERS

Various studies have indicated a substantial association of antisocial personality disorder with various substance use disorders (Grande, Wolf, Schubert, Patterson, & Brocco, 1984). Interpretation of this research, however, has been complicated by the questionable independence of the diagnoses (Gerstley, Alterman, Woody, & McLellan, 1990; Sutker, Bugg, & West, 1993; Widiger, Corbitt, & Millon, 1992). For example, the DSM-III-R antisocial personality disorder diagnosis includes an inability to sustain consistent work behavior, failure to conform to social norms with respect to lawful behavior, failure to honor financial obligations, failure to plan ahead, recklessness in regard to safety, and inability to function as a responsible parent (American Psychiatric Association, 1987, pp. 345–346). The diagnosis of substance dependence includes hazardous behavior, theft, and difficulties in fulfilling major role obligations at home, school, or work (American Psychiatric Association, 1987, p. 168). It is apparent that some of the diagnostic criteria are almost equivalent. It is then difficult to determine which (if any) direction of causality has occurred when one assesses the covariation of the presence of at least 4 of any of the 10 adult antisocial criteria (the threshold for an antisocial personality disorder diagnosis) with at least three of any of the nine substance dependence criteria (the threshold for the substance dependence diagnosis), even with the requirement of the childhood antisocial criterion (Gerstley et al., 1990).

The Research Diagnostic Criteria (RDC) for antisocial personality disorder (Spitzer et al., 1978) emphasize that antisocial behaviors can result from or be exacerbated by a substance use disorder. RDC raters count only those manifestations of antisocial personality disorder that cannot clearly be attributed to a drug use disorder. In DSM-III, on the other hand, it was stated that the antisocial personality disorder criteria would count "regardless of the extent to which some of the antisocial behavior may be a consequence of the Substance Use Disorder, e.g., illegal selling of drugs, or the assaultive behavior associated with Alcohol Intoxication" (American Psychiatric Association, 1980, p. 319) (no revision to this statement was made in DSM-III-R; American Psychiatric Association, 1987). Williams and Spitzer (1982) suggested that the RDC and DSM-III antisocial personality disorder criteria sets would identify virtually the same group of persons. Hesselbrock, Stabenau, Hesselbrock, Mirkin, and Meyer (1982) did report a kappa of .79 for the agreement between RDC and DSM-III (assessed by the DIS) in a sample of 42 alcoholic inpatients. Rounsaville, Eyre, Weissman, and Kleber (1983), however, reported that 54% of 533 opiate dependents met the DSM-III criteria for antisocial personality disorder, whereas only 27% did so with the RDC. Rounsaville et al. concluded "that the key difference in the two systems . . . is in the RDC requirement that antisocial activity be independent of the need to obtain drugs" (p. 38). Woody, McLellan, Luborsky, and O'Brien (1985) likewise reported that 45% of their 110 opiate-dependent subjects met the DSM-III criteria for antisocial personality disorder, but only 19% met RDC criteria. Hasin and Grant (1987) reported a kappa for the agreement between RDC and DSM-III antisocial personality disorder diagnoses of only .05 in a sample of 120 substance abuse patients.

Alterman and Cacciola (1991) and Gerstley et al. (1990) have suggested that the DSM-III(-R) antisocial personality disorder criteria overdiagnose antisocial personality disorder in substance use patients because of a "focus on behavioral patterns rather than underlying personality dynamics" (Gerstley et al., 1990, p. 173), as well as the absence of an exclusion criterion to rule out substance abuse. They recommended as an alternative the PCL, which places relatively more emphasis on psychopathic personality traits. Additional emphasis on more general traits (e.g., lack of remorse or guilt, superficial charm, and callous lack of empathy) would presumably be more successful in assessing antisocial/psychopathic personality traits independent of a substance use disorder than an emphasis on more specific behaviors (e.g., being reckless regarding safety as indicated by driving while intoxicated; American Psychiatric Association, 1987). On the other hand, it is also possible that in the assessment of such personality traits as manipulativeness, poor behavior controls, and proneness to boredom (Hare, 1991), one might still use specific acts and behaviors that are secondary to a substance use disorder (Widiger & Shea, 1991).

Cooney, Kadden, and Litt (1990) compared DSM-III antisocial personality disorder (assessed by the DIS) and PCL psychopathy assessments in a sample of 118 alcoholic inpatients. Correlation between total PCL and DIS scores was significant but low ($r = .34$, $p < .001$); point-biserial correlation with the DIS antisocial personality disorder diagnosis was insignificant ($r = .14$). However, these results may not have been attributable to an overdiagnosis of antisocial personality disorder by the DSM-III, as only 25% of the subjects met the DSM-III criteria. Cooney et al. acknowledged that the low correlation could have resulted in part from inadequate training with the PCL, but they concluded instead that it was attributable to differences in the content of the respective interviews. Their content analysis suggested that the DIS emphasized criminal and childhood conduct problems (50% of the interview), whereas the PCL placed relatively more emphasis on affective poverty (37% of the interview).

## COMPLEXITY OF THE CRITERIA SET

Hare et al. (1991), Rogers and Dion (1991), and Vaillant (1984) have suggested that the increased behavioral specificity of the DSM-III(-R) antisocial personality disorder criteria has been problematic to clinical utility. It is no coincidence that the personality disorder criteria set that is the most specific is also the longest and most complex. The DSM-III-R antisocial personality disorder criteria set consists of 10 adult items and 1 childhood item. Three of the 10 adult items include subitems (parental irresponsibility has 6 subitems), and the childhood conduct disorder item involves 12 subitems, resulting in a total of 30 items to assess (see Table 6.1 for a summary of the 10 adult items).

The DSM-III(-R) criteria for antisocial personality disorder may have been constructed primarily for the benefit and concerns of the researcher, rather than for those of the practicing clinician (Frances, Pincus, Widiger, Davis, & First, 1990). Researchers may have little difficulty with lengthy and complex criteria sets, but it is unlikely that clinicians adhere closely to the DSM-III-R antisocial personality disorder criteria during routine clinical practice. A systematic and comprehensive assessment of the personality disorders can require 2 hours of interviewing; as a result, clinicians may often fail to follow the criteria closely when making their diagnoses (Morey &

Ochoa, 1989). Ford and Widiger (1989) suggested that sex biases in the diagnosis of antisocial personality disorder might be attributable in part to a
failure of clinicians to adhere closely to the diagnostic criteria.

The length of the DSM-III-R criteria set is a result of the effort to
minimize the occurrence of inferences and judgments in assessment. For
example, the clinician and researcher employing these criteria are not free
to use their own judgment in assessing whether a patient has been unable
to sustain consistent work behavior; they must, instead, assess whether there
has been significant unemployment for 6 months or more within 5 years
when the patient was expected to work and work was available, whether there
has been repeated absences from work that were unexplained by illness in
the patient or the patient's family, and whether there has been an abandonment of several jobs without a realistic plan for subsequent employment.
Likewise, the clinician and researcher do not assess whether a patient fails
to plan ahead or is impulsive; they assess, instead, whether the patient has
traveled from place to place without a prearranged job, clear goal, or clear
idea when the travel would terminate and whether the patient has lacked
a fixed address for at least 1 month. This specificity has resulted in tremendous improvements in the reliability of the diagnosis in clinical practice (a
reliability that is not evident in the clinical diagnoses for the other personality disorders; Mellsop, Varghese, Joshua, & Hicks, 1982), but it is also cumbersome and constraining. To a large extent, the DSM-III-R antisocial
personality disorder criteria attempt to provide a comprehensive or at least
sufficient list of the ways in which each of the antisocial traits are expressed,
thereby indicating explicitly how each must be assessed. However, this may
not be particularly realistic (Widiger & Trull, 1987). It is evident that impulsivity (or a failure to plan ahead) can be expressed by behaviors other than
traveling from place to place without a clear goal or the absence of a fixed
address for a month or more. Even the list of the six specific ways in which
one can be an irresponsible parent is incomplete. The specificity is, then,
very helpful in obtaining reliable diagnoses; however, it may not be realistic
to attempt to specify all of the ways in which one can fail to sustain consistent work behavior, fail to plan ahead, or fail to be a responsible parent,
as well as all of the qualifications to each of the acts that are listed (e.g., to
rule out illness in self and family and absence of available jobs when assessing periods of unemployment).

It might be possible to simplify the antisocial personality disorder criteria
by deleting or collapsing items to construct a more practical and user-friendly
set that would not result in any change in who is diagnosed. For example,
in studies of the DSM-III-R antisocial personality disorder criteria by Freiman and Widiger (1989), Millon and Tringone (1989), Morey and Heumann
(1988), and Pfohl and Blum (1990), solicited by the DSM-IV Personality Disorders Work Group, the item with the lowest correlation with the diagnosis
of antisocial personality disorder was typically irresponsibility as a parent
(phi coefficients = .03, −.03, .22, and −.02, respectively), in large part be-

because of its rarity (e.g., it cannot be scored if the person is not a parent, and it is difficult to document as present when the person is a parent). The next worst-performing item was usually failure to sustain a monogamous relationship (phi coefficients = .04, .13, .25, and −.03, respectively). The worst performing item in a study by Zanarini (1989) using DSM-III criteria was also irresponsibility as a parent (phi coefficient = .27). It is conceivable that the parental irresponsibility and monogamous relationship items (and others) could be deleted without significantly affecting who receives the diagnosis.

Simplification without any effect on diagnosis would appear to be an unassailable proposal. On the other hand, if specific criteria do provide an overly narrow representation of the construct (Hare et al., 1991), resulting in the need to include a substantial number of items to represent the construct fully, it may not be possible to reduce the number of items without affecting the diagnosis (Widiger & Trull, 1987). A brief list of very specific items would provide an even more narrow representation of psychopathy than is provided by the 30 DSM-III-R items.

Empirical support for the perception that the DSM-III(-R) criteria set is cumbersome and unwieldy may also be somewhat limited. The finding that antisocial personality disorder is the only personality disorder diagnosis that consistently demonstrates adequate to good levels of interrater reliability in routine clinical practice (Mellsop et al., 1982), and adequate to good convergent validity with semistructured interview and self-report assessments (Hyler et al., 1989; Skodol et al., 1991), suggests that practicing clinicians may be able to use the criteria set in a consistent and valid manner.

Perry, Lavori, Cooper, Hoke, and O'Connell (1987) have suggested that DSM-III-R antisocial personality disorder may provide an overdiagnosis as a result of the "constriction of clinical judgment" (p. 130). Whenever a subject reported a behavioral symptom of antisocial personality disorder, it was scored as positive on the DIS in their study of 70 clinical, criminal, and community subjects, whereas during a clinical interview administered by an experienced clinician, further inquiry was provided to assess whether the reported behaviors were clinically meaningful. Kappa for the agreement between the clinical and DIS diagnoses was equal to only .54, with the DIS diagnosing antisocial personality disorder in 49% of the 70 cases and the clinical interview diagnosing 29%. Robins et al. (1981) and Robins, Helzer, Ratcliff, and Seyfried (1982), however, reported somewhat better results in their original validation studies of the DIS. For example, lay interviewers' antisocial personality disorder diagnoses agreed with psychiatrists' diagnoses in a sample of 216 patients, with kappa equaling .63 (Robins et al., 1981). Robins et al. (1982) concluded that the DIS, administered by lay interviewers, "agrees well with results when the same interview is given blindly by a psychiatrist instructed to use his clinical experience in scoring and pursuing answers" (p. 869). Robins et al. (1981) did not find the psychiatrists to be particularly constrained or dissatisfied with the specific and explicit criteria (in only 7% of 204 cases did they indicate that they had doubts about their diagnoses). Helzer et al. (1985) reported similar results in a subsequent study (kappa was only .52, but Yule's Y was .71), and Helzer, Spitznagel, and McEvoy (1987) reported that DIS diagnoses of antisocial personality disorder had somewhat better predictive validity than the psychiatrists' DSM-III assessments.

Morey and Ochoa (1989) reported that clinicians' diagnoses were often in disagreement with the diagnoses that would be given if the diagnoses had been based on the clinicians' assessments of each of the DSM-III personality disorder criteria. In other words, the diagnoses provided by the clinicians were often inconsistent with their own assessments of the individual criteria. This disagreement was lowest for the borderline and antisocial personality disorder diagnoses (the clinicians diagnosed 6.8% of 291 cases with antisocial personality disorder, whereas 5.8% would have been diagnosed with antisocial personality disorder based on their ratings of the antisocial personality disorder criteria; kappa = .53, $p$ < .001). However, Morey and Ochoa (1989) did conclude that "a history of criminal acts may lead a diagnostician to assign the antisocial diagnosis even though other criteria are not met" (p. 190). In other words, clinicians may not find the criteria set to be particularly cumbersome because they focus on only a subset of the criteria (i.e., overt criminal acts), resulting in high reliability, consistent usage, and convergent validity with other measures that have a similar emphasis.

## ALTERNATIVES TO DSM-III-R
## ANTISOCIAL PERSONALITY DISORDER

Two viable alternatives to DSM-III-R antisocial personality disorder are provided by the PCL-R (Hare, 1991) and by the research criteria for dyssocial personality disorder from the 10th revision of the *International Classification of Diseases* (IDC-10; World Health Organization, 1990). Both of these alternatives place more emphasis on such personality traits as lack of remorse or guilt, callous lack of empathy, and failure to accept responsibility for one's actions.

Compatibility with the forthcoming ICD-10 is both desirable and perhaps to some extent necessary (Frances et al., 1990). Deviations from the international nomenclature should at least be supported by empirical documentation. This concern is particularly important in the case of antisocial personality disorder, given the relatively greater emphasis that ICD-10 will place on personality traits of psychopathy. Table 6.2 presents the original draft of the ICD-10 research criteria for dyssocial personality disorder (the final version will not be equivalent). A major limitation of the ICD-10 alternative, however, is that no data concerning its reliability or validity have yet been published, nor is there any explanation of the source and rationale for the items.

The original PCL was developed by Hare (1980) to provide a systematic

TABLE 6.2. ICD-10 Research Criteria for Dyssocial Personality Disorder

1. Callous unconcern for the feelings of others and lack of the capacity for empathy
2. Gross and persistent attitude of irresponsibility and disregard for social norms, rules, and obligations
3. Incapacity to maintain enduring relationships
4. Very low tolerance to frustration and a low threshold for discharge of aggression, including violence
5. Incapacity to experience guilt and to profit from experience, particularly punishment
6. Marked proneness to blame others, or to offer plausible rationalizations for the behavior bringing the subject into conflict with society
7. Persistent irritability

*Note.* From World Health Organization (1990, pp. 103–104). Copyright 1990 by the World Health Organization. Reprinted by permission. (A revised version of these research criteria was published in 1993 by the World Health Organization.)

means by which to assess psychopathy as described originally by Cleckley (1941). The PCL-R is a revision of the PCL based on the substantial amount of research conducted with the original instrument (Hare, 1991). For example, drug and alcohol abuse that was not a direct cause of antisocial behavior was deleted, because it was considered to be too difficult to score (a deletion that is somewhat ironic in the context of the suggestions of Gerstley et al., 1990, with respect to the differentiation of antisocial personality disorder from substance use disorders). The PCL item concerning irresponsible behavior as a parent was found to be too specific and was broadened to irresponsibility in general.

Hare and his colleagues have consistently obtained good to excellent reliability in the assessment of the personality traits of psychopathy (Hare, 1991; Hare et al., 1991), a finding replicated by independent researchers (e.g., Raine, 1985; Smith & Newman, 1990). There is also substantial empirical support for the PCL(-R) formulation of psychopathy (Hare, 1991; Hart, Hare, & Harpur, in press). For example, Hart, Kropp, and Hare (1988) reported that the PCL was more predictive of recidivism subsequent to prison release than was the DSM-III antisocial personality disorder diagnosis. The PCL predicted postrelease behavior in their sample of 231 federal offenders even when prior criminal history, previous conditional-release violations, and demographic variables were controlled. Similar findings have been reported by Serin, Peters, and Barbaree (1990). Laboratory tests of hypothesized correlates of psychopathy, including abnormal processing of the affective components of language, selective attention, disinhibition, and passive-avoidance learning, have also consistently supported the construct validity of the PCL(-R) (Hart et al., in press).

However, the research reviewed above concerning the overdiagnosis, underdiagnosis, and differential diagnosis of DSM-III(-R) antisocial personality disorder has not been consistently negative. In addition, DSM-III(-R) antisocial personality disorder has substantial empirical support, including epidemiological, psychophysiological, longitudinal, childhood antecedent, family history, and treatment studies (Robins et al., 1991; Sutker et al., 1993). Research cited in support of the DSM-III(-R) diagnosis has at times concerned studies that used earlier or alternative diagnostic criteria, but the empirical support includes many studies that used the DSM-III, DSM-III-R, or sufficiently comparable criteria (e.g., Cadoret, O'Gorman, Troughton, & Heywood, 1985; Grove et al., 1990; Lewis, Rice, Andreasen, Clayton, & Endicott, 1985; Regier et al., 1988; Robins et al., 1984). Finally, DSM-III(-R) antisocial personality disorder is the only personality disorder diagnosis to demonstrate adequate to good levels of interrater reliability consistently in clinical practice (Mellsop et al., 1982). Any revision of the antisocial personality disorder criteria set that required more subjective judgment and inferences could undermine the only clinically reliable personality disorder diagnosis (Skodol et al., 1991).

## THE DSM-IV ANTISOCIAL PERSONALITY DISORDER FIELD TRIAL

Proposals to simplify the criteria set and to place greater emphasis on personality traits of psychopathy were reasonable options to consider for DSM-IV. These proposals reflected criticisms of DSM-III(-R) antisocial personality disorder, as well as the empirical literature. However, the threshold for revisions to the nomenclature was necessarily higher for DSM-IV than was the case for DSM-III or DSM-III-R (Frances et al., 1990). The DSM-III-R criteria set for antisocial personality disorder is lengthy and complex, and fails to provide substantial representation of the personality traits of psychopathy included within the ICD-10 and the PCL-R; however, it has performed well in clinical practice, it is supported by empirical data, and any revision would probably be disruptive to both research and clinical practice. It was therefore important to field-test any proposed revisions, to document that the proposed revisions would in fact represent an improvement (Widiger, Frances, Pincus, Davis, & First, 1991).

The field trial conducted for DSM-IV compared three criteria sets: (1) the DSM-III-R antisocial personality disorder criteria (American Psychiatric Association, 1987); (2) the seven-item research criteria set that was at the time proposed for ICD-10 dyssocial personality disorder (World Health Organization, 1990); and (3) a 10-item criteria set developed through data reanalyses of the PCL-R by Hare (presented in Table 6.3, and hereafter referred to as the PCL-R-derived criteria set). Data were collected from five populations: (1) male prisoners in Vancouver, Canada (Hare); (2) psychiatric inpatients in Belmont, Massachusetts (Zanarini); (3) substance use disorder patients in Philadelphia, Pennsylvania (Alterman); (4) adopted-away offspring in Iowa (Cadoret); and (5) a mixed sample from a public mental hospital, drug treatment program, and homeless shelter in St. Louis, Missouri (Robins). The three

TABLE 6.3.  Field Trial Criteria Set Derived from the Psychopathy Checklist—Revised (PCL-R)

1. *Early behavior problems* (enduring pattern of serious behavioral problems that starts prior to age 12, persists through age 17, and is evident in a variety of settings. Such problems are not limited to isolated incidents occurring as a result of physical, sexual, or emotional abuse, such as running away from home to escape an abusive parent).

2. *Adult antisocial behaviors* (a serious and persistent disregard for explicit social norms; has engaged in frequent or varied antisocial behaviors that are grounds for arrest, whether arrested or not).

3. *Impulsive* (individual does things on the spur of the moment, without adequately considering the consequences of his or her behavior; frequently changes employment, sexual partners, or residence; and frequently engages in risky and exciting activities).

4. *Poor behavioral controls* (easily angered or frustrated; frequently responds with verbal or physical aggression which may be sudden, unprovoked and short-lived; may be exacerbated by drug or alcohol use).

5. *Lacks remorse* (rationalizes, minimizes, or denies the negative effects of own behavior on others; any statements of remorse are made in an insincere manner or are inconsistent with the individual's behavior).

6. *Lacks empathy* (callous and cynical; contemptuous of or indifferent to the feelings, rights, and suffering of others).

7. *Deceitful and manipulative* (lies excessively, often for no apparent reason; deceives or manipulates in order to achieve personal gratification, such as money, sex, or power, without concern for others; a con or fraud artist).

8. *Irresponsible* (individual's tendency to enter into and then violate explicit or implicit social contracts and obligations to others; individual consistently fails to meet obligations and commitments to others or frequently causes others hardship or puts them at risk, in two or more areas: unreliable at work, drives while impaired, fails to provide financial support for dependents, fails to adequately care for children, fails to honor debts).

9. *Inflated and arrogant self-appraisal* (arrogant, opinionated, and has an inflated view of self and abilities; unrealistically conceited or acts unconcerned or indifferent about present problems or the future, such as not anticipating being adversely affected by current legal or clinical problems).

10. *Glib and superficial* (individual presents as a glib, voluble, verbally facile person who exudes an insincere and superficial charm; e.g., attempts to make a favorable impression on others by telling clever and entertaining stories that put self in good light, provides many convincing but unlikely excuses for past behavior, uses technical terms or jargon to impress interviewer with only superficial knowledge, and/or presents with pleasant charm or wit that appears to be inappropriate to the current problems or interview).

*Note.* From Hare (1991). Copyright 1991 by Multi-Health Systems. Adapted by permission.

criteria sets and their respective items were compared with respect to interrater reliability, descriptive validity, and correlations with a variety of external validators, including self-report measures of antisocial personality disorder and psychopathy; clinicians' and interviewers' subjective impressions of antisocial personality disorder/psychopathy; self-report measures of empathy, Machiavellianism, and trait anxiety; indicators of personality dysfunction (e.g., number of arrests and duration of longest job); and family history of drug abuse, alcohol abuse, and antisocial behaviors.

The report from this field trial is currently under editorial review (Widiger et al., 1993). It would be premature to present actual findings, but it may be safe to describe our impressions based on the initial findings. The results indicated that many of the PCL-R-derived and ICD-10 items could be assessed as reliably as the DSM-III-R items, although most of the sites did have difficulty with "lacks empathy" and "irresponsible" derived from the PCL-R. It should be noted, however, that perhaps any criteria set can be assessed reliably when it is supplemented by a semistructured interview that provides explicit and specific questions and scoring guidelines. All of the DSM-III-R personality disorders have been diagnosed reliably when the assessment was conducted by trained interviewers using a semistructured interview (Widiger & Frances, 1987). Only DSM-III-R antisocial personality disorder has consistently been assessed reliably in the absence of this support. It then remains questionable whether the PCL-R or ICD-10 items would be assessed reliably in general clinical practice unless they were supplemented by more specific guidelines.

There were few significant differences among the criteria sets with respect to their association with the external validators. One exception occurred with respect to clinicians' and interviewers' subjective impressions. The research interviewer and a clinician closely familiar with the interviewee were asked to rate the extent to which they believed the interviewee manifested or exemplified the characteristics of someone with an antisocial/psychopathic personality disorder. They were to use their own formulation or conceptualization, which might or might not be consistent with the DSM-III-R, PCL-R, or ICD-10. Across four of the five sites, there was a tendency for the greatest association to be with the PCL-R-derived criteria set. However, the PCL-R-derived items that obtained the highest correlations were those that overlapped in content with the DSM-III-R (i.e., "early behavior problems" and "adult antisocial behaviors"). The difference between these PCL-R-derived items and the respective items from the DSM-III-R is that the former assess the same content in a broader, more global manner. Items that are confined to more specific manifestations of a trait may not be providing an adequate representation of the trait; as a result, they may fail to correlate as highly with the construct than items that are more comprehensive in their description.

Items with content unique to the PCL-R (e.g., "lacks empathy," "inflated and arrogant self-appraisal," and "glib and superficial" ) correlated more highly with the interviewers' impressions of antisocial personality disorder/psychopathy in the Vancouver prison site. This may have been attributable in part to a bias of interviewers experienced with and trained with the PCL-R. However, the finding may also reflect the fact that the PCL-R-derived items are more useful indicators of antisocial personality disorder/psychopathy than DSM-III-R items within a prison setting. One of the more interesting findings was that the number of arrests and convictions correlated substantially with all of the criteria sets in all but the Vancouver prison site. Arrests and convictions correlated substantially with the PCL-R-derived criteria set in clinical settings, wherein arrests and convictions are fairly specific to psychopathic tendencies; however, arrests and convictions did not correlate with the DSM-III-R antisocial personality disorder or PCL-R-derived criteria sets within the prison setting, wherein arrests and convictions are normative and not specific to antisocial personality disorder/psychopathy. To the extent that the DSM-III-R criteria set emphasizes acts of criminality and delinquency, it would probably overdiagnose antisocial personality disorder within a prison setting and fail to perform as well as the PCL-R (Hare et al., 1991). On the other hand, this would be less problematic in general clinical settings.

Two of the items with content unique to the PCL-R ("lacks empathy" and "inflated and arrogant self-appraisal") were significantly associated with the DSM-III-R antisocial personality disorder diagnosis and with the external validators of antisocial personality disorder (e.g., clinicians' and interviewers' impressions and the self-report measures of antisocial personality disorder/psychopathy), but these items were included within the DSM-III-R criteria for narcissistic personality disorder. The field trial suggested that their inclusion within the DSM-IV antisocial personality disorder criteria set would increase the overlap of the antisocial and narcissistic personality disorders and complicate their differentiation.

The field trial data also addressed the proposal to simplify the DSM-III-R antisocial personality disorder criteria set. Deletion of the items pertaining to parental irresponsibility, failure to sustain a monogamous relationship, and inconsistent work (and lowering the threshold to three of the remaining seven adult items) did not have an appreciable effect on the diagnosis. At least 98% of the subjects in each of the five sites continued to receive the same diagnosis with this simplified version. Parental irresponsibility was an obvious item to delete, because it obtained the weakest association with the full criteria set (consistent with prior studies); it was rarely present; and it is the most cumbersome of the DSM-III-R adult items (containing six subitems). The failure to sustain a monogamous relationship has also obtained a relatively weak association with the diagnosis in prior studies (e.g., Pfohl & Blum, 1990). In the field trial, it obtained a low prevalence rate and a weak association with the full criteria set across most of the sites.

The decision to delete any additional items was less clear. The item on inconsistent work obtained the second weakest interrater reliability, and it contains three subitems; however, it was also highly correlated with the full criteria set. An alternative item for deletion would be the one concerning failure to honor financial obligations, because it showed a low association with the full criteria set in two of the four sites.

The DSM-IV Personality Disorders Work Group also considered replacing some DSM-III-R items with items from the PCL-R and/or the ICD-10. Replacing the DSM-III-R item "fails to plan ahead . . ." (which contains two subitems) with the similar (but broader) PCL-R-derived "impulsive" item resulted in the same diagnosis being given to 96% of the cases in each of the five sites. Replacing the DSM-III-R item "repeatedly fails to honor financial obligations . . . " with the PCL-R-derived item "irresponsible" still maintained substantial agreement with the original antisocial personality disorder diagnosis, with the worst agreement rate still 94% in two of the sites (St. Louis and Belmont). The PCL-R irresponsibility item provides an obvious choice because it involves similar content to the deleted DSM-III-R items concerning parental irresponsibility, inconsistent work, and failure to honor financial obligations. However, the PCL-R-derived item on irresponsibility was not assessed reliably in most of the sites.

## CHANGES MADE IN DSM-IV

The DSM-IV (American Psychiatric Association, 1994) criteria set incorporating the revisions described above is presented in Table 6.4. The criteria as originally proposed differed slightly in wording from the published criteria.

A review of the published literature does support further revisions, particularly the inclusion of additional traits of psychopathy (Hare et al., 1991). However, the field trial results did not indicate that items unique to the PCL-R or ICD-10 (e.g., "lacks empathy," "inflated and arrogant self-appraisal," and "glib and superficial") significantly improved the validity of the diagnosis,

---

TABLE 6.4. DSM-IV Diagnostic Criteria for Antisocial Personality Disorder

---

A. There is a pervasive pattern of disregard for and violation of the rights of others occurring since age 15 years, as indicated by three (or more) of the following:

   (1) failure to conform to social norms with respect to lawful behaviors as indicated by repeatedly performing acts that are grounds for arrest
   (2) deceitfulness, as indicated by repeated lying, use of aliases, or conning others for personal profit or pleasure
   (3) impulsivity of failure to plan ahead
   (4) irritability and aggressiveness, as indicated by repeated physical fights or assaults
   (5) reckless disregard for safety of self or others
   (6) consistent irresponsibility, as indicated by repeated failure to sustain consistent work behavior or honor financial obligations
   (7) lack of remorse, as indicated by being indifferent to or rationalizing having hurt, mistreated, or stolen from another

B. The individual is at least age 18 years.

C. There is evidence of Conduct Disorder . . . with onset before age 15 years.

D. The occurence of antisocial behavior is not exclusively during the course of Schizophrenia or a Manic Episode.

---

Note. From APA (1994, pp. 649–650). Copyright 1994 by the American Psychiatric Association. Reprinted by permission.

and their addition could complicate the differentiation of antisocial personality disorder from narcissistic personality disorder. Given the reliability and validity of the DSM-III-R criteria set within clinical practice and empirical studies, and the mandate to be conservative with respect to revisions (Frances et al., 1990), additional revisions were not as clearly justifiable.

The criteria set presented in Table 6.4, however, is closer to the PCL-R and ICD-10 in its use of more general representations of the traits rather than specific behavioral manifestations (e.g., "consistent irresponsibility . . ." rather than "repeatedly fails to honor financial obligations . . ."). A shift to more general trait concepts, though, should be supplemented by a description of explicit, behavioral manifestations of the traits to facilitate reliable assessments. For example, the DSM-IV text expands on the criteria set by stating that a failure to conform to social norms can be indicated by such behaviors as destroying property, harassing others, stealing, or pursuing an illegal occupation (American Psychiatric Association, 1994, p. 646). It also states that childhood conduct disorder is suggested by frequent truancy, running away from home overnight at least twice, frequently initiating fights, using a weapon in more than one fight, and so forth, with more exact specification provided by the DSM-IV criteria for conduct disorder (American Psychiatric Association, 1994, pp. 90–91). The text also indicates that beating one's spouse or child counts for the "irritability and aggressiveness" item, whereas physical fights required by one's job or to defend oneself or someone else do not count (American Psychiatric Association, 1994, p. 646). In other words, all of the behaviorally specific criteria provided in DSM-III-R are still included in DSM-IV, but placing them within the text discussion allows for additional examples and qualifications to be presented without further complicating the criteria set and constraining the assessment. More detailed specification is clearly necessary for the irresponsibility item, given the poor reliability of its assessment in the field trial. For example, the DSM-IV text indicates that such behaviors as significant periods of unemployment when work was available, repeated absences from work unexplained by illness in self or family, or abandonment of several jobs without realistic plans for others would qualify for this item, as would defaulting on debts, failure to provide child support, or failure to support other dependents (American Psychiatric Association, 1994, p. 646).

The "Associated Features and Disorders" section of the DSM-IV text (American Psychiatric Association, 1994, p. 647) indicates how additional or supplementary items might be particularly relevant in a prison or forensic setting (e.g., items unique to the PCL-R and ICD-10, such as lack of empathy, inflated self-appraisal, and glib, superficial charm). In DSM-III and DSM-III-R, items that were considered but for various reasons failed to be included within the criteria set were often included within the "Associated Features" section; however, items unique to the PCL-R and ICD-10 were not included in this section in DSM-III-R. This omission has been remedied, and the relevance of these items in prison or court contexts indicated, in DSM-IV.

These changes in the DSM-IV text are consistent with the broader DSM-IV decision to include a new text section for each disorder that discusses cross-cultural, age-associated, and gender-related features. The purpose of these new sections is to discuss how items might be revised when they are applied across particular cultural, ethnic, age, or gender groups. In the case of antisocial personality disorder, the existing criteria even in DSM-IV may be too heavily weighted toward antisocial behaviors that are seen most often in males. Antisocial personality disorder does occur more often in males than in females, but this differential sex prevalence can contribute to a male-biased description if one selects items simply on the basis of their overall diagnostic efficiency. Most studies on antisocial personality disorder are largely confined to males. Therefore, data concerning the diagnostic efficiency of the criteria set based on these studies will be biased in favor of items that perform best for diagnosing the disorder in males, and may not be successful in identifying the best items for diagnosing the disorder in females. For example, forced sexual activity is unlikely to be seen in antisocial females, but it is included within the DSM-III-R and DSM-IV conduct disorder criteria sets because it is diagnostic of conduct disorder in males. A study that was confined to conduct disorder within females would probably find that the item is a very weak predictor of conduct disorder (and antisocial personality disorder). Sexual promiscuity and prostitution, on the other hand, might be more specific to and diagnostic of conduct disorder in females (the DSM-IV antisocial personality disorder field trial data were analyzed separately for males and females; Widiger et al., 1993).

## ACKNOWLEDGMENTS

The opinions expressed herein are our own and do not necessarily represent the American Psychiatric Association or its Task Force on DSM-IV. We express our appreciation to Drs. Blum, Freiman, Heumann, Millon, Morey, Pfohl, Tringone, and Zanarini for providing unpublished data.

## REFERENCES

Alterman, A. I., & Cacciola, J. S. (1991). The antisocial personality disorder diagnosis in substance abusers: Problems and issues. *Journal of Nervous and Mental Disease, 179,* 401–409.

American Psychiatric Association. (1980). *Diagnostic and statistical manual of mental disorders* (3rd ed.). Washington, DC: Author.

American Psychiatric Association. (1987). *Diagnostic and statistical manual of mental disorders* (3rd ed., rev.). Washington, DC: Author.

American Psychiatric Association. (1994). *Diagnostic statistical manual of mental disorders* (4th ed.). Washington, DC: Author.

Bland, R. C., Newman, S. C., Dyck, R. J., & Orn, H. (1990). Prevalence of psychiatric disorders and suicide attempts in a prison population. *Canadian Journal of Psychiatry, 35,* 407–413.

Bland, R. C., Orn, H., & Newman, S. C. (1988). Lifetime prevalence of psychiatric disorders in Edmonton. *Acta Psychiatrica Scandinavca, 77*(Suppl. No. 338), 24–32.

Blashfield, R. K., & Breen, M. J. (1989). Face validity of the DSM-III-R personality disorders. *American Journal of Psychiatry, 146.* 1575–1579.

Cadoret, R. J., O'Gorman, T. W., Troughton, E., & Heywood, E. (1985). Alcoholism and antisocial personality: Interrelationships, genetic and environmental factors. *Archives of General Psychiatry, 42,* 161–167.

Cleckley, H. (1941). *The mask of sanity.* St. Louis, MO: Mosby.

Cooney, N. L., Kadden, R. M., & Litt, M. D. (1990). A comparison of methods for assessing sociopathy in male and female alcoholics. *Journal of Studies on Alcohol, 51,* 42–48.

Cote, G., & Hodgins, S. (1990). Co-occurring mental disorders among criminal offenders. *Bulletin of the American Academy of Psychiatry and Law, 18,* 271–281.

Feighner, J. P., Robins, E., Guze, S. B., Woodruff, R. A., Winokur, G., & Munoz, R. (1972). Diagnostic criteria for use in psychiatric research. *Archives of General Psychiatry, 26,* 57–63.

Ford, M. R., & Widiger, T. A. (1989). Sex bias in the diagnosis of histrionic and antisocial personality disorders. *Journal of Consulting and Clinical Psychology, 57,* 301–305.

Frances, A. J. (1980). The DSM-III personality disorders section: A commentary. *American Journal of Psychiatry, 137,* 1050–1054.

Frances, A. J., Pincus, H. A., Widiger, T. A., Davis, W. W., & First, M. B. (1990). DSM-IV: Work in progress. *American Journal of Psychiatry, 147,* 1439–1448.

Freiman, K, & Widiger, T.A. (1989). [Co-occurrence and diagnostic efficiency statistics.] Unpublished raw data.

Gerstley, L. J., Alterman, A. I., McLellan, A. T., & Woody, G.E. (1990). Antisocial personality disorder in patients with substance abuse disorders: A problematic diagnosis? *American Journal of Psychiatry, 147,* 173–178.

Grande, T. P., Wolf, A. W., Schubert, D. S., Patterson, M. B., & Brocco, K. (1984). Associations among alcoholism, drug abuse, and antisocial personality: A review of the literature. *Psychological Reports, 55,* 455–474.

Grove, W. M., Eckert, E. D., Heston, L., Bouchard, T. J., Segal, N., & Lykken, D. T. (1990). Heritability of substance abuse and antisocial behavior: A study of monozygotic twins reared apart. *Biological Psychiatry, 27,* 1293–1304.

Gunderson, J. G. (1983). DSM-III diagnoses of personality disorders. In J. Frosch (Ed.), *Current perspectives on personality disorders* (pp. 20–39). Washington, DC: American Psychiatric Press.

Guze, S. B., Goodwin, D. W., & Crane, J. B. (1969). Criminality and psychiatric disorders. *Archives of General Psychiatry, 20,* 583–591.

Hare, R. D. (1980). A research scale for the assessment of psychopathy in criminal populations. *Personality and Individual Differences, 1,* 111–117.

Hare, R. D. (1983). Diagnosis of antisocial personality disorder in two prison populations. *American Journal of Psychiatry, 140,* 887–890.

Hare, R. D. (1985). A comparison of procedures for the assessment of psychopathy. *Journal of Consulting and Clinical Psychology, 53,* 7–16.

Hare, R. D. (1991). *The Hare Psychopathy Checklist—Revised.* New York: Multi-Health Systems (908 Niagra Falls Blvd., North Tonawanda, NY, 14120-2060, [800] 456-3003).

Hare, R. D., Hart, S. D., & Harpur, T. J. (1991). Psychopathy and the proposed DSM-IV criteria for antisocial personality disorder. *Journal of Abnormal Psychology, 100,* 391–398.

Hart, S. D., & Hare, R. D. (1989). Discriminant validity of the Psychopathy Checklist in a forensic psychiatric population. *Psychological Assessment: A Journal of Consulting and Clinical Psychology, 1,* 211–218.

Hart, S. D., Hare, R. D., & Harpur, T. J. (in press). The Psychopathy Checklist: An overview for researchers and clinicians. In J. Rosen & P. McReynolds (Eds.), *Advances in psychological assessment* (Vol. 8). New York: Plenum.

Hart, S. D., Kropp, P. R., & Hare, R. D. (1988). Performance of male psychopaths following conditional release from prison. *Journal of Consulting and Clinical Psychology, 56,* 227–232.

Hasin, D. S., & Grant, B. F. (1987). Psychiatric diagnosis of patients with substance abuse problems: A comparison of two procedures, the DIS and the SADS-L. *Journal of Psychiatric Research, 2,* 17–22.

Helzer, J. E., Robins, L. N., McEvoy, L. T., Spitznagel, E. L., Stoltzman, R. K., Farmer, A., & Brockington, I. F. (1985). A comparison of clinical and Diagnostic Interview Schedule Diagnoses. *Archives of General Psychiatry, 42,* 657–666.

Helzer, J. E., Spitznagel, E. L., & McEvoy, L. (1987). The predictive validity of lay Diagnostic Interview Schedule diagnoses in the general population. *Archives of General Psychiatry, 44,* 1069–1077.

Hesselbrock, V., Stabenau, J., Hesselbrock, M. N., Mirkin, P., & Meyer, R. (1982). A comparison of two interview schedules. *Archives of General Psychiatry, 39,* 674–677.

Hyler, S. E., Rieder, R. O., Williams, J. B. W., Spitzer, R. L., Lyons, M., & Hendler, J. (1989). A comparison of clinical and self-report diagnoses of DSM-III personality disorders in 552 patients. *Comprehensive Psychiatry, 30,* 170–178.

Kernberg, O. F. (1989). The narcissistic personality disorder and the differential diagnosis of antisocial behavior. *Psychiatric Clinics of North America, 12,* 553–570.

Lewis, C. E., Rice, J., Andreasen, N., Clayton, P., & Endicott, J. (1985). Alcoholism in antisocial and nonantisocial men with unipolar major depression. *Journal of Affective Disorders, 9,* 253–263.

Livesley, W. J., Reiffer, L. I., Sheldon, A. E. R., & West, M. (1987). Prototypicality ratings of DSM-III criteria for personality disorders. *Journal of Nervous and Mental Disease, 175,* 395–401.

Loranger, A. W. (1988). The impact of DSM-III on diagnostic practice in a university hospital: A comparison of DSM-II and DSM-III in 10,914 patients. *Archives of General Psychiatry, 47,* 672–675.

McCord, W., & McCord, J. (1964). *The psychopath: An essay on the criminal mind.* Princeton, NJ: Van Nostrand.

Mellsop, G., Varghese, F. T. N., Joshua, S., & Hicks, A. (1982). Reliability of Axis II of DSM-III. *American Journal of Psychiatry, 139,* 1360–1361.

Millon, T. (1981). *Disorders of personality: DSM-III, Axis II.* New York: Wiley–Interscience.

Millon, T. (1983). The DSM-III: An insider's perspective. *American Psychologist, 38,* 804–814.

Millon, T., & Tringone, R. (1989). [Co-occurrence and diagnostic efficiency statistics]. Unpublished raw data.

Morey, L. C., & Heumann, K. (1988). [Co-occurrence and diagnostic efficiency statistics]. Unpublished raw data.

Morey, L. C., & Ochoa, E. S. (1989). An investigation of adherence to diagnostic criteria:

Clinical diagnosis of the DSM-III personality disorders. *Journal of Personality Disorders, 3,* 180–192.

Perry, J. C. (1990). Challenges in validating personality disorders: Beyond description. *Journal of Personality Disorders, 4,* 273–289.

Perry, J. C., Lavori, P. W., Cooper, S. H., Hoke, L., & O'Connell, M. E. (1987). The Diagnostic Interview Schedule and DSM-III antisocial personality disorder. *Journal of Personality Disorders, 1,* 121–131.

Pfohl, B., & Blum, N. (1990). [Internal consistency statistics for the DSM-III-R personality disorder criteria.] Unpublished raw data.

Raine, A. (1985). A psychometric assessment of Hare's checklist for psychopathy on an English prison population. *British Journal of Clinical Psychology, 24,* 247–258.

Regier, D. A., Boyd, J. H., Burke, J. D., Rae, D. S., Myers, J. K., Kramer, M., Robins, L. N., George, L. K., Karno, M., & Locke, B. Z. (1988). One-month prevalence of mental disorders in the United States. *Archives of General Psychiatry, 45,* 977–986.

Reid, W. H. (1987). Antisocial personality. In R. Michels & J. O. Cavenar (Eds.), *Psychiatry* ((pp. 1–13). Philadelphia: J. B. Lippincott.

Robins, L. N. (1966). *Deviant children grown up.* Baltimore: Williams & Wilkins.

Robins, L. N., Helzer, J. E., Croughan, J., & Ratcliff, K. S. (1981). The NIMH Diagnostic Interview Schedule: Its history, characteristics, and validity. *Archives of General Psychiatry, 38,* 381–389.

Robins, L. N., Helzer, J. E., Ratcliff, K. S., & Seyfried, W. (1982). Validity of the Diagnostic Interview Schedule, Version II: DSM-III diagnoses. *Psychological Medicine, 12,* 855–870.

Robins, L. N., Helzer, J. E., Weissman, M. M., Orvaschel, H., Gruenberg, E., Burke, J. D., & Regier, D. A. (1984). Lifetime prevalence of specific psychiatric disorders in three sites. *Archives of General Psychiatry, 41,* 949–958.

Robins, L. N., Tipp, J., & Przybeck, T. (1991). Antisocial personality. In L. N. Robins & D. A. Regier (Eds.), *Psychiatric disorders in America* (pp. 258–280). New York: Free Press.

Rogers, R., & Dion, K. (1991). Rethinking the DSM-III-R diagnosis of antisocial personality disorder. *Bulletin of the American Academy of Psychiatry and Law, 19,* 21–31.

Rounsaville, B. J., Eyre, S. L., Weissman, M. M., & Kleber, H. D. (1983). The antisocial opiate addict. In B. Stimmeo (Ed.), *Psychosocial constructs: Alcoholism and substance abuse* (pp. 29–42). New York: Haworth Press.

Serin R., Peters, R. D., & Barbaree, H. E. (1990). Predictors of psychopathy and release outcome in a criminal population. *Psychological Assessment: A Journal of Consulting and Clinical Psychology, 2,* 419–422.

Skodol, A. E. (1989). *Problems in differential diagnosis: From DSM-III to DSM-III-R in clinical practice.* Washington, DC: American Psychiatric Press.

Skodol, A. E., Oldham, J. M., Rosnick, L., Kellman, H. D., & Hyler, S. E. (1991). Diagnosis of DSM-III-R personality disorders: A comparison of two structured interviews. *Methods in Psychiatric Research, 1,* 13–26.

Smith, S. S., & Newman, J. P. (1990). Alcohol and drug abuse–dependence disorders in psychopathic and nonpsychopathic criminal offenders. *Journal of Abnormal Psychology, 99,* 430–439.

Spitzer, R. L., Endicott, J., & Robins, E. (1978). Research Diagnostic Criteria: Rationale and reliability. *Archives of General Psychiatry, 35,* 773–782.

Sutker, P. B., & Allain, A. N. (1983). Behavior and personality assessment in men labelled adaptive sociopaths. *Journal of Behavioral Assessment, 5,* 65–79.

Sutker, P. B., Bugg, F., & West, S. A. (1993). Antisocial personality disorder. In P.B. Sutker & H. Adams (Eds.), *Comprehensive handbook of psychopathology* (2nd ed., pp. 337-369). New York: Plenum.

Tennent, G., Tennent, D., Prins, H., & Bedford, A. (1990). Psychopathic disorder—a useful clinical concept? *Medicine, Science, and Law, 30,* 39-44.

Vaillant, G. E. (1984). The disadvantages of DSM-III outweigh its advantages. *American Journal of Psychiatry, 141,* 542-545.

Widiger, T. A., Cadoret, R., Hare, R. D., Robins, L., Rutherford, M., Zanarini, M., Alterman, A., Apple, M., Corbitt, E. M., Forth, A., Hart, S. D., Kultermann, J., & Woody, G. (1993). *DSM-IV antisocial personality disorder field trial.* Manuscript under editorial review, University of Kentucky.

Widiger, T. A., Corbitt, E. M., & Millon, T. (1992). Antisocial personality disorder. In A. Tasman & M. Riba (Eds.), *Review of psychiatry* (Vol. 11, pp. 63-79). Washington, DC: American Psychiatric Press.

Widiger, T. A., & Frances, A.J. (1987). Interviews and inventories for the measurement of personality disorders. *Clinical Psychology Review, 7,* 49-75.

Widiger, T. A., Frances, A. J., Pincus, H. A., Davis, W. W., & First, M. B. (1991). Toward an empirical classification for the DSM-IV. *Journal of Abnormal Psychology, 100,* 280-288.

Widiger, T. A., & Shea, T. (1991). Differentiation of Axis I and Axis II disorders. *Journal of Abnormal Psychology, 100,* 399-406.

Widiger, T. A., & Trull, T. J. (1987). Behavioral indicators, hypothetical constructs, and personality disorders. *Journal of Personality Disorders, 1,* 82-87.

Widom, C. S. (1977). A methodology for studying noninstitutionalized psychopaths. *Journal of Consulting and Clinical Psychology, 45,* 674-683.

Widom, C. S., & Newman, J. P. (1985). Characteristics of noninstitutionalized psychopaths. In J. Gunn & D. Farrington (Eds.), *Current research in forensic psychiatry and psychology* (Vol. 2, pp. 57-80). New York: Wiley.

Williams, J. B. W., & Spitzer, R. L. (1982). Research Diagnostic Criteria and DSM-III: An annotated comparison. *Archives of General Psychiatry, 39,* 1283-1289.

Woody, G. E., McLellan, A. T., Luborsky, L., & O'Brien, C. P. (1985). Sociopathy and psychotherapy outcome. *Archives of General Psychiatry, 42,* 1081-1086.

World Health Organization. (1990). *The ICD-10 Chapter V. Mental and behavioural disorders: Diagnostic criteria for research.* Geneva: Author.

World Health Organization. (1993). *The ICD-10 classification of mental and behavioral disorders: Diagnostic criteria for research.* Geneva: Author.

Wulach, J. S. (1983). Diagnosing the DSM-III antisocial personality disorder. *Professional Psychology: Research and Practice, 14,* 330-340.

Zanarini, M. (1989). [Co-occurrence and diagnostic efficiency statistics]. Unpublished raw data.

Zimmerman, M., & Coryell, W. (1989). DSM-III personality disorder diagnoses in a nonpatient sample. *Archives of General Psychiatry, 46,* 682-689.

# Commentary on Antisocial Personality Disorder: The DSM-IV Field Trial

Robert D. Hare
Stephen D. Hart

In Chapter 6, Tom Widiger and Elizabeth Corbitt have written an excellent review of the issues surrounding the DSM-III(-R) criteria for antisocial personality disorder and the DSM-IV field trial for this disorder. In our commentary, we discuss what we perceive to be major problems with the field trial and the antisocial personality disorder criteria adopted for DSM-IV: their failure to address adequately the reliability and content-related validity of the criteria. This discussion is based on Widiger and Corbitt's chapter (see also Widiger & Corbitt, 1993) and on the recently published DSM-IV text and criteria for antisocial personality disorder (American Psychiatric Association [APA], 1994).

## THE DSM-IV CRITERIA: HOW RELIABLE ARE THEY?

### "Shortening" versus "Rewriting" the Criteria

The DSM-IV Personality Disorders Work Group made its goals for the field trial clear (Widiger, Frances, Pincus, Davis, & First, 1991): to shorten and reduce the complexity of the antisocial personality disorder criteria set; to increase its compatibility with the 10th revision of the *International Classification of Diseases* (ICD-10); and to improve its coverage of traditional symptoms of psychopathy as reflected in the Psychopathy Checklist—Revised (PCL-R; Hare, 1991), an instrument with demonstrated reliability and validity, but one that required a considerable amount of time and effort to complete. The field trial compared three sets of items: the DSM-III-R criteria for antisocial personality disorders; the ICD-10 research criteria for dyssocial personality disorder (World Health Organization, 1990); and a 10-item psychopathy set derived from the PCL-R (Hare, Hart, & Harpur, 1991). The only explicit conditions were that changes for DSM-IV should be conservative and should not be made at the expense of interrater reliability.

Although the results of the field trial provided the basis for attaining each of the work group's goals, its primary recommendations were to shorten the list of adult items for antisocial personality disorder from 10 to 7 and, in line with the ICD-10 and PCL-R, to make the representations of some of these items more general than they were before. Although such changes might have been possible without a significant reduction in interrater reliability of the criteria set, *this issue was not actually addressed in the field trial.* This is because the field trial evaluated the DSM-III-R adult criteria for antisocial personality disorder, not the DSM-IV adult criteria. The 7-item DSM-IV set was derived from the 10-item DSM-III-R set; this derivation was logical rather than empirical, and involved, among other things, transferring the specific examples for each item from the criterion set to the text description of the disorder. For example, one of the seven adult items in DSM-IV is criterion A3: "impulsivity or failure to plan ahead" (American Psychiatric Association, 1994, p. 650). The DSM-III-R item from which it was derived is C5:

> Fails to plan ahead or is impulsive, as indicated by one or both of the following:
>     (a) travelling from place to place without a prearranged job or clear goal or clear idea about when the travel will terminate
>     (b) lack of a fixed address for a month or more. (American Psychiatric Association, 1987, p. 345)

Exemplars of the item are now contained in the "Diagnostic Features" section of the DSM-IV text: "A pattern of impulsivity may be manifested by a failure to plan ahead.... Decisions are made on the spur of the moment, without forethough, and without consideration for the consequences of self or others; this may lead to sudden changes of jobs, residences, or relationships" (American Psychiatric Association, 1994, p. 646). The point here is that this item, *as written,* was not evaluated in the field trial. What *was* evaluated was the DSM-III-R precursor to the item. As a result, we do not know whether clinicians, on seeing "impulsive or failure to plan ahead" in DSM-IV, will interpret the item in the same way as they would if the examples were an integral part of the item rather than being buried in the text. The same criticism applies to other items in the adult criteria set. The fact is, the DSM-IV criteria for antisocial personality disorder have not yet been empirically evaluated. We do not know how reliable or valid the seven-item set is, given that the items, in their present form, were not actually used in the field trial.

## Criterion C: Conduct Disorder

Most critiques of the DSM-III and DSM-III-R criteria for antisocial personality disorder — including our own (e.g., Hare et al., 1991) — have focused on adult antisocial behavior (criterion C in DSM-III-R; criterion A in DSM-IV). In fact, it has become commonplace to refer to the antisocial personality disorder criteria as polythetic or as comprising, in DSM-III-R, 10 symptoms. This is misleading. The four major criteria in DSM-III-R and DSM-IV are monothetic. In DSM-III-R, these criteria are as follows: (A) age 18 or older; (B) conduct disorder before age 15; (C) adult antisocial behavior; and (D) the exclusion criterion. The order of these criteria is changed in DSM-IV: (A) adult antisocial behavior; (B) age 18 or older; (C) conduct disorder before age 15; (D) the exclusion criterion. Each criterion is necessary, and together they are jointly sufficient, to diagnose antisocial personality disorder. The symptoms (or subcriteria) within DSM-III-R criteria B and C, and DSM-IV criteria A and C, are the ones that are polythetic.

Ignoring the impact of the conduct disorder criterion on antisocial personality disorder diagnoses can be risky. To illustrate, we recently analyzed DSM-III-R antisocial personality disorder ratings for 363 prison inmates and 51 forensic psychiatric outpatients, all men aged 18 or older (Hart, Forth, & Hare, 1992). (We also studied 50 undergraduates, but we will not discuss these subjects further, as they were younger and included both men and women.) The prevalence of antisocial personality disorder was 64.2% in the prisoners (a figure consistent with that found in a number of previous studies in the United States and Canada) and 15.7% in the patients. However, these overall prevalence rates masked a marked disparity in the prevalence of childhood and adult antisocial behavior. On average, the prisoners and patients had, respectively, 5.53 ($SD$ = 1.87) and 3.37 ($SD$ = 1.96) adult antisocial symptoms. Only four symptoms are required to meet the criteria for adult antisocial behavior; 85.7% of prisoners and 45.1% of patients met or exceeded this cutoff. On the other hand, the average number of conduct disorder (childhood) symptoms was 3.69 ($SD$ = 2.27) for prisoners and 1.57 ($SD$ = 1.71) for patients; only 68.0% of prisoners and 31.4% of patients met or exceeded the cutoff of three or more symptoms. Clearly, the childhood symptoms had the greater influence on the final diagnosis. If a prisoner met conduct disorder, he was virtually certain (about 95%) to be diagnosed as having antisocial personality disorder, whereas only 75% of those meeting adult antisocial behavior criterion were so diagnosed. For patients, 50% of those who met conduct disorder criterion were diagnosed as having antisocial personality disorder, compared to 34.8% of those who met the adult antisocial behavior criterion.

As might be expected from the figures presented above, the association between childhood and adult antisocial behaviours was quite modest. The kappa coefficient of agreement for the presence versus absence of conduct disorder and adult antisocial behavior was only .32 in prisoners and .15 in patients. The correlation between symptom counts for conduct disorder and adult antisocial behavior was .47 in prisoners, but only .26 in patients. Although statistically significant, these kappas and correlations are low to moderate in magnitude. Conduct disorder and adult antisocial behavior symptom counts also had different external correlates. Adult antisoical behavior symptom counts showed a good pattern of concurrent validity: In the prisoners, they correlated .54 with PCL-R Factor 1 scores (a measure of the interpersonal and affective features of psychopathy); the correlation in patients was .48. In contrast, the correlation between conduct disorder symptoms and Factor 1 was only .27 in the prisoners, and −.02 in the patients.

These findings are disquieting. It is apparent from Widiger and Corbitt's chapter that the analysis of the antisocial personality disorder field trial focused solely on the adult antisocial behavior criterion and its subcriteria. As a consequence, these analyses reveal less than half of the antisocial personality disorder picture. Reanalyses of the field trial data, taking the conduct disorder criterion into account, would appear to be an obvious solution to this problem. Regrettably, the Personality Disorders Work Group's recommendations concerning the DSM-IV criteria had to be limited to the adult antisocial behavior criterion, as the symptoms for conduct disorder in DSM-IV differ from those found in DSM-III-R. In light of the strong impact the conduct disorder criterion has on the diagnosis of antisocial personality disorder, and the lack of association between this criterion and the adult antisocial behavior criterion, it is clear that the field trial tells us little about the reliability or validity of antisocial personality disorder in DSM-IV.

## WHAT ABOUT CONTENT-RELATED VALIDITY?

The field trial indicated that most of the ICD-10 and PCL-R items reflecting the traditional symptoms of psychopathy had interrater reliabilities at least as high as those of the more behaviorally specific antisocial personality disorder items. The Personality Disorders Work Group therefore had a firm basis for increasing the content-related validity of antisocial personality disorder without a reduction in interrater reliability, thereby meeting one of its stated goals for DSM-IV: to increase compatibility of antisocial personality disorder with ICD-10 and to improve coverage of traditional symptoms of psychopathy. Yet it did so only in a very limited way.

### Reliability of Traditional Items

Widiger and Corbitt (Chapter 6, pp. 118–119) argue that the PCL-R and ICD-10 items were reliable only because the interviewers were trained and used a semistructured interview. They state, "It then remains questionable whether [these] items would be assessed reliably in general clinical practice unless they were supplemented by more specific guidelines." This raises several questions. As there is little information concerning the reliability of individual DSM-III-R symptoms in clinical practice, does not the same criticism apply to those symptoms? If the reliability of symptoms in the field trials can be dismissed or explained away on the basis of the procedures used to evaluate them, why were these procedures used in the first place? If explicit

guidelines are needed to help clinicians make reliable inferences of personality traits—a reasonable assumption, and one that is fundamental to the
PCL-R—why not simply provide them in DSM-IV?

## Too Much Emphasis on Concurrent Validity

Another reason given for not improving coverage in the DSM-IV criteria
is that the inclusion of PCL-R/ICD-10 items did not significantly increase
correlations with a variety of external validators, including several self-report
personality inventories, clinicians' and interviewers' impressions, and indicators of "personality dysfunction." This is not surprising; there is no reason
to assume that the clinically based PCL-R and ICD-10 symptoms *should* have
been more strongly correlated with self-report measures of personality than
was the case. Indeed, the correlations between criteria sets and external validators were very similar in magnitude (about .20 to .35) to those reported
in past research examining the association between clinical/behavioral and
self-report measures of psychopathy (e.g., Hare, 1985, 1991). In any case, we
wonder why the issue of content-related validity did not enter the picture.
That is, although the PCL-R or ICD-10 symptoms did not significantly *increase* the correlations of the criteria set with the external validators used
in the field trial, they did not result in a *decrease*, and their inclusion would
have greatly improved the content-related validity of the criteria set. As things
stand, the coverage of traditional symptoms of psychopathy is little better
in DSM-IV than it was in DSM-III-R.

It appears that both the DSM-IV Task Force and those involved in the
field trial are well aware of the limited coverage of the antisocial personality disorder criteria. For example, Widiger and Corbitt suggest in Chapter
6 that the interpersonal and affective symptoms measured by Factor 1 of
the PCL-R may be useful indicators of antisocial personality disord-
er/psychopathy in prison settings. The "Associated Features and Disorders"
section of the DSM-IV text, to which they refer, uses words, phrases and constructs derived from the clinical literature, the PCL-R manual, and the 10-item
list of criteria for psychopathy used in the field trial:

> Individuals with Antisocial Personality Disorder frequently lack empathy and
> tend to be callous, cynical, and contemptuous of the feelings, rights, and suffer-
> ing of others. They may have an inflated and arrogant self-appraisal . . . and may
> be excessivley opinionated, self-assured, or cocky. The may display a glib, su-
> perficial charm and can be quite voluble and verbally facile. . . . Lack of empa-
> thy, inflated self-appraisal, and supperficial charm are features that have
> commonly been included in traditional conceptions of psychopathy and may
> be particularly distinguishing of Antisocial Personality Disorder in prison or
> forensic settings where criminal, delinquent, and aggressive acts are likely to
> be nonspecific. (American Psychiatric Association, 1994, p. 647)

Curiously, however, clinicians are left to their own devices when it comes
to operationalizing the associated features; no guidelines are provided, nor

are clinicians referred to an instrument (such as the PCL-R) that does provide explicit guidelines for each symptom. In any case, it appears that DSM-
IV is proposing two sets of criteria (DSM-IV items; DSM-IV items plus some
undefined personality traits) for what should be the same disorder. If the
personality traits mentioned in the "Associated Features and Disorders" section of the text are considered important for the diagnosis of antisocial personality disorder in forensic settings, they should be just as useful in more
general settings.

Given the problems with the DSM-III-R criteria for antisocial personality disorder, the Personality Disorders Work Group set a surprisingly high
and narrowly defined threshold for revisions to the criteria. The major de-
terminant of whether or not this threshold had been reached was the incre-
ment in concurrent validity that changes would produce. As we have
indicated above, there are problems with this emphasis on concurrent validity and in the way in which it was measured. Had reliability and content-
related validity also been used to determine the threshold for revisions, it
is likely that the DSM-IV diagnostic criteria for antisocial personality disorder would have included more of the traditional symptoms of psychopathy.
As things stand, DSM-III-R and DSM-IV identify much the same individuals
as having antisocial personality disorder. However, the formal and explicit
inclusion in DSM-IV of traditional symptoms of psychopathy would have
altered substantially who receives a diagnosis of antisocial personality
disorder—a situation that the work group may not have been comfortable with.

## Concerns about a Possible Increase in Comorbidity

Widiger and Corbitt express concerns in Chapter 6 that increasing the coverage of traditional psychopathy symptoms might complicate the differential
diagnosis of antisocial personality disorder and narcissistic personality disorder. This argument appears to be based on the assumption that these two
disorders should be largely independent. But diagnostic overlap among Axis
II disorders is the rule rather than the exception. Indeed, the "Associated
Mental Disorders" section of the DSM-IV text states, "Individuals with Antisocial Personality Disorder also often have personality features that meet
criteria for other Personality Disorders, particularly Borderline, Histrionic,
and Narcissistic Personality Disorders" (American Psychiatric Association,
1994, p. 647). Moreover, it is quite possible that the overlap between antisocial and narcissistic personality disorders reflects a failure to "carve nature
at its joints." As several investigators have shown, cluster and factor analyses
of the symptoms that define DSM-III-R personality disorders often produce
results that are not congruent with the DSM-III-R criteria sets for antisocial
and narcissistic personality disorders. Instead, symptoms from several personality disorders, including antisocial and narcissistic, coalesce to form a
cluster of symptoms that is consistent with the traditional category of psy-

chopathy as measured by the PCL-R (e.g., Harpur, Hare, Zimmerman, & Coryell, 1990; Livesley, Jackson, & Schroeder, 1989, 1992; Livesley & Schroeder, 1991; Morey, 1988).

From a methodological perspective, we wonder why the items in each of the three criteria sets (DSM-III-R, ICD-10, PCL-R) were not put into one large pot, to determine whether natural factors or clusters of items would emerge. It is quite possible, even likely, that we would have ended up with a reliable combination of items from several criteria sets—a combination that would have looked a lot like the PCL-R and that would have been considerably more valid than the criteria found in DSM-IV.

## SUMMARY AND CONCLUSIONS

We have identified what we believe to be some serious problems with the development of the DSM-IV criteria for antisocial personality disorder. In light of these problems, we find it difficult not to question the value of the field trail. The failure to include traditional symptoms of psychopathy explicitly and formally in the criteria for antisocial personality disorder lays the groundwork for a continuation of the sort of criticism that has marked the last decade or more (e.g., Gerstley, Alterman, McLellan, & Woody, 1990; Hare et al., 1991; Millon, 1981; Rogers & Dion, 1991; Wulach, 1983). It also ensures that some clinicians will continue to believe that antisocial personality disorder (as measured by DSM-III-R and DSM-IV) and psychopathy (as measured by ICD-10 and the PCL-R) are synonymous disorders.

## REFERENCES

American Psychiatic Association. (1987). *Diagnostic and statistical manual of mental disorders* (3rd ed., rev.). Washington, DC: Author.

American Psychiatric Association. (1994). *Diagnostic and statistical manual of mental disorder* (4th ed.). Washington, DC: Author.

Gerstley, L. J., Alterman, A. I., McLellan, A. T., & Woody, G. E. (1990). Antisocial personality disorder in substance abusers: A problematic diagnosis? *American Journal of Psychiatry, 147,* 173–178.

Hare, R. D. (1985). Comparison of procedures for the assessment of psychopathy. *Journal of Consulting and Clinical Psychology, 53,* 7–16.

Hare, R. D. (1991). *Manual for the Hare Psychopathy Checklist—Revised.* Toronto, Multi-Health Systems.

Hare, R. D., Hart, S. D., & Harpur, T. J. (1991). Psychopathy and the proposed DSM-IV criteria for antisocial personality disorder. *Journal of Abnormal Psychology, 100,* 391–398.

Harpur, T. J., Hare, R. D., Zimmerman, M., & Coryell, W. (1990, August). *Dimensions underlying DSM-III personality disorders: Cluster 2.* Paper presented at the annual meeting of the American Psychological Association, Boston.

Hart, S. D., Forth, A. E., & Hare, R. D. (1992, March). *Psychometric Analysis of the DSM-III-R Criteria for Antisocial Personality Disorder.* Paper presented at the mid-year meeting of the American Psychology–Law Society (APA Division 41), San Diego.

Livesley, W. J., Jackson, D. N., & Schroeder, M. (1989). A study of the factorial structure of personality pathology. *Journal of Personality Disorders, 3,* 292–306.

Livesley, W. J., Jackson, D. N., & Schroeder, M. (1992). Factorial structure of traits delineating personality disorders in clinical and general population samples. *Journal of Abnormal Psychology, 101,* 432–440.

Livesley, W. J., & Schroeder, M. (1991). Dimensions of personality disorder: The DSM-III-R Cluster B diagnoses. *Journal of Nervous and Mental Disease, 179,* 320–328.

Millon, T. (1981). *Disorders of personality: DSM-III, Axis II.* New York, Wiley–Interscience.

Morey, L. C. (1988). The categorical representation of personality disorder: A cluster analysis of the DSM-III-R personality features. *Journal of Abnormal Psychology, 97,* 314–321.

Rogers, R., & Dion, K. (1991). Rethinking the DSM-III-R diagnosis of antisocial personality disorder. *Bulletin of the American Academy of Psychiatry and Law, 19,* 21–31.

Widiger, T. A., & Corbitt, E. M. (1993). Antisocial personality disorder: Proposals for DSM-IV. *Journal of Personality Disorders, 7,* 63–77.

Widiger, T. A., Frances, A. J., Pincus, H. A., Davis, W. W., & First, M. B. (1991). Toward an empirical classification for DSM-IV. *Journal of Abnormal Psychology, 100,* 280–288.

World Health Organization. (1990). *ICD-10 Chapter V. Mental and behavioural disorders: Diagnostic criteria for research.* Geneva: Author.

Wulach, J. S. (1983). Diagnosing the DSM-III antisocial personality disorder. *Professional Psychology: Research and Practice, 14,* 330–340.

# Commentary on Antisocial Personality Disorders

LEE ROBINS

To begin with, let me say that I think Tom Widiger and Elizabeth Corbitt's chapter on the issues raised concerning the changes in criteria for antisocial personality disorder in DSM-IV (American Psychiatric Association, 1994) and the level of evidence for deciding on these changes is masterful. But they give me more credit than is my due. I did not invent the criteria for sociopathy used in the study on which my 1966 book, *Deviant Children Grown Up*, was based. At the time Dr. Patricia O'Neal and I chose those criteria, the first edition of DSM (American Psychiatric Association, 1952) was about 3 years old. It did not yet have the status of the Bible that DSM-III (American Psychiatric Association, 1980) achieved, having been written mainly to give hospitals a common coding system. We were not greatly impressed with its four-sentence discussion of sociopathic personality — antisocial reaction, and decided to ask my husband, Eli, what criteria he had been using in what was then called the Washington University Department Interview. The 19 criteria he recommended appear as Appendix D in my book (Robins, 1966). Our study did not attempt to validate these criteria; it simply used them. The diagnosing psychiatrists were told not to consider the diagnosis unless at least 5 of 19 criteria had been met, but no number of symptoms obligated them to award it.

The original criteria in DSM-I and DSM-II did not inlude childhood behavior problems, but when the study was complete, we found that some childhood antisocial behavior appeared in the clinic records of almost all those who received the diagnosis. This finding became the basis for the DSM-III requirement for a history of substantial antisocial behavior before the age of 15 years. But the rest of the DSM-III criteria had only a modest dependence on our study. Between the publication of my book and the creation of DSM-III, two reformulations of the criteria for antisocial personality were published that were in the same lineage but substantially modified: the Feighner et al. (1972) criteria and the Research Diagnostic Criteria (Spitzer, Endicott, & E. Robins, 1975). I played no direct role in creating either.

DSM-III was a third reformulation. This time I was on the committee, along with many others. Of the 18 criteria not specific to childhood in our study, only 10 appeared in DSM-III, and some of those were transformed considerably. Dropped altogether were our criteria of drug use, heavy drinking, financial dependency, poor military record, somatic complaints, suicide attempts, lack of friends, and lack of guilt. DSM-III also added two new symptoms — parental irresponsibility (which has now been discarded from the DSM-IV criteria set) and financial default. DSM-III-R (American Psychiatric Association, 1987) put lack of guilt back.

I have forgotten how the symptoms were selected for DSM-III but there was no attempt comparable to that guiding the construction of DSM-IV criteria to identify a minimum criterion set that dropped items not needed to include persons given the diagnosis according to earlier manuals. Two of the five most common symptoms were dropped (financial dependence and heavy drinking), and two of the rarest were kept (the use of aliases and pathological lying).

This history will explain, I hope, that I have no reason to feel a proprietary interest in the antisocial personality criteria in DSM-III or DSM-III-R. I did translate those criteria, along with criteria for many other diagnoses, into questions that would allow the Diagnostic Interview Schedule (DIS) to make DSM-III and DSM-III-R diagnoses. I was also one of five principal investigators who used the DIS in the Epidemiologic Catchment Area study. It was not until I found that antisocial personality compared very favorably with other diagnoses in test–retest reliability (Robins, Helzer, Croughan, & Ratcliff, 1981) and in meeting two validity criteria (Helzer et al., 1985; Robins, 1989) — agreement with a clinician's assessment and prediction of responses a year later — that I began to develop a bit of affection for the criteria.

If they had not performed well, I would have been eager to replace them in DSM-IV, but my experience with epidemiological research made me conservative. The old criteria were easily translated into simple questions. Symptoms like those suggested for adoption in DSM-IV, such as inability to form meaningful relationships and manipulativeness, did not suit my need as an author of interviews to write questions that both unequivocally operationalize diagnostic criteria and will be answered correctly by respondents. "Can you form meaningful relationships?" would operationalize the first, but would not be answered correctly by respondents who have never had a meaningful relationship; without the experience, they have no yardstick against which to judge the quality of their relationships. And might not a manipulative respondent be able to manipulate the interviewer into believing that the respondent is responding sincerely? Such symptoms create for the author something like that classic problem in logic: "If all Cretans are liars and all others tell the truth, what question could you ask to discover whether you are talking to a Cretan?" If the critical question does not exist, lay interviewers, even though they have been shown to be able to get admissions of discreditable behavior, cannot be expected to judge the veridicality of a respondent's assessment of his or her own personality traits.

If a lay interviewer cannot assess such criteria, can clinicians? During training in the use of the Psychopathy Checklist—Revised (PCL-R) for the DSM-IV antisocial personality field trials, we were shown a tape in which a school teacher who had been fired for sexually molesting his students admitted to heavy drinking, barroom fights, and frequent casual sexual encounters, but he said he was very sorry for his behavior and really loved his wife. His clinician examiners did not give him an antisocial personality diagnosis because he professed a meaningful relationship. As a skeptical empiricist, I thought that if he truly cared for his wife, he would have acted differently. How could our disagreement be resolved? Surely not simply by appeal to the superiority of clinical judgment. Authority alone has no standing in scientific endeavors.

Widiger and Corbitt do an excellent job in Chapter 6 of explaining the arguments offered in favor of adding these more psychological criteria. One argument has been that the DSM-III and DSM-III-R antisocial personality criteria are more crime-centered than are criteria describing the psychological substrate; another is that clinicians do not feel as comfortable with the DSM-III(-R) criteria as with the older criteria; and, finally, it is argued that DSM criteria should be compatible with the 10th revision of the *International al Classification of Diseases* (ICD-10).

The claim that the DSM-III-R criteria are crime-centered has chiefly been argued by showing that when a recommended cutoff was used for the PCL or PCL-R, fewer incarcerated felons received the diagnosis than with the DSM criteria. Still, it is ironic that in one study (Hart, Kropp, & Hare, 1988) done by a group that has claimed that the DSM criteria are too crime-centered, the superiority of the PCL over the DSM diagnosis was demonstrated by finding that the PCL was the better predictor of criminal recidivism subsequent to release from prison!

It would be possible to have the two systems identify the same proportion of a prison population as antisocial personalities without having to add criteria from the PCL-R to DSM. Since no strong argument has been made for the cutoff used for either the PCL-R or DSM-III-R criterion lists, either lowering the PCL-R cutoff or raising the number of symptoms required for a DSM-IV diagnosis could achieve parity. But if DSM criteria were raised to match the prevalence determined by the PCL-R, would the felons who no longer met the DSM criteria be considered well? They would still clearly fulfill the general criteria for DSM-III-R personality disorders, in that their traits are inflexible and maladaptive, and cause significant impairment in social or occupational functioning and subjective distress. Furthermore, as DSM-III-R suggests is typical, these traits begin by adolescence or earlier and continue throughout most of their adult lives. Yet DSM users would have no category applicable to those displaced by raising the number of criteria required. In the event, very little has been done about this in the published DSM-IV: The diagnostic threshold for the adult behavior criteria has been changed from 4 of 10 to 3 of 7, and no items from the PCL-R have been added (though the usefulness of some of these items in a prison or forensic setting is discussed in the "Associated Features and Disorders" section).

What about clinician discomfort as an argument for reversion to the earlier symptoms? Clinicians can be uncomfortable with criteria for at least three reasons: They do not see cases who fit the criteria; the criteria are not sufficiently broad to include people they feel belong; or the criteria do not capture what they believe is the "essence" of the disorder. The first would certainly be reasonable grounds for revision. But the research Widiger and Corbitt cite in Chapter 6 shows little evidence for difficulties in applying the DSM-III or DSM-III-R criteria in clinical settings.

Criteria are seen as overly specific when they do not allow clinicians to give the diagnosis to people whom they cannot distinguish qualitatively from those who do qualify. Imagine, for example, a man who would qualify for the diagnosis of antisocial personality if he met the recklessness criterion, but who does not drive and therefore is not at risk of speeding or drunk driving. Should he not be labeled reckless because he frequently has unprotected sex with people who may be infected with AIDS? Certainly recklessness should be broadened to include more varied and less culture-bound behaviors. Broadening criteria by giving more examples and instances seems a fine idea, but there have also been pressures to broaden them by not specifying examples at all. Unfortunately (to my mind), these pressures have been yielded to in the formation of the DSM-IV criteria, though there has been an attempt to specify examples in the accompanying texts. This loss of definition may make it impossible to settle on a universally accepted operationalization of the criteria. Well-defined criteria are essential for replication across studies. The detailed definitions in DSM-III and DSM-III-R have been very important to the scientific achievements of psychiatry since 1980.

The third reason for clinicians' discomfort—that the DSM-III(-R) criteria do not capture what they feel to be the "essence" of the disorder—is an important concern. No matter how precise a description may be, if it does not match the reality it is supposed to be measuring, it is useless. But it is hard to know how much the protesting clinicians' sense of the "essence" of antisocial personality is a distillation of clinical experience, and how much it is fidelity to what they were taught as students and residents. One way to judge this might have been to compare the feelings of younger but experienced clinicians trained on DSM-III and DSM-III-R with the feelings of older clinicians trained on the first and second DSM editions. Nothing like this was attempted in the DSM-IV revision process, and it remains to be seen whether the shorter and less specific DSM-IV criteria set will capture the "essence" of the disorder with greater success than its predecessor.

The final argument—that DSM-IV and ICD-10 should agree—is a powerful argument. Yet most research on antisocial personality since World War II has been done by Americans. The epidemiological instruments popular in Europe, the General Health Questionnaire and the Present State Examination, include none of its symptoms. Research on this disorder in Europe has been limited, in part because the disorder became tainted with Naziism. It is not clear to me why antisocial personality was thus singled out among psychiatric disorders, since the Nazis judged all their psychiatric patients to have defective protoplasm, and starved them indiscriminately. Perhaps it is because antisocial personality was once called "constitutional psychopathic inferiority," with that term's echoes of a genetic taint.

A final comment with respect to the task force's consideration of recommending different symptoms or different numbers of symptoms for women and prisoners. I think that this would be a big mistake, and I am pleased that it has not been done in DSM-IV. If different criteria are used for different groups, comparing their prevalences and risk factors becomes meaningless. It would be far better in future editions to expand the criteria for all to include symptoms that are believed to be particularly common among women. One definition per diagnosis, please, in the interest of communication, science, and sanity!

## REFERENCES

American Psychiatric Association. (1952). *Diagnostic and statistical manual of mental disorders* (1st ed.). Washington, DC: Mental Hospitals Service.

American Psychiatric Association. (1980). *Diagnostic and statistical manual of mental disorders* (3rd ed.). Washington, DC: Author.

American Psychiatric Association. (1987). *Diagnostic and statistical manual of mental disorders* (3rd ed., rev.). Washington, DC: Author.

American Psychiatric Association. (1994). *Diagnostic and statistical manual of mental disorders* (4th ed.). Washington, DC: Author.

Feighner, J. P., Robins, E., Guze, S. B., Woodruff, R. A., Winokur, G., & Munoz, R. (1972). Diagnostic criteria for use in psychiatric research. *Archives of General Psychiatry, 26,* 57–63.

Hart, S. D., Kropp, P. R., & Hare, R. D. (1988). Performance of male psychopaths following conditional release from prison. *Journal of Consulting and Clinical Psychology, 56,* 227–232.

Helzer, J. E., Robins, L. N., McEvoy, L. T., Spitznagel, E. L., Stoltzman, R. K., Farmer, A., & Brockington, I. F. (1985). A comparison of clinical and Diagnostic Interview Schedule diagnoses: Physician reexamination of lay interviewed cases in the general population. *Archives of General Psychiatry, 42,* 657–666.

Robins, L. N. (1966). *Deviant children grown up: A sociological and psychiatric study of sociopathic personality.* Baltimore: Williams & Wilkins.

Robins, L. N. (1989). Diagnostic grammar and assessment: Translating criteria into questions. In L. Robins & J. Barrett (Eds.), *The validity of diagnosis* (pp. 263–278). New York: Raven Press.

Robins, L. N., Helzer, J. E., Croughan, J., & Ratcliff, K. S. (1981). National Institute of Mental Health Diagnostic Interview Schedule: Its history, characteristics, and validity. *Archives of General Psychiatry, 38,* 381–389.

Spitzer, R. L., Endicott, J., & Robins, E. (1975). Clinical criteria for psychiatric diagnosis and DSM-III. *American Journal of Psychiatry, 132*(11), 1187–1192.

# CHAPTER 7

## Borderline Personality Disorder

JOHN G. GUNDERSON
MARY C. ZANARINI
CASSANDRA L. KISIEL

This chapter reviews the available literature and data that bear on the issue of revisions to the DSM-III-R (American Psychiatric Association [APA], 1987) account of borderline personality disorder in DSM-IV (American Psychiatric Association, 1994). The emphasis is on empirical evidence assembled since the introduction of this category in DSM-III (American Psychiatric Association, 1980), but the review necessarily moves into the earlier literature that gave rise to the disorder's recognition and into the nonempirical resources offered by the accumulated expertise of advisors. Readers are invited to consider, as did the DSM-IV Personality Disorders Work Group, how to reconcile the value of sustaining a definition of borderline personality disorder that has now received partial validation with the value of modifications that might better reflect the borderline personality disorder construct. The issues addressed by the work group and covered here are as follows: (1) Is the diagnosis distinct from other disorders? (2) Are the criteria effective in identifying the disorder? (3) Do the criteria accurately identify the intended constructs? (4) Are the criteria congruent with the descriptive literature? (5) Are the polythetic format and diagnostic threshold appropriate? (6) Should the essential feature be altered?

This chapter condenses a review prepared for use by the DSM-IV Personality Disorders Work Group. It updates an earlier version published in the *Journal of Personality Disorders*, 1991, 5, 340–352. Copyright 1991 by The Guilford Press. Adapted by permission. It is not an official document of that group or of the American Psychiatric Association.

## LITERATURE REVIEW

Potential sources were identified through a computer search of all English-language journal articles published since 1975 using the index terms "borderline personality," "borderline conditions," and "borderline states," a review of the tables of contents since 1983 of 15 major psychiatry and psychology journals; and a review of major review articles and books (e.g., Gunderson, 1984; Gunderson & Zanarini, 1987; Skodol & Spitzer, 1987). The resulting list of approximately 1,300 articles, chapters, and books was reduced by deleting those that primarily concerned children and/or adolescents, were not empirical, sampled fewer than five cases, and/or failed to address descriptive issues. In reports that involved identical or overlapping data sets (approximately 7% of the total), weight was given to results based on the largest sample size and DSM-III-R criteria. In addition, researchers who had developed structured interviews for the diagnosis of personality disorders and who had unpublished data were solicited for personality disorders. Tables 7.1 and 7.2 give background information on the major data sources used in this review to address the issues of overlap and diagnostic efficiency.

In addition to these efforts to canvas the relevant data and literature, input from a range of advisors was used. Efforts were made to include people with varied professional, conceptual, and clinical orientations.

### Is the Diagnosis Distinct from Other Disorders?

The comorbidity with other Axis II disorders observed in 10 samples of borderline patients indicates that borderline personality disorder was rarely the only personality disorder diagnosis. The percentage of single-diagnosis cases ranged from a low of 3% (Dahl, 1986) to a high of only 10% (Millon & Tringone, 1989; Pfohl, Coryell, Zimmerman, & Stangl, 1986). In contrast, clinicians in practice rarely employ multiple diagnoses of the personality disorders (Pfohl et al., 1986; Widiger & Frances, 1987).

In studies using the DSM-III criteria, the most serious overlap was with histrionic personality disorder (Table 7.3). Three studies found that more that 50% of the patients who met criteria for borderline personality disorder also met criteria for histrionic personality disorder (Dahl, 1986; Pfohl et al., 1986; Zanarini, 1989). As intended, the changes in the DSM-III-R definitions of the disorders significantly lowered the levels of overlap with histrionic personality disorder. In seven studies, using DSM-III-R criteria, the mean overlap fell to 23%.

Table 7.3 also shows that the overlap with antisocial personality disorder was also reduced in DSM-III-R based studies. On the other hand, DSM-III-R introduced a significant overlap issue *vis-à-vis* self-defeating personality disorder and increased the overlap with avoidant personality disorder. Two studies (Freiman & Widiger, 1989; Skodol, Rosnick, Kellman, Oldham, & Hyler, 1988) found that more than 50% of their borderlines fulfilled criteria

TABLE 7.1. Major Data Sources

| Study | Tot-n | Nom | Meth | Loc | Int | CompG | %M |
|---|---|---|---|---|---|---|---|
| Clarkin et al. | 76 | 3 | AI | O | MC | PD | 21 |
| Cowdry et al. | 59 | 3 | CI | I | MC | DEP | — |
| Dahl | 103 | 3 | SI | I | MC | PD | 58 |
| Dubro et al. | 56 | 3 | SI | I | VA | PD/NOR | 93 |
| Jacobsberg et al. | 64 | 3 | SI | O/I | MC | PD | 39 |
| Kass | 367 | 3R | CI | O | PP/Cl | — | 39 |
| Kass et al. | 59 | 3R | CI | O | PP/Cl | MXD | 36 |
| Mallow | 163 | 3 | SI | I | VA | DRG | 100 |
| McGlashan | 109 | 3 | CT | I | PRH | BPD/SZT | 36 |
| Millon/Tringone | 584 | 3R | CI | MXD | MXD | — | — |
| Modestin | 129 | 3 | CI | I | MC | PD | 50 |
| Morey | 37 | 3 | CT | I | MC | MXD | 55 |
| Morey/Heumann | 291 | 3R | CI | O/I | MXD | PD | 46 |
| Nurnberg | 37 | 3 | SI | I | MC | NOR | 46 |
| Perry et al. | 19 | 3 | SI | O | MXD | BPD/BA | — |
| Pfohl et al. | 137 | 3 | SI | I/O | MC | PD | 24 |
| Plakun | 63 | 3 | CT | I | PRH | NAR | 38 |
| Reich | 159 | 3 | INV | O | MXD | MXD/AN | 37 |
| Ronningstam | 51 | MXD | SI | MXD | PRH | — | 51 |
| Skodol | 97 | 3R | SI | I | MC | PD | — |
| Spitzer et al. | 1,616 | 3 | CI | I/O | MXD | MXD | 64 |
| Widiger et al. | 84 | 3 | SI | I | PUB | PD | — |
| Widiger & Freiman | 50 | 3R | SI | I | PUB | PD | 70 |
| Zanarini | 253 | 3 | SI | MXD | MXD | PD | 55 |

*Note.* Tot-*n*, total *n* in sample; Nom, nomenclature (DSM-III [3], DSM-III-R [3R], or mixed [MXD]); Meth, methodology (semistructured interview [SI], unstructured clinical interview [CI], chart review [CT], or self-report interview [INV]); Loc, location (outpatient [O], inpatient [I], or mixed [MXD]); Int, institution (medical center [MC], Department of Veterans Affairs hospital [VA], private practice [PP], clinic [Cl], private hospital [PRH], or public hospital [PUB]); CompG, comparison group (personality disorders [PD], depressives [DEP], normals [NOR], drug abusers [DRG], bipolar affective disorders [BA], anxiety disorders [AN], schizotypals [SZT], narcissists [NAR], or mixed [MXD]); %M, percent male.

TABLE 7.2. Prototypicality Studies

| Study | Total *n* | Nature of sample | Metric |
|---|---|---|---|
| Hilbrand | 30 | MXD | % listed |
| Livesley | 938 | MD | M ratings |
| Blashfield | 61 | MXC/NAT | % coded |
| Burns | 467 | MD/SWEDE | % listed |

*Note.* MD, psychiatrists'; NAT, national sample; SWEDE, Swedish sample; MXD, mixed; % listed, percentage of subjects who included items; % coded, percent of subjects who coded items correctly; M rating, mean prototypicality rating.

TABLE 7.3. Percentage of Borderline Personality Disorder Patients with Other Personality Disorder Diagnoses

| Study | Criteria | n | ASPD | HPD | NPD | AVPD | STPD | SDPD |
|-------|----------|---|------|-----|-----|------|------|------|
| Dahl (1986)[a] | III | 38 | 68 | 61 | 5 | 3 | 45 | — |
| Pfohl (1986)[b] | III | 29 | 24 | 69 | 14 | 21 | 21 | — |
| Zanarini (1989)[c] | III | 179 | 46 | 62 | 24 | 24 | 40 | — |
| Morey (1988)[d] | III-R | 96 | 8 | 36 | 31 | 9 | 36 | — |
| Skodol (1988)[e] | III-R | 61 | 10 | 25 | 34 | 59 | 23 | 30 |
| Skodol (1988)[f] | III-R | 60 | 13 | 35 | 23 | 55 | 20 | 50 |
| Freiman & Widiger (1989)[g] | III-R | 17 | 59 | 24 | 29 | 59 | 35 | 24 |
| Millon & Tringone (1989)[d] | III-R | 118 | 7 | 124 | 7 | 9 | 3 | 19 |
| Millon & Tringone (1989)[h] | III-R | 95 | 2 | 12 | 2 | 12 | 9 | 22 |
| Millon & Tringone (1989)[i] | III-R | 40 | 20 | 15 | 5 | 25 | 3 | 38 |

Note. Key to personality disorder abbreviations: ASPD, antisocial; HPD, histrionic; NPD, narcissistic; AVPD, avoidant; STPD, schizotypal; SDPD, self-defeating.
[a]Diagnoses made with Schedule for Affective Disorders and Schizophrenia and the Personality Disorder Examination.
[b]Diagnoses made with the Structural Interview for Diagnosing Personality.
[c]Diagnoses made with Diagnostic Interviews for Personality Disorders.
[d]Diagnoses made by clinicians.
[e]Diagnoses made with Personality Disorder Examination.
[f]Diagnoses made with Structured Clinical Interview for DSM-III-R, Axis II.
[g]Diagnoses made with the Personality Interview Questionnaire.
[h]Diagnoses made via checklist.
[i]Diagnoses made with Millon Clinical Multiaxial Inventory.

for avoidant personality disorder. The high levels of overlap with avoidant personality disorder may be partly attributable to the change in a borderline personality disorder criterion (i.e., DSM-III's "intolerance of aloneness" [American Psychiatric Association, 1980] criterion for borderlin personality disorder may have been more able to distinguish borderline patients from avoidant ones than its DSM-III-R replacement "frantic efforts to avoid real or imagined abandonment" [see Table 7.7, below]). But the more likely causes for the increased overlap in DSM-III-R are the radical shifts that took place in the avoidant personality disorder conceptualization and criteria (Millon, 1991). Shifts in the avoidant criteria set have greatly enlarged the number of patients who meet its diagnostic requirements (Morey, 1988).

The assembled data were next examined from the "reverse overlap" perspective: That is, which other types of Axis II disorder are most frequently apt to fulfill criteria for borderline personality disorder as well? Despite much variation among studies, several generalizations emerge. The overlap with the other "dramatic cluster" (Cluster B) personality disorders (antisocial, narcissistic, and histrionic) was uniformly high; each category had borderline personality disorder among its top five overlapping Axis II conditions in seven or eight studies. Schizotypal personality disorder also frequently appeared, but in the lower rank of the top five, whereas when self-defeating personality disorder was assessed (it was absent in DSM-III), it usually appeared amongst the highest in overlap.

These studies on overlap with other Axis II disorders showed the Personality Disorders Work Group that DSM-IV might usefully sharpen the boundaries (i.e., improve the discriminability) of borderline personality disorder, and that this would be most important *vis-à-vis* the other Cluster B disorders and the avoidant, schizotypal, and self-defeating disorders.

The data sources shown in Tables 7.1 and 7.2 do not address the overlap of borderline personality disorder with Axis I. Yet a very extensive literature has arisen regarding the overlap of borderline personality disorder with mood disorders (Gunderson & Elliot, 1985; Gunderson & Phillips, 1991). This literature indicated to the work group that it would be useful if DSM-IV could more clearly distinguish the affective problems seen in borderline patients from those that belong on Axis I. Another conceptually complex overlap involves posttraumatic stress disorder (Gunderson & Sabo, 1993; Herman, Perry, & van der Kolk, 1989). Here too, it was felt that the DSM-IV criteria should aspire to help clinicians make this distinction.

## Are the Criteria Effective in Identifying the Disorder?

The many studies available to examine the diagnostic efficiency of specific criteria reveal a generally high profile of efficiency. This satisfactory performance by all of the criteria argues for a conservative approach to the consideration of change. Nonetheless, two other considerations — the overlap problems noted above, and the potential advantages of new criteria — give cause to examine each criterion's psychometric efficiency in more detail.

Item × diagnosis (criterion) analyses, in which each criterion is correlated with the later total score for its own diagnosis and all other diagnoses, help identify which of the borderline personality disorder criteria contribute most to the problem of diagnostic overlap (see Tables 7.4, 7.5, and 7.6). These analyses show that although several criteria contribute to the heavy overlap with Cluster B disorders, DSM-III-R criterion 3 ("affective instability . . . ") is especially problematic. Affective instability is very prevalent in borderline samples but lacks specificity. It contributes especially to diagnostic overlap with schizotypal and histrionic personality disorders, and, most dramatically, with the self-defeating disorder. Although similar item × diagnosis analyses are not available for the affective disorders, it seems very likely that criterion 3 also contributes to the overlap with depression and bipolar disorders. To retain the focus on affective instability but diminish these overlap problems, the criterion as reviesed (see Table 7.7, DSM-IV criterion 6) which continues to cite the presence of anxiety and irritability, but replaces "depression" with "dysphoria" and emphasizes that the affects are reactive.

TABLE 7.4. Phi Coefficients for DSM-III Borderline Personality Disorder Criteria

| Study | Sample size | UIR | IMP | AFF | ANG | PSD | IDD | EMP | INT |
|---|---|---|---|---|---|---|---|---|---|
| Clarkin et al. | 20 | .59 | .63 | .55 | .43 | .57 | .46 | .59 | .34 |
| Cowdry et al. | 59 | .14 | .66 | .35 | .40 | .42 | — | .57 | .32 |
| Dahl | 38 | .64 | .43 | .59 | .27 | .41 | .52 | .33 | .29 |
| Dubro et al. | 10 | .37 | .59 | .57 | .57 | .47 | .52 | .33 | .29 |
| Jacobsberg et al. | 22 | .18 | .14 | .30 | .33 | .46 | .20 | .16 | .28 |
| McGlashan & Fenton | 99 | .29 | .43 | .44 | .39 | .34 | .36 | .31 | .21 |
| Mallow & Donnelly | 38 | .56 | .29 | .57 | .56 | .41 | .50 | .43 | — |
| Modestin | 33 | .45 | .44 | .42 | .38 | .34 | .39 | .35 | .48 |
| Morey | 21 | .28 | .67 | .32 | .32 | .61 | .45 | .14 | .13 |
| Morey & Heumann | 97 | .50 | .52 | .50 | .35 | .54 | .47 | .55 | .42 |
| Nurnberg et al. | 17 | .84 | .84 | .46 | — | .56 | .68 | .56 | — |
| Pfohl et al. | 29 | .63 | .66 | .53 | .54 | .77 | .63 | .51 | .28 |
| Plakun | 44 | .30 | .52 | .36 | .35 | .36 | .35 | .30 | .34 |
| Spitzer et al. | 808 | .12 | .11 | .08 | .11 | .11 | .11 | .09 | .05 |
| Widiger et al. | 53 | .39 | .53 | .06 | .44 | .58 | .36 | .41 | .30 |
| Zanarini | 179 | .66 | .47 | .42 | .50 | .36 | .33 | .40 | .33 |

*Note.* Criteria abbreviations: UIR, unstable/intense relationships; IMP, impulsivity; AFF, affective instability; ANG, inappropriate/intense anger; PSD, physically self-damaging acts; IDD, identity disturbance; EMP, emptiness or boredom; INT, intolerance of being alone.

These changes should help differentiate the borderline's unstable affect from the mood lability seen in cyclothymic disorder, while also improving the discrimination between borderline patients and unipolar depressives.

## Do the Criteria Accurately Identify the Intended Constructs?

DSM-III-R criterion 6 ("marked and persistent identity disturbance...") has been found to be the least reliable criterion for assessment (Widiger & Frances, 1989). It has also been considered unclear and/or hard to assess by the *International Classification of Diseases* (ICD) representatives. It reads like Erikson's identity crisis of adolescence. In particular, vacillations in sexual

TABLE 7.5. Correlations between Individual Criteria and Total Criteria Scores in Prototypicality Studies Using DSM-III Criteria

| Study | Sample size | UIR | IMP | AFF | ANG | PSD | IDD | EMP | INT |
|---|---|---|---|---|---|---|---|---|---|
| Burns | 467 | — | .20 | — | .06 | .20 | .71 | .58 | — |
| Hilbrand | 30 | .73 | .50 | .70 | .60 | .53 | <.50 | .57 | <.50 |
| Livesley | 45 | 6.3 | 5.3 | 5.5 | 5.9 | 5.6 | 6.0 | 5.6/4.9 | 4.8 |

*Note.* Criteria abbreviations as in Table 7.4 footnote.

TABLE 7.6. Phi Coefficients for DSM-III-R Borderline Personality Disorder Criteria

| Study | Sample size | UIR | IMP | AFF | ANG | SCD | IDD | EMP | ABN |
|---|---|---|---|---|---|---|---|---|---|
| Millon & Tringone (1989) | 118 | .28 | .43 | .44 | .21 | .46 | .29 | .19 | .14 |
| Freiman & Widiger (1989) | 17 | .32 | .38 | .41 | .30 | .36 | .32 | .43 | .47 |
| Morey & Heumann (1988) | 97 | .51 | .52 | .51 | .36 | .50 | .48 | .53 | .41 |
| Blashfield (prototypicality study) | 61 | .79 | .75 | .73 | .50 | .84 | .80 | .84 | .45 |

*Note.* Criteria abbreviations as in Table 7.4 footnote, except PSD changed to SCD, recurrent suicidal threats, etc.; and INT changed to ABN, efforts to avoid abandonment.

orientation, goals, careers, values, and types of friends are all aspects of more general identity problems. Consistent with this conceptual broadness, item × diagnosis analyses show that it lacks specificity for borderline personality disorder. Although it is prevalent in borderline samples, it is also common in most other Axis II disorders, particularly the antisocial, narcissistic, and self-defeating disorders—categories where the need for better differentiation is documented. Thus it was considered a candidate for deletion in DSM-IV.

In favor of deletion was the fact that "caseness" would not be affected by removing this criterion, and, as we describe below, a strong candidate for a new criterion existed ("transient, stress-related paranoid ideation or severe dissociative symptoms"; see Table 7.7, DSM-IV criterion 9) that could replace it and offer better specificity. The reason for the inclusion of an identity criterion in DSM-III was its centrality in Kernberg's seminal description of "borderline personality organization" (e.g., Kernberg, 1967). Yet, consistent with the broad prevalence noted above, Kernberg's construct was intended to apply to all severe personality disorders. The argument for retaining identity disturbance as a criterion rested upon the question of whether it could be revised so as to improve its reliability and specificity. The eventual revision of the criterion (see Table 7.7, DSM-IV criterion 3) was derived from the clinical experience of the DSM-IV Personality Disorders Work Group and its expert advisors. The revision highlights the aspect of identity that is introduced as part of the essential features for borderline personality disorder (i.e., instability of self-image), and the accompanying text (American Psychiatric Association, 1994, p. 651) gives more specific examples. The revised criterion may thereby help to distinguish the identity problems of borderline patients from the identity problems found in other disorders and in adolescents. (The criterion as originally proposed was "identity disturbance: persistent and markedly disturbed, distorted, or unstable self-image and/or sense of self, e.g., feeling like one doesn't exist or embod-

TABLE 7.7. DSM-III-R and DSM-IV Diagnostic Criteria for Borderline Personality Disorder

| DSM-III-R criteria | DSM-IV criteria |
|---|---|
| A pervasive pattern of instability of mood, interpersonal relationships, and self-image, beginning by early adulthood and present in a variety of contexts, as indicated by at least *five* of the following: | A pervasive pattern of instability of interpersonal relationships, self-image, and affects, and marked impulsivity beginning by early adulthood and present in a variety of contexts, as indicated by five (or more) of the following: |
| (1) a pattern of unstable and intense interpersonal relationships characterized by alternating between extremes of overidealization and devaluation | (1) frantic efforts to avoid real or imagined abandonment. **Note:** Do not include suicidal or self-mutilating behavior covered in Criterion 5 |
| (2) impulsiveness in at least two areas that are potentially self-damaging, e.g., spending, sex, substance use, shoplifting, reckless driving, binge eating (Do not include suicidal or self-mutilating behavior covered in [5].) | (2) a pattern of unstable and intense interpersonal relationships characterized by alternating between extremes of idealization and devaluation |
| (3) affective instability: marked shifts from baseline mood to depression, irritability, or anxiety, usually lasting a few hours and only rarely more than a few days | (3) identity disturbance: markedly and persistently unstable self-image or sense of self |
| (4) inappropriate, intense anger or lack of control of anger, e.g., frequent displays of temper, constant anger, recurrent physical fights | (4) impulsivity in at least two areas that are potentially self-damaging (e.g., spending, sex, substance abuse, reckless driving, binge eating). **Note:** Do not include suicidal or self-mutilating behavior covered in Criterion 5. |
| (5) recurrent suicidal threats, gestures, or behavior, or self-mutilating behavior | (5) recurrent suicidal behavior, gestures, or threats, or self-mutilating behavior |
| (6) marked and persistent identity disturbance manifested by uncertainty about at least two of the following: self-image, sexual orientation, long-term goals or career choice, type of friends desired, preferred values | (6) affective instability due to a marked reactivity of mood (e.g., intense episodic dysphoria, irritability, or anxiety usually lasting a few hours and only rarely more than a few days) |
| (7) chronic feelings of emptiness or boredom | (7) chronic feelings of emptiness |
| (8) frantic efforts to avoid real or imagined abandonment (do not include suicidal or self-mutilating behavior covered in [5].) | (8) inappropriate, intense anger or difficulty controlling anger (e.g., frequent displays of temper, constant anger, recurrent physical fights) |
|  | (9) transient, stress-related paranoid ideation or severe dissociative symptoms |

*Note.* From APA (1987, pp. 347–348) and APA (1994, p. 654). Copyright 1987 and 1994 by the American Psychiatric Association. Reprinted by permission.

ies evil" [American Psychiatric Association, 1991, p. R:9]. However, this proved controversial — particularly the phrase "embodies evil" — and so the criterion was simplified as shown in Table 7.7.)

Another change made in DSM-IV involved dropping reference to chronic boredom from DSM-III-R criterion 7 (i.e., "chronic feelings of emptiness or boredom"). Boredom was initially linked to emptiness because they were combined into one characteristic in the original version of the Diagnostic Interview for Borderlines, which was shown to be discriminating (Gunderson & Kolb, 1978; Gunderson, Kolb, & Austin, 1981). It subsequently became clear to users of the Diagnostic Interview for Borderlines that boredom was not particularly useful. As a result, a specific analysis (comparing 43 borderline personality disorder patients to 58 patients with other personality disorders) was conducted. It revealed that emptiness was highly discriminating for the borderline personality disorder diagnosis ($p < .001$), whereas boredom was not (Zanarini, 1989). Because boredom is more prevalent in narcissistic or antisocial patients than in borderlines, its removal from the borderline criteria set should improve differentiation.

## Are the Criteria Congruent with the Descriptive Literature?

The centrality of brief psychotic regression experiences in seminal descriptions of borderlines (i.e., Friedman, 1973; Kernberg, 1967; Knight, 1953; Masterson, 1972; Zetzel, 1971) and empirical reports that these experiences are associated with a borderline diagnosis (Grinker, 1968; Gunderson & Kolb, 1978; Sheehy, Goldsmith, & Charles, 1980; Singer & Larsen, 1978) provided strong arguments for including this feature as a criterion in the DSM-III definition of borderline personality disorder. The decision to include stress-related psychotic symptoms only as an "associated feature" stirred controversy (Gunderson & Siever, 1979; Rosenthal, 1979; Spitzer & Endicott, 1979). Since then, multiple studies (see Table 7.8) have shown that cognitive/perceptual dysfunctions not only are common among borderline patients (most studies indicating about 75%), but statistically discriminate borderline patients from others (in six of the eight studies that had comparative prevalence rates). These studies show that dissociative experiences and nondelusional paranoia are the most common symptoms of this sort. Moreover, between about 20% and 40% of DSM-III or DSM-III-R borderlines experience transient, circumscribed, and/or atypical delusions and hallucinations (Silk, Lohr, Westen, & Goodrich, 1989; Widiger, Trull, Hurt, Clarkin, & Frances, 1987; Zanarini, Gunderson, & Frankenburg, 1990). This type of cognitive/perceptual dysfunction is nearly pathognomonic; that is, it is rarely found in any other diagnostic group (Zanarini, Gunderson, & Frankenburg, 1990; Zanarini, Gunderson, Frankenburg, & Chauncey, 1990). If borderline patients were found who experienced prolonged, widespread, and/or more bizarre delusions and hallucinations, it was attributable to a concurrent affective or sub-

TABLE 7.8. Prevalence of Cognitive/Perceptual Symptoms in Samples of Patients with Borderline Personality Disorder

| Cognitive/perceptual problem | Study[a] | Range |
|---|---|---|
| Depersonalization | 1,3,5,7,8,9 | 30–85% |
| Derealization | 1,3,4,7,8,9 | 30–92% |
| Paranoid experiences | 3,5,6,7,8,9 | 32–100% |
| Hopelessness/worthlessness | 3,7,8 | 77–88% |
| Visual illusions | 4,5,6,7,9 | 24–42% |
| Muddled thinking | 4 | 52% |
| Magical thinking | 5,6,9 | 34–68% |
| Ideas of reference | 5,6,9 | 49–74% |
| Odd speech | 5,6 | 30–59% |
| Disturbed thoughts | 2,9 | 39–68% |

[a]Key to study numbers:
   1. Frances et al. (1984)
   2. Pope et al. (1985)
   3. Chopra and Beatson (1986)
   4. George and Soloff (1986)
   5. Jacobsberg et al. (1986)
   6. Widiger et al. (1987)
   7. Links et al. (1989)
   8. Silk et al. (1989)
   9. Zanarini, Gunderson, & Frankenburg (1990)

stance use disorder (Pope, Jonas, Hudson, Cohen, & Tohen, 1985; Zanarini, Gunderson, & Frankenburg, 1990).

This literature shows that borderline patients have cognitive/perceptual problems that can be distinguished from the psychotic experiences found in other diagnostic groups. This empirical evidence for the diagnostic efficiency of such a feature joined the fact of its clinical importance (i.e., failures in reality testing) to support the addition of a cognitive/perceptual criterion to the borderline personality disorder definition. Indeed, when asked about such an addition, 15 of the 21 advisors endorsed this plan. Most of the advocates, in line with the arguments by Gunderson (1979, 1984) and Frosch (1988), felt strongly that this feature is central to the borderline construct and that its addition would helpfully capture one of the most discriminating features and thereby diminish the current confusion over usage of this diagnosis.

The controversy surrounding the addition of such a criterion is reflected in reactions from the remaining six advisors. Notably, none were contributors to the pre-DSM-III literature on this subject upon which the construct was established. Two objected because this feature did not conform to their concept or usage of borderline personality disorder. The other four objected because they felt that better empirical substantiation was needed. The most telling empirical objection was that the cognitive/perceptual disturbances seen in borderline patients may be caused by comorbid schizotypal personality disorder. This argument is supported by the fact that all four studies comparing "pure" borderlines to those who were "mixed" (borderline plus schizotypal) and/or to "pure" schizotypals found that the "pure" borderlines had fewer cognitive difficulties than either the "mixed" patients or the "pure" schizotypal patients (George & Soloff, 1986; McGlashan, 1987; Perry, 1988; Widiger et al., 1987). Yet the comorbidity rate between borderline and schizotypal personality disorders in these four studies was significantly increased (i.e., 6–55%, with the range in the three non-chart-review studies being 38–55%) because they used DSM-III and not DSM-III-R criteria. The comorbidity for schizotypal personality disorder in borderlines was significantly lowered (to between 7% and 20%) when DSM-III-R criteria replaced DSM-III criteria (Morey, 1988; Vaglum, Friis, Vaglum, & Larsen, 1989; Silk, Westen, Lohr, Benjamin, & Gold, 1990).

Two initiatives were undertaken to address the issue of whether the cognitive/perceptual problems observed in borderline patients can be differentiated from those seen in schizotypal personality disorder. First, a series of vignettes describing the cognitive/perceptual problems of either "pure" borderline or "pure" schizotypal patients was solicited and subjected to careful ratings by clinicians (Sternbach, Judd, Sabo, McGlashen, & Gunderson, 1992). The results indicated that the borderline personality disorder sample had more dissociative experiences, and generally more transient and interpersonally reactive perceptual distortions. The second initiative was a multisite field trial to assess prospectively whether the DSM-IV modifications in criteria for the cognitive/perceptual problems of schizotypals (i.e., ideas of reference, odd beliefs, and unusual percepts) make them more distinct from those observed in borderline personality disorder (Siever, & Zanarini, 1991). The results show that the DSM-IV changes in the schizotypal criteria will modestly diminish their association with borderline personality disorder. Unfortunately, this study did not examine how the changes to the borderline personality disorder criteria in DSM-IV will affect the overlap with schizotypal personality disorder. Insofar as these disorders overlap because of a shared underlying biogenetic disposition to cognitive/perceptual dysfunctions (Kavoussi & Siever, 1992), it may be that further efforts to sharpen their descriptive distinctions are unwarranted.

## Are the Polythetic Format and Diagnostic Threshold Appropriate?

The generally high diagnostic efficiency of all eight of the borderline criteria in both the DSM-III and DSM-III-R data sets is impressive. The high quality of the criteria is also reflected in the series of studies reporting that a smaller set of criteria, three to five, can attain the same efficiency as the entire set of eight (McGlashan & Fenton, 1990; Nurnberg, Hurt, Feldman, & Suh, 1987; Reich, 1990). Regrettably, since the preferred subgroup of criteria found in each of these studies was different, they failed to distinguish certain core criteria that should receive heavier weighting. These results support the retention of a polythetic format for the borderline criteria set. This corresponds with the current era of diverse theories about the nature of that core feature. The results also indicate that dropping any criterion would have little affect on "caseness."

A recent study indicates that the overlap with other personality disorders could be reduced by increasing the diagnostic threshold from five to six criteria (Zanarini, Gunderson, Frankenburg, Chauncey, & Glutting, 1991). However, this change still seems imprudent without replication, in view of the fact that the diagnostic threshold for this category has been one of the very few derived from empirical results. Yet the addition of a ninth criterion in DSM-IV without an increase in the threshold may fail to give this diagnosis the desired specificity that is intended.

## Should the Essential Feature Be Altered?

The essential feature identified in DSM-III-R is a "pervasive pattern of instability of mood, interpersonal relationships, and self-image." Nineteen experts responded to the request for a critique of it. A minority of the advisors favored a proposed alternative essential feature: "fear of and angry intolerance for being alone. [Typically this fear leads to behavioral markers such as the repetitive use of self-destructiveness, substance abuse, promiscuity, and other desperate impulsive actions]." Those who favored this alternative did so because it offers more explanation for the interrelationship of the descriptive characteristics (Adler, 1985; Gunderson, 1984; Masterson, 1971); because it conveys more meaning in terms of both etiology and treatment; and because it could usefully help differentiate borderline personality disorder from posttraumatic stress disorder, narcissistic personality disorder, and depression. Nonetheless, the majority of the advisors felt that the emphasis in the DSM-III-R definition on instability links it with an a theoretical descriptive tradition; that it is satisfactorily apt; and that its change should await empirical validation of what is "core."

Yet the essential feature should correspond with what the empirical evidence indicates is central to diagnosis. As noted earlier, the DSM-III-R essential feature highlights three criteria, two of which (i.e., those pertaining to unstable self-image and mood) were found to be problematic criteria where revisions were proposed for DSM-IV (i.e., DSM-III-R criteria and 6), because they lacked specificity and/or reliability. Criterion 6 was even considered for omission. Moreover, there is growing evidence that dyscontrol over impulses (as reflected in DSM-III-R criteria 2, 4, and 5) may be more "essential" to this diagnosis than mood (Gunderson & Zanarini, 1989; Coccaro, Siever, Klar, Maurer, & Cochrane, 1989; Nurnberg et al., 1991; Zanarini, 1993). As such, impulsivity has been added to the essential feature in DSM-IV.

## DISCUSSION

The generally good performance of all the DSM-III-R criteria for borderline personality disorder does little to resolve the competing claims for intolerance of aloneness, excessive aggression, affective instability, impulsivity, or interpersonal instability as the central organizing dysfunction that defines this personality type. The new DSM-IV definition provides a platform from which the validity of these competing claimants can and should be tested. Clearly, the extensive descriptive literature should now be supplemented by an equally extensive turn toward methodologically sophisticated studies that will demonstrate how alterations in the criteria will improve or diminish the predictive power with regard to such meaningful external validators.

Existing studies highlight the need to sharpen the boundaries between borderline personality disorder and other diagnoses. Multiple diagnoses are accepted in DSM-III-R, but the extent of overlap is problematic to establishing their validity, and it clearly does not reflect clinical practice (Dahl, 1986; Morey, 1988; Pfohl et al., 1986; Zanarini, Frankenburg, Chauncery, & Gunderson, 1987). More specifically, the results point to the value of increasing the differentiation of borderline personality disorder from other "dramatic cluster" disorders and from the schizotypal and self-defeating disorders. Less obvious in this review, but apparent to most readers of the literature, is the need to clarify the boundaries between of borderline personality disorder and recurrent and labile mood disorders (Akiskal et al., 1985; Gunderson & Elliot, 1985). DSM-IV criteria 6 and 7 are designed to achieve this objectives.

The addition of criterion 9 is expected to be useful to clinicians and to reduce overlap with other disorders. Yet, despite the overwhelming consensus of the advisors and its imposing empirical support, this revision has been the most controversial. Because it touches upon the nature of the borderline construct itself, there is an ongoing effort to investigate the issues empirically.

Another disorder whose boundary with borderline personality disorder is becoming an important conceptual and perhaps clinical issue is post-traumatic stress disorder (Herman et al., 1989; Ogata, Silk, & Goodrich, 1990; Gunderson & Sabo, 1993). Because trauma can readily account for the needy dependency, disoriented and unstable self identity, and self-destructiveness associated with borderline personality disorder, this boundary involves questions of how personality development is conceptualized. The next generation of research will undoubtedly clarify both the conceptualization and the criteria by which this boundary can be distinguished.

This review should be understood within its historical perspective. Borderline personality is a recent addition to psychiatric nosology. It has engendered far more study than any other new category, and in some respects more than all the other old categories combined. It represents a creative melding of psychiatry's dynamic traditions with its newer empiricism. Yet this chapter suggests that this empirical development has not altogether mirrored the disorder's clinical base. This category began with conceptualizations of what causes clinically troublesome signs and symptoms to co-occur. Now that the disorder is defined by what is expected to be a representative listing of those signs and symptoms on whose basis the disorder was conceptualized, research into etiology and treatment will necessarily be confounded by the accuracy of their selection and the quality of their description. We are concerned that the diagnosis of borderline personality disorder is now overused and that the DSM-III and DSM-III-R definitions may have contributed to this overuse. Insofar as the revisions made in DSM-IV help to anchor this category's definition by emphasizing its connection with core problems with impulse regulation and childhood abuse, they should help to define a more discrete and specific diagnostic entity.

## ACKNOWLEDGMENT

Appreciation is due to Drs. Freiman, Goodman, Millon, Morey, Skodol, Tringone, Trull, Widiger, and Zanarini for providing access to their unpublished data.

## REFERENCES

Adler, G. (1985). *Borderline psychopathology and its treatment.* New York: Jason Aronson.

Akiskal, H. S., Chen, S. E., Davis, G. C., Puzantian, V. R., Kashgarian, M., & Bolinger, J. M. (1985). Borderline: An adjective in search of a noun. *Journal of Clinical Psychiatry, 46,* 41–48.

American Psychiatric Association. (1980). *Diagnostic and statistical manual of mental disorders* (3rd ed.). Washington, DC: Author.

American Psychiatric Association. (1987). *Diagnostic and statistical manual of mental disorders* (3rd ed., rev.). Washington, DC: Author.

American Psychiatric Association. (1991). *DSM-IV options book: Work in progress.* Washington, DC: Author.

American Psychiatric Association. (1994). *Diagnostic and statistical manual of mental disorders* (4th ed.). Washington, DC: Author.

Coccaro, E. F., Siever, L. J., Klar, H. M., Maurer, G., & Cochrane, K. (1989). Serotonergic studies in patients with affective and personality disorders: Correlates with suicidal and impulsive aggressive behavior. *Archives of General Psychiatry, 46,* 587–599.

Dahl, A. (1986). Some aspects of the DSM-III personality disorders illustrated by a consecutive sample of hospitalized patients. *Acta Psychiatrica Scandinavica, 73*(Suppl. 328), 61–66.

Friedman, H. (1975). Psychotherapy of borderline patients: Influences of theory and technique. *American Journal of Psychiatry, 132,* 1048–1052.

Freiman, K., & Widiger, T. (1989). [Co-occurrence and diagnostic efficiency statistics]. Unpublished raw data.

Frosch, J. (1988). Psychotic character versus borderline (Part 1). *International Journal of Psycho-Analysis, 69,* 347–357.

George, A., & Soloff, P. (1986). Schizotypal symptoms in patients with borderline personality disorders. *American Journal of Psychiatry, 143,* 313–215.

Grinker, R. (1968). *The borderline syndrome.* New York: Basic Books.

Gunderson, J. G. (1979). The relatedness of borderline and schizophrenic disorders. *Schizophrenic Bulletin, 5*(1), 17–22.

Gunderson, J. G. (1984). *Borderline personality disorder.* Washington, DC: American Psychiatric Press.

Gunderson, J. G., & Elliot, G. (1985). The interface between borderline personality and affective disorder. *American Journal of Psychiatry, 142,* 277–288.

Gunderson, J. G., & Kolb, J. E. (1978). Discriminating features of borderline patients. *American Journal of Psychiatry, 135,* 792–796.

Gunderson, J. G., Kolb, J. E., & Austin, V. (1981). The Diagnostic Interview for Borderline Patients. *American Journal of Psychiatry, 138,* 896–903.

Gunderson, J. G., & Phillips, K. A. (1991). Borderline personality disorder and depression: A current overview of the interface. *American Journal of Psychiatry, 148,* 967–975.

Gunderson, J. G., & Sabo, A. (1993). Borderline personality disorder and PTSD: Conceptual, phenomenologic, and treatment distinctions. *American Journal of Psychiatry, 150,* 19–27.

Gunderson, J. G., & Zanarini, M. C. (1987). Current overview of the borderline diagnosis. *Journal of Clinical Psychiatry, 48*(8), 5–11.

Gunderson, J. G., & Zanarini, M. C. (1989). Pathogenesis of borderline personality, In A. J. Frances, R. E. Hales, & A. Tasman (Eds.), *Review of psychiatry* (Vol. 8). Washington, DC: American Psychiatric Press.

Herman, J., Perry, C., & van der Kolk, B. (1989). Childhood trauma in borderline personality disorder. *American Journal of Psychiatry, 146,* 490–495.

Kavoussi, R. J., & Siever, L. J. (1992). Overlap between borderline and schizotypal personality disorders. *Comprehensive Psychiatry, 33*(1), 7–12.

Kernberg, O. (1967). Borderline personality organization. *Journal of the American Psychoanalytic Association, 15,* 641–685.

Knight, R. (1953). Borderline states. *Bulletin of the Menninger Clinic, 17,* 1–12.

Masterson, J. (1971). Treatment of the adolescent with borderline syndrome (a problem in separation–individuation). *Bulletin of the Menninger Clinic, 35,* 5–18.

Masterson, J. (1972). *Treatment of the borderline adolescent: A developmental approach.* New York: Wiley.

McGlashan, T. H. (1987). Testing DSM-III symptom criteria for schizotypal and borderline personality disorders. *Archives of General Psychiatry, 44,* 143–148.

McGlashan, T. H., & Fenton, W. (1990). Diagnostic efficiency of DSM-III borderline personality disorder and schizotypal disorder. In J. Oldham (Ed.), *Personality disorders: New perspectives on diagnostic validity.* Washington, DC: American Psychiatric Press.

Millon, T. (1991). Avoidant personality disorder: A brief review of issues and data. *Journal of Personality Disorders, 5,* 353–362.

Millon, T., & Tringone, R. (1989). [Co-occurrence and diagnostic efficiency statistics]. Unpublished raw data.

Morey, L. C. (1988). Personality disorders in DSM-III and DSM-III-R: An examination of convergence, coverage, and internal consistency. *American Journal of Psychiatry, 145,* 573–577.

Morey, L. C., & Heumann, K. (1988). [Co-occurence and diagnostic efficiency statistics]. Unpublished raw data.

Nurnberg, H. G., Hurt, S., Feldman, A., & Suh, R. (1987). Efficient diagnosis of borderline personality dsorder. *Journal of Personality Disorders, 1*, 307–315.

Nurnberg, H. G., Raskin, M., Levine, P. E., Pollack, S., Siegel, O., & Prince, R. (1991). The co-morbidity of borderline personality disorder and other DSM-III-R Axis II personality disorders. *American Journal of Psychiatry, 148*, 1371–1377.

Ogata, S., Silk, K., & Goodrich, S. (1990). The childhood experience of the borderline patient. In P. Links (Ed.), *The family environment and borderline personality disorder*. Washington, DC: American Psychiatric Press.

Perry, J. C. (1988). A prospective study of life stress, defenses, psychotic symptoms, and depression in borderline and antisocial personality disorders and bipolar type II affective disorder. *Journal of Personality Disorders, 2*, 49–59.

Pfohl, B., Coryell, W., Zimmerman, M., & Stangl, D. (1986). DSM-III personality disorders: Diagnostic overlap and internal consistency of individual DSM-III criteria. *Comprehensive Psychiatry, 27*, 21–34.

Pope, H., Jonas, J., Hudson, J., Cohen, B., & Tohen, M. (1985). An empirical study of psychosis in borderline personality disorder. *American Journal of Psychiatry, 142*, 1285–1290.

Reich, J. (1990). Criteria for diagnosing DSM-III borderline personality disorders. *Annals of Clinical Psychiatry, 2*, 189–197.

Rosenthal, D. (1979). Was Thomas Wolfe a borderline? *Schizophrenia Bulletin, 5*, 87–94.

Sheehy, M., Goldsmith, L., & Charles, E. (1980). A comparative study of borderline patients in a psychiatric outpatient clinic. *American Journal of Psychiatry, 376*, 1374–1379.

Siever, L., & Gunderson, J. G. (1979). Genetic determinants of borderline conditions. *Schizophrenia Bulletin, 1*, 59–86.

Siever, L., & Zanarini, M. C. (1991). *DSM-IV field trials for schizotypal personality disorder*. Unpublished manuscript.

Silk, K., Lohr, N., Westen, D., & Goodrich, S. (1989). Psychosis in borderline patients with depression. *Journal of Personality Disorders, 3*, 92–100.

Silk, K., Westen, D., Lohr, N., Benjamin, J., & Gold, L. (1990). DSM-III and DSM-III-R schizotypal symptoms in borderline personality disorder. *Comprehensive Psychiatry, 31*, 103–110.

Singer, M., & Larson, D. (1981). Borderline personality and the Rorschach test. *Archives of General Psychiatry, 38*, 693–702.

Skodol, A., Rosnick, L., Kellman, D., Oldham, J. M., & Hyler, S. E. (1988). Validating structured DSM-III-R personality disorder assessments with longitudinal data. *American Journal of Psychiatry, 145*, 1297–1299.

Skodol, A., Rosnick, L., & Kellman, D. (1988). *The validity of structured assessments of Axis II*. Paper presented at the 141st Annual Meeting of the American Psychiatric Association, Montreal.

Skodol, A., & Spitzer, R. (Eds.). (1987). *An annotated bibliography of DSM-III*. Washington, DC: American Psychiatric Press.

Spitzer, R., & Endicott, J. (1979). Justification for separating schizotypal and borderline personality disorders. *Schizophrenia Bulletin, 5*, 95-104.

Spitzer, R., Endicott, J., & Gibbon, M. (1979). Crossing the border into borderline personality and borderline schizophrenia: The development of criteria. *Archives of General Psychiatry, 36*, 17–24.

Sternbach, S., Judd, A., Sabo, A., McGlashen, T., & Gunderson, J. G. (1992). Cognitive and perceptual distortions in borderline personality disorder and schizotypal personality disorder in a vignette sample. *Comprehensive Psychiatry, 33,* 186–189.

Vaglum, P., Friis, S., Vaglum, S., & Larsen, F. (1981). Comparison between personality disorder diagnoses in DSM-III and DSM-III-R: Reliability, diagnostic overlap, predictive validity. *Psychopathology, 22,* 309–314.

Widiger, T. A., & Frances, A. J. (1987). Interviews and inventories for the measurement of personality disorders. *Clinical Psychology Review, 7,* 49–75.

Widiger, T. A., & Frances, A.J. (1989). Epidemiology, diagnosis and comorbidity of borderline personality disorder. In A. J. Frances, R. E. Hales, & A. Tasman (Eds.), *Review of psychiatry* (Vol. 8). Washington, DC: American Psychiatric Press.

Widiger, T., Sanderson, C., & Warner, L. (1986). The MMPI, prototypal typology, and borderline personality disorder. *Journal of Personality Assessment, 50,* 540–553.

Widiger, T. A., Trull, T., Hurt, S., Clarkin, J. F., & Frances, A. J. (1987). A multidimensional scaling of the DSM-III personality disorders. *Archives of General Psychiatry, 44,* 557–563.

Zanarini, M. C. (1989). [Co-occurrence and diagnostic efficiency statistics]. Unpublished raw data.

Zanarini, M. C. (1993). Borderline personality disorder as an impulse spectrum disorder. In J. Paris (Ed.), *Borderline personality disorder: Etiology and treatment* (pp. 67–85). Washington, DC: American Psychiatric Press.

Zanarini, M. C., Frankenburg, F. R., Chauncey, D. L., & Gunderman, J. G. (1987). The Diagnostic Interview for Personality Disorders: Interrater and test–retest reliability. *Comprehensive Psychiatry, 28,* 467–480.

Zanarini, M. C., Gunderson, J. G., & Frankenburg, F. R. (1990). Cognitive features of borderline personality disorder. *American Journal of Psychiatry, 147,* 57–63.

Zanarini, M. C., Gunderson, J. G., Frankenburg, F. R., & Chauncey, D. L. (1990b). Discriminating borderline personality disorder from other Axis II disorders. *American Journal of Psychiatry, 147,* 161–167.

Zanarini, M. C., Gunderson, J. G., Frankenburg, F. R., Chauncey, D. L., & Glutting, B. A. (1991). The validity of the DSM-III and DSM-III-R criteria sets for borderline personality disorder. *American Journal of Psychiatry, 148,* 870–874.

Zetzel, E. (1971). A developmental approach to the borderline patient. *American Journal of Psychiatry, 128,* 867–871.

# Commentary on Borderline Personality Disorder

Alv A. Dahl

Borderline personality disorder has been conceptualized in various ways, which influenced the way the disorder was defined in DSM-III (American Psychiatric Association, 1980) and D⁻M-III-R (American Psychiatric Association, 1987) (see Dahl, 1985; Widiger, Miele, & Tilly, 1992). When DSM-IV (American Psychiatric Assocation, 1994) was developed, three stages of empirical documentation (Frances, Pincus, Widiger, Davis, & First, 1990) were required for all disorders: (1) a comprehensive and systematic review of the published literature; (2) reanalyses of the existing data sets; and (3) field trials to assess the proposed revisions. In Chapter 7, Gunderson, Zanarini, and Kisiel address the first two issues and consider the following basic issues: "how to reconcile the value of sustaining a definition of borderline personality disorder that has now received partial validation with the value of modifications that might better reflect the borderline personality disorder construct" (p. 141). They ask six questions that I comment on below, but let me start with the conclusion: Basically, few changes in the diagnostic criteria set for borderline personality disorder have been made in DSM-IV, and changes to the essential features, have been minimal. The same is true for the individual criteria pertaining to impulsivity, interpersonal relationships, anger, suicidality/self-mutilation, and efforts to avoid abandonment. The criteria pertaining to identity disturbance and affective instability have been reformulated; boredom has been dropped from the criteria pertaining to feelings of emptiness; and a criterion covering transient, stress-related cognitive/perceptual symptoms has been added.

## IS THE DIAGNOSIS DISTINCT FROM OTHER DISORDERS?

Chapter 7 has disclosed that in various studies, borderline personality disorder was rarely the only personality disorder diagnosis a patient received.

When DSM-III criteria were used, borderline personality disorder most frequently overlapped with histrionic personality disorder. The revision of criteria in DSM-III-R reduced this overlap and that with antisocial personality disorder. On the other hand, the overlap with schizotypal and avoidant personality disorder changed less. It is an open question whether rearrangement and rewording of criteria can really make borderline personality disorder a distinct diagnosis because of underlying basic personality dimensions (Grove & Tellegen, 1991). Gunderson and colleagues state that DSM-IV should improve the discriminability of borderline personality disorder versus other personality disorder diagnoses, but it is hard to see how this can be achieved, given the moderate changes to the criteria set. Behind the descriptive diagnoses, there is also a level of hampered ego functioning that borderline personality disorder has in common with the other Cluster B and the Cluster A disorders, and that makes increased discrimination problematic.

An extensive overlap of borderline personality disorder with Axis I disorders, especially mood disorders, has also been demonstrated (Gunderson & Phillips, 1991). It would have been useful if DSM-IV had more clearly distinguished the affective problems seen in patients with borderline personality disorder from those seen in patients with Axis I mood disorders. The actual DSM-IV criteria hardly achieve this result. The difference between a chronic feeling of emptiness in borderline personality disorder and the feeling of worthlessness or excessive or inappropriate guilt in major depression is an example of specification of criteria that should have been carried further in DSM-IV.

As Gunderson and colleagues state, there is a conceptually complex overlap between borderline personality disorder and posttraumatic stress disorder (PTSD). The occurrence of intrusive recollections, avoidance, and increased arousal in patients with borderline personality disorder has not been systematically studied. Such a study would be of interest, because a history of sexual and physical abuse is common in women with PTSD and borderline personality disorder. The obvious question is this: What predisposes individuals to develop PTSD and borderline personality disorder respectively?

## ARE THE CRITERIA EFFECTIVE
## IN IDENTIFYING THE DISORDER?

Chapter 7 confirms that the DSM-III-R criteria for borderline personality disorder are efficient in identifying a disorder. Although the affective instability criterion is problematic, the introduction in DSM-IV of the nebulous concept of "marked reactivity of mood" (American Psychiatric Association, 1994, p. 654), although possibly helpful in relation to Axis I mood disorder, does not seem helpful in regard to the other personality disorders. As pointed out by Millon (1981), "marked reactivity" is a basic feature of the personality disorders, compared to the normal personality's ability to demonstrate smooth mastery and competence under stress.

Although the chapter points to the high diagnostic efficiency of all DSM-III-R borderline personality disorder criteria, it does not touch on the idea that specific criteria are either necessary or sufficient to diagnose borderline personality disorder. Hurt and colleagues (1990) reported that the presence of three of four criteria (those pertaining to impulsivity, unstable interpersonal relationships, affective instability, and identity disturbance) was adequate to diagnose borderline personality disorder in inpatients. I have reported similar results, except that the criterion describing emptiness or boredom performed better than the one describing unstable relationships (Dahl, 1987).

## DO THE CRITERIA ACCURATELY IDENTIFY THE INTENDED CONSTRUCTS?

Identity disturbance is the least reliable component of the DSM-III-R borderline personality disorder concept. This emphasizes the difference between developing observable behavioral criteria (e.g, the one for recurring suicidal threats) and subjectively experienced ones (e.g., the ones for identity disturbance or chronic feelings of emptiness). It also brings up the question of the informant's role in making valid diagnoses of a personality disorder. DSM-IV still relies only on self-report and the interviewer's interpretation, and not on confirmation by an informant (see Tyrer, Chapter 2, this volume). The DSM classification system from DSM-III on has never really made the basic distinction between ego-syntonic and ego-dystonic features when compiling the diagnostic criteria for personality disorders. "Frantic efforts to avoid real or imagined abandonment" (retained in DSM-IV as criterion 1; American Psychiatric Assóciaion, 1994, p. 654) for example, can be a highly ego-syntonic type of behavior, which can really only be judged validly by an informant.

The identity disturbance criterion is one that has been repeatedly reformulated since DSM-III. Identity diffusion is essential to Kernberg's (1967) concept of "borderline personality organization" which embraces all the severe personality disorders of Clusters A and B. As pointed out by Akhtar (1984), Kernberg's concept of identity diffusion is quite broad and concerns both self and object. Sexual orientation, long-term goals, types of friends preferred, and preferred values all refer to repression of both self and object. When DSM-IV defines identity disturbance only in terms of self-image and sense of self, the concept is considerably narrowed and brought closer to the self pathology of narcissistic disorders.

## ARE THE CRITERIA CONGRUENT
## WITH THE DESCRIPTIVE LITERATURE?

The inclusion of a criterion covering brief regressive psychotic experiences in the criteria set for borderline personality disorder fulfills the long-held opinion of Gunderson (1984), and is the only major innovation for borderline personality disorder in DSM-IV. This is a radical step taken by the Personality Disorders Work Group, but it is a controversial one. The conceptual issue is whether psychotic symptoms are an inherent part of the borderline personality disorder concept or constitute an associated feature. According to the work group, the pervasive pattern of instability that is the essential feature of borderline personality disorder also pertains to reality testing. However, the group only describes "paranoid ideation and severe dissociative symptoms" (American Psychiatric Association, 1994, p. 654) as examples of impaired reality testing. It is unclear what is meant by "severe dissociative symptoms," since these include amnesia, fugue, and depersonalization as well as multiple personality disorder in the DSM-IV section on dissociative disorders. There is also a need for specification of the pervasive pattern of severe dissociative symptoms and paranoid ideation reactions; the trait–state distinction is not clear here.

An alternative definition of DSM-IV borderline personality disorder criterion 9 that would include instability of reality testing would be the following: "Reality testing instability: transient, stress-related impairment of reality testing shown as brief episodes of psychotic symptoms (hallucinations, delusions, thought disorder, or confusion)."

My own study (Dahl, 1987) of hospitalized patients showed that brief psychotic episodes occurred significantly more frequently in patients with schizotypal personality disorder than in those with borderline personality disorder (67% vs. 24%, respectively), while patients with combined schizotypal and borderline personality disorders were in between (59%). In my experience, psychotic episodes are particularly frequent after abrupt losses or long-term substance abuse in all severe personality disorders, not just borderline personality disorder. Besides paranoid ideation, auditory hallucinations of less than 1 week's duration were significantly more frequent in borderline personality disorder and/or in other personality disorders in my study. Other investigators have also taken a reserved stance as to whether the borderline personality disorder concept would be improved by including brief psychotic episodes as a criterion (Widiger et al., 1992).

## ARE THE POLYTHETIC FORMAT
## AND DIAGNOSTIC THRESHOLDS APPROPRIATE?

DSM's polythetic format for diagnosis, with multiple optional criteria, creates considerable heterogeneity among patients with a borderline diagnosis.

No rules are given in DSM-IV for coding this heterogeneity. As Reich (1992) points out, several studies indicate that a combination of two or three borderline personality disorder criteria gives a high degree of diagnostic accuracy. This suggests that the cutoff level could be reduced to four criteria without false negatives. However, this would mean that the total number of criteria would have to be reduced to seven, to avoid the possibility that some borderline patients would have no criteria in common.

## SHOULD THE ESSENTIAL FEATURE BE ALTERED?

The essential feature should be consistent with empirical evidence regarding the central feature of the diagnosis. This evidence seems to indicate clearly that instability is the central feature of borderline personality disorder, and that this should be reflected in all the criteria. Chronic feelings of emptiness constitue a stable rather than an unstable pattern, even though such feelings often lead to impulsiveness. Efforts to avoid abandonment also seem to contradict the instability of interpersonal relationships, since such efforts represent a pervasive pattern of clinging behavior. Thus, because there is a consensus that instability is the essential feature of borderline personality disorder, these two criteria should be reconsidered for their failure to fit that feature.

## SOME EMPIRICAL ISSUES NOT ADDRESSED IN CHAPTER 7

Several important issues concerning borderline personality disorder are not touched on in Chapter 7, although relevant data exist. One is the issue of whether equal diagnostic weight should be assigned to all criteria. DSM-IV follows this principle, although the borderline personality disorder criteria differ considerably in diagnostic efficiency. Differential weighting would obviously create problems for busy clinicians, but for research differential weights could be important. The chapter also only considers the criteria in the context of cross-sectional diagnosis of borderline personality disorder. There are data, however, on the temporal stability of the borderline personality disorder criteria that are relevant to the issue of revision (Grueneich, 1992).

Finally, Gunderson and colleagues evaluate the efficiency of the diagnostic criteria for borderline personality disorder without considering the basic issue of whether borderline personality disorder as defined by DSM-III and DSM-III-R really is a valid disorder or whether alternative conceptualizations are appropriate. Elsewhere (Dahl, 1990), I have argued for a broad borderline concept that includes all severe personality disorders (Clusters A and B); this is similar to Kernberg's (1967) concept of borderline personality organization.

## THE RELATIONSHIP TO ICD-10

The creators of the 10th revision of the *International Classification of Diseases* (ICD-10; World Health Organization, 1992) originally did not think of borderline personality disorder as a valid diagnosis. Considerable pressure from several quarters, however, led to the diagnosis of "emotionally unstable personality disorder, borderline type." The description of that disorder contains all the DSM-IV borderline personality disorder criteria except for brief psychotic episodes. The overlap between the DSM-IV and ICD-10 concepts of borderline personality disorder remains to be studied.

## CONCLUSIONS

Again, Gunderson et al. state in Chapter 7 that borderline personality disorder "has now received partial validation." In my view, face validity and procedural validity have been demonstrated. Some family studies of borderline personality disorder have supported construct validity (Dahl, 1993), but that is all. Considerable research has shown that borderline personality disorder overlaps with other personality disorders and with mood disorders. Thus the amount of nonredundant information provided by a borderline personality disorder diagnosis is still modest. If borderline personality disorder is to survive in DSM-V, more construct and predictive validity must be demonstrated by the DSM-IV concept.

## REFERENCES

Akhtar, S. (1984). The syndrome of identity diffusion. *American Journal of Psychiatry, 141,* 381–1385.

American Psychiatric Association. (1980). *Diagnostic and statistical manual of mental disorders* (3rd ed.). Washington, DC: Author.

American Psychiatric Association. (1987). *Diagnostic and statistical manual of mental disorders* (3rd ed., rev.). Washington, DC: Author.

American Psychiatric Association. (1994). *Diagnostic and statistical manual of mental disorders* (4th ed.). Washington, DC: Author.

Dahl, A. (1985). A critical examination of empirical studies of the diagnosis of borderline disorders in adults. *Psychiatric Developments, 3,* 1–29.

Dahl, A. (1987). *Borderline disorders: A comparative study of hospitalized patients.* Oslo: Faculty of Medicine, University of Oslo.

Dahl, A. (1990). Empirical evidence for a core borderline syndrome. *Journal of Personality Disorders, 4,* 192–202.

Dahl, A. (1993). The personality disorders: A critical review of family, twin, and adoption studies. *Journal of Personality Disorders, 7*(Suppl.), 86–99.

Frances, A., Pincus, H., Widiger, T., Davis, W., & First, M. (1990). DSM-IV: Work in progress. *American Journal of Psychiatry, 147,* 1439–1448.

Grove, W., & Tellegen, A. (1991). Problems in the classification of personality dis-
orders. *Journal of Personality Disorders, 5,* 31–41.
Grueneich, R. (1992). The borderline personality disorder diagnosis: Reliability, di-
agnostic efficiency, and covariation with other personality disorder diagnoses.
*Journal of Personality Disorders, 6,* 197–212.
Gunderson, J. (1984). *Borderline personality disorder.* Washington, DC: American Psy-
chiatric Press.
Gunderson, J., & Phillips, K. (1991). Borderline personality disorders and depression:
A current overview of the interface. *American Journal of Psychiatry, 148,* 967–975.
Hurt, S., Clarkin, J., Widiger, T., Fyer, M., Sullivan, T., Stone, M. H., & Frances, A.
(1990). Evaluation of DSM-III decision rules for case detection using joint con-
ditional probability structures. *Journal of Personality Disorders, 4,* 121–130.
Kernberg, O. (1967). Borderline personality organization. *Journal of the American Psychoanalytic Association, 15,* 641–685.
Millon, T. (1981). *Disorders of personality: DSM-III, Axis II.* New York: Wiley–Interscience.
Reich, J. (1992). Measurement of DSM-III and DSM-III-R borderline personality dis-
order. In J. Clarkin, E. Marziali, & H. Munroe-Blum (Eds.), *Borderline personality
disorder: Clinical and empirical perspectives.* New York: Guilford Press.
Widiger, T., Miele, G., & Tilly, S. (1992). Alternative perspectives on the diagnosis
of borderline personality disorder. In J. Clarkin, E. Marziali, & H. Munroe-Blum
(Eds.), *Borderline personality disorder: Clinical and empirical perspectives.* New York:
Guilford Press.
World Health Organization. (1992). *The ICD-10 classification of mental and behavioural
disorders: Clinical descriptions and ddagnostic guidelines.* Geneva: Author

# Commentary on Borderline Personality Disorder

Steven Taylor

Borderline personality disorder is one of the most controversial of the Axis II disorders; the reliability and validity of the diagnostic criteria have been criticized, and the utility of the borderline construct has been called into question. Gunderson, Zanarini, and Kisiel, in Chapter 7, have sought to address these concerns by discussing the revisions proposed for and actually made in the borderline personality disorder criteria in DSM-IV (American Psychiatric Association, 1994). The purpose of the present commentary is to examine these revisions, as well as their relationship to the essential feature of borderline personality disorder. A further aim is to determine whether the revisions meet the Personality Disorders Work Group's aim of limiting changes to ones that are conservative and explicitly justified. Gunderson et al. describe four main changes; three are amendments to existing criteria, and the fourth is the inclusion of a new criterion. Each is considered here in turn.

## IDENTITY DISTURBANCE

According to DSM-III-R (American Psychiatric Association, 1987), the essential feature of borderline personality disorder is "a pervasive pattern of instability of mood, interpersonal relationships, and self-image, beginning by early adulthood and present in a variety of contexts" (p. 346). In DSM-III-R, instability of self-image is operationalized as "identity disturbance," manifested in uncertainty about two or more facets of the self (i.e., "self-image, sexual orientation, long-term goals or career choice, type of friends desired, preferred values" [American Psychiatric Association, 1987, p. 347]). This is one of the least reliable criteria (Widiger & Frances, 1989). It has been criticized for being too vague; it is also nonspecific to the borderline diagnosis, since identity disturbance is often found in other personality disorders, such as the antisocial, narcissistic, and self-defeating personality disorders (Gunderson et al., Chapter 7). Recent evidence suggests that identity disturbance is associated with a variety of Axis I and II psychopathology (Taylor & Goritsas, 1994). This nonspecific criterion should perhaps have been omitted from the DSM-IV specification of borderline personality disorder. Gunderson et al. note that the reason for its inclusion in DSM-IV (American Psychiatric Association, 1980) was its importance in Kernberg's seminal description of "borderline personality organization."

This rationale seems unsound, because borderline personality organization and borderline personality disorder are different constructs. Borderline personality organization is a broad construct, encompassing several forms of serious personality disturbance, including borderline personality disorder and antisocial, narcissistic, and histrionic personalities (Kernberg, 1967, 1975). Identity disturbance is central to borderline personality organization, which is consistent with the lack of specificity of this criterion. Could borderline personality disorder be replaced with borderline personality organization? This would address the substantial comorbidity associated with borderline personality disorder (see below). Of course, it would mean that borderline personality disorder and many other personality disorders would cease to exist as discrete categories. Given the substantial overlap among the personality disorders, it would be of interest to determine whether there are any advantages to replacing some of the DSM-III-R personality disorders with borderline personality organization. Unfortunately, like borderline personality disorder, there is little empirical evidence that borderline personality organization constitutes a discrete syndrome.

Both the originally proposed revision and the one eventually adopted for the identity disturbance criterion in DSM-IV, however, present further problems. Both were derived from the clinical experience of the Personality Disorders Work Group, and were intended to improve the reliability and specificity of the criterion. However, the initially proposed revision would greatly broaden the criterion by defining it as a "persistent and markedly disturbed, distorted, or unstable self-image and/or sense of self, e.g., feeling like one doesn't exist or embodies evil" (quoted in Gunderson et al., Chapter 7, pp. 147, 149). This definition focuses directly on identity instability, and its examples suggest that it refers to identity deficit ("feeling like one doesn't exist") and low self-esteem ("embodies evil"). Thus, the proposed revision would replace the DSM-III-R focus on specific instances of identity uncertainty (e.g., uncertainty regarding goals, sexual orientation, etc.) with a broad and imprecise description of identity disturbance. The revision as it actually appears in DSM-IV (criterion 3) is even less precise: "identity disturbance: markedly and persistently unstable self-image or sense of self" (American Psychiatric Association, 1994, p. 654). It is difficult to see how this revision will increase specificity or interrater reliability. The revision is likely to increase the overlap between borderline personality disorder and other disorders in which low self-esteem is prominent, such as major depression or dysthymia.

Gunderson et al. have suggested that the revision to this criterion and the accompanying text may help to distinguish the identity problems of borderline patients from the identity problems that are found in other disorders and in adolescents. This begs the question of whether such differences exist in the first place. There appear to be no published empirical studies on this issue, although the descriptive literature (e.g., Kernberg, 1975, 1984) suggests that identity disorder in borderline personality disorder is qualitatively similar to identity disturbance in other conditions, such as schizoid personality disorder (Deutsch, 1942) and adolescent, midlife, and other phase-of-life crises (Baumeister, Shapiro, & Tice, 1985; Erikson, 1968; Levinson, Darrow, Klein, Levinson, & McKee, 1978). Uncertainty, instability, and deficits in identity have been reported in all these conditions. Identity disturbance in borderline personality may be quantitatively different from that found in these other conditions, in that it is associated with greater chronicity and severity, but there is no empirical evidence to support this idea.

## AFFECTIVE INSTABILITY

Another aspect of the essential feature of borderline personality disorder is assessed by the criterion defined in DSM-III-R as "affective instability: marked shifts from baseline mood to depression, irritability, or anxiety, usually lasting a few hours and only rarely more than a few days" (American Psychiatric Association, 1987, p. 347). This criterion assesses an aspect of the essential feature of borderline personality disorder, yet it also is nonspecific to this disorder. Affective instability is found in a variety of other personality disorders and Axis I conditions, particularly histrionic personality disorder, schizotypal personality disorder, self-defeating personality disorder, and cyclothymia. The revision, appearing in DSM-IV as criterion 6, is as follows: "affective instability due to a marked reactivity of mood (e.g., intense episodic dysphoria, irritability, or anxiety . . . " [American Psychiatric Association, 1994, p. 654]. Thus, the term "depression" (in the DSM-III-R version) has been replaced with "dysphoria" for the DSM-IV revision, and the affects have been specified as reactive. According to Gunderson et al., these changes should help differentiate the borderline's unstable affect from the mood lability found in cyclothymia, while also improving the discrimination between borderline patients and unipolar depressives.

Despite the work group's mandate to justify its revisions, this amendment is presented without a conceptual or empirical rationale. There is little evidence that affects in borderline personality disorder are predominantly reactive, or that the reactive–endogenous distinction separates borderline personality disorder from cyclothymia. Some theorists consider the affective features of borderline personality disorder to be endogenous (e.g., Millon, 1981). Borderline personality disorder patients often report that their overwhelming affects (e.g., anger, anxiety, depression) seem to come "out of the blue." Although this may be an indication of the patients' failure to identify precipitating events, it questions the assumption that the borderline personality disorder's affective instability is necessarily reactive. Moreover, there is little evidence that cyclothymic mood swings are entirely or even largely endogenous in nature; such swings may be precipitated or exacerbated by environmental stressors. The same applies to the mood shifts seen in major depression and dysthymia. There are also practical problems in determining what is endogenous and what is reactive. The diagnostician may fail to identify stressors, or may overemphasize the causal significance of a given stressor. Thus, the stipulation of reactive affects is likely to reduce the reliability of DSM-IV criterion 6.

With regard to the second amendment to the affective instability criterion, the replacement of "depression" with "dysphoria" is an amendment that is trivial at best, and counterproductive at worst. Dysphoria has been defined as "the condition of being ill at ease ... bodily discomfort ... fidgetiness ... morbid restlessness" (Critchley, 1980, p. 554). English and English (1958) regard dysphoria as "a generalized feeling of anxiety, restlessness, and depression" (p. 167). Hinsie and Campbell (1976) consider dysphoria to be "dejection; disaffection; misery in various degrees; perhaps the most frequent and widespread of all disorders of the mind, and that with numerous associations with other disorders" (p. 240). These definitions vary in their breadth and emphasis. Yet they all consider dysphoria to encompass a mixture of states, including anxiety, depression, and agitation.

Replacing "depression" with "dysphoria" does not help to distinguish borderline personality disorder from the mood disorders, since anxiety and agitation are common secondary features of major depression and cyclothymia (Katon & Roy-Byrne, 1991). Dysphoria is a nonspecific feature of many forms of psychopathology, and marked shifts in dysphoric mood is a common stress response for a variety of disorders. Thus, it is difficult to see how DSM-IV criterion 6 will help differentiate borderline personality disorder from other disorders. It seems more likely that it will further blur the distinction between borderline personality disorder and other personality or mood disorders.

## EMPTINESS AND BOREDOM

According to DSM-III-R, the borderline's instability of self-image is often experienced as "chronic feelings of emptiness or boredom" (American Psychiatric Association, 1987, p. 347). In DSM-III-R, these states were specified as criterion 7. Gunderson et al. claimed that Zanarini's unpublished data show that emptiness was highly discriminating for borderline personality disorder, whereas boredom was not. Since boredom is prevalent in narcissistic and antisocial personalities, Gunderson et al. proposed that boredom be deleted from this criterion, and this has been done in DSM-IV (the criterion number remains 7).

This revision does not meet the work group's mandate of making conservative changes, since the change in criterion is based on the findings of a single unpublished study. Moreover, the revised criterion remains problematic, since the meaning of "chronic emptiness" is unclear. When patients describe themselves as feeling empty, they are often speaking metaphorically about any of a variety of states, such as feelings of anhedonia, a lack of direction in life, a sense of unfulfillment, a lack of identity, or a lack of something that they perceive they need (e.g., an intimate relationship). "Chronic emptiness" may be discriminating, but its meaning is ambiguous.

## TRANSIENT QUASI-PSYCHOTIC EPISODES

A ninth criterion has been added to the borderline criteria set in DSM-IV: "transient, stress-related paranoid ideation or severe dissociative experiences" (American Psychiatric Association, 1994, p. 654). This inclusion is consistent with the early formulations of borderline personality disorder (e.g., Grinker, 1968; Kernberg, 1967; Knight, 1953). However, it will probably increase the overlap between borderline personality disorder and other disorders, such as schizotypal personality disorder, brief reactive psychosis, and posttraumatic stress disorder. In response to this, Gunderson et al. claim in Chapter 7 that the cognitive/perceptual distortions in borderline personality disorder tend to be transient (i.e., to last no more than a few days), whereas those in schizotypal personality disorder tend to be stable and chronic. The distortions in borderline personality disorder are also said to be more likely to be associated with affective disturbance and to be interpersonally reactive. Several studies fail to support these arguments. Silk, Lohr, Westen, and Goodrich (1989) concluded from their results that "the criterion 'brief or prolonged altered experiences of reality' rather than 'brief psychosis' (should) be considered as a prototypic borderline symptom" (p. 92; emphasis added). McGlashan (1987) reported that "transient psychoses and brief paranoid experiences and/or regression in treatment . . . fit better as SPD [schizotypal personality disorder] criteria" (p. 143). George and Soloff (1986) found that "it is difficult to separate the schizotypal and . . . borderline syndromes using any psychotic-like symptoms" (p. 215). Thus, several studies challenge the claim that quasi-psychotic episodes in borderline personality disorder are transient whereas those in schizotypal personality disorder are chronic.

## ESSENTIAL FEATURE AND DIAGNOSTIC CRITERIA

Each DSM-III-R diagnostic category consists of two levels of description: an essential feature and diagnostic criteria. According to Gunderson et al., the

Personality Disorder Work Group explored the possibility of altering the essential feature, but decided to retain the one in DSM-III-R with only one change in DSM-IV—the addition of "marked impulsivity." This addition does bring the essential feature more into line with the empirical evidence on what is important in diagnosis. However, only three diagnostic criteria directly embody the aspects of this feature retained from DSM-III-R: DSM-IV criteria 2 (unstable, intense relationships), 3 (identity disturbance), and 6 (affective instability). As noted above, criterion 6 is one of the main contributors to the overlap of borderline personality disorder with other disorders, and criterion 3 also typifies many forms of serious personality disturbance. Thus, two out of four aspects of borderline personality disorder's "essential" feature are found in many other disorders. This raises further doubt about the construct validity of borderline personality disorder.

## THE MEANING OF COMORBIDITY

The overlap among personality disorders is considerable and well documented (e.g., Pfohl, Coryell, Zimmerman, & Stangl, 1986), and borderline personlity disorder is present as the only form of personality disturbance in only 3–10% of cases. Gunderson et al. claim that the unacceptably high comorbidity highlights the need to sharpen the boundaries between borderline personality disorder and other disorders, and they suggest that the revisions in DSM-IV should help to achieve this result. Thus, they interpret the extensive comorbidity as merely a problem of sharpening boundaries by tightening the diagnostic criteria. It seems unlikely that the substantial comorbidity can be addressed by such a strategy. Even if there is a decrease in comorbidity, it is likely to be at the cost of an increased incidence of cases that fall between diagnostic categories ("mixed" personality disorders).

The strategy of "boundary sharpening" rests on several questionable assumptions. First, there is the assumption that meaningful boundaries exist (cf. Trull, Widiger, & Guthrie, 1990). Second, it implies that the extensive comorbidity as merely "noise" in a categorical classificatory system. Yet it may indicate that something is fundamentally wrong with the categorical system for classifying personality disorders. The fact that borderline personality disorder occurs as a single diagnosis in only 3–10% of cases raises the question of whether cases diagnosed as having a single personality disorder represent Type I errors (i.e., failures to detect other personality disorders when they are actually present). Notably absent in Chapter 7 is a discussion of the considerable evidence that personality disorders are dimensional and do not fall into the categories specified in DSM-III-R (see Widiger, 1992, for a review). Several studies, for example, suggest that borderline personality disorder is not a discrete category (e.g., Trull et al., 1990) and may be better defined as severe neuroticism, with minor contributions from other personality dimensions (e.g., Costa & McCrae, 1990; O'Boyle & Holzer, 1992;

Schroeder, Wormworth, & Livesley, 1992; Trull, 1992). This possibility is considered in further detail elsewhere (Taylor, 1993).

## CONCLUSIONS

The DSM-IV revisions described by Gunderson et al. in Chapter 7 were intended to decrease comorbidity and increase in reliability, but it seems that they will have the opposite effect. The revisions embodied in criterion 3 (covering identity disturbance) and criterion 6 (covering affective instability) make the criteria broader or less precise, and hence they are likely to become less reliable. The addition of criterion 9 (describing transient, stress-related quasi-psychotic episodes) will probably increase the comorbidity with schizotypal personality disorder and other disorders, such as brief reactive psychosis. Some revisions are lacking in an empirical justification, and so fail to meet the Personality Disorders Work Group's goal of limiting changes to conservative and explicitly justified ones. Perhaps the time has come to discard the concept of borderline personality disorder altogether, and to consider borderline personality disorder largely as an expression of extreme neuroticism, with minor contributions from other personality dimensions. Although such a shift may seem a radical departure from the DSM-III-R version of borderline personality disorder, it at least has a stronger empirical foundation. The same cannot be said for the categorical conception of borderline personality disorder. Proponents of the categorical scheme may counter that borderline personality disorder should be retained as a diagnostic category because it serves the clinical function of demarcating a region of psychopathology. If this is the case, however, it would be simpler and more accurate to define these individuals as having high neuroticism rather than to use the borderline personality disorder label to imply (falsely) a distinct psychopathological entity.

## REFERENCES

American Psychiatric Association. (1980). *Diagnostic and statistical manual of mental disorders* (3rd ed.). Washington, DC: Author.

American Psychiatric Association. (1987). *Diagnostic and statistical manual of mental disorders* (3rd ed., rev.). Washington, DC: Author.

American Psychiatric Association. (1994). *Diagnostic and statistical manual of mental disorders* (4th ed.). Washington, DC: Author.

Baumeister, R. F., Shapiro, J. P., & Tice, D. M. (1985). Two kinds of identity crisis. *Journal of Personality, 53,* 407–424.

Costa, P. T., & McCrae, R. R. (1990). Personality disorders and the five-factor model of personality. *Journal of Personality Disorders, 4,* 362–371.

Critchley, M. (1980). *Butterworths medical dictionary.* London: Butterworths.

Deutsch, H. (1942). Some forms of emotional disturbance and their relationship to schizophrenia. *Psychoanalytic Quarterly, 11,* 301–321.

English, H. B., & English, A. C. (1958). *Comprehensive dictionary of psychological and psychoanalytical terms.* New York: Longmans, Green.

Erikson, E. H. (1968). *Identity: Youth and crisis.* New York: Norton.

George, A., & Soloff, P. H. (1986). Schizotypal symptoms in patients with borderline personality disorders. *American Journal of Psychiatry, 143,* 212–215.

Grinker, R. (1968). *The borderline syndrome.* New York: Basic Books.

Hinsie, L. E., & Campbell, R. J. (1967). *Psychiatric dictionary* (4th ed.). New York: Oxford University Press.

Katon, W., & Roy-Byrne, P. P. (1991). Mixed anxiety and depression. *Journal of Abnormal Psychology, 100,* 337–345.

Kernberg, O. (1967). Borderline personality organization. *Journal of the American Psychoanalytic Association, 15,* 641–685.

Kernberg, O. (1975). *Borderline conditions and pathological narcissism.* New York: Aronson.

Kernberg, O. (1984). *Severe personality disorders: Psychotherapeutic strategies.* New Haven, CT: Yale University Press.

Knight, R. (1953). Borderline states. *Bulletin of the Menninger Clinic, 17,* 1–12.

Levinson, D. J., Darrow, C. N., Klein, E. B., Levinson, M. H., & McKee, B. (1978). *The seasons of a man's life.* New York: Ballantine.

McGlashan, T. H. (1987). Testing DSM-III symptom criteria for schizotypal and borderline personality disorders. *Archives of General Psychiatry, 44,* 143–148.

Millon, T. (1981). *Disorders of personality: DSM-III, Axis II.* New York: Wiley–Interscience.

O'Boyle, M., & Holzer, C. (1992). DSM-III-R personality disorders and Eysenck's personality dimensions. *Personality and Individual Differences, 13,* 1157–1159.

Pfohl, B., Coryell, W., Zimmerman, M., & Stangl, D. (1986). DSM-III personality disorders: Diagnostic overlap and internal consistency of individual DSM-III criteria. *Comprehensive Psychiatry, 27,* 21–34.

Schroeder, M. L., Wormworth, J. A., & Livesley, W. J. (1992). Dimensions of personality disorder and their relationships to the big five personality dimensions. *Psychological Assessment, 4,* 47–53.

Silk, K. R., Lohr, N. E., Westen, D., & Goodrich, S. (1989). Psychosis in borderline patients with depression. *Journal of Personality Disorders, 3,* 92–100.

Taylor, S. (1993). DSM-IV criteria for borderline personality disorder: A critical evaluation. *Journal of Psychopathology and Behavioral Assessment, 15,* 97–112.

Taylor, S., & Goritsas, E. (1994). Dimensions of identity diffusion. *Journal of Personality Disorders, 8,* 229–239.

Trull, T. J. (1992). DSM-III-R personality disorders and the five-factor model of personality: An empirical comparison. *Journal of Abnormal Psychology, 99,* 40–48.

Trull, T. J., Widiger, T. A., & Guthrie, P. (1990). Categorical versus dimensional status of borderline personality disorder. *Journal of Abnormal Psychology, 101,* 553–560.

Widiger, T. A. (1992). Categorical versus dimensional classification: Implications from and for research. *Journal of Personality Disorders, 6,* 287–300.

Widiger, T. A., & Frances, A. J. (1989). Epidemiology, diagnosis and comorbidity of borderline personality disorder. In A. Frances, R. Hales, & A. Tasman (Eds.), *American Psychiatric Press review of psychiatry* (Vol. 8). Washington, DC: American Psychiatric Press.

# CHAPTER 8

# Histrionic Personality Disorder

BRUCE PFOHL

The concept of histrionic personality disorder has evolved over many decades. DSM-I (American Psychiatric Association [APA], 1952) had no category for hysterical personality, although some traits were encompassed by a broader category called "emotionally unstable personality." DSM-II (American Psychiatric Association, 1968) included "hysterical personality," with "histrionic personality disorder" in parentheses. The definition stated:

> These behavior patterns are characterized by excitability, emotional instability, overreactivity, and self-dramatization. This self-dramatization is always attention-seeking and often seductive, whether or not the patient is aware of its purpose. These personalities are also immature, self-centered, often vain, and usually dependent on others. This disorder must be differentiated from Hysterical neurosis. (American Psychiatric Association, 1968, p. 43)

DSM-III (American Psychiatric Association, 1980) drew on the DSM-II concept as a starting point for the operational criteria, although seductiveness was not included. Later research indicated that the DSM-III criteria for histrionic personality disorder overlapped semantically and empirically with those for borderline personality disorder. Thus DSM-III-R (American Psychiatric Association, 1987) omitted several DSM-III criteria: those pertaining to craving for activity and excitement; irrational, angry outbursts or tantrums; and proneness to manipulative suicide attempts. DSM-III-R added two new criteria that actually represent a return to the historical roots of the diagnosis: "is inappropriately sexually seductive in appearance and behavior," and "has a style of speech that is excessively impressionistic and lacking in detail."

An earlier version of this chapter was published in the *Journal of Personality Disorders*, 1991, *5*, 150–166. Copyright 1991 by The Guilford Press. Adapted by permission.

## SIGNIFICANT ISSUES

A review of the histrionic personality disorder diagnosis for DSM-IV (American Psychiatric Association, 1994) raised several issues. The concerns noted most often in the literature and by the DSM-IV consultants and Personality Disorders Work Group members related to the extent to which the diagnosis incorporates a sex bias (Blashfeld, Sprock, & Fuller, 1990; Chodoff, 1982; Kaplan, 1983), adequately represents the clinical concept of hysterical personality (Cooper, 1987; Gunderson, 1983; Kernberg, 1988), and lacks adequate descriptive validity (Pfohl, Coryell, Zimmerman, & Stangl, 1986; Siever & Klar, 1986). These issues can be operationalized as follows: Are the criteria congruent with the descriptive literature? Are the criteria internally consistent? Are the criteria supported by external validators? Is the diagnosis used in a manner prejudicial to patients? Is the diagnosis distinct from other disorders? Are the structure of the diagnostic criteria and the threshold for diagnosis appropriate?

## LITERATURE REVIEWS

Relevant empirical studies of the DSM-III or DSM-III-R criteria for histrionic personality disorder were identified through Medline searches and consultations with committee advisors and other interested researchers. Investigators with relevant data sets were asked to provide information on internal consistency of the criteria and overlap with other psychiatric disorders. Research reports using non-DSM approaches to diagnosing histrionic personality disorder and suggestions from consultants not based on empirical data were also considered.

### Are the Criteria Congruent with the Descriptive Literature?

Although clinical tradition and theoretical constructs do not establish validity, they do provide a useful starting point. In particular, concepts traditionally associated with histrionic or hysterical personality that are missing from the DSM-III-R criteria might be studied to determine whether they might improve predictive and descriptive validity.

The roots of histrionic personality can be traced to cases of hysterical neurosis described by Freud. These cases would be classified with somatization or conversion disorders in DSM-III-R. According to Easser and Lesser (1965), Freud recognized a relationship (though not a 1:1 correlation) between these disorders and what he called the "erotic personality, whose major goal in life is the desire to love or above all to be loved" (quoted by Easser & Lesser, 1965, p. 391). The authors commented: "The terms, hysteria, hysterical character, etc., are so loosely defined and applied so promiscuously that their application to diagnostic categories has become meaningless"

(p. 392). In a similar vein, Lazare (1971) wrote, "Hysterical is commonly used in a pejorative sense to describe a patient who is self-engrossed, incapable of loving deeply, lacking depth, emotionally shallow, fraudulent in affect, immature, emotionally incontinent, and a great liar.... The presence, of just one of these traits together with a tired resident, may result in the diagnosis of 'just hysterical' (p. 131).

Table 8.1 indicates a variety of different but overlapping descriptive traits and features to describe histrionic (or hysterical) personality. Kernberg (1967) attempted to outline those features that distinguished histrionic personality disorder from related disorders; several of these are not represented by the DSM-III-R criteria for histrionic personality disorder (see Table 8.2). The next entry in Table 8.1 summarizes traits from a comprehensive review of the literature on hysterical personality prior to 1966 by Lazare, Klerman, and Armor (1966). In a later publication, Lazare (1971) noted that psychoanalytic theorists often distinguished between a "healthier" (genital) and "sicker" (oral) hysteric personality. Several traits of the "sicker" variant appear to overlap with borderline personality disorder.

Lazare and colleagues were the first to use factor analysis to examine the clustering of traits in hysterical personality (Lazare, Klerman, & Armor, 1966, 1970). They began with a series of traits representing the oral, obsessive, and hysterical personality constructs, and used a 200-item self-report rating scale to operationalize measurement of the underlying traits. The scale (later called the Lazare–Klerman Trait Scale) was given to a series of female psychiatric patients. A hysterical factor emerged (Table 8.1) that included aggression, emotionality, oral aggression, exhibitionism, egocentricity, and sexual provocativeness. Dependence and obstinacy had a moderate loading on this factor. The hypothesized association with fear of sexuality, suggestibility, superego, and lack of perseverance did not load on this self-report-based hysterical factor. Similar results were obtained by Torgersen and Psychol (1980), using the same instrument—this time with a mixed-gender, nonpatient sample.

Table 8.1 shows that the label "histrionic personality" or "hysterical personality" has been used by different authors to describe somewhat different but overlapping syndromes, some of which are captured in whole or in part by various personality disorders in DSM-III-R, such as histrionic, borderline, and dependent personality disorder. The syndrome defined by Lazare et al. (1966, 1970) through factor analysis strongly resembles DSM-III-R histrionic personality, in that most of the eight traits of the hysterical factor are captured in some way by the DSM-III-R histrionic personality disorder criteria. The factor analysis can thus be seen as providing some construct validity for the DSM-III-R formulation.

## Are the Criteria Internally Consistent?

"Internal consistency" is used here to describe how well the components of a criteria set cluster together in individual patients and discriminate the syn-

TABLE 8.1. Prototypical Traits for Histrionic Personality Disorder

*DSM-III-R (American Psychiatric Association, 1987) histrionic personality disorder*
  Seeking of reassurance/approval
  Seductiveness
  Concern with physical attractiveness
  Exaggerated expression of emotion
  Discomfort if not center of attention
  Shifting/shallow expression of emotion
  Self-centeredness/immediate gratification
  Vague speech

*Kernberg (1967)*
  Emotional lability
  Overinvolvement (superficial resonance with others)
  Dependent and exhibitionistic needs
  Pseudohypersexuality
  Sexual inhibition
  Competititiveness (Oedipal rivalry)*
  Masochism (strict punitive superego)*

*Lazare et al. (1966) (literature review)*
  Dependence*
  Egocentricity
  Emotionality
  Exhibitionism
  Fear of sexuality*
  Sexual provocativeness
  Suggestibility

*Lazare (1971) (after Easser & Lesser, Kernberg, Zetzel)*
  Healthier (genital) histrionic:
    Seductive
    Ambitious, competitive*
    Buoyant and energetic*
    Experiences guilt (punitive superego) and obsessional traits*
    Stable object relations though sexually frigid*
  Sicker (oral) histrionic:
    Self-absorption*
    Crude socially disapproved sexual behavior
    Generalized impulsivity
    Generalized lability
    Weaker superego, little guilt*
    Unstable object relations

*Lazare et al. (1966, 1970) (factor analysis)*
  Aggression*
  Emotionality
  Oral aggression*
  Exhibitionism
  Egocentricity
  Sexual provocativeness
  Dependence
  Obstinacy

*(cont.)*

TABLE 8.1. (cont.)

*Additions suggested by Personality Disorders Work Group advisors\**
  Naiveté\*
  Denial of dysphoric affects
  Disingenuous interpersonal interaction
  Desire to be taken care of by strong but controllable person
  Manipulative suicide gestures
  Lack of interest in developing personal competence in tasks or logic
  Helplessness and dependence
  Profound lack of self-esteem

*Note.* Asterisk (\*) indicates a trait not represented by DSM-III-R histrionic personality disorder criteria.

drome in question from other syndromes. Rather than referring to external validators, this analysis represents a "bootstrap" procedure in which the criteria as a whole are assumed to approximate a real diagnostic entity, and patients are categorized as cases or noncases according to the criteria set taken as a whole. Individual criteria can be examined according to their frequency among cases ("sensitivity") and rarity among noncases ("specificity"). It is also useful to examine the frequency of the diagnosis among individuals scoring positive on a specific criterion ("positive predictive value"). Such information can help to identify which criteria enhance discrimination from other disorders, and which are not discriminating or are not strongly related to the syndrome defined by the remaining criteria.

Only limited data are available for DSM-III-R. Data from four unpublished data sets are discussed. The Freiman and Widiger (1989) data set is based on a study of 50 hospitalized psychiatric patients who received a structured interview for personality assessment. The Millon and Tringone (1989) data set is based on 584 patients described by clinicians as part of a mail survey; DSM-III-R criteria were paraphrased in this study. The Morey and Heumann (1988) data set is based on a mixed group of 291 patients who received an unstructured clinical interview. A final data set is based on the use of the Structured Interview for DSM-III-R Personality Disorders with a mixed group of 112 nonpsychotic inpatients, outpatients, and normal controls (Pfohl & Blum, 1990). The numbers of patients with DSM-III-R histrionic personality disorder in the four groups were 9, 44, 63, and 26, respectively.

Statistics for these four studies are presented in Table 8.3. Sensitivity for all eight DSM-III-R criteria averaged approximately .50 or better across the four studies, with the possible exception of criterion 8 (impressionistic speech). Given that only four criteria are required for diagnosis, this should be more than adequate. The first criterion for histrionic personality disorder in DSM-III-R reads, "constantly seeks or demands reassurance, approval, or praise." When compared to the other seven criteria, this criterion had the lowest specificity in the Freiman and Widiger study (.63) and the Morey

TABLE 8.2. DSM-III-R and DSM-IV Diagnostic Criteria for Histrionic Personality Disorder

| DSM-III-R criteria | DSM-IV criteria |
|---|---|
| A pervasive pattern of excessive emotionality and attention-seeking, beginning by early adulthood and present in a variety of contexts, as indicated by at least *four* of the following: | A pervasive pattern of excessive emotionality and attention seeking, beginning by early adulthood and present in a variety of contexts, as indicated by five (or more) of the following: |
| (1) constantly seeks or demands reassurance, approval, or praise | (1) is uncomfortable in situations in which he or she is not the center of attention |
| (2) is inappropriately sexually seductive in appearance or behavior | (2) interaction with others is often characterized by inappropriate sexually seductive or provocative behavior |
| (3) is overly concerned with physical attractiveness | (3) displays rapidly shifting and shallow expression of emotions |
| (4) expresses emotion with inappropriate exaggeration, e.g., embraces casual acquaintances with excessive ardor, uncontrollable sobbing on minor sentimental occasions, has temper tantrums | (4) consistently uses physical appearance to draw attention to self |
| (5) is uncomfortable in situations in which he or she is not the center of attention | (5) has a style of speech that is excessively impre ssionistic and lacking in detail |
| (6) displays rapidly shifting and shallow expression of emotions | (6) shows self-dramatization, theatricality, and exaggerated expression of emotion |
| (7) is self-centered, actions being directed toward obtaining immediate satisfaction; has no tolerance for the frustration of delayed gratification | (7) is suggestible, i.e., easily influenced by others or circumstances |
| (8) has a style of speech that is excessively impressionistic and lacking in detail, e.g., when asked to describe mother, can be no more specific than, "She was a beautiful person." | (8) considers relationships to be more inti mate than they actually are |

*Note.* From APA (1987, p. 349) and APA (1994, pp. 657–658). Copyright 1987 and 1994 by the American Psychiatric Association. Reprinted by permission.

and Heumann study (.71), and the second lowest in the Millon and Tringone study (.78) and the Pfohl and Blum study (.66). Positive predictive value ranged from .22 to .45 across the four studies. The Pfohl and Blum study reported this criterion in 92% of histrionic patients, 88% of patients with dependent personality disorder, 80% of patients with borderline personality disorder, and 79% of patients with passive–aggressive personality disor-

TABLE 8.3. Internal-Consistency-Based Diagnostic Statistics for DSM-III-R Histrionic Personality Disorder Criteria

| Study | Freq[b] | Criteria[a] | | | | | | | |
|---|---|---|---|---|---|---|---|---|---|
| | | 1 | 2 | 3 | 4 | 5 | 6 | 7 | 8 |
| *Sensitivity* | | | | | | | | | |
| Freiman & Widiger (1989) | 9 | .56 | .78 | .67 | .56 | .78 | (.33)[c] | .89 | (.44) |
| Millon & Tringone (1989) | 44 | .77 | .55 | (.32) | .55 | — | .55 | .68 | (.34) |
| Morey & Heumann (1988) | 63 | .75 | .65 | (.60) | .68 | (.54) | .73 | .81 | .71 |
| Pfohl & Blum (1990) | 26 | 92 | (.54) | .62 | .73 | (.54) | .81 | .81 | (.23) |
| *Specificity* | | | | | | | | | |
| Freiman & Widiger | 9 | (.63) | .95 | .98 | .76 | .81 | .98 | (.51) | .85 |
| Millon & Tringone | 44 | (.78) | .88 | .87 | .85 | — | .85 | (.74) | .91 |
| Morey & Heumann | 63 | (.71) | .91 | .85 | .86 | .94 | .93 | (.74) | .78 |
| Pfohl & Blum | 26 | (.66) | .87 | .79 | .83 | .98 | .84 | (.59) | .98 |
| *Positive predictive value* | | | | | | | | | |
| Freiman & Widiger | 9 | (.25) | .78 | .86 | .33 | .47 | .75 | (.29) | .40 |
| Millon & Tringone | 44 | .22 | .26 | (.18) | .23 | — | .23 | (.18) | .24 |
| Morey & Heumann | 63 | (.42) | .67 | .53 | .58 | .72 | .73 | (.46) | .47 |
| Pfohl & Blum | 26 | (.45) | .56 | .47 | .56 | .88 | .60 | (.38) | .75 |

[a]Numbers for criteria corresponds to those in the DSM-III-R column in Table 8.2.
[b]Frequency of histrionic personality disorder diagnosis in each study. Total sample size for each study was $n = 50$ (Freiman & Widiger), $n = 584$ (Millon & Tringone), $n = 291$ (Morey & Heumann), and $n = 112$ (Pfohl & Blum),
[c]Parentheses indicate the two worst-performing items in each study.

der. Criterion 7 in DSM-III-R reads "is self-centered, actions being directed toward obtaining immediate satisfaction; has no tolerance for the frustration of delayed gratification." When compared to the other seven criteria, this criterion had the lowest specificity in the Freiman and Widiger (.51) and the Pfohl and Blum (.59) studies, and the second lowest specificity in the Millon and Tringone (.74) and the Morey and Heumann studies (.74). In the Pfohl and Blum study, this criterion was present among 81% of histrionic patients, 85% of borderline patients, 83% of passive–aggressive patients and 80% of dependent patients.

The evaluation of criterion 7 is complicated, because it contains two separate items—self-centeredness and no tolerance for delayed gratification. The latter is captured to some extent by a phrase in the Millon and Tringone study, "has penchant for momentary excitements." The phrase received a moderately high specificity of .87, and was scored positive in 48% of histrionic, 36% of antisocial, and 31% of narcissistic cases. In contrast, the factor-analytic studies by Lazare et al. (1966, 1970), mentioned earlier, found no evidence of a negative loading for perseverance on the hysterical factor. The old DSM-III criterion, "egocentric, self-indulgent, and inconsiderate of others"

(American Psychiatric Association, 1980), captures the essence of self-centeredness. This criterion had a specificity of .60 in a study of ours (Pfohl et al., 1986) and .75 in a study by Zanarini (1989). These results place self-centeredness in the average range for both studies. However, these two studies used DSM-III criteria to define histrionic personality disorder, not DSM-III-R.

With the exclusion of criteria 1 and 7, the remaining DSM-III-R histrionic personality disorder criteria appear to have reasonable internal consistency. To the extent that overlap between the personality disorder diagnoses is viewed as undesirable, the performance of criteria 1 and 7 must be considered a weakness in the diagnostic criteria.

### Are the Criteria Supported by External Validators?

Few studies have examined the predictive and external validity of DSM-III and DSM-III-R criteria for histrionic personality disorder. Therefore, studies using other assessment schemes are considered briefly here. Pollak (1981) reviewed empirical research supporting the construct of hysterical personality. Most studies used some type of self-report measure to assess hysterical personality, such as the Lazare–Klerman Trait Scale (Lazare et al., 1966) or the Hysteroid–Obsessoid Questionnaire (Caine & Hawkins, 1963). Compared to controls, individuals who scored high on hysterical personality were more likely to have depression and somatization symptoms and emotional liability rated prospectively over a 2-week time period; were less likely to perform well in a learning task involving sexual words when tested by a flirtatious examiner; and were more sensitive to unfavorable judgments made about their sex-role adequacy. Pollak (1981) concluded that the research literature was "rather modest in size and scope" (p. 96), but that it would be premature to dismiss the concept.

Since 1981, there has been a modest increase in empirical studies of the histrionic dimension. Magaro, Smith, and Ashbrook (1983) studied female college students and found that those who scored high on a self-report measure of the histrionic dimension performed more poorly on detailed visual search tasks than those scoring high on the compulsive dimension. This might support the predisposition to a vague, impressionistic cognitive style with lack of attention to detail that is captured to some extent by DSM-III-R criterion 8 (the one pertaining to impressionistic speech). On the other hand, "vagueness" (as rated by a clinician/observer) was not strongly associated with other histrionic traits in a study of 100 patients with unexplained medical symptoms (Slavney & Chase, 1985).

Kernberg (1967) stated that the emotionality of the hysteric is really a pseudoemotionality; it is a defensive operation reinforcing repression. Von der Lippe and Torgersen (1984) examined correlations between a self-report measure of hysterical personality and a projective measure of defensive style in 33 pregnant women. The hysterical character pattern correlated weakly with repression, but the results did not reach statistical significance ($r = .23$,

$p < .10$). The authors did not indicate whether assessment of defensive style was done blindly to personality assessment.

Standage, Bilsby, Subhash, and Smith (1984) compared female patients they diagnosed as having histrionic personality disorder with controls on several operationalized measures designed to detect impaired ability to view social situations from the perspective of others ("role taking"). This variable might relate to DSM-III-R criterion 7 (self-centeredness). The authors found only limited support for their hypothesis.

Familial and genetic links have been suggested as one useful validator of psychiatric diagnosis (Goodwin & Guze, 1989). Torgersen and Psychol (1980) studied 99 predominantly "normal" twins, using the Lazare–Klerman self-report measure. By comparing the correlations for monozygotic and dizygotic twins, they found evidence that the hysterical dimension is genetically influenced among women but not among men.

Since personality diagnoses are common in patients with Axis I disorders (Pfohl, 1990), it is possible to examine predictive validity with respect to the influence of Axis II diagnosis on the outcome of an Axis I disorder. There are data to suggest that a comorbid personality diagnosis speaks for a worse outcome among patients with major depression (Pfohl, Stangl, & Zimmerman, 1984; Pilkonis & Frank, 1988). However, no studies have examined whether histrionic personality disorder has different implications for patients than do other Cluster B personality diagnoses.

The situation today is similar to that summarized by Pollak in 1981: The empirical research is rather modest, but the available data and nonsystematized clinical observations suggest that the concept of histrionic personality disorder should not be dismissed.

## Is the Diagnosis Used in a Manner Prejudicial to Patients?

Historically, the typical patient with hysterical personality has been described as female, and there is concern that the diagnosis may be prejudicial to women. This raises several questions: Are women truly at higher risk for receiving this diagnosis than men? Are any sex-related differences in rates of diagnosis accounted for by sex-related differences in underlying psychopathology? Does the diagnosis result in inappropriate treatment of patients?

Depending on the approach to diagnosis, it is not clear that women are at higher risk than men for a DSM-III or DSM-III-R diagnosis of histrionic personality disorder. Reich (1987) assessed DSM-III personality diagnosis, using a variety of instruments in a sample of nonpsychotic, nonorganic psychiatric outpatients. Sixty-four percent of the sample was female. Of 31 cases diagnosed via the Structured Interview for DSM-III Personality Disorders as having histrionic personality disorder, 20 (65%) were women; this finding indicated no sex bias. Using the same interview, Zimmerman and Coryell (1989) reported similar results with a series of 797 relatives of inpatients, of whom 56% were women. Twenty-five received a diagnosis of histrionic personality disorder, and 58% of these were women.

The structured interview may reduce sex bias by requiring the interviewer simply to note the presence or absence of certain traits. An objective paradigm specified by the diagnostic criteria determines the final diagnosis. This explanation is supported by a study by Ford and Widiger (1989), in which clinicians' ratings of individual histrionic personality disorder criteria were unrelated to the patients' sex; however, final diagnosis of histrionic personality disorder was significantly more frequent for female patients. Slavney and Chase (1985) used male and female actors, who followed identical patient scripts, to create videos of dramatic and nondramatic behavior. In an experimental setting, the sex of the actor did not bias clinician ratings of self-dramatizing behavior. In contrast, Warner (1978) used identical written clinical vignettes in which only the patients' stated sex was varied, and found significant bias when clinicians were asked to judge the presence of a histrionic personality disorder diagnosis. Thompson and Goldberg (1987) completed a chart review and concluded that clinicians frequently diagnosed hysterical personality disorder (according to the ninth revision of the *International Classification of Diseases*) in the absence of documented features of the disorder. It appears that although the criteria for diagnosis may not be sex-biased, the application of the diagnosis may indeed be.

These findings still leave open the question as to whether clinicians' predilection for making this diagnosis in women is justified by sex-related differences in underlying psychopathology. It is possible that the same configuration of symptoms may indicate a different underlying pathology in men than it does in women. For example, baldness is more likely to be a sign of significant underlying pathology when it occurs in women than when it occurs in men. I have previously noted the Torgersen and Psychol (1980) twin study, which found a genetic association for histrionic personality disorder in women but not in men. This finding is not unprecedented in psychiatry. Similar findings have been reported in a family study of somatization disorder, which is at least historically related to histrionic personality (Cloninger, Martin, Guze, & Clayton, 1986). It is apparent that more research is needed to determine whether DSM histrionic personality disorder, as a syndrome, has the same meaning when it is diagnosed in women as when it is diagnosed in men. In the meantime, there are insufficient data to justify the use of different thresholds for diagnosis in men and women.

There are even fewer data available on what may be the most important question regarding prejudice: Does the diagnosis result in inappropriate treatment of patients? Anecdotal experience suggests the need to consider several questions. Are patients with the diagnosis less likely to be offered psychotherapy because histrionic personality disorder is considered resistant to treatment? Do nurses and other support staff members give a patient less time and support when the diagnosis of histrionic personality disorder is in the chart? Are patients with a medication-responsive depression less

likely to receive antidepressant treatment when the clinician diagnoses histrionic personality disorder?

Two studies suggest that these concerns are not just hypothetical. Slavney and McHugh (1974) found that patients diagnosed as having hysterical
personality (by DSM-II) with depressive symptoms were less likely to receive
tricyclic antidepressants than were other depressed patients. My colleagues
and I (Pfohl, Coryell, Zimmerman, & Stangl, 1987) found that depressed patients meeting DSM-III criteria for any personality diagnosis were less likely
to be taking antidepressants during a 6-month follow-up period, although
the study design did not evaluate whether this was the patients' or the physicians' decision. On the other hand, more limited use of antidepressants in
this population might be justified by the fact that depressed patients with
personality disorders appear less responsive to antidepressants (Pfohl et al.,
1984; Pilkonis & Frank, 1988; Tyrer, Casey, & Gall, 1983). These questions
clearly deserve further study.

## Is the Diagnosis Distinct from Other Disorders?

This question raises the issue as to whether the criteria are too broadly or
too narrowly defined. Does histrionic personality disorder overlap so often
with other diagnoses that it is not a clearly distinguishable entity? Is histrionic personality disorder better conceptualized as being on a continuum
with other disorders? Freud initially described hysterical personality features
in women with conversion symptoms. There is current evidence that somatization disorder and histrionic personality are more frequently comorbid than
might be expected by chance (Kaminsky & Slavney, 1983; Lilienfeld, Van
Valkenburg, Larntz, & Akiskal, 1986; Pollak, 1981).

Several studies using a structured approach to ensure that all diagnostic criteria are evaluated on their own merits have found a great deal of overlap between histrionic personality disorder and other Axis II personality
disorders, defined according to both DSM-III and DSM-III-R criteria. This
is not necessarily true of studies where clinicians apply the criteria in a global
manner. In Table 8.4 the overlap of histrionic with borderline personality
ranges from 44% to 95% in various studies. This finding is compatible with
at least two different hypotheses: Either borderline and histrionic personality disorder are distinct entities with operational criteria that provide inadequate discrimination, or the two disorders represent slightly different
manifestations of the same underlying psychopathology. No empirical studies
have compared borderline personality disorder with histrionic personality
disorder on such variables as childhood history of sexual abuse and other
significant events, family history of psychiatric disorder, rates of comorbid
Axis I disorders, social and occupational functioning, and other variables
that might validate the independence of these two diagnoses.

It has been suggested that borderline personality disorder and histrionic personality disorder might represent part of a continuum of personal-

TABLE 8.4. Percentages of Histrionic Personality Disorder Patients with Comorbid
Axis II Cluster B Diagnoses

| | | | Comorbid diagnoses (%) | | |
| --- | --- | --- | --- | --- | --- |
| Study | Criteria | Sample size | Antisocial | Borderline | Narcissistic |
| Pfohl et al. (1986) | DSM-II | 131 | 10 | 67 | 13 |
| Zanarini (1989) | DSM-III | 253 | 49 | 95 | 34 |
| Dahl (1986) | DSM-III | 103 | 36 | 64 | 8 |
| Freiman & Widiger (1989) | DSM-III-R | 50 | 44 | 44 | 33 |
| Skodol (1989) | DSM-III-R | 97 | 31 | 94 | 44 |

ity pathology. Kernberg (1988) suggests that there may be a continuum from
more mild psychopathology to more severe; he would capture this continuum with the labels "hysterical personality disorder" (no equivalent in DSM-
III-R), "histrionic personality disorder," and "borderline personality disorder." He describes hysterical personality disorder as characterized by "an essentially intact sense of identity; the capacity for stable, discriminating,
emotionally rich and empathic, internal and interpersonal relations with
others, including the capacity to tolerate ambivalence and complexity; and
a predominance of defense mechanisms centering on repression" (p. 19:1).
At the other extreme, the borderline personality disorder is characterized
by "inability to differentiate relationships with other people and to evaluate
others in depth, and the consequently inappropriate selection of sexual and
marital partners . . . [with a ] . . . predominance of primitive defensive operations centering around the mechanism of splitting" (p. 19:1). This relates
to the historical division between "sicker" and "healthier" hysterics (see Table
8.1). Similarly, Stone (1981) hypothesized that increasing levels of biological predisposition and "negative parenting" lead to increasing degrees of psychopathology, ranging from milder "neurotic" derangements to borderline
personality disorder.

     To complicate the picture further, others have used family history and
comorbidity data to argue that a common underlying psychopathological
process may express itself as histrionic personality disorder (and/or somatization disorder) in women and as antisocial personality disorder in men
(Robins, Purtell, & Cohen, 1952; Lilienfeld et al., 1986). The possibility of
organizing histrionic and borderline (and possibly antisocial and narcissistic personality disorders) on a continuum of related diagnoses remains an
idea deserving empirical research. However, there are currently insufficient
data to conclude that such a scheme would truly be an improvement over
DSM-III-R.

     It might be argued that the overlap among personality diagnoses is not
a problem. If personality disorder diagnoses are viewed as selections from
a descriptive catalogue of behavior, the fact that many patients meet criteria for multiple overlapping diagnoses is of no great consequence. On the

other hand, if the diagnoses are intended to operationalize the diagnosis of a set of personality syndromes that are at least theoretically distinguishable on the basis of etiology, course, and treatment response, a high rate of overlap greatly complicates the problem of validating the distinctions between disorders.

## Are the Structure of the Diagnostic Criteria and the Threshold for Diagnosis Appropriate?

The DSM-III-R personality committee elected to use a "polythetic" format for criteria in which no single criterion is absolutely required, although a certain minimum number of criteria are needed for diagnosis. Implicit in this format is an assumption that individual patients are unlikely to represent perfect examples of a given personality disorder; rather, individuals approximate the prototype to a greater or lesser degree. Features considered most central to the personality disorder can be weighted more by incorporating them into several different criteria. For example, DSM-III-R states that the essential feature of histrionic personality disorder is "a pervasive pattern of excessive emotionality and attention-seeking"; criteria 4 and 6 deal with the former feature, and criteria 1 and 5 (and probably 2) capture the latter.

There has been little comment in either the empirical literature or from the DSM-IV Personality Disorders Work Group consultants regarding the minimum number of criteria required for a diagnosis of histrionic personality disorder. DSM III-R requires at least four of eight. This question would probably best be addressed using data sets based on structured interview and systematic criteria rating, because it is likely that clinicians would tend to correct automatically for any problems with the threshold automatically by letting clinical judgment influence how the criteria are elicited, interpreted, and rated.

Most alternative structures for the diagnostic criteria involve giving certain key criteria greater weight or withholding a diagnosis altogether in their absence. Such an alternative would require a decision as to what features are most important to the diagnosis. The work group's consultants were surveyed as to what features are most essential to the diagnosis. There was a marked diversity of opinion.

Several consultants suggested that not only the behavior but the goal of the behavior ought to be part of the essential feature and criteria ratings. This presents an interesting challenge to the clinician, since, according to psychoanalytic theory, the goal of a behavior may often be unconscious and may not even be clear to the clinician until after many months of psychoanalysis. Short of psychoanalysis, a clinician could perhaps decide the goal of the behavior by looking at the result of the behavior and then assessing whether the patient appeared pleased or displeased by the result. For example, if a patient dressed and behaved seductively but was very upset when a sexual invitation was returned, it might be assumed that the goal of the behavior was not sexual intercourse. At present, there are no data indicating whether clinicians can agree on rating the goals of behaviors. Before a "goal-oriented" approach can be considered for inclusion in a diagnostic system, further thought on how to operationalize the concept and further empirical research will be needed. The present diversity of opinion and lack of data fail to provide a clearly superior approach to the weighting and structure of the criteria for histrionic personality disorder in DSM-III-R. The same can be said for the statement of the essential feature.

## CHANGES PROPOSED FOR AND MADE IN DSM-IV

The DSM-III-R criteria set for histrionic personality disorder must be viewed primarily as a good-faith attempt to operationalize a rather polymorphic concept rooted in the descriptive literature and clinical tradition, rather than as a valid diagnosis whose implications are supported by empirical research. Enough empirical research exists to suggest that the diagnosis has fair internal consistency and at least some external validity. The biggest problem with the DSM-III-R criteria is the overlap with other personality disorders. Another is the limited test–retest reliability, especially when a general clinical interview rather than a structured clinical interview is used. There appear to be important sex-related differences in the application of this diagnosis, but the clinical implications of this are not clear.

Although the Personality Disorders Work Group felt it had reason to conclude that improvements were needed, there was disagreement about how much data should be accumulated before a change was accepted as a valid improvement. The DSM-IV review process adopted a high threshold for recommending changes in the criteria and a low threshold for suggesting alternatives needing further research. The former was necessary, since the varied history of this diagnostic concept and lack of empirical research created an almost irresistible temptation to make changes that reflected the composition of the DSM-IV committee more than any real progress in knowledge about the disorder. The latter was necessary, because the need for progress in this area mandates that future investigators explore a richer variety of alternatives, along with the DSM criteria, in order simultaneously to illuminate weaknesses and to identify which of many plausible alternatives are truly better. Changes in DSM-IV affecting some DSM-III-R criteria, and a new DSM-IV criterion, are described below. Explications of the criteria are also provided in the text of DSM-IV, to further amplify the intention of each criterion. Finally, the threshold for diagnosis has been raised from four to five criteria.

The first change in DSM-IV involves DSM-III-R criterion 1: "constantly seeks or demands reassurance, approval, or praise." It was originally proposed that this item be omitted from DSM-IV. Although this criterion was frequently present in patients with this disorder, it was also frequent in patients with several other personality disorders, resulting in low specificity scores. After considering several revisions, a majority of the committee recommended dropping the criterion. The proposal to drop the criterion, however, had to be weighed against the fact that, in the absence of field trials, it was not clear whether the omission of this criterion would substantially reduce overlap with other personality diagnoses; nor was it clear whether the change would have undesirable effects on the prevalence of the diagnosis. In the end, a version of the item was retained in DSM-IV as criterion 7, but it has been reworded as follows: "is suggestible, i.e., easily influenced by others or circumstances."

The second DSM-IV change involves DSM-III-R criterion 7: "is self-centered, actions being directed toward obtaining immediate satisfaction; has no tolerance for the frustration of delayed gratification." It was originally proposed that this item be revised as follows: "is intolerant of, or frustrated by, situations involving delayed gratification." DSM-III-R criterion 7 was plagued by low specificity scores across four separate studies. Drawing on clinical experience, only two out of eight consultants considered the criterion highly useful. Finally, since this criterion is really two criteria (it covers both self-centeredness and need for immediate satisfaction), available studies cannot clarify whether one or both of the criteria might be responsible for the poor performance. Splitting the one criterion into two separate criteria might have the unfortunate effect of doubling the impact of this low-specificity criterion. There was no consensus among the consultants as to which of the two concepts was more discriminating. The proposed change would at least guarantee that a single trait would be rated. The main argument against this change was that, in the absence of further research, it was difficult to be confident that the disruption to the DSM-III-R criteria would be compensated for by any substantial improvement in applying this diagnosis. It was ultimately decided to drop this item altogether from DSM-IV.

Yet another change introduced in DSM-IV is a completely new criterion. It was originally proposed that this item read as follows: "Views relationships as possessing greater intimacy than is actually the case, e.g., refers to someone he or she recently met as a 'dear, dear friend'; uses first name and talks about 'special' relationships when referring to a doctor known on a casual professional level." This criterion is based on concepts in the historical literature and was favorably rated by the expert consultants. In addition, since a criterion was being dropped, adopting this item would keep the number of criteria at eight. The criterion was eventually adopted in the following form: "considers relationships to be more intimate than they really are." The examples provided in the criterion as originally proposed have been moved to the explication of the criterion in the "Diagnostic Features" section of the text.

## CRITERIA PROPOSED FOR RESEARCH

As noted earlier, several concepts suggested by advisors or found in the descriptive literature are not represented in the DSM-III-R criteria set. Many of these were not thought to have sufficient data to justify incorporation into DSM-IV, but they may deserve further research. In order to translate suggestions on various concepts into testable hypotheses, operational criteria are provided below, along with ratings from a minisurvey of expert consultants. Eight of 12 expert advisors returned a survey form on which they rated whether each experimental criterion had "high," "medium," or "low" likelihood of discriminating patients with histrionic personality disorder. However, the best way to evaluate any new criteria is a prospective study of actual patients. Researchers are invited to test and improve on these experimental criteria.

1. Remains superficially cheerful and denies being upset by situations or events that most people would find upsetting, e.g., tells therapist that relationship with boyfriend is going "just super," and later describes having had a major fight the night before. (High, 2; medium, 3; low, 3.)

2. Tends to view relationships as possessing a greater level of intimacy than is actually the case, e.g., refers to someone he or she recently met as a "dear, dear friend"; refers to doctors and other professionals by first name. (High, 4; medium, 4; low, 0.)

3. Finds it hard to imagine that anyone would want to harm or take advantage of him or her and maintains an idealized view of people even when they are uncaring or abusive. (High, 1; medium, 2; low, 5.)

4. Interaction with others (including superficial acquaintances) is remarkable for behavior that tends to elicit attention and nurturance, e.g., discusses his or her horrible nightmares with computer repair person. (High, 4; medium, 4; low, 0.)

5. Socially naive in judging the intent and devotion of others, e.g., assumes that an owner of an advertising firm will be a big help in finding him or her a job based on a few friendly words of encouragement exchanged at a cocktail party. (High, 2; medium, 4; low, 2.)

6. Seeks relationships in which a strong individual can take care of major decision making and daily problems for him or her and appears confident that he or she can control and maintain the devotion of this individual, i.e., rarely worries about abandonment. (High, 3; medium, 1; low, 4.)

7. Despite adequate time and intelligence, refuses to learn how to do a wide variety of tasks, but instead persuades others to help with such things as balancing a checkbook, using self-service gas pump, sewing on a button, etc. (High, 3; medium, 3; low, 2.)

8. Reacts to situations that most people would find emotional with an inappropriate emotion, e.g., laughs hysterically when someone gets hurt, or

cries uncontrollably in a situation where someone he or she has been flirting with makes sexual advances. (High, 2; medium, 3; low, 3.)

9. Prone to manipulative suicidal threats, gestures, or attempts [from DSM-III]. (High, 3; medium, 2; low, 3.)

10. Cognitive style dominated by formation of poorly delineated global impressions without consideration of details that support or contradict their opinion, e.g., believes a particular professor is a fantastic teacher but cannot provide details about how the professor's technique differs from others, and is unable to identify areas that could use improvement. (High, 5; medium, 3; low, 0.)

11. Finds it difficult to discuss personal needs and wants and exert overt control in a relationship, but instead accomplishes goals indirectly by such means as disguising them as altruistic concern for others, persuading others that it was their own idea, seductive behavior, or complaining of physical symptoms that justify special treatment: e.g., a patient might express her own desire to join a club by commenting to her husband, "Mrs. Smith has no right to brag about her husband's acceptance into the country club when you have done so much more for this community then he ever did." (High, 1; medium, 3; low, 4.)

12. Is inappropriately seductive in style of dress or behavior such that the person feels insecure when the flirtation fails to get a response and/or is frequently surprised and upset when the flirtation is interpreted as a sexual invitation. (High, 4; medium, 3; low, 1.)

13. Constantly seeks or demands reassurance, approval, or praise from others who are viewed as stronger and more competent. (High, 4; medium, 3; low, 1.)

14. Overly concerned with physical attractiveness as demonstrated by expenditures of time and money that go beyond requirements of occupation, or by hypersensitivity to comments critical of his or her appearance. (High, 6; medium, 1; low, 1.)

15. Is self-centered, unable to weigh own needs against those of significant others, e.g., does not understand that a friend must study for an exam instead of taking him or her to a movie. (High, 1; medium, 6; low, 1.)

16. Has difficulty working for long-term goals; actions are directed toward obtaining immediate satisfaction; has no tolerance for the frustration of delayed gratification. (High, 0; medium, 6; low, 2.)

17. Interactions with others often characterized by a seductive style of dress and behavior, including interactions with people in whom the patient denies any potential sexual/romantic interest or from whom a sexual invitation is a source of discomfort and surprise. Do not rate if the seductive behavior is limited to individuals from whom the patient is seeking money, a job, or other material gain. (High, 5; medium, 3; low, 0.)

18. Naive about effort required or problems to be surmounted to attain worthy goals, e.g., patient announces decision to work as a free-lance

novelist, unaware of the difficulties and without any substantial experience as a writer. (High, 1; medium, 5; low, 2.

## REFERENCES

American Psychiatric Association. (1952). *Diagnostic and statistical manual of mental disorders* (1st ed.). Washington, DC: Mental Hospitals Service.

American Psychiatric Association. (1968). *Diagnostic and statistical manual of mental disorders* (2nd ed.). Washington, DC: Author.

American Psychiatric Association. (1980). *Diagnostic and statistical manual of mental disorders* (3rd ed.). Washington, DC: Author.

American Psychiatric Association. (1987). *Diagnostic and statistical manual of mental disorders* (3rd ed., rev.). Washington, DC: Author.

American Psychiatric Association. (1994). *Diagnostic and statistical manual of mental disorders* (4th ed.). Washington, DC: Author.

Barrash, J., Pfohl, B., Blum, N., Zimmerman, M., & Stangl, D. (1989). *Prognostic implications of unstable personality disorders for major depression: A 3-year follow-up study.* Manuscript submitted for publication.

Blashfield, R., Sprock, J., & Fuller, A. (1990). Suggested guidelines for including/excluding categories in the DSM IV. *Comprehensive Psychiatry, 31,* 15–19.

Caine, T., & Hawkins, L. (1963). Questionnaire measure of the hysteroid obsessoid component of personality. *Journal of Consulting Psychology, 27,* 206–209.

Chodoff, P. (1982). Hysteria and women. *American Journal of Psychiatry, 139,* 545–551.

Chodoff, P., & Lyons, H. (1958). Hysteria—personality in hysterical conversion. *American Journal of Psychiatry, 114,* 734–740.

Cloninger, C., Martin, R., Guze, S., & Clayton, P. (1986). A prospective follow-up and family study of somatization in men and women. *American Journal of Psychiatry, 143,* 873–878.

Cooper, A. (1987). Histrionic, narcissistic, and compulsive personality disorders. In G. Tischler (Ed.), *Diagnosis and classification in psychiatry* (pp. 20–39). Washington, DC: American Psychiatric Press.

Dahl, A. (1986). Some aspects of the DSM-III personality disorders illustrated by a consecutive sample of hospitalized patients. *Acta Psychiatrica Scandinavica, 73*(Suppl. 328), 61–66.

Easser, B., & Lesser, S. (1965). Hysterical character and psychoanalysis. *Psychoanalytic Quarterly, 34,* 390–405.

Ford, M., & Widiger, T. (1989). Sex bias in the diagnosis of histrionic and antisocial personality disorders. *Journal of Consulting and Clinical Psychology, 57,* 301–305.

Freiman, K., & Widiger, T. (1989). [Co-occurrence and diagnostic efficiency statistics]. Unpublished raw data.

Goodwin, D., & Guze, S. (1989). *Psychiatric diagnosis.* New York: Oxford University Press.

Gunderson, J. (1983). DSM-III diagnosis of personality disorders. In J. Frosch (Ed.), *Current perspectives on personality disorders* (pp. 20–39). Washington, DC: American Psychiatric Press.

Kaminsky, M., & Slavney, P. (1983). Hysterical and obsessional features in patients with Briquet's syndrome (somatization disorder). *Psychological Medicine, 13,* 111–120.

Kaplan, M. (1983). A woman's view of DSM III. *American Psychologist, 38,* 786–792.

Kernberg, O. (1967). Borderline personality organization. *Journal of the American Psychoanalytic Association, 15,* 641–685.

Kernberg, O. (1988). Hysterical and histrionic personality disorders. In A. Cooper, A. Frances, & M. Sacks (Eds.), *The personality disorders and neuroses.* Philadelphia: J. B. Lippincott.

Lazare, A. (1971). The hysterical character in psychoanalytic theory. *Archives of General Psychiatry, 25,* 131–137.

Lazare, A., Klerman, G., & Armor, D. (1966). Oral, obsessive and hysterical personality patterns. *Archives of General Psychiatry, 14,* 624–630.

Lazare, A., Klerman, G., & Armor, D. (1970). Oral, obsessive and hysterical personality patterns: Replication of factor analysis in an independent sample. *Journal of Psychiatric Research, 7,* 275–279.

Lilienfeld, S., Van Valkenburg, C., Larntz, K., & Akiskal, H. (1986). The relationship of histrionic personality disorder to antisocial personality and somatization disorder. *American Journal of Psychiatry,143,* 718–722.

Magaro, P., Smith, P., & Ashbrook, R. (1983). Personality style differences in visual search performance. *Psychiatry Research, 10,* 131–138.

Millon, T., & Tringone, R. (1989). [Co-occurrence and diagnostic efficiency statistics]. Unpublished raw data.

Morey, L. (1988). Personality disorders in DSM-III and DSM-III-R: Convergence, coverage, and internal consistency. *American Journal of Psychiatry, 145,* 573–577.

Morey, L., & Heumann, K. (1988). [Co-occurrence and diagnostic efficiency statistics]. Unpublished raw data.

Paykel, E., & Prusoff, B. (1973). Relationships between personality dimensions: Neuroticism and extraversion against obsessive, hysterical and oral personality. *British Journal of Social and Clinical Psychology, 12,* 309–318.

Pfohl, B. (1990). Axis I/Axis II comorbidity findings: Implications for validity. In J. Oldham (Ed.), *Personality disorders: New perspectives on diagnostic validity* (pp. 146–161). Washington, DC: American Psychiatric Press.

Pfohl, B., & Blum, N. (1990). [Co-occurrence and diagnostic efficiency statistics]. Unpublished raw data.

Pfohl, B., Coryell, W., Zimmerman, M., & Stangl, D. (1986). DSM-III personality disorders: Diagnostic overlap and internal consistency of individual DSM-III criteria. *Comprehensive Psychiatry, 27,* 21–34.

Pfohl, B., Coryell, W., Zimmerman, M., & Stangl, D. (1987). Prognostic validity of self-report and interview measures of personality in depressed patients. *Journal of Clinical Psychiatry, 48,* 468–472.

Pfohl, B., Stangl, D., & Zimmerman, M.(1984). The implications of DSM-III personality disorders for patients with major depression. *Journal of Affective Disorders, 7,* 309–318.

Pilkonis, P., & Frank, E. (1988). Personality pathology in recurrent depression: Nature, prevalence, and relationship to treatment response. *American Journal of Psychiatry, 145,* 435–441.

Pollak, J. (1981). Hysterical personality: An appraisal in light of empirical research. *Genetic Psychology Monographs, 104,* 71–105.

Reich, J. (1987). Sex distribution of DSM-III personality disorders in psychiatric outpatients. *American Journal of Psychiatry, 144,* 485–488.

Robins, E., Purtell, J., & Cohen, M. (1952). "Hysteria" in men. *New England Journal of Medicine, 246,* 677–685.

Siever, L., & Klar, H. (1986). A review of DSM-III criteria for the personality disorders. In A. Frances & R. Hales (Eds.), *Psychiatry update* (pp. 279–314). Washington, DC: American Psychiatric Press.

Skodol, A. (1989). [Co-occurrence and diagnostic efficiency statistics]. Unpublished raw data.

Slavney, P., & Chase, G. (1985). Clinical judgments of self-dramatization: A test of the sexist hypothesis. *British Journal of Psychiatry, 146,* 614–617.

Slavney, P., & McHugh, P. (1974). The hysterical personality. *Archives of General Psychiatry, 30,* 325–329.

Slavney, P., Teitelaum, M., & Chase, G. (1989). Referral for medically unexplained somatic complaints: The role of histrionic traits. *Psychosomatics, 26,* 103–109.

Standage, K., Bilsbury, C., Subhash, J., & Smith, D. (1984). An investigation of role taking in histrionic personalities. *Canadian Journal of Psychiatry, 29,* 407-411.

Stone, M. (1981). Borderline syndromes: A consideration of subtypes and an overview of directions for research. *Psychiatry Clinics of North America, 4,* 3–24.

Thompson, D., & Goldberg, D. (1987). Hysterical personality disorder: The process of diagnosis in clinical and experimental settings. *British Journal of Psychiatry, 150,* 241–245.

Torgersen, S., & Psychol, C. (1980). The oral, obsessive and hysterical personality syndromes: A study of hereditary and environmental factors by means of the twin method. *Archives of General Psychiatry, 37,* 1272–1277.

Tyrer, P., Casey, P., & Gall, J. (1983). Relationship between neurosis and personality disorder. *British Journal of Psychiatry, 142,* 404–408.

Von der Lippe, A., & Torgersen, S. (1984). Character and defense: Relationships between oral, obsessive and hysterical character traits and defense mechanisms. *Scandinavian Journal of Psychology, 25,* 258–264.

Warner, R. (1978). The diagnosis of antisocial and hysterical personality disorders: An example of sex bias. *Journal of Nervous and Mental Diseases, 166,* 839–845.

Zanarini, M. (1989). [Co-occurrence and diagnostic efficiency statistics]. Unpublished raw data.

Zanarini, M., Frankenburg, F., Chauncey, D., & Gunderson, J. (1987). The Diagnostic Interview for Personality Disorders: Interrater and test–retest reliability. *Comprehensive Psychiatry, 28,* 467–480.

Zimmerman, M., & Coryell, W. (1989). DSM-III personality disorder diagnosis in a nonpatient sample. *Archives of General Psychiatry, 46,* 682–689.

# Commentary on Histrionic Personality Disorder: Where Should We Go with Hysteria?

HAROLD MERSKEY

It is obvious, but necessary, to state that there is an immense gap between the modern studies of histrionic personality disorder and the scattered and diverse comments from which the concept arose. However, the roots of the modern concepts are rather older than Pfohl acknowledges in Chapter 8. Elements of these prior concepts are worth tracing, if only to show the difference between the casual and incidental labels from which a large part of the concept has grown and the most recent effort (well represented in Pfohl's chapter) to produce organized, reliable data from which to diagnose histrionic personality disorder. When we struggle today with the effort to establish a core concept for histrionic personality disorder and to demonstrate reliability and validity, it may seem as if we are involved in a disheartening exercise. Yet looking back may encourage us in the belief that we have actually made some progress.

## ORIGINS

As early as the late 17th century, Sydenham described some familiar phenomena as characteristics of what he called the "hysterical" patient:

> Tears and laughter succeed each other. Neither from any ostensible cause.... Fear, anger, jealousy, suspicion, and the worst passions of the mind arise without cause. Joy, hope and cheerfulness, if they find place at all in their spirits, find it at intervals "few and far between," and then take their leave quickly.... All is caprice. They love without measure those whom they will soon hate without reason. Now they will do this, now that; never receding from their purpose. (Sydenham, 1682, pp. 88–89)

It has been pointed out (Alam & Merskey, 1992) that the lack of moderation observed by Sydenham, together with emotional lability, was frequently restated by others as exaggeration and as a "want of control over the emotions" (Savill, 1909, p. 18) or "the predominance of the emotions over the intellect, and especially over the will" (Hammond, 1886, p. 761). Theatricality began to be specified by Du Saulle (1883). Preston (1897, p. 31) suggested that the "demonstrativeness" of Southern peoples increased their disposition to hysteria. Suggestibility as a notion culminated with Babinski and Froment (1918), who wanted to call hysteria "pithiatism" (meaning "suggestibility") and abandon the whole concept of hysteria.

These traits and a series of others, emerged strongly during the 19th century (Alam & Merskey, 1992). Dependency, immaturity, egocentricity, self-centeredness, attention seeking, deceitfulness, lack of control or responsibility, simulation and imagination were all held to characterize hysteria. Williams (1990) has pointed out that eroticism was linked with what was called hysteria as early as 1665, and that by 1840, "erotic passion" had become an instrument capable of exciting hysteria (e.g., Laycock, 1840). It is interesting to note the words of Richer (1885): "Erotic ideas often have an important place in the hysterical delusions. However, they are far from playing the exclusive role there that former theories tended to attribute to them. They can even be completely absent" (p. 245). But other 19th-century authors were quite prolific in their recognition of sexual disturbances. Griesinger (1867) wrote of hysterics having nymphomaniacal attacks, and Du Saulle (1883) described hysteria and nymphomania as accessory to hysterical delirium. Janet (1907) mentioned erotic crises, and German authors cited them as well (Steyerthal, 1911; Voss, 1909). There were many before and about the time of Freud who attributed hysteria to sexual problems.

The growth in the number of traits characterized as hysterical was clearly largest in the 19th century. The author who mentioned the largest number before then was Blackmore (1725), with 9. Axenfeld (1864) described 12, but then Charcot and his school gradually extended the number of traits mentioned as occurring with hysteria, until Janet (1907) reached the maximum of 23. At this time, the last word was still left with Reynolds (1880), who wrote that, "the employment of the word 'hysterical' may sometimes be found indicative of the state of mind of the practitioner rather than that of the patient's health" (p. 631).

Reynolds's conclusion was not surprising, in view of the negative interactions that the various attributes of hysterical personality have often implied. Moreover, while all these developments in listing hysterical traits were going on, the notion of what constitutes the illness was evolving steadily. In the 18th century, "hypochondriasis" was being used for what we now call depression; anxiety was not distinguished; and hysteria was conceived of as organic, whether it was uterine or cerebral in its seat and whether or not psychological factors could provoke or modify it. In the 19th century, degeneration was held to be the basic sinister problem underlying the disorder. The disorder itself was understood to be an episodic condition with paroxysmal fits and very varied interictal phenomena (Briquet, 1859). (However, Briquet himself never described the patterns that were later to be called Briquet's syndrome, out of respect for him.) In fact, the usage was broader: Hirschmuller (1989) points out that in the mid-1800s "hysteria" described any general neurosis without specific localization, and that this was the concept taught to Breuer and Freud in their student days. Thus, the evolving notions of hysteria that we have inherited were a kaleidoscope of traits that were slowly distinguished from patterns of depression, organic disease (that could only be done once the techniques of neurology improved in the 19th century), hypochondriasis, and anxiety. The pattern of this illness is well captured by Kraepelin (1904), whose graphic description of multiple symptoms, capricious and inconstant behavior, histrionic exaggeration, and a life of illness has never been bettered. It was from these origins that the usual adjectives—or epithets—matured into the DSM-II (American Psychiatric Association, 1968) version that Pfohl has cited.

Berrios (1993) gives a masterly description of the relationships among efforts at psychiatric diagnosis, the intellectual background of the concepts, and the way in which psychiatrists—who had at first thought of character types and disorders as forms of attenuated insanity—later made them into a separate group. The most influential person in this regard was Kurt Schneider (1923), who chose the term "personality" and thus contributed to making the words "temperament" and "character" obsolete. It was his description of personality disorders that became the model for the great majority of subsequent attempts at the classification of personality, especially those relying upon the description of behavioral traits to separate the groups of individuals.

## PROBLEMS

The contrast of this evolution with our present situation is clear, and the justification for the systematic approach is unquestioned. How much further has it gotten? Although the reliability of the diagnosis of personality disorders was among the lowest to be found in DSM-III (American Psychiatric Association, 1980), the intervening years have led to a steady improvement of techniques and studies, so that we can assume with confidence that the reliable evaluation of any criteria sets or groups of traits will be feasible. Going beyond that to internal consistency, we find that the sophistication of Pfohl's Table 8.3 is more than adequate for the refinement of individual criteria. Coupled with his careful analysis of different criteria, attention to the most apt phrasing of each trait, and attention to each trait's separation from others, we can expect clear progress in the future in defining those things that we intend to define, so long as we are able to agree upon what ought to be thus specified.

Occasionally one might quibble with some of the criteria proposed by Pfohl for further research. For example, it is possible to object to the very first in his list of experimental criteria, inasmuch as the change from the bad state the day before to the present state on the day of assessment may be objectively characterized by the words "just super." Similarly, one can object to item 4: The discussion of horrible feelings or experiences with a relative stranger is quite a characteristic phenomenon for individuals who need to confide, and they can do this better with people who are not going to return or be found much in their personal lives than with people to whom they are close. The phenomenon of talking in an old-fashioned railway compartment comes to mind as a good example of strangers' unburdening themselves beneficially as if to a therapist, fairly comfortable in the belief that they will not have to deal with the "therapist" on other matters. But these are small points and not of material importance to the general argument.

There is more reason for concern with the general failure of current attempts to delineate personality types that are individualized and distinctive from others. Livesley and Jackson (1991) point out that current attempts suffer from the absence of an accompanying rationale for the inclusion of specific clinical features; a lack of distinctiveness among features relevant to different disorders, and criteria sets that mark specific behaviors, such as truancy (one of the childhood criteria for antisocial personality disorder), versus more global stylistic behaviors and traits, such as rapidly shifting and shallow expression of emotions (histrionic personality disorder) or interpersonally exploitative behavior (narcissistic personality disorder). Where do we stop and where should we stop?

One answer comes from Ekselius, Lindstrom, Von Knorring, Bodlund, & Kullgren (1993), who have investigated the question of whether the personality disorders are to be regarded as extreme variants of normal personality, or whether they should be regarded as categories (i.e., psychopathological entities that can be quantitatively set apart from normal personality)—a problem of which Pfohl is clearly aware. The evidence of Ekselius and colleagues, of Dowson and Berrios (1991), and of Schroeder and Livesley (1991) demonstrates that DSM-III-R (American Psychiatric Association, 1987) criteria for personality disorders do not distinguish independent categories. The lack of such categories reduces the support for DSM-III-R diagnostic concepts, and these authors' findings are consistent with the observations by Widiger (1991) from a series of investigations that a number of the DSM-III-R categories are frequently found together in patients, particularly those who are more ill. Pfohl emphasizes most of this argument in Chapter 8:

> If personality disorder diagnoses are viewed as selections from a descriptive "catalogue" of behavior, the fact that many patients meet criteria for multiple overlapping diagnoses is of no great consequence. On the other hand, if the diagnoses are intended to operationalize the differentiation of a set of personality syndromes that are at least theoretically distinguishable on the basis of etiology,

course, and treatment response, a high rate of overlap greatly complicates the problem of validating the distinctions between disorders. (pp. 184–185)

Dowson and Berrios (1991) conclude from this that the most important derivative of the DSM-III-R classification of personality disorders is the total number of criteria scored as positive for a personality disorder. In other words, perhaps we should be looking simply at a large number of traits that will be added up to determine how severely individuals are disturbed, notwithstanding the pattern. Or perhaps we could take an index of severity and look at profiles as well, but not think that we are looking at islands of organized personality phenomena.

The idea that we should rely simply upon an index of severity is supported by the finding of Mulder (1991) that the diagnoses of personality disorder (made according to the categories of the *International Classification of Diseases,* ninth revision) in New Zealand were constant as a proportion of hospital admissions from 1980 to 1986, and that the commonest diagnosis was "personality disorder" without any further specification. This diagnosis accounted for 45% of the total sample. Of course, the value of epidemiological data from hospital admission statistics is much less than that of data from organized research studies in terms of reliability, specificity, and the other exacting demands we place upon systematic investigations. On the other hand, an effective classification of conditions for general use should be generally usable and generally used. DSM-III-R and DSM-IV (American Psychiatric Association, 1994) may be fine, and indeed are fine, for many research investigations that add to the validity of fundamental concepts (or change them), but perhaps we need something different for regular practice and the accumulation of national data. Each type of category—that is, either highly refined or uncommonly broad—has its justification and place in the scheme of things. Comorbidity presents another problem, but not one that cannot be resolved.

Psychiatric diagnosis began to look very tidy with DSM-III and even perhaps efficient. It is not a criticism of DSM-III to say that it was carving out definable islands of phenomena that would conveniently serve to impose standards of comparability upon practicing psychiatrists (particularly in North America), and that, being proudly atheoretical, it did not necessarily account either for the etiology of disorders or for the whole range of phenomena that might have been identified. It was inevitable that psychiatry—and especially the study of personality disorder—would not be limited to this tidy arrangement. The varieties of human behavior are understandably harder to pin down than even the varieties of a bunch of butterflies. Thus, as each syndrome was defined successively, it began to be obvious that other syndromes occurred with it; today, for instance, a major affective disorder may be found concomitantly with a variety of other diagnoses. We will have comorbidity on Axis I disorders, and we are bound to have comorbidity with Axis II disorders. This need not be a problem to us.

The only need is to be ready to treat both sets of phenomena whenever they manifest themselves in patients.

So where should we go now with hysteria, which is also histrionic personality disorder? The answer is fairly simple. We should do as Pfohl has recommended, which is to patiently organize the evaluation of sets of subjects and gradually try to establish which phenomena sort themselves out best together and which are better discriminated separately. There will be no perfect answer to this, but there will be several workable answers of which one or another will begin to stand out. In the nature of things, psychiatric diagnosis (and indeed medical diagnosis in general) is never complete and never perfect; at the same time, it cannot be ignored.

We may well decide in time that certain disorders should be grouped together—for example, histrionic personality disorder and borderline personality disorder. Although borderline personality disorder is still very popular (for bad reasons related to historical sentiment among psychiatrists who grew up with it), it lacks logical justification, despite its striking place in North American psychiatry. A recent review by a student (Lapensee, 1992) observed that

> the majority of patients diagnosed as having borderline personality disorder also suffer from an affective disturbance, and show similar family histories and biological markers to those of patients with affective disorders. Subcategories of intractable borderline patients have been found to suffer from neurological disturbances such as epilepsy, learning disabilities, or residual minimal brain dysfunction. . . . The validity of the borderline category has been questioned by a number of authors, and the [present] findings suggest that this is not a useful diagnostic category.

In the face of such weaknesses of borderline personality disorder, it might as well be merged with its neighbors, particularly histrionic personality disorder. Of course, we may find that histrionic personality disorder is just as bad, but Pfohl has not demonstrated that.

## SOLUTIONS?

In clinical practice and in the few research studies that have looked at personality in relation to conversion symptoms, there is no doubt that the classical hysterical personality disorder is found at an increased rate with conversion symptoms. About 20% of patients are so affected with conversion disorder, and much smaller numbers have hysterical personality features in association with other psychiatric symptoms (Merskey & Trimble, 1979). A similar percentage with immature or passive–dependent personalities is also found among patients with conversion symptoms (Merskey & Trimble, 1979). These phenomena too are less frequent in control patients. We should look at the possibility of combining passive, immature, and dependent personalities with what now pass for borderline personality disorder and histrionic personality disorder. A dimension of severity would probably have to be added to the evaluation.

The frequency with which histrionic personality disorder seems to occur also means that it merits continuing preservation. In the four studies of DSM-III-R criteria that Pfohl has cited, the percentage of patients diagnosed ranged from 7.5% to 23.2%. This last figure may also be an underestimate, since some controls were included in the total number there. The only qualification that one ought to express (although one assumes that appropriate precautions were taken) is that most of the subjects reported were patients in or out of hospitals, and that if the evaluation of personality disorders was not undertaken in terms of the long-term state of the patients, but only based upon the current findings, the results may well have been misleading. One would not expect workers of this sophistication to overlook such a consideration. Nevertheless, the occurrence of traits that indicate disturbance in individuals who are already depressed or otherwise suffering from an Axis I disorder is well known, and relief from or remission of some of these traits when the patients improve is likewise well recognized.

In the end, no obligatory policy can be offered on how to organize the phenomena of personality disorders. The consensus will presumably still favor retaining clusters of traits with a familiar shape, and further work may be expected on their details. Perhaps adding a dimension of intensity would also prove popular, and this may well give an effective overall arrangement of the data.

## REFERENCES

Alam, C. N., & Merskey, H. (1992). The development of the hysterical personality. *History of Psychiatry, 3,* 135–165.

American Psychiatric Association. (1968). *Diagnostic and statistical manual of mental disorders* (2nd ed.). Washington, DC. Author.

American Psychiatric Association. (1980). *Diagnostic and statistical manual of mental disorders* (3rd ed.). Washington, DC: Author.

American Psychiatric Association. (1987). *Diagnostic and statistical manual of mental disorders* (3rd ed., rev.). Washington, DC: Author.

American Psychiatric Association. (1994). *Diagnostic and statistical manual of mental disorders* (4th ed.). Washington, DC: Author.

Axenfeld, A. (1864). *Des néuroses,* Paris: Germer Baillière Libraire-Éditeur.

Babinski, J., & Froment, J. (1918). *Hysteria or pithiatism* (E. F. Buzzard, Ed. & J. D. Rolleston, Trans.). London: University of London Press.

Berrios, G. E. (1993). European views on personality disorders: A conceptual history. *Comprehensive Psychiatry, 34,* 14–30.

Blackmore, R. (1725). *A Treatise of the spleen and vapours: Or hypochondriacal and hysterical affections.* London: J. Pemberton.

Briquet, P. (1885). *Traité clinique et thérapeutique de l'hystérie.* Paris: J. B. Baillière et Fils. 1885.

Dowson, J. H., & Berrios, G. E. (1991). Factor structure of DSM-III-R personality disorders shown by self-report questionnaire: Implications for classifying and assessing personality disorders. *Acta Psychiatrica Scandinavica, 84,* 555-560.

Du Saulle, L. (1883). *Les hystériques: État physique et états analogues.* Paris: J. B. Baillière et Fils.

Ekselius, L., Lindstrom, E., Von Knorring, L., Boldlund, O., & Kullgren, G. (1993). Personality disorders in DSM-III-R as categorical or dimensional. *Acta Psychiatrica Scandinavica, 88,* 183-187.

Griesinger, W. (1867). *Mental pathology and therapeutics* (C. L. Robertson & J. Rutherford, Trans.). London: New Sydenham Society.

Hammond, W. A. (1886). *A treatise on the diseases of the nervous system.* New York: D. Appleton.

Hirschmuller, A. (1989). *The life and work of Joseph Breuer: Physiology and psychoanalysis.* New York: New York University Press.

Janet, P. (1907). *The major symptoms of hysteria.* London: Macmillan.

Kraepelin, E. (1904). Hysterical insanity. In E. Kraepelin, *Lectures on clinical psychiatry* (T. Johnstone, Trans.). New York: William Wood.

Lapensee, M. (1992). *Borderline personality disorder: Still a heterogeneous category.* Unpublished manuscript.

Laycock, T. (1840). *A treatise on the nervous disease of women: Comprising an inquiry into the nature, causes and treatment of spinal and hysterical disorders.* London: Longmans, Orme, Brown, Green & Longmans.

Livesley, W. J., & Jackson, D. N. (1991). Construct validity and the classification of personality disorders. In J. Oldham (Ed.), *DSM-III-R Axis II: Perspectives in validity.* Washington, DC: American Psychiatric Press.

Merskey, H., & Trimble, M. (1979). Personality, sexual adjustment and brain lesions in patients with conversion symptoms. *American Journal of Psychiatry, 136,* 179-192.

Mulder, R. T. (1991). Personality disorders in New Zealand hospitals. *Acta Psychiatrica Scandinavica, 84,* 197-202.

Preston, G. J. (1897). *Hysteria and certain allied conditions.* Philadelphia: P. Blakiston, Son.

Reynolds, J. R. (Ed.). (1880). *A system of medicine.* New York: William Wood.

Richer, P. (1885). *Études cliniques sur la grande hystérie, ou hystéro-épilepsie* (C. N. Alam & H. Merskey, Trans.). Paris: Adrien Delahaye et Émile Lecrosnier.

Savill, T. D. *Lectures on hysteria and allied vaso-motor conditions.* London: Henry J. Glaisher.

Schneider, K. (1923). *Clinical psychopathology.* (M. W. Hamilton, Trans.). London: Grune & Stratton, 1959.

Schroeder, M. L., & Livesley, W. J. (1991). An evaluation of DSM-III-R personality disorders. *Acta Psychiatrica Scandinavica, 84,* 512-519.

Steyerthal, A. (1911). *Hysterie und kein Ende!* Halle A. S., Carl Marhold.

Sydenham, T. (1682). Letter to Dr. Cole. In R. G. Latham (Ed.), *The works of Thomas Sydenham* (Vol. 2, pp. 88-89). London: New Sydenham Society, 1850.

Voss, G. (1909). *Klinische Beiträge zur Lehre von der Hysterie.* Jena, Germany: Gustav Fischer.

Widiger, T. A. (1991). DSM-IV reviews of the personality disorders: Introduction to special series. *Journal of Personality Disorders, 5,* 122-134.

Williams, K. E. (1990). Hysteria in seventeenth-century case records and unpublished manuscripts. *History of Psychiatry, 1,* 383-401.

CHAPTER 9

# Narcissistic Personality Disorder

JOHN G. GUNDERSON
ELSA RONNINGSTAM
LAUREN E. SMITH

Narcissistic personality disorder was introduced into our diagnostic system in DSM-III (American Psychiatric Association [APA], 1980). There was no precedent in earlier DSMs or in the *International Classification of Diseases* for a narcissistic category. The stimulus for its inclusion was the widespread usage of the term by psychodynamically informed clinicians. The DSM-III definition of narcissistic personality disorder arose out of that committee's summary of the pre-1978 literature and was modified after additional expert input.

Notable among the changes that were made in moving from DSM-III to DSM-III-R (American Psychiatric Association, 1987) were the following:

1. The format for the criteria was changed from a mixed polythetic monothetic format to a polythetic one.
2. DSM-III had interpersonal relationship features as one criterion, with the requirement that patients have two out of the four listed options. In DSM-III-R, these four options were made into three separate criteria: criterion 2 (describing exploitativeness), criterion 6 (describing feelings of entitlement), and criterion 8 (describing absence of empathy). The fourth option in DSM-III (i.e., relationships characterized by idealization and devaluation) was dropped in DSM-III-R because it overlapped with a similar criterion for borderline personality disorder.
3. Criterion 3 in DSM-III related to both grandiosity and uniqueness. It was subdivided into two criteria in DSM-III-R: Criterion 3 retained the focus on grandiosity per se, while criterion 4 took up the focus on uniqueness.

An earlier version of this chapter was published in the *Journal of Personality Disorders*, 1991, 5, 167–177. Copyright 1991 by The Guilford Press. Adapted by permission.

4. A new criterion (criterion 9) related to preoccupation with feelings of envy was added in DSM-III-R.

## SIGNIFICANT ISSUES

This chapter examines available empirical data about both the DSM-III and DSM-III-R descriptions of narcissistic personality disorder, with respect to the following issues confronted by the Personality Disorders Work Group in the DSM-IV (American Psychiatric Association, 1994) revision process:

1. Prevalence—does this disorder apply to a significant subsample in clinical populations?
2. Overlap (comorbidity)—can the disorder, as defined in DSM-III and DSM-III-R, be distinguished from other disorders?
3. Criterion performance (diagnostic efficiency)—what is the relative contribution of the DSM-III(-R) criteria to the capturing of prototypical features and/or to the problems in overlap?
4. Phenomenological studies—are there alternative criteria that perform as well as or better than the DSM-III(-R) ones?
5. The essential feature—is it clearly stated, is it congruent with the literature, and does it capture the disorder's most prototypical features?

## LITERATURE REVIEW

The review of the literature began with the already published reviews and commentaries on the DSM-III and DSM-III-R descriptions of narcissistic personality disorder (Akhtar, 1989; Akhtar & Thomson, 1982; Bursten, 1982, 1989; Cooper, 1982, 1987; Emmons, 1987; Frances, 1980; Goldstein, 1985; Gunderson, 1983; Kernberg, 1984, 1987; Lerner, 1985; Vaillant & Perry, 1985, Ronningstam, 1988; Widiger, Frances, Spitzer, & Williams, 1988). The literature search was then extended by a computer search using the key term "narcissism" with modifiers that included "pathological," "personality," and "character," covering the period from 1978 to 1989. This search of the post-DSM-III literature located 789 documents on narcissism, 397 on narcissistic personality, 77 on narcissistic personality disorder, 64 on narcissistic character, and 45 on pathological narcissism. It also indicated that despite the continued widespread interest in this category, much of the literature has continued to be theoretical and therapeutic, with relatively few descriptive analyses.

Nonpublished sources for this review included 46 major contributors to the personality disorder literature, who were invited to provide advice about the essential feature of this disorder. A smaller group of advisors with special interest in this disorder offered comments and/or references relevant to its revision in DSM-IV. In addition, 20 researchers who collected relevant data were solicited to provide unpublished data that could be used in conjunction with the published reports to examine overlap, diagnostic efficiency, and item × diagnosis analyses.

## Prevalence

The use of narcissistic personality disorder as the primary clinical diagnosis is probably relatively unusual in both outpatient and inpatient settings. The shifts from DSM-III to DSM-III-R greatly increased the number of patients diagnosable by the narcissistic personality disorder criteria (Morey, 1988a). In the studies assessing clinical populations, the prevalence of patients meeting criteria varied from 2.0% (Dahl, 1986) to 16% (Frances, Clarkin, Gilmore, Hurt, & Brown, 1984; Zanarini, Frankenburg, Chauncey, & Gunderson, 1987; Skodol, 1989). Given the extensive literature within psychoanalytic or psychotherapeutic journals, its usage seems to increase in outpatient private practice settings. Prevalence in the general population is estimated to be less than 1% (Reich, Yates, & Nduaguba, 1989; Zimmerman & Coryell, 1990).

## Comorbidity

Data from 11 studies (Blashfield & Breen, 1989; Dahl, 1986; Frances et al., 1984; Freiman & Widiger, 1989; Loranger, Susman, Oldham, & Russakoff, 1987; Millon & Tringone, 1989; Morey, 1988a; Pfohl, Coryell, Zimmerman & Stangl, 1986; Skodol, 1989; Widiger, Trull, Hurt, Clarkin, & Frances, 1987; Zanarini et al., 1987) using structured DSM-III or DSM-III-R assessments indicate that patients meeting criteria for this disorder rarely failed to meet criteria for other Axis II disorders. At its highest rate, Millon and Tringone (1989) found that the single diagnosis of narcissistic personality disorder appeared in 21% of patients receiving personality disorder diagnoses. These studies also indicated that patients meeting criteria for narcissistic personality disorder had especially high overlap with other "dramatic cluster" disorders; the overlap actually exceeded 50% in most studies. When DSM-III-R criteria were used, the overlap with "dramatic cluster" disorders fell about 25% and was never above 50%, but other personality disorders that emerged with significant overlap included passive–aggressive, schizotypal, and paranoid. The fact that overlap occurred with diagnoses from all three clusters speaks to the diversity of overlap, and the degree to which the overlap varied from study to study speaks to the power of idiosyncrasies in the samples and in the assessment instruments.

Although many studies on clinical populations have documented the prevalence of patients diagnosed as having narcissistic personality disorder, these studies do not provide evidence of whether these patients conformed to diagnostic criteria—which was the incentive for including the narcissistic personality disorder diagnosis in DSM-III. Morey and Ochoa (1989) showed that clinicians used the narcissistic personality disorder diagnosis twice as often as the patients actually met DSM-III criteria. Both Millon and Tringone (1989) and we ourselves (Ronningstam & Gunderson, 1990) found that even the more inclusive DSM-III-R criteria frequently failed to identify patients who were clinically given primary diagnosis of narcissistic personality disorder. In the latter study, only 10 of 24 prototypical narcissistic personality disorder patients met the threshold for the DSM-III-R diagnosis for narcissistic personality disorder. In general, these results indicate that the correspondence of DSM-III-R criteria for narcissistic personality disorder with clinical diagnosis is not very high, and that its distinction from other Axis II disorders (especially other "dramatic cluster" types) is not very sharp.

## Criteria Performance Characteristics (Diagnostic Efficiency)

Phi correlation coefficients between individual criteria and the total diagnosis were similar in two DSM-III-based studies (Plakun, 1987; Zanarini, 1989); both found that the three worst-performing criteria were those covering poor response to criticism, alternating attitudes, and lack of empathy. The DSM-III criterion about disturbed interpersonal relationships, which required two out of four interpersonal features to be present, was the best-performing criterion in one study (Zanarini 1989) but was untested in the other.

DSM-III-R criteria are shown in Table 9.1. Three studies using these criteria (Morey & Heumann, 1988; Freiman & Widiger, 1989; Millon & Tringone, 1989) found that criterion 3 ("has a grandiose sense of self-importance . . . "), criterion 5 ("is preoccupied with fantasies of unlimited success . . . "), and criterion 7 ("requires constant attention and admiration . . . ") performed best. As in the DSM-III-based studies, the criteria related to reactions to criticism (criterion 1) and absence of empathy (criterion 8) were among the worst performers. The new DSM-III-R criterion ("is preoccupied with feelings of envy"), which replaced a previous poor performer (the DSM-III criterion pertaining to alternating attitudes), also showed a low correlation with the total diagnosis. In general, these studies show considerable variability in the quality of narcissistic personality disorder criteria, and highlight the fact that the criteria related to grandiosity have usually been the best performers.

DSM-III-R criterion 1 (pertaining to reactions to criticism) was found to be a sufficiently poor performer that omission or radical revision in DSM-IV was indicated. Item × diagnosis analyses indicate that the criterion had similar (or higher) sensitivity, specificity, and positive predictive power for paranoid personality disorder (First & Spitzer, 1989; Morey & Goodman, 1989; Skodol, 1989) and borderline personality disorder (Freiman & Widiger, 1989; Morey & Goodman, 1989; Skodol, 1989). Morey (1988b) also found that it was more highly correlated with paranoid and borderline personality disorders. Advisor input and our own work (Ronningstam & Gunderson, 1990) suggested that adding defeat and rejection to criticism as precipitants

TABLE 9.1. DSM-III-R and DSM-IV Diagnostic Criteria for Narcissistic Personality Disorder

| DSM-III-R criteria | DSM-IV criteria |
|---|---|
| A pervasive pattern of grandiosity (in fantasy or behavior), lack of empathy, and hypersensitivity to the evaluation of others, beginning by early adulthood and present in a variety of contexts, as indicated by at least *five* of the following: | A pervasive pattern of grandiosity (in fantasy or behavior), need for admiration, and lack of empathy, beginning by early adulthood and present in a variety of contexts, as indicated by five (or more) of the following: |
| (1) reacts to criticism with feelings of rage, shame, or humiliation (even if not expressed) | (1) has a grandiose sense of self-importance (e.g., exaggerates achievements and talents, expects to be recognized as superior without commensurate achievements) |
| (2) is interpersonally exploitative: takes advantage of others to achieve his or her own ends | (2) is preoccupied with fantasies of unlimited success, power, brilliance, beauty, or ideal love |
| (3) has a grandiose sense of self-importance, e.g., exaggerates achievements and talents, expects to be noticed as "special" without appropriate achievement | (3) believes that he or she is "special" and unique and can only be understood by, or should associate with, other special or high-status people (or institutions) |
| (4) believes that his or her problems are unique and can be understood only by other special people | (4) requires excessive admiration |
| (5) is preoccupied with fantasies of unlimited success, power, brilliance, beauty, or ideal love | (5) has a sense of entitlement, i.e., unreasonable expectations of especially favorable treatment or automatic compliance with his or her expectations |
| (6) has a sense of entitlement: unreasonable expectation of especially favorable treatment, e.g., assumes that he or she does not have to wait in line when others must do so | (6) is interpersonally exploitative, i.e., takes advantage of others to achieve his or her own ends |
| (7) requires constant attention and admiration, e.g., keeps fishing for compliments | (7) lacks empathy: is unwilling to recognize or identify with the feelings and needs of others |
| (8) lack of empathy: inability to recognize and experience how others feel, e.g., annoyance and surprise when a friend who is seriously ill cancels a date | (8) is often envious of others or believes that others are envious of him or her |
| (9) is preoccupied with feelings of envy | (9) shows arrogant, haughty behaviors or attitudes |

*Note.* From APA (1987, p. 351) and APA (1994, p. 661). Copyright 1987 and 1994 by the American Psychiatric Association. Reprinted by permission.

for the narcissistic reactions might improve the functions of this criterion. Moreover, "rage" as a type of reaction to criticism, as suggested in DSM-III-R, does not differentiate narcissistic from other "dramatic cluster" personality disorders. Reactions of disdain, shame, and humiliation are more likely to be pathognomonic (Morey & Goodman, 1989). These observations suggested that the criterion might be improved as follows: "reacts to criticism, defeat, or rejection with sustained feelings of disdain, shame, or humiliation (even if not expressed)." This effort to salvage "narcissistic injury," a prototypical feature in the analytic literature (Kohut, 1972; Kernberg, 1984), ultimately gave way to the advantages of adding a new criterion (see below).

DSM-III-R criterion 8 ("lack of empathy . . . ") reflects a frequently cited feature of narcissistic persons in the clinical literature (Kohut, 1971). Whatever its clinical utility, we (Ronningstam & Gunderson, 1989) have argued that it is sufficiently difficult to achieve valid judgments about the presence or absence of lack of empathy from single interviews that the item should be ignored or omitted when rated from single assessments or research-based diagnoses. Closer examinations of its poor efficiency, using item × diagnosis analyses, showed that it was equally associated with antisocial and passive–aggressive personality disorders (Morey, 1988b; First & Spitzer, 1989; Skodol, 1989) and strongly associated with histrionic and schizoid personality disorders (Morey, 1988b). This suggested that overlap might be diminished by revising the criterion to specify that the narcissist's empathic failures are due to an unwillingness, not an inability, to identify with the feelings and needs of others. This would emphasize the contrast with the lack of empathy in antisocial personality disorder, which is due to uncaring callousness, and with that in passive–aggressive personality disorder, which is due to obstructionism. Such a revision has been made in DSM-IV (see DSM-IV criterion 7, Table 9.1)

Existing research indicates that the third problematic criterion, criterion 9 (describing preoccupation with envy), is not observed very often and that it is not necessarily seen in subjects with narcissistic personality disorder. In one study, more than half of a sample of clinicians assigned this criterion to other categories (Blashfield & Breen, 1989). Item × diagnosis analyses showed that this criterion was strongly associated with histrionic (First & Spitzer, 1989) and avoidant (Morey & Goodman, 1989) personality disorders, and significantly associated with seven other personality disorders (Morey, 1988b). These problems appear to be attributable to the particular wording of the criterion and difficulty in its assessment. We (Ronningstam & Gunderson, 1990) found that although preoccupation with envy was not useful in distinguishing a prototypic narcissistic personality disorder sample, such people frequently inferred envy about themselves in others. Personality Disorders Work Group advisors agreed that narcissistic patients may more readily acknowledge resentment then envy per se toward others who have privileges, achievements, or loyalties that they feel are better deserved by themselves. Hence revisions in the envy criterion were proposed and adopted (see DSM-IV criterion 8, Table 9.1) to increase the likelihood of positive responses, and perhaps also the specificity of the feature.

## Phenomenological Studies

Several investigators evaluated features related to pathological narcissism beyond those found in DSM-III-R. Those features that functioned better than some (or all) of the DSM-III-R narcissistic personality disorder criterion were noted as possible additions or replacements in DSM-IV. Using a structured diagnostic interview for narcissism (Gunderson, Ronningstam, & Bodkin, 1990) to assess 33 characteristics imputed to narcissistic personality from the literature, we found that three non-DSM features emerged as helpful possible criteria: (1) boastful and/or pretentious behavior, (2) arrogant and haughty attitude or behavior, and (3) self-centeredness and self-reference (Ronningstam & Gunderson, 1990). Morey's survey of how DSM-III and DSM-III-R personality disorder criteria corresponded with clinician diagnoses of narcissistic personality disorder in a sample of 291 personality-disordered patients pointed toward the advantages of the following alternative characteristics: egocentricity, dominance, interpersonal disdain, preoccupation with status, petulant anger, and fragile self-concept (L. C. Morey, personal communication). Millon and Tringone (1989) used the Millon Personality Disorder Checklist (Millon, 1987) to assess a sample of 49 patients diagnosed as having narcissistic personality disorder. This work supported the possible use of four new features: "acts arrogantly self-assured and confident," "has sense of high self-worth," "is viewed as vain and self-indulgent," and "views self as gregarious and charming."

These studies suggested that an alternative criterion to be considered for DSM-IV should be "shows arrogant, haughty behaviors or attitudes." This criterion has both cognitive and interpersonal dimensions. It captures the personal disdain or even contempt toward others that is indirectly reflected in the criteria pertaining to sense of entitlement and insensitivity toward others (DSM-III-R criteria 6 and 8, respectively). We (Ronningstam & Gunderson, 1990) found that this observable item was useful in distinguishing narcissistic patients and could be more readily identified in single interviews than several DSM-III-R criteria (i.e., criteria 8 and 9). A related item, "acts arrogantly self-assured and confident," was clearly the best item in Millon and Tringone's (1989) study of pathological narcissism, and it surpassed even very good DSM criteria (those related to sense of entitlement and grandiose self-image). The proposed criterion also helpfully differentiates narcissists from histrionics, antisocials, and borderlines, who are self-centered but coquettish, distant but callous, and entitled but needy, respectively.

A few other revisions have been made in DSM-IV that incorporate some of the alternative criteria, while at the same time clarifying the clinical phenomena of narcissistic personality disorder in ways that should help to diminish overlap, especially with histrionic personality disorder (see Table

9.1). For example, although DSM-III-R criterion 3 ("has a grandiose sense of self-importance . . . ") generally functioned satisfactorily, item × diagnosis analyses indicated that this criterion was equally closely associated with histrionic personality disorder (First & Spitzer, 1989; Morey & Goodman, 1989; Zanarini, 1989) and strongly associated with other personality disorders (Morey, 1988b). Replacing "expects to be noticed as 'special'" with "expects to be recognized as superior" (see DSM-IV criterion 1, Table 9.1) seemed likely to diminish the overlap with histrionic personality disorder, while at the same time capturing an aspect of grandiosity. Superiority was the single best-performing item in studies using the Diagnostic Interview for Narcissistic Patients (Ronningstam & Gunderson, 1990) and the Millon Personality Disorder Checklist (Millon & Tringone, 1989). Likewise, although DSM-III-R criterion 7 ("requires constant attention and admiration . . . ") did not perform badly, the "attention" component seemed to encourage the overlap noted earlier with histrionic and borderline personalities, and the example provided ("keeps fishing for compliments") implies more manifest insecurity than is typical for narcissists. In fact, this criterion regularly correlated more highly with histrionic personality disorder than with narcissistic personality disorder (Freiman & Widiger, 1989; First & Spitzer, 1989; Morey, 1988b; Morey & Goodman, 1989; Skodol, 1989). Thus, it was decided that changing "constant attention and admiration" to "excessive admiration" (see DSM-IV criterion 4, Table 9.1) might improve differentiation from other diagnoses.

## Essential Feature

The DSM-III-R description of the essential feature for narcissistic personality disorder is "A pervasive pattern of grandiosity (in fantasy or behavior), lack of empathy, and hypersensitivity to the evaluation of others" (see Table 9.1). The responses from 20 advisors about the essential feature(s) of this disorder generally supported this statement. However, concern was expressed that grandiosity may not be overt and therefore may easily be overlooked by descriptors that do not attend to subjective experience, internal fantasies, and more covert behaviors. An alternative statement of the essential feature that was considered was "A persistent and unrealistic overvaluation of one's own importance and achievements." This simpler and more restrictive version would emphasize grandiosity—a feature that is central to many descriptions of narcissistic personality disorder (e.g., Kohut, 1971; Kernberg, 1984; Masterson, 1981), and one that emerged as the most discriminating feature for patients with this diagnosis. Nonetheless, this proposal was not considered desirable by most advisors. The reason was that other diagnostic groups, such as hypomanics and obsessives,, can also be grandiose. There was no clear consensus for other modifications to the essential feature. When it became clear, however, that "hypersensitivity . . . " performed very poorly, the committee decided that it should be replaced by "need for the admiration."

## DISCUSSION

The empirical data that have accumulated on the DSM-III and DSM-III-R criteria sets for narcissistic personality disorder represent significant progress in efforts to describe this disorder. Nonetheless, these data are marked by two fundamental limitations. First, although the criteria that appeared in DSM III and DSM-III-R were meant to capture what informed clinical judgments would identify as narcissistic psychopathology, most of the research on narcissistic personality disorder has not evaluated the degree to which DSM-III-R criteria capture the essential features of the diagnosis. To do this would require the use of clinicians with expertise on narcissistic psychopathology to serve as standards of reference, or the use of the "longitudinal, expert, all data" (LEAD) standard proposed by Spitzer (1983). A second, related limitation is the absence of validation studies to determine whether a diagnosis of narcissistic personality disorder predicts etiology, course, and/or treatment response. In the absence of such studies, the value of including this diagnosis in DSM rests solely upon the attributions of clinical utility from a widely recognized, psychodynamically informed clinical literature and tradition.

Existing data bear largely on the descriptive validity of the diagnosis, based on systematic assessment of patient populations using structured clinical interviews to assess all Axis II disorders. These data, assembled on several thousand patients, indicate that narcissistic personality disorder as defined in DSM rarely occurs in patients who do not fulfill criteria for other Axis II disorders. Although DSM-III-R significantly reduced the overlap with the other "dramatic cluster" disorders that occurred when DSM-III criteria were used, overlap continued to occur. Assessments of diagnostic efficiency especially highlighted problems with DSM-III-R criteria 8 and 9. Item × diagnosis analyses indicated that these criteria were important sources of overlap with other Axis II disorders. Phenomenological studies, as well as advisor input, suggested ways in which the revision of these problematic criteria might increase their specificity. Phenomenological studies also identified more subtle ways in which changes could be made to other criteria so as to increase their specificity.

## ACKNOWLEDGMENT

Appreciation is due to Drs. Freiman, Goodman, Millon, Morey, Skodol, Tringone, Widiger, and Zanarini for providing access to their unpublished data.

## REFERENCES

Akhtar, S. (1989). Narcissistic personality disorder: Descriptive features and differential diagnosis. *Psychiatric Clinics of North America, 12,* 505–529.

Akhtar, S., & Thomson, J. (1982). Overview: Narcissistic personality disorder. *American Journal of Psychiatry, 139,* 12–20.

American Psychiatric Association. (1980). *Diagnostic and statistical manual of mental disorders* (3rd ed.). Washington, DC: Author.

American Psychiatric Association. (1987). *Diagnostic and statistical manual of mental disorders* (3rd ed., rev.). Washington, DC: Author.

American Psychiatric Association. (1994). *Diagnostic and statistical manual of mental disorders* (4th ed.). Washington, DC: Author.

Blashfield, R. K., & Breen, M. J. (1989). Face validity of the DSM-III-R personality disorders. *American Journal of Psychiatry, 146,* 1575–1579.

Bursten, B. (1982). Narcissistic personalities in DSM-III. *Comprehensive Psychiatry, 23,* 409–420.

Bursten, B. (1989). The relationship between narcissistic and antisocial personalities. *Psychiatric Clinics of North America, 12,* 571–584.

Cooper, A. (1982). Narcissistic disorders within psychoanalytic theory. In L. Grinspoon (Ed.), *Psychiatry* (Vol. 1, pp. 487–498). Washington, DC: American Psychiatric Press.

Cooper, A. (1987). Histrionic, narcissistic, and compulsive personality disorders. In G. Tischler (Ed.), *Diagnosis and classification in psychiatry: A critical appraisal of DSM-III* (pp. 290–299). New York: Cambridge University Press.

Dahl, A. A. (1986). Some aspects of the DSM-III personality disorders illustrated by a consecutive sample of hospitalized patients. *Acta Psychiatrica Scandinavica, 73*(Suppl. 328), 61–66.

Emmons, R. (1987). Narcissism: Theory and measurement. *Journal of Personality and Social Psychology, 52,* 11–17.

First, M., & Spitzer, R. (1989). [Diagnostic efficiency statistics]. Unpublished raw data.

Frances, A. (1980). The DSM-III personality disorders section: A commentary. *American Journal of Psychiatry, 137,* 1050–1054.

Frances, A., Clarkin, J., Gilmore, M., Hurt, S., & Brown, R. (1984). Reliability of criteria for borderline personality disorder: A comparison of DSM-III and the Diagnostic Interview for Borderline Personality Disorder. *American Journal of Psychiatry, 141,* 1080–1084.

Freiman, K., & Widiger, T. (1989). [Co-occurrence and diagnostic efficiency statistics]. Unpublished raw data.

Goldstein, W. (1985). DSM-III and the narcissistic personality. *American Journal of Psychotherapy, 39,* 4–16.

Gunderson, J. G. (1983). DSM-III diagnosis of personality disorders. In J. Frosch (Ed.), *Current perspectives on personality disorders* (pp. 20–39). Washington, DC: American Psychiatric Press.

Gunderson, J. G., Ronningstam, E., & Bodkin, A. (1990). The Diagnostic Interview for Narcissistic Patients. *Archives of General Psychiatry, 47,* 676–680.

Kernberg, O. (1984). *Severe personality disorders.* New Haven, CT: Yale University Press.

Kernberg, O. (1987). Narcissistic personality disorder. In R. Michels & J. Cavenar (Eds.), *Psychiatry* (Vol. 1, Chap. 18). Philadelphia: J. B. Lippincott.

Kohut, H. (1971). *The analysis of the self.* New York: International Universities Press.

Kohut, H. (1972). Thoughts on narcissism and narcissistic rage. *Psychoanalytic Study of the Child, 27,* 360–400.

Lerner, P. (1985). Current psychoanalytic perspectives on the borderline and narcissistic concepts. *Clinical Psychology Review, 5,* 199–214.

Loranger, A. W., Susman, V. L., Oldham, J. M., & Russakoff, L. M., (1987). The Personality Disorders Examination: A preliminary report. *Journal of Personality Disorders, 1*, 1–13.

Masterson, J. F. (1981). *The narcissistic and borderline disorders.* New York: Brunner/Mazel.

Millon, T. (1987). *Millon Clinical Multiaxial Inventory—II: Manual.* Minneapolis: National Computer Systems.

Millon, T., & Tringone, R. (1989). [Co-occurrence and diagnostic efficiency statistics]. Unpublished raw data.

Morey, L. C. (1988a). Personality disorders in DSM-III and DSM-III-R: Convergence, coverage, and internal consistency. *American Journal of Psychiatry, 145*(5), 573–577.

Morey, L. C. (1988b). A psychometric analysis of the DSM-III-R personality disorder criteria. *Journal of Personality Disorders, 2*, 109–124.

Morey, L. C., & Goodman, R. (1989). [Diagnostic efficiency statistics]. Unpublished raw data.

Morey, L. C., & Heumann, K. (1988). [Co-occurrence and diagnostic efficiency statistics]. Unpublished raw data.

Morey, L. C., & Ochoa, E. S. (1989). An investigation of adherence to diagnostic criteria: Clinical diagnosis of the DSM-III personality disorders. *Journal of Personality Disorders, 3*(3), 180–192.

Pfohl, B., Coryell, W., Zimmerman, M., & Stangl, D. (1986). DSM-III personality disorders: Diagnostic overlap and internal consistency of individual DSM-III criteria. *Comprehensive Psychiatry, 27*, 21–34.

Plakun, E. (1987). Distinguishing narcissistic and borderline personality disorders using DSM-III criteria. *Comprehensive Psychiatry, 28*, 437–443.

Reich, J., Yates, W., & Nduaguba, M. (1989). Prevalence of DSM-III personality disorders in the community. *Social Psychiatry and Psychiatric Epidemiology, 24*, 12-16.

Ronningstam, E. (1988). Comparing three systems for diagnosing narcissistic personality disorder. *Psychiatry, 51*, 300–211.

Ronningstam, E., & Gunderson, J. G. (1989). Descriptive studies on narcissistic personality disorder. *Psychiatric Clinics of North America, 12*(3), 585–601.

Ronningstam, E., & Gunderson, J. G. (1990). Identifying criteria for NPD. *American Journal of Psychiatry, 147*, 918–922.

Skodol, A. (1989). [Co-occurrence and diagnostic efficiency statistics]. Unpublished raw data.

Spitzer, R. L. (1983). Psychiatric diagnosis: Are clinicians still necessary? *Comprehensive Psychiatry, 24*, 399–411.

Vaillant, G., & Perry, C. (1985). Personality disorders. In H. Kaplan & B. Sadock (Eds.), *Comprehensive textbook of psychiatry* (4th ed., Vol. 1, pp. 958–986). Baltimore: Williams & Wilkins.

Widiger, T., Frances, A., Spitzer, R., & Williams, J. (1988). The DSM-III-R personality disorders: An overview. *American Journal of Psychiatry, 145*, 786–795.

Widiger, T., Trull, T., Hurt, S., Clarkin, J., & Frances, A. (1987). A multidimensional scaling of the DSM-III personality disorders. *Archives of General Psychiatry, 44*, 557–563.

Zanarini, M. (1989). [Co-occurrence and diagnostic efficiency statistics]. Unpublished raw data.

Zanarini, M., Frankenburg, F., Chauncey, D., & Gunderson, J. G. (1987). The Diagnostic Interview for Personality Disorders: Interrater and test–retest reliability. *Comprehensive Psychiatry, 28,* 467–480.

Zimmerman, M., & Coryell, W. (1990). Diagnosing personality disorders in the community: A comparison of self-report and interview measures. *Archives of General Psychiatry, 47,* 527–531.

# Commentary on Narcissistic Personality Disorder

JOEL PARIS

Narcissism is a construct that derives from psychoanalytic theory. When Freud (1914) introduced the term, it referred not to a personality type, but to a psychodynamic process characterized by excessive self-love. Reich (1933) who introduced the concept of character pathology to analytic theory, included a category of "phallic–narcissistic" character. Horney (1937) also described some of the features of narcissism in her construct of an "aggressive–expansive" personality type.

After a long hiatus, two theorists emerged who stimulated strong interest in the dynamics of narcissism. Kohut (1971, 1977) popularized the term "narcissistic personality disorder," but made its identification contingent on characteristic forms of transference in analysis. Needless to say, this method was not designed as a practical scheme for pretreatment diagnosis; rather, Kohut's theories led to a revised form of analytic theory called "self psychology." On the other hand, Kernberg's (1976) ideas on narcissism, although rooted in complex metapsychological constructs drawn from object relations theory, did include a fairly precise description of the behavioral characteristics of narcissistic personality disorder. In fact, the criteria that were eventually adopted for DSM-III (American Psychiatric Association, 1980) showed a strong resemblance to Kernberg's clinical descriptions.

Narcissistic personality disorder was accepted as a valid diagnosis for the first time in DSM-III. It has still not been accepted in the personality disorders section of the *International Classification of Diseases,* 10th revision (ICD-10; World Health Organization, 1992). Some of the new categories on Axis II, such as narcissistic and borderline personality disorders, had a tradition in the psychoanalytic literature but not in descriptive psychiatry. Their acceptance may have been in part a concession to dynamic psychiatry, whose adherents felt excluded by the neo-Kraepelinian perspective that pervaded Axis I (Gunderson, 1985). However, the diagnostic criteria that were used for the Axis II personality disorders had, for the most part, never been studied empirically. Nor was the revision in DSM-III-R (American Psychiatric Association, 1987) based on systematic investigation. This situation was redressed by the preparatory work for Axis II in DSM-IV (American Psychiatric Association, 1994), in which all descriptive criteria for each personality disorder were carefully reviewed for their diagnostic efficiency.

The clinical descriptions for Axis II categories could fall into two general groups. The first consists of disorders characterized by clear-cut behavioral changes. The phenomena that are described in the criteria are clearly psychopathological, and the categories have relationships with Axis I diagnoses (Siever & Davis, 1991). This group would include the Cluster A disorders, as well as borderline personality disorder. The second group consists of disorders that are essentially exaggerated and maladaptive versions of personality traits. Since such traits are widely distributed, these disorders blend more closely into normality (Livesley, Jackson, & Schroeder 1992). Most of the disorders in Clusters B, including narcissistic personality disorder, and all the disorders in Cluster C could fall into this group.

This distinction might shed light on why it may prove more difficult to operationalize criteria for narcissistic personality disorder than, for example, for borderline personality disorder. Gunderson's development of a diagnostic instrument, the Diagnostic Interview for Narcissistic Patients (Gunderson, Ronningstam, & Bodkin, 1990), is modeled on the process that led to the Diagnostic Interview for Borderlines (DIB), now revised as the DIB-R (Zanarini, Gunderson, Frankenburg, & Chauncey, 1989). The DIB reliably separates borderline personality disorder from major psychiatric disorders (Gunderson & Kolb, 1978), while the DIB-R separates BPD from other Axis II disorders (Zanarini, Gunderson, Frankenburg, & Chauncey, 1990). In contrast to the DSM-III criteria for narcissistic personality disorder, many of the DSM-III-R criteria for borderline personality disorder are observable and in spite of all the problems with the validity of this diagnosis, are phenomenologically grounded. Of the four subscales of the DIB-R, three (those covering affect, cognition, and impulse–action) describe symptoms that are measured in rating scales for the major psychiatric disorders, and only one subscale (the one covering relationships) requires a major level of inference. On the other hand, the DSM-III-R descriptions of narcissistic phenomena require significant introspection by patients, as well as inferences about mental processes by the clinician. For example, the overall construct of narcissism describes a grandiose concept of oneself that requires constant external support and interferes with the perception of other people's needs. Narcissism may be a continuously distributed trait that can be observed in everyone and that can be adaptive under many circumstances. Narcissistic personality disorder would therefore be a maladaptive extreme on this hypothetical personality dimension.

Grandiosity seems to have both observable and nonobservable components. Gunderson, Ronningstam, and Smith note in Chapter 9 that some of the advisors for DSM-IV suggested using fantasies as clinical descriptors; this could overstretch the construct. An emphasis on inner dynamics rather than behavioral observations is precisely what has led to overdiagnosis of narcissistic personality disorder by clinicians.

The description of the disorder in DSM-III-R uses several other terms that are difficult to operationalize. How can we reliably measure phenomena such as lack of empathy or hypersensitivity? Of the nine DSM-III-R criteria, only one could readily be interpreted as describing observable behavior ("requires constant attention and admiration . . ."; American Psychiatric Association, 1987, p. 351).

Considering all these obstacles, the work for DSM-IV as described in Chapter 9 is an admirable first step. At the very least, we should be sure that our criteria have a high "hit rate" for narcissistic personality disorder, and a low one for near-neighbor disorders on Axis II. Narcissistic personality disorder is in fact particularly problematic in its overlap with other personality disorders (Livesley & Schroeder, 1991).

As Gunderson et al. point out, the problems in defining precise criteria for narcissistic personality disorder make estimates of its prevalence treacherous. It is entirely possible, for example, that the diagnosis is applied more often in centers that are interested in the dynamics of self psychology. The same patients might receive other diagnoses elsewhere.

The problem of comorbidity among the Axis II disorders is a serious threat to the validity of all categories (Pfohl, Coryell, Zimmerman, & Stangl, 1986; Nurnberg et al., 1991). But the clinical significance of the comorbidity problem could depend on the type of disorder under consideration. For disorders with clear-cut behavioral pathology and a relatively known treatment course, such as schizotypal or borderline personality disorders, most clinicians would not be unduly disturbed in practice by comorbidity. Most likely, they would simply consider the more serious diagnosis as the primary one. The same consideration would not apply to narcissistic personality disorder. This problem requires sharpening of the criteria for this category.

Two approaches to achieving this goal are described in Chapter 9. One has been to measure the diagnostic efficiency of the DSM-III-R criteria. It is worth noting that the worst performers (reactions to criticism, lack of empathy, envy) are those requiring highly inferential judgments about mental events. These criteria seem to be the source of some of the problems encountered in making narcissistic personality disorder distinct from its neighbors.

The other approach has involved a fresh start: working to build a more useful set of criteria from clinical descriptions of narcissistic patients. Drawing on findings using their own Diagnostic Interview for Narcissistic Patients, as well as Millon's Personality Disorder Checklist, Gunderson and colleagues describe a new criterion for DSM-IV that may be more specific to narcissistic personality disorder: "shows arrogant, haughty behaviors or attitudes" (American Psychiatric Association, 1994, p. 661). They describe this criterion as "observable" and find that it can differentiate narcissists from other patients in Cluster B who are overtly needy. Although there is good empirical evidence for the criterion, it is not clear whether the reliability of observers scoring arrogance would be as high for the average clinician as for personality disorder researchers. A series of other revisions for DSM-IV involve changes of wording that may make the criteria more precise by further reducing comorbidity.

As Gunderson et al. acknowledge, the greatest problem with narcissistic personality disorder is its lack of validation through such external criteria as a specific etiological pathway, a specific course, or a specific treatment response (Robins & Barrett, 1989). In this respect, narcissistic personality disorder is a weaker category than other Axis II disorders such as antisocial personality disorder (Robins, 1966), in which, although the etiology is unknown, there is at least some knowledge about course and treatment. It is the ability to predict clinical phenomena that makes these categories clinically useful. Until such validation is available for narcissistic personality disorder, it may tend to reflect not so much a diagnosis as a particular constellation of psychodynamic perspectives.

## REFERENCES

American Psychiatric Association. (1980). *Diagnostic and statistical manual of mental disorders* (3rd ed.). Washington, DC: Author.

American Psychiatric Association. (1987). *Diagnostic and statistical manual of mental disorders* (3rd ed., rev.). Washington, DC: Author.

American Psychiatric Association. (1994). *Diagnostic and statistical manual of mental disorders* (4th ed.). Washington, DC: Author.

Freud, S. (1914). On narcissism: An introduction. In J. Strachey (Ed. and Trans.) *The standard edition of the complete psychological works of Sigmund Freud* (Vol. 14, pp. 73–104). London: Hogarth Press, 1957.

Gunderson, J. G. (1985). Conceptual risks of the Axis I–II division. In H. Klar & L. J. Siever (Eds.), *Biological response styles: Clinical implications* (pp. 81–95). Washington DC: American Psychiatric Press.

Gunderson, J. G., & Kolb, J. E. (1978). Discriminating features of borderline patients. *American Journal of Psychiatry, 135,* 792–796.

Gunderson, J. G., Ronningstam, E., & Bodkin, A. (1990). The Diagnostic Interview for Narcissistic Patients. *Archives of General Psychiatry, 47,* 676–680.

Horney, K. (1937). *The neurotic personality of our time.* New York: Norton.

Kernberg, O. F. (1976). *Borderline conditions and pathological narcissism.* New York: Jason Aronson.

Kohut, H. (1971). *The analysis of the self.* New York: International Universities Press.

Kohut, H. (1977). *The restoration of the self.* New York: International Universities Press.

Livesley, W. J., Jackson, D. N., & Schroeder, M. L. (1992). Factorial structure of traits delineating personality disorders in clinical and general population samples. *Journal of Abnormal Psychology, 101,* 432–440.

Livesley, W. J., & Schroeder, M. L. (1991). Dimensions of personality disorder: The DSM-III-R Cluster B diagnoses. *Journal of Nervous and Mental Disease, 179,* 320–328.

Nurnberg, G., Raskin, M., Levine, P. E., Pollack, S., Siegel, O., & Prince, R. (1991). The comorbidity of borderline personality disorder with other DSM-III-R Axis II personality disorders. *American Journal of Psychiatry, 148,* 1311–1317.

Pfohl, B., Coryell, W., Zimmerman, M., & Stangl, D. (1986). DSM-III personality disorders: Diagnostic overlap and internal consistency of individual DSM-III criteria. *Comprehensive Psychiatry, 27,* 21–34.

Reich, W. (1933). *Character analysis.* New York: Farrar, Straus & Giroux, 1972.

Robins, E. R., & Barrett, J. E. (Eds.). (1989). *The validity of psychiatric diagnosis.* New York: Raven Press.

Robins, L. N. (1966). *Deviant children grown up.* Baltimore: Williams & Wilkins.

Siever, L. J., & Davis, K. L. (1991). A psychobiological perspective on the personality disorders. *American Journal of Psychiatry, 148,* 1647–1658.

World Health Organization. (1992). *The ICD-10 classification of mental and behavioural disorders: Diagnostic criteria for research.* Geneva: Author.

Zanarini, M. C., Gunderson, J. G., Frankenburg, F. R., & Chauncey. (1989). The Revised Diagnostic Interview for Borderlines. *Journal of Personality Disorders, 3,* 10–18.

Zanarini, M. C., Gunderson, J. G., Frankenburg, F. R., & Chauncey. (1990). Discriminating borderline personality disorder from other Axis II disorders. *American Journal of Psychiatry, 147,* 161–167.

# CHAPTER 10

# Avoidant Personality Disorder

THEODORE MILLON
ALEXANDRA MARTINEZ

Avoidant personality disorder represents a category named in 1969 by Millon and included for the first time in DSM-III (American Psychiatric Association [APA], 1980), although parallels may be found in the writings of numerous clinical theorists. Among the earliest portrayals to approximate the character of the avoidant personality was that presented by Eugen Bleuler in his classic text *Dementia Praecox: Or the Group of Schizophrenias* (1911). Here, Bleuler depicted patients who "quite consciously shun contact with reality because their affects are so powerful that they must avoid everything which might arouse their emotions" (1950, p. 65). In 1923, Schneider described his conception of the "aesthetic personality," which also resembles the avoidant trait constellation. Some of Schneider's descriptions are as follows: "Feelings do not seem genuine, relationships appear lifeless and voided. . . . All human activity needs a certain psychic half light or chiaroscuro if it is to be experienced as an integral part of the self" (1950, p. 141). Ernst Kretschmer (1925) proposed two polarities within the schizoid temperament, the "anaesthetic" and the "hyperaesthetic." Attributes that gravitate toward anaesthetic polarity appear to resemble the DSM-III-R (American Psychiatric Association, 1987) description of schizoid personality disorder, whereas the hyperaesthetic extreme closely resembles the DSM-III-R avoidant pattern. According to Kretschmer, for the hyperaesthetic "life is composed of a chain of tragedies. . . . [the patient] behaves shyly, or timidly, or distrustfully . . . seeks as far as possible to avoid and deaden all stimulation from the outside" (1925, p. 172). In 1945, Karen Horney's book *Our Inner Conflicts* characterized a pattern akin to avoidant personality disorder, which she termed the "detached type," referring to it as exhibiting a "moving away from" interpersonal style.

An earlier version of this chapter was published in the *Journal of Personality Disorders*, 1991. 5, 353–362. Copyright 1991 by The Guilford Press. Adapted by permission.

She notes that for these personalities "there is intolerable strain in associating with people and solitude becomes primarily a means of avoiding it . . . the underlying principle here is never to become so attached to anybody or anything so that it becomes indispensable . . . better to have nothing matter much" (1945, p. 79). Horney later described self-hate and self-contempt among the central features that illustrate the detached style.

Psychoanalytic theorists such as Fairbairn (1940), Winnicott (1956), Arieti (1955), Guntrip (1952), and Laing (1960) have also formulated concepts corresponding to the characteristics of the avoidant personality, which were referred to by this group as "schizoid" and "false self." Other parallels may be found in Fenichel's (1945) elaboration of the "phobic character." He posited that these individuals circumscribe their reactive behavior "to the avoidance of situations originally wished for" (1945, p. 527). Along similar lines, MacKinnon and Michels (1971) proposed a set of criteria that they termed "phobic character traits." Central to the phobic character is "the use of avoidance and inhibition as characterological defenses. . . . [It] is recognized as defensive avoidance only when the person's life situation exposes his inhibition as maladaptive" (1971, p. 149). Early object relations theorists spoke of a "need–fear dilemma" as the primary symptomatology of this group (Burnham, Gladstone, & Gibson, 1969). Burnham et al. stated: "His very psychological existence depends on his maintaining contacts with objects, whether as individuals or as part of a social structure. . . . The very excessiveness of his need for objects also makes them inordinately dangerous and fearsome since they can destroy him through abandonment" (1969, pp. 27–28). The symptom constellation of avoidant personality disorder as conceived in DSM-III-R has its origins in biosocial learning theory (Millon, 1969), which depicts the avoidant personality as an actively detached character type.

Reservations have been expressed as to whether avoidant personality disorder deserves its own designation and whether it is encountered with sufficient clinical frequency to justify being considered a distinctive disorder. Despite these concerns, there was apparently an increasing recognition of its prevalence as clinicians became more acquainted with its criterion features following the publication of DSM-III in 1980. Nevertheless, significant changes were introduced in the avoidant personality disorder criteria with the publication of DSM-III-R — changes in line with the psychoanalytic concept of the phobic character. Minimized were features associated with low self-esteem and hypersensitivity to rejection; added were fears of being inappropriate or embarrassed, as well as tendencies to exaggerate dangers and risks.

## SIGNIFICANT ISSUES

The major issues confronted by the Personality Disorders Work Group in regard to the revision of avoidant personality disorder for DSM-IV (American Psychiatric Association, 1994) may be separated into five questions:

1. What prototypical traits should be selected for the category's essential feature?
2. As a relatively new category, does avoidant personality disorder display evidence of an adequate prevalence level and frequency of diagnostic usage?
3. Can avoidant personality disorder be differentiated from other disorders with which it shares certain features?
4. Do the DSM-III-R avoidant personality disorder criteria achieve satisfactory levels of diagnostic efficiency and validity?
5. Are there DSM-III-R criteria that should be omitted in DSM-IV, and alternate criteria that may add important features beyond those on the DSM-III-R list?

## LITERATURE REVIEW

Computer-based literature searches were employed to locate articles, chapters, and books from 1968 to 1992 in which terms such as "avoidant," "shy," "withdrawn," "phobic," and the like were associated. Related references (mostly under the designation "schizoid") prior to this period were also obtained. Because of the category's recency, the literature is quite sparse; only a few publications were of an empirical nature. In addition, useful views were offered by advisors and consultants, and data (largely unpublished) relevant to prevalence, comorbidity, and descriptive validity were supplied by Blashfield (1988), Dahl (1986), Freiman and Widiger (1989), Millon and Tringone (1989), Morey and Heumann (1988), Pfohl and Blum (1990), Reich (1990), and Zanarini (1989).

### What Prototypical Criteria Should Be Used for the Category's Essential Feature?

The following characteristics were proposed by the work group's advisors:

1. "There is intense fear of social derogation, humiliation, and rejection. The baseline position is to avoid social contact, to wall off socially, and to restrain self-expression tightly."
2. "There is fearful avoidance of situations in which one is observed by others and where there is a risk of failure, rejection, or revelation of strong feelings."
3. "Accompanying the fearful avoidance is a strong desire for interpersonal affiliation."
4. "Important . . . is the wish for relationships to help distinguish it from the schizoid."
5. "The essential feature is low self esteem and a chronic state of social anxiety, especially in situations where there is a risk of rejection or fail-

ure. . . . These fearful and self-demeaning attitudes coexist with strong desires for affection and acceptance."

6. "[There] is the simultaneous existence . . . of strong wishes for relationships and challenges and of fearful avoidance of people and situations where there is a risk of failure, rejection, or strong feelings, resulting in a pervasive pattern of social discomfort, fear of negative evaluation, and timidity."

As a final guide, the criteria formulated for the 10th revision of the *International Classification of Diseases* (ICD-10; World Health Organization, 1992) were examined:

> F60.6 Anxious (Avoidant) Personality Disorder: Personality disorder characterized by: (i) persistent and pervasive feelings of tension and apprehension; (ii) habitual self-consciousness and feelings of insecurity and inferiority; (iii) continuous yearning to be liked and accepted; (iv) hypersensitivity to rejection and criticism; (v) refusal to enter into relationships unless receiving strong guarantees of uncritical acceptance; very restricted personal attachments; (vi) habitual proneness to exaggerate the potential dangers or risks in everyday situations, to the extent of avoiding certain activities, not amounting to phobic avoidance; (vii) restricted lifestyle because of need to have certainty and security.

In contrast to decisions regarding the diagnostic criteria, where efficiency and validity statistics could be drawn upon, judgments here were of a qualitative nature. The proposed essential feature description for this section was phrased as follows: "A pervasive pattern of social discomfort and reticence, low self-esteem, and hypersensitivity to negative evaluation." For publication, this was revised to read: "A pervasive pattern of social inhibition, feelings of inadequacy, and hypersensitivity to negative evaluation" (American Psychiatric Association, 1994, p. 664).

## Does the Disorder Achieve a Satisfactory Prevalence Level and Frequency of Diagnostic Usage?

An issue raised in some quarters following the publication of DSM-III pertained to whether cases described as avoidant personality disorder were, in fact, found in clinical settings (e.g., Kernberg, 1984). As of this date, we do not have a fully representative epidemiological study of personality disorders among the general population or among patients (Weissman, 1990). However, a review of several studies on DSM-III personality disorder prevalence found that the range for avoidant personality disorder was .05 to .55 (see Widiger, 1991). Even if the upper extremes (where multiple diagnoses were encouraged) are excluded, the prevalence of avoidant personality disorder appears to average about 10% — substantial enough to justify confidence in its clinical authenticity. However, the advent of avoidant personality disorder (and also schizotypal personality disorder) has resulted in a drop in the prevalence of schizoid personality disorder, to the extent that questions have arisen as to the latter's viability as a diagnostic entity.

## Can the Disorder Be Differentiated from Other Disorders?

Although overlap data are based on diverse methodologies and patient samples, a measure of consistency for avoidant personality disorder does appear. Except for borderline personality disorder (where overlap can be attributed in great part to that disorder's high prevalence), avoidant personality disorder shows up most frequently with schizoid, schizotypal, dependent, paranoid, and self-defeating personality disorders—a wide variety, but each understandable in terms of particular shared features.

To expect each personality disorder to be a wholly distinct entity with defining features (or diagnostic criteria) that do not overlap with those characterizing other such disorders is to expect a level of symptomatological uniqueness rarely found in medicine at large. Numerous "diseases" share symptoms in common, yet may be differentiated by the unique configuration of their symptoms. Prototypal avoidants share typical social withdrawal with both schizoids and schizotypals, low self-esteem (as per DSM-III) with dependents, social anxiety with social phobics, and so on. A brief elaboration of this theme may be useful in regard to this last-mentioned, somewhat problematic Axis I syndrome.

Social phobia is an anxiety disorder in which the DSM-III-R defining feature is a persistent fear of and immediate anxiety reaction to social situations (circumscribed or generalized). Social phobia may covary with avoidant personality disorder, but the two can be distinguished on several grounds. First, avoidant personality disorder exhibits a wider range of anxiety precipitants than social phobia. Social phobics may have a multitude of satisfying social/personal relationships with others. Avoidants are socially withdrawn and have few close relationships; they desire such relationships, but do not trust others sufficiently to relate closely without assurances of acceptance. Avoidant personality is essentially a problem of relating to persons, whereas social phobia is largely a problem of performing in situations. Avoidant disorder involves a feeling of low self-esteem; social phobia implies no such self-critical judgment.

In part, the overlap problem between avoidant personality disorder and social phobia was created by DSM-III-R committee actions. These decisions, it should be noted, were guided not by empirical data, but by an epistemological reversal in DSM principles—namely, that of favoring a particular theoretical viewpoint. As noted earlier, trait criteria considered central to the DSM-III avoidant formulation were deleted (e.g., those pertaining to desire for acceptance and low self esteem); simultaneously, several new criteria were added (e.g., "fears being embarrassed by blushing . . ."). These latter not only represented a theoretically based shift, but created an overlap with the expanded construct of social phobia. By dropping differentiating DSM-III criteria for avoidant personality disorder and introducing common phobia criteria, DSM-III-R committees inadvertently made avoidant personality disorder and social phobia highly comparable—a similarity further compounded by the decision to introduce a "generalized type" of social phobia. Several studies have reflected the existence of the overlap between these diagnostic categories. For example, Herbert, Hope, and Bellak (1992) investigated the discriminant validity of these categories by examining the comorbidity of generalized social phobia and avoidant personality disorder. The results indicated that all subjects who met the criteria for avoidant personality disorder met the criteria for generalized social phobia, suggesting a high rate of comorbidity between the two disorders. The authors propose that these categories do not reflect distinct taxa, but rather "quantitative variants of the same spectrum of psychopathology" (p. 337). Holt, Heimberg, and Hope (1992) also suggest that the criteria for avoidant personality disorder and generalized social phobia do not define distinct disorders. By contrast, Greenberg and Stravynski (1983) and Turner, Beidel, Dancee, and Keys (1986) propose that the avoidant and social phobia constructs can and should be distinguished on both empirical and clinical grounds. In their reports, avoidant personalities are a more severely impaired individuals who exhibit greater deficits in social skills, interpersonal sensitivity, and avoidant behaviors, and who experience a greater measure of distress, anxiety, and depression.

To turn to Axis II disorders, Reich (1990) assessed 170 psychiatric outpatients using the Personality Diagnostic Questionnaire and found only minor differences between avoidant and dependent personalities. The results suggest that dependents and avoidants show low self-esteem. However, among dependents this stems from a feeling of inadequate competence, which leads to a fear of performing on their own. They do not share the avoidants' broad-ranging fear of relating to others; on the contrary, they feel most secure when they do affiliate. The general level of anxiety in the dependent is not a notable feature, as it is in the avoidant. Most central to the dependent's anxieties is interpersonal loss, in contrast to the avoidant's, which derive from fears of becoming too close (Trull, Widiger, & Frances, 1987).

The distinction between schizoid and avoidant personality disorders has also been called into question, as they share the trait of social disengagement or distancing. Similarly, other investigators feel that the active detachment characteristic of the avoidant disorder is essentially a variant of the schizoid disorder (Livesley & West, 1986). According to Livesley and West, carving two distinct personality disorders, schizoid and avoidant, from Kretschmer's original definition of the schizoid personality is conceptually incorrect. They propose that the two characterological qualities are not distinct, but rather are present at the same time in different proportions in a given schizoid patient, so that they form a continuous series. They also suggest that to separate these two qualities into distinct categories would render the essential definition of "schizoid" meaningless. However, the Personality Disorders Work Group's decision to differentiate the two categories is based on basic qualitative differences, as well as on the underlying motivation driving the observable behavior. For example, in the avoidant, social distancing stems from interpersonal anxiety; in the schizoid, it reflects interpersonal indifference. The avoidant desires (but does not trust) affection and closeness, whereas the schizoid has little interest in affection and closeness. The avoidant personality disorder devalues himself or herself and has low self-esteem; the schizoid does not. Finally, the avoidant is self-conscious and hyperalert to the meaning of others' communications; the schizoid is quite un-self-conscious and rather insensitive to the feelings and intents conveyed in the communications of others.

Despite the foregoing, the Work Group concluded that problems could be avoided by rewriting the criteria for avoidant personality disorder so as to differentiate them more clearly from similar characteristics seen among schizoids, dependents, social phobics, and others.

## Do the DSM-III-R Criteria Achieve Satisfactory Levels of Diagnostic Efficiency and Validity?

Recent published and unpublished studies carried out by members and advisors were submitted to the Personality Disorders Work Group; they provided a reasonable body of data and statistics to guide the following review. More extensive studies with a variety of representative samples and alternate methodologies should be undertaken in the future to confirm the following analysis of the DSM-III-R avoidant personality disorder construct and criteria. Additional concurrent studies and projects on experimental criterion items are in progress and may provide some empirical grounds for expanding the DSM-III-R list. The following summarizes the results of the aforementioned studies; the reader should be advised that these findings exhibited only modest consistency from project to project.

Diagnostic efficiency statistics, both internal and external, suggested that DSM-III-R criterion 1 ("is easily hurt by criticism or disapproval") was not only highly consistent with other avoidant criteria, but did not overlap appreciably with the criteria of other disorders. It fared poorly, however, when examined against clinicians' avoidant personality disorder diagnoses (low specificity was the problem). DSM-III-R criterion 2 ("has no close friends or confidants . . . ") showed high consistency with avoidant personality disorder but also with schizoid and schizotypal; in fact, according to this gauge, it was a superior item for the latter two. As far as external validity was concerned, it proved reasonably efficient. Criterion 2 ("is unwilling to get involved with people . . . ") was also an excellent item, in that it was highly consistent internally and also showed good external validity. Criterion 4 ("avoids social or occupational activities that involve interpersonal contact . . . ") overlapped somewhat with schizoid and schizotypal disorders, but showed better internal consistency with avoidant personality disorder than with the former two. Its strength was its excellent correspondence with external diagnoses of avoidant personality disorder. Criterion 5 ("is reticent in social situations . . . ") proved a poor item both internally and externally, as did criterion 6 ("fears being embarrassed by blushing . . . "). Although criterion 7 ("exaggerates the potential difficulties . . . invloved in doing something ordinary but outside his or her usual routine . . . ") obtained reasonable results, it proved the weakest criterion on the important sensitivity statistic.

Although the overall efficiency statistics for avoidant personality disorder were adequate, the work group concluded that revisions in the form of criterion condensations, sharpening distinctions from overlapping disorders, greater concordance with ICD-10 anxious (avoidant) personality disorder, and the addition of trait criteria that would broaden the descriptive range of avoidant personality disorder would all be worthwhile undertakings.

### Are There Criteria That Should Be Omitted, and Alternate Criteria That May Add Important Diagnostic Features?

To turn first to the last consideration just noted, a major criterion of DSM-III was inadvisably deleted from DSM-III-R, according to suggestions from several work group consultants — namely, that relating to low self-esteem. Evidence favoring the reintroduction of this general criterion was also obtained in a study of new or "experimental" diagnostic criteria (Millon & Tringone, 1989). Moreover, this characteristic is related to a new ICD-10 criterion for anxious (avoidant) personality disorder: "habitual self-consciousness and feelings of insecurity and inferiority" (see the ICD-10 criteria set given earlier). Work group discussions considered data, advisor input, descriptive literature, and consonance with ICD-10 in fashioning a new DSM-IV avoidant personality disorder criterion; this is discussed in more detail below.

As for the option of pruning items from the DSM-III-R list that demonstrated empirically poor diagnostic efficiency, it was decided that two criteria should be omitted (again, these decisions are discussed further below). It was also felt that both of these deletions should reduce overlap with other disorders, attributable to highly similar criteria in DSM-III-R.

## CHANGES PROPOSED FOR AND MADE IN DSM-IV

The following paragraphs outline the rationale and suggestions made by the Personality Disorders Work Group to increase the diagnostic clarity of the criteria for avoidant personality disorder in DSM-IV, as well as to facilitate their distinction from criteria for similar disorders and syndromes. Table 10.1 lists DSM-III-R and DSM-IV criteria.

TABLE 10.1. DSM-III-R and DSM-IV Diagnostic Criteria for Avoidant Personality Disorder

| DSM-III-R criteria | DSM-IV criteria |
|---|---|
| A pervasive pattern of social discomfort, fear of negative evaluation, and timidity, beginning by early adulthood and present in a variety of contexts, as indicated by at least *four* of the following: | A pervasive pattern of social inhibition, feelings of inadequacy, and hypersensitivity to negative evaluation, beginning by early adulthood and present in a variety of contexts, as indicated by four (or more) of the following: |
| (1) is easily hurt by criticism or disapproval | (1) avoids occupational activities that involve significant interpersonal contact, because of fears of criticism, disapproval, or rejection |
| (2) has no close friends or confidants (or only one) other than first-degree relatives | (2) is unwilling to get involved with people unless certain of being liked |
| (3) is unwilling to get involved with people unless certain of being liked | (3) shows restraint within intimate relationships because of the fear of being shamed or ridiculed |
| (4) avoids social or occupational activities that involve significant interpersonal contact, e.g., refuses a promotion that will increase social demands | (4) is preoccupied with being criticized or rejected in social situations |
| (5) is reticent in social situations because of a fear of saying something inappropriate or foolish, or of being unable to answer a question | (5) is inhibited in new interpersonal situations because of feelings of inadequacy |
| (6) fears being embarrassed by blushing, crying, or showing signs of anxiety in front of other people | (6) views self as socially inept, personally unappealing, or inferior to others |
| (7) exaggerates the potential difficulties, physical dangers, or risks involved in doing something ordinary but outside his or her usual routine, e.g., may cancel social plans because she anticipates being exhausted by the effort of getting there | (7) is unusually reluctant to take personal risks or to engage in any new activities because they may prove embarrassing |

*Note.* From APA (1987, p. 353) and APA (1994, pp. 654–665). Copyright 1987 and 1994 by the American Psychiatric Association. Reprinted by permission.

## Modifications and Deletions of DSM-III-R Criteria

*Criterion 1: "Is Easily Hurt by Criticism or Disapproval"*

*Explication.* The special sensitivity and touchiness of avoidant personalities about the judgments that others make of them is one of their more frequently referred-to traits. Although sensitivity statistics for this item were satisfactory, those for specificity were quite problematic, owing in part to the fact that the same criterion is employed in the DSM-III-R dependent personality disorder list.

*Changes Proposed and Made.* To reduce overlap and draw attention to the anticipatory and ruminative character of the avoidant personality's sensitivity, the following modification was suggested in work group discussions: "frequently anticipates and worries about being criticized or disapproved in social situations." In DSM-IV as published, this has been revised as follows: "is preoccupied with being criticized or rejected in social situations." It is now criterion 4 in the DSM-IV list (see Table 10.1)

### Criterion 2: "Has No Close Friends or Confidants (or Only One) Other than First-Degree Relatives"

*Explication.* Although this criterion is likely to be factually true, it fails to characterize the personality trait that this consequence exemplifies. Also, the phrasing is identical to that of DSM-III-R schizoid criterion A(6), which derives its consequence from a rather different trait characteristic, that of indifference to social relationships. Empirically, this criterion proved to be among the weakest of the avoidant personality disorder set; adding further to its questionable status, it correlated higher with schizoid and schizotypal disorders than with avoidant personality disorder. Finally, ICD-10 does not include this item in its set for anxious (avoidant) personality disorder.

*Changes Proposed and Made.* Recognizing the avoidant personality's discontent over his or her lack of friends, as differentiated from, for example, the schizoid's apparent indifference, the work group evolved the following alternative, which has similarities to the ICD-10 anxious (avoidant) personality disorder criterion that speaks of a "continuous yearning to be liked and accepted": "has few friends despite the desire to relate to others." In the end, however, this criterion was dropped altogether from the published version of DSM-IV.

### Criterion 3: "Is Unwilling to Get Involved with People Unless Certain of Being Liked"

*Explication.* This descriptor gets at the "reason" that accounts for the consequence described in item 2, and is therefore more useful in directing clinicians to its root source than to one of its several outcomes (which will vary in its expression by virtue of circumstance). It is similar to criterion 1, but goes an important step further in that it touches on how the avoidant personality copes interpersonally with "being hurt." Empirically, this criterion's statistics were among the highest in the avoidant personality disorder set; furthermore, it did not correlate particularly highly with schizoid or schizotypal disorders. Finally, ICD-10 does include this item in its anxious (avoidant) personality disorder list.

Changes Proposed and Made. This criterion has been retained intact in DSM-IV' only the numbering has been changed (it is now criterion 2).

### Criterion 4: "Avoids Social or Occupational Activities That Involve Significant Interpersonal Contact: e.g., Refuses a Promotion That Will Increase Social Demands"

*Explication.* This interpersonal characteristic relates again to a core form of behavior of the prototypical avoidant personality. Like criterion 3, it achieved one of the better levels of diagnostic efficiency in the empirical studies.

*Changes Proposed and Made.* Work group discussions suggested that the example given in the criterion ("refuses a promotion . . . ") was too infrequent and unauthentic an event to be useful. An alternative was proposed, to wit: "avoids social or occupational activities that involve significant interpersonal contact; for example, is unwilling to attend a party because he or she does not know many of those likely to be there." In the published version of DSM-IV, however, this example too has been discarded, and the item has been rephrased as follows: "avoids occupational activities that involve significant interpersonal contact, because of fears of criticism, disapproval, or rejection" (social situations are covered in other DSM-IV criteria). It is now criteria 1 in the DSM-IV list (see Table 10.1).

### Criterion 5: "Is Reticent in Social Situations Because of a Fear of Saying Something Inappropriate or Foolish, or of Being Unable to Answer a Question"

*Explication.* This criterion was new to DSM-III-R, added to reflect the phobic quality of avoidant personality disorder. Although efficiency statistics for this criterion were satisfactory, it overlaps in meaning and focus with the simultaneously introduced notion in DSM-III-R of a "generalized" type of social phobic; as noted above, a spurious, committee-generated commonality between the two disorders was thereby created. Along with criterion 6 (see below), this criterion overlaps with social phobia criteria in DSM-III-R—an overlap that has fostered confusion and led to the assumption that a comorbidity exists, when it is essentially a result of common phrasing.

*Changes Proposed and Made.* In an effort to distinguish these two disorders, work group discussions concluded that the quality avoidant personalities possess, beyond mere reticence in social situations, is a fear of establishing intimate personal relationships. The following phrasing was an attempt to capture this distinction (it subsumed criterion 6 as well): "development of intimate relationships is inhibited (despite desire), owing to the fear of being foolish and ridiculed, or being exposed and shamed." In DSM-IV as published, this criterion reads: "shows restraint within intimate relationships because of the fear of being shamed or ridiculed." However, the idea of social reticence has been retained in an additional criterion: "is inhibited in new interpersonal situations because of feelings of inadequacy." These are criteria 3 and 5, respectively, in the DSM-IV list (see Table 10.1).

### Criterion 6: "Fears Being Embarrassed by Blushing, Crying, or Showing Signs of Anxiety in Front of Others"

*Explication.* Efficiency statistics were relatively poor, for criterion 6, with specificity especially low (i.e., overlap was quite high). The similarity to criterion 5 is notable, both being examples of the fear of being foolish by virtue of one's own inadequacies, and both resembling criteria for DSM-III-R Axis I social phobia, generalized type (hence contributing to differential diagnostic difficulties). As expressed above, the work group felt that an effort should be made to shift the focus in avoidant personality disorder away from the main theme of social phobia—that of public embarrassment and humiliation—to that of a fear of intimate relationships. Of course, some avoidant personalities, like other disordered personalities, exhibit an Axis I disorder (in this case, social phobia) in addition to their Axis II diagnosis.

*Changes Proposed and Made.* See comments on criterion 5, above. Criterion 6 per se has been omitted from DSM-IV.

### Criterion 7: "Exaggerates the Potential Difficulties, Physical Dangers, or Risks Involved in Doing Something Ordinary but Outside His or Her Usual Routine . . ."

*Explication.* Item 7 was also added to reflect DSM-III-R to the phobic quality of these patients. However, it is phrased in a manner more like situations that would prompt anxiety among obsessive–compulsive personalities; in addition, it correlated quite highly with both dependent and schizotypal personality disorders. Furthermore, this criterion exhibited the poorest level of sensitivity among the avoidant personality disorder criterion set and was among the most infrequently assigned criteria.

*Changes Proposed and Made.* The work group originally proposed that criterion 7 be deleted from DSM-IV. However, an altered version of the criterion that stresses the element of feared embarrassment has been included in the published criteria set: "is unusually reluctant to take personal risks or to engage in any new activities because they may prove embarrassing." This remains criterion 7 in DSM-IV (see Table 10.1).

## Addition of a Criterion

The major reason for considering "new" criteria was to facilitate distinctions between the avoidant personality disorder construct and other personality disorders of a similar cast (e.g., dependent, paranoid, schizoid), as well as the DSM-III-R introduced social phobia, generalized type. As noted previously, a number of avoidant personality disorder criteria were dropped in the change from DSM-III to DSM-III-R; the wisdom of these decisions is debatable, particularly in light of added criteria that have created overlap with the new social phobia variant. The Personality Disorders Work Group felt that is "new" criterion for DSM-IV (actually, one reinstated from DSM-III) might remedy some of these difficulties. An additional and not unimportant goal was to bring DSM-IV more in line with the ICD-10.

This additional criterion relates to the DSM-III criterion "low self-esteem, for example, devalues self achievements and is overly dismayed by personal shortcomings." This diagnostic feature is not in DSM-III-R but is in ICD-10, phrased there as "habitual self-consciousness and feelings of insecurity and inferiority." The ICD phrasing may be too general and likely to fit several other personality disorders (e.g., dependent). By sharpening the focus on attitudes not usually found among dependent personalities (who do have low self-esteem), such as being socially inept and personally unattractive (views often held by avoidants but not dependents), the work group felt that an important trait might be included and a potentially complicating overlap might be avoided. Blending the ICD theme with the original DSM-III statement resulted in this proposed wording: "possesses low self-esteem because he or she feels socially inept and/or unappealing." The criterion as published, although not referring explicitly to "low self-esteem," retains the sharpened focus: "views self as socially inept, personally unappealing, or inferior to others." ("Low self-esteem" was judged to be too broad ranging.) It is criterion 6 in the DSM-IV set (set Table 10.1).

## CONCLUDING COMMENTS AND REMAINING ISSUES

The concerns raised when DSM-III was first published regarding the prevalence of the then-new avoidant personality disorder appear to have faded by virtue of its increasing acceptability in the literature, its generally satisfactory efficiency statistics, and its frequent diagnostic usage among clinicians. Problems remain for some in differentiating aspects of the disorder from several other syndromes, notably schizoid and dependent personality disorders within Axis II and social phobia within Axis I. Meaningful distinctions can be made in each case, although certain commonalities are inevitable, as they are with most complex disorders. This chapter has described various changes made in DSM-IV: phrasing changes, condensation or deletion of DSM-III-R criteria, and a new criterion in line with the original DSM-

III as well as ICD-10. ICD-10 includes this disorder under the title "anxious (avoidant) personality disorder. Though not identical, the criteria for these two disorders are highly similar.

It should be noted that two alternative designations to the "avoidant" label have been considered: the "phobic personality," a name emerging from analytic quarters, and the "anxious personality," in line with ICD-10. In both of these, emphasis is given to a single feature that corresponds to a diagnostic category in Axis I. The "anxious personality" designation raises, among other matters, the same issue with which the Personality Disorders Work Group has been struggling in its discussions of the "depressive personality—namely, the identification of a wide-ranging personality disorder by a label that may be a valid description but is in no way distinctive to that personality disorder (both anxiety and depression are key elements in more than a few personality disorders). As for the "phobic personality," this label may introduce a psychoanalytic interpretive implication twist that may not be worth the negative reaction it fosters.

The shift in DSM-III-R to a polythetic format for the avoidant personality disorder criteria is consonant with the logically defensible prototypical character of personality disorders, but it does raise questions as to the number of criteria that should be required; as to whether an absolute, "in or out" cutoff makes sense (as opposed to a quantitative gradation); and as to whether the differential weighting of criteria may not prove useful in identifying "authentic" avoidant personality disorder types. Unfortunately, there is little in the empirical literature on avoidant personality disorder (or other personality disorders, for that matter) to aid us in addressing these issues with confidence.

The lack of a substantial empirical basis for refining our conception of the avoidant personality disorder is matched, in our judgment, by a parallel failure to clarify the theoretical grounding that gives meaning to the construct. A foundation of latent psychological principles is needed, so that the character of the disorder can be understood as a logically derivable form of personality pathology. On the other hand, a major principle guiding the DSM is that of eschewing theoretical principals and favoring observable data; this principle is understandable in light of current controversies, but it may ultimately prove fruitless and misguided.

## REFERENCES

American Psychiatric Association. (1980). *Diagnostic and statistical manual of mental disorders* (3rd ed.). Washington, DC: Author.

American Psychiatric Association. (1987). *Diagnostic and statistical manual of mental disorders* (3rd ed., rev.). Washington, DC: Author.

American Psychiatric Association. (1994). *Diagnostic and statistical manual of mental disorders* (4th ed.). Washington, DC: Author.

Arieti, S. (1955). *Interpretation of schizophrenia.* New York: Brunner/Mazel.

Blashfield, R. (1988). [Similarity matrix for personality disorders]. Unpublished raw data.

Bleuler, E. (1911). *Dementia praecox: Or the group of schizophrenias* (J. Zinkin, Trans.). New York: International Universities Press.

Burnham, D. L., Gladstone, A. O., & Gibson, R. W. (1969). *Schizophrenia and the need–fear dilemma.* New York: International Universities Press.

Dahl, A. (1986). Some aspects of the DSM-III personality disorders illustrated by a consecutive sample of hospitalized patients. *Acta Psychiatrica Scandinavica, 73*(Suppl. 328), 61–66.

Fenichel, O. (1945). *The pychoanalytic theory of neurosis.* New York: Norton.

Fairbairn, W. R. D. (1940). Schizoid factors in the personality. In W. R. D. Fairbairn, *Psychoanalytic studies of the personality.* London: Tavistock, 1952.

Freiman, K., & Widiger, T. (1989). [Co-occurrence and diagnostic efficiency statistics]. Unpublished raw data.

Greenberg, D., & Stravynski, A. (1983). Social phobia [Letter]. *British Journal of Psychiatry, 143,* 526.

Guntrip, H. (1952). A study of Fairbairn's theory of schizoid reactions. *British Journal of Medical Psychology, 25,* 86–104.

Herbert, J. D., Hope, D. A., & Bellak, A. S. (1992). Validity of the distinction between generalized social phobia and avoidant personality disorder. *Journal of Abnormal Psychology, 101,* 332–338.

Holt, C. S., Heimberg, R. G., & Hope, D. A. (1992). Avoidant personality disorder and the generalized subtype of social phobia. *Journal of Abnormal Psychology, 101,* 318–325.

Horney, K. (1945). *Our inner conflicts.* New York: Norton.

Kernberg, O. (1984). *Severe personality disorders.* New Haven, CT: Yale University Press.

Kretschmer, E. (1925). *Physique and character.* London: Kegan Paul, 1926.

Laing, R. D. (1960). *The divided self.* Chicago: Quadrangle.

Livesley, J. W., & West, M. (1986). The DSM-III distinction between schizoid and avoidant personality disorders. *Canadian Journal of Psychiatry, 31,* 59–62.

MacKinnon, R. A., & Michels, R. (1971). *The psychiatric interview in clinical practice.* Philadelphia: W. B. Saunders.

Millon, T., (1969). *Modern psychopathology.* Philadelphia: W. B. Saunders.

Millon, T., & Tringone, R. (1989). [Co-occurrence and diagnostic efficiency statistics]. Unpublished raw data.

Morey, L., & Heumann, K. (1988). [Co-occurrence and diagnostic efficiency statistics]. Unpublished raw data.

Pfohl, B., & Blum, N. (1990). [Internal consistency statistics for the DSM-III-R personality disorder criteria]. Unpublished raw data.

Reich, J. (1990). The relationship between DSM-III avoidant and dependent personality disorders. *Psychiatry Research, 34,* 218–292.

Schneider, K. (1923). *Die psychopathischen personlichkeiten.* Vienna: Deuticke.

Trull, T. J., Widiger, T. A., & Frances, A. (1987). Covariation of criteria sets for avoidant, schizoid, and dependent personality disorder. *American Journal of Psychiatry, 144,* 767–772.

Turner, S. M., Beidel, D. C., Dancee, C. V., & Keys, D. J. (1986). Psychopathology of social phobia and comparison to avoidant personality disorder. *Journal of Abnormal Psychology, 95,* 389–394.

Weissman, M. M. (1990). *The epidemiology of personality disorder: A 1990 update.* Paper presented at the Conference on the Personality Disorders, Williamsburg, VA.

World Health Organization. (1992). *The ICD-10 classification of mental and behavioral disorders: Diagnostic criteria for research.* Geneva: Author.

Widiger, T. A. (1991). DSM-IV reviews of the personality disorders: Introduction to special series. *Journal of Personality Disorders, 5,* 122–134.

Winnicott, D. W. (1956). Primitive emotional development. In D. W. Winnicott, *Collected papers.* London: Tavistock, 1958.

Zanarini, M. (1989). [Co-occurrence and diagnostic efficiency statistics]. Unpublished raw data.

# Commentary on Avoidant Personality Disorder: Temperament, Shame, or Both?

Paul A. Pilkonis

In Chapter 10, Millon and Martinez describe the varied concepts that can be related in one fashion or another to "avoidant personality disorder." The mixture usually includes a blend of avoidant, schizoid, schizotypal, dependent, self-defeating, and "phobic" traits (Pilkonis, 1984). The fact that this is a "fuzzy set" is itself a commentary on the potential limitations of categorical classification, especially for categories whose prototypes include many different, equally salient features rather than a smaller number of distinctive, pathognomonic indicators (Livesley, 1985). It is ironic that the category is probably less controversial (although perhaps not less fuzzy) for the layperson than for the mental health professional: The common term, "shyness," has a rich set of connotations with which most people feel they have some firsthand experience (Jones, Briggs, & Smith, 1986; Zimbardo, 1977).

As Millon and Martinez point out, there has been an ebb and flow in the professional nomenclature from a position emphasizing poor self-esteem (DSM-III; American Psychiatric Association, 1980) to one describing other aspects of the "phobic character" (DSM-III-R; American Psychiatric Association, 1987) to a concept that again focuses on a deficient sense of self (DSM-IV; American Psychiatric Association, 1994). An alternative summary for the current "gestalt" might be avoidant personality disorder as an impaired sense of self that leads to an approach–avoidance conflict about relationships with others. Various phrases in the DSM-IV criteria presume a certain degree of relatedness; for example, "restraint within intimate relationships" requires that some such relationships be present, and "inhibited in new interpersonal situations" presumes that such situations are not avoided entirely. More striking, however, is the emphasis of the new criteria on shame and diminished self-esteem in relationships: "fear of being shamed or ridiculed," "feelings of inadequacy," a view of self as "inferior to others," and reluctance to take personal risks "because they may prove embarrassing" (all quotes from American Psychiatric Association, 1994, pp. 664–665). All these fears, of course, lead to some inhibition and withdrawal, and they create the conflicts about relationships that avoidant people describe.

The strongest arguments (theoretical and empirical) have been made for links between avoidant personality disorder and Axis I anxiety disorders in general, usually with the implication that avoidant personality is a subclinical or "spectrum" disorder on the same continuum. According to this reasoning, an avoidant person is one who is primarily motivated by harm avoidance and less influenced by reward dependence or novelty seeking (Cloninger, 1987). In the same vein, it is easy to imagine that the young children described by Kagan (1989) as "inhibited to the unfamiliar" carry some of this temperamental constraint into interpersonal relationships later in life. This anxious prototype is also consistent with the criteria of the *International Classification of Diseases,* 10th revision (ICD-10; World Health Organization, 1992), for "anxious (avoidant) personality disorder."

I emphasize the themes of shame and problems in self-esteem, however, because they alert us to one connection that has been neglected in the descriptive literature on personality disorders (although there is some discussion of the topic in the psychodynamic literature). This connection is the link between avoidant personality and narcissism—that is, narcissistic problems understood generically as resulting from flawed self-esteem that precludes a modulated, generally positive view of self, others, and self in relation to others. In the terms of object relations theory, the interpersonal "script" internalized by the avoidant person is that of a diminished self wishing for some contact with a loving and respectful other whose endowments the person hopes to share; at the same time, the person assumes that the likely reaction from this significant other will be criticism, scorn, or derision, leading to still further humiliation and shame. There is some limited empirical support for this model: Stravynski, Elie, and Franche (1989) report data from a small sample describing the perceptions that avoidant patients have of their parents as "shaming, guilt-engendering, and intolerant" (p. 415). In the terms of attachment theory, such parental behavior would be a recipe for the development of "anxious–ambivalent" attachments; the crucial ingredient is early experience with parents who are affectively engaged but primarily in hostile, critical, or (at best) inconsistent modes.

If we hypothesize at least two subgroups of avoidant personalities—one that is temperamentally overanxious, and a second that is narcissistically vulnerable—distinctions between them could be made on the basis of early developmental histories and adult attachment styles. If truly temperamentally driven, members of the first group should have a more varied (and potentially more normative) attachment history. They may have "taken in" even reasonably benign experiences through a sensitive temperamental filter, but, to the extent that these early experiences were benign, they should be associated with a better history of success in adult intimate relationships. The second group is likely to have had more developmental adversity and should have a more uniformly negative attachment pattern later in life.

Again, there are some data to support such a position. Wink (1992), for example, describes a "hypersensitivity" subscale for narcissism derived from the California Q-Sort and defines such hypersensitivity as a "frequent but 'atypical' form of narcissism in which overt inhibition, introversion, and lack of self-confidence mask an underlying (covert) grandiose sense of self-importance, entitlement, and exhibitionism" (p. 9). His results demonstrate more negative retrospective reports of parenting and a more negative prognosis in midlife for women displaying these features.

Other discussions from the psychoanalytic literature of a "vulnerable" narcissistic person (who might be labeled "shy" or "avoidant") deserve mention. Kaplan (1972) provides an interesting account of shyness as both an everyday experience and a more pervasive symptom. Kernberg (1970, 1974) and Akhtar and Thomson (1982) describe vulnerable as well as grandiose presentations of narcissism, and Kohut (1971; Kohut & Wolf, 1978), of course, explicates in considerable detail covert aspects of narcissism associated with compliance, idealization, and a manifestly anxious presentation.

Any attempt to diagnose these variants of avoidant personality disorder differentially is not intended to split hairs, but rather to have direct treatment implications. There are clear differences between focusing on hyperarousal and avoidant behavior based on the need to cope with a "temperamental" vulnerability (i.e., a lowered threshold for anxiety), and focusing on an impaired sense of self with the goal of generating greater self-esteem. The former point of view would promote behavioral interventions based on social learning principles: exposure to feared situations, desensitization of interpersonal anxiety, social skills training, and practice of a new behavioral repertoire. The latter would focus on interventions designed to enhance a positive sense of self. Some of this enhancement might arise naturally out of "good enough" individual therapy (through processes of modeling and internalization, familiar to readers of Kohut), as well as a more overt behavioral focus on experiences of mastery and competence likely to promote self-esteem. From the point of view of attachment theory, stronger internal psychological structures are likely to develop out of the dialectic between attachment and separation inherent in most extended interpersonal encounters and transacted in the relationship in individual therapy (Blatt & Shichman, 1983). With this model, however, there needs to be a prescribed therapeutic sequence. Attachment must come first; that is, the therapist must be able to communicate (verbally or nonverbally) a spirit of consistency, availability, and positive affective engagement (a "secure base"), even in the face of realistic boundaries and limits ("optimal frustration"), if appropriate attachment needs are to be validated. Only when these needs are validated will the capacity for genuine self-esteem, autonomy, and unconflicted separation emerge.

Finally, in any discussion of the descriptive diagnostic criteria of the DSMs, I believe that there should be some comment about the alleged need to forsake "theory." In Chapter 10, Millon and Martinez criticize this approach, decrying the lack of a theoretical structure in the nosology. I endorse this comment. Whether as nosologists, as researchers on psychopathology, or as clinicians, we need to have "models" that consider the phenomenology and motivations underlying the overt markers we assess. Without such explicit conceptual models, we do get into hair-splitting debates about the appropriate application of descriptive criteria, because of different implicit (unarticulated) models of the meaning of the criteria. Not all criteria are equal in all contexts; their meanings will vary depending on both the internal environment of the actor and the external environment provided by different settings and interpersonal transactions. Measuring such things is, of course, difficult, but there is much interesting work being done on case formulation methods (Horowitz, 1991; Luborsky & Crits-Christoph, 1990; Persons, 1991). Also, an increasingly influential system that blends dynamic and interpersonal theory with a rigorous empirical approach is Benjamin's (1974, 1987) Structural Analysis of Social Behavior, which is useful because it helps us to explicate "scripts" focused on self, others, and self in relation to others in ways that are more transparent than many less empirical psychodynamic discussions.

## ACKNOWLEDGMENT

Support for this work was provided, in part, by National Institute of Mental Health Grant No. R01 MH44672.

## REFERENCES

Akhtar, S., & Thomson, J. A. Jr. (1982). Overview: Narcissistic personality disorder. *American Journal of Psychiatry, 139,* 12–20.

American Psychiatric Association. (1980). *Diagnostic and statistical manual of mental disorders* (3rd ed.). Washington, DC: Author.

American Psychiatric Association. (1987). *Diagnostic and statistical manual of mental disorders* (3rd ed., rev.). Washington, DC: Author.

American Psychiatric Association. (1994). *Diagnostic and statistical manual of mental disorders* (4th ed.). Washington, DC: Author.

Benjamin, L. S. (1974). Structural Analysis of Social Behavior. *Psychological Review, 81,* 392–425.

Benjamin, L. S. (1987). Use of the SASB dimensional model to develop treatment plans for personality disorders: I. Narcissism. *Journal of Personality Disorders, 1,* 43–70.

Blatt, S. J., & Shichman, S. (1983). Two primary configurations of psychopathology. *Psychoanalysis and Contemporary Thought, 6,* 187–254.

Cloninger, C. R. (1987). A systematic method for clinical description and classification of personality variants: A proposal. *Archives of General Psychiatry, 44,* 573–588.

Horowitz, M. J. (Ed.). (1991). *Person schemas and maladaptive interpersonal patterns.* Chicago: University of Chicago Press.

Jones, W. H., Briggs, S. R., & Smith, T. G. (1986). Shyness: Conceptualization and measurement. *Journal of Personality and Social Psychology, 51,* 629–639.

Kagan, J. (1989). Temperamental contributions to social behavior. *American Psychologist, 44,* 668–674.

Kaplan, D. (1972). On shyness. *International Journal of Psycho-Analysis, 53,* 439–453.

Kernberg, O. F. (1970). Factors in the treatment of narcissistic personalities. *Journal of the American Psychoanalytic Association, 18,* 51–85.

Kernberg, O. F. (1974). Further contributions to the treatment of narcissistic personalities. *International Journal of Psycho-Analysis, 55,* 215–240.

Kohut, H. (1971). *The analysis of the self.* New York: International Universities Press.

Kohut, H., & Wolf, E. (1978). The disorders of the self and their treatment. *International Journal of Psycho-Analysis, 59,* 413–425.

Livesley, W. J. (1985). The classification of personality disorder: I. The choice of category concept. *Canadian Journal of Psychiatry, 30,* 353–358.

Luborsky, L., & Crits-Christoph, P. (Eds.). (1990). *Understanding transference: The CCRT method.* New York: Basic Books.

Persons, J. B. (1991). Psychotherapy outcome studies do not accurately represent current models of psychotherapy: A proposed remedy. *American Psychologist, 46,* 99–107.

Pilkonis, P. A. (1984). Avoidant and schizoid personality disorders. In H. E. Adams & P. B. Sutker (Eds.), *Comprehensive handbook of psychopathology* (pp. 479–494). New York: Plenum.

Stravynski, A., Elie, R., & Franche, R. L. (1989). Perception of early parenting by patients diagnosed avoidant personality disorder: A test of the overprotection hypothesis. *Acta Psychiatrica Scandinavica, 80,* 415–420.

Wink, P. (1992). Three types of narcissism in women from college to mid-life. *Journal of Personality, 60,* 7–30.

World Health Organization. (1992). *The ICD-10 classification of mental and behavioural disorders: Diagnostic criteria for research.* Geneva: Author.

Zimbardo, P. G. (1977). *Shyness: What it is, what to do about it.* Reading, MA: Addison-Wesley.

# CHAPTER 11

# Dependent Personality Disorder

ROBERT M. A. HIRSCHFELD
M. TRACIE SHEA
RICHARD WEISE

The concept of "dependency" has its roots in psychoanalytic theory, social-psychological theory, and ethological theory (Hirschfeld, Klerman, Chodoff, Korchin, & Barrett, 1976). Psychoanalytic theory emphasizes the attainment of instinctual aims through interaction with social objects, such as the mother, as the source of dependency. Social learning theories consider dependency to be a learned behavior—that is, one acquired in experience rather than instinctual in the organism. More specifically, dependency refers to a class of behaviors stemming from the infant's initial reliance on the mother; these learned behaviors subsequently generalize to interpersonal relations in general. In ethological theory, the concept of attachment has been proposed to refer to the affectionate bond that one person forms to another specific individual. This bond is manifested by behaviors fostering proximity to and contact with the love object, and by behavioral disruptions if separation occurs.

These three theoretical roots (psychoanalytic, social learning, and ethological) share certain elements but are far from identical. The psychoanalytic viewpoint emphasizes intrapsychic mechanisms, both motivational and cognitive. Social learning theory emphasizes behavior and is much less concerned with internal events. Also, from the standpoint of social learning theory, dependent behaviors are contingent upon reinforcements and therefore may vary over time and situation. The ethological approach blends intrapsychic and behavioral aspects. Attachments are intrapsychic but lead to quite specific behavioral manifestations; attachments are enduring and specific.

These theoretical roots have contributed to the concept of dependent

An earlier version of this chapter was published in the *Journal of Personality Disorders*, 1991, 5, 135–149. Copyright 1991 by The Guilford Press. Adapted by permission.

personality disorder as defined in the *Diagnostic and Statistical Manual of Mental Disorders* (DSM) of the American Psychiatric Association (APA). The essential feature of this mental disorder has been abnormal dependency, which causes subjective distress and/or impairment in functioning for the individual. The definition and criteria of dependent personality disorder have shifted in the different versions of the DSM. In DSM-I (American Psychiatric Association, 1952), passive–dependent personality was defined as a subtype of passive–aggressive personality and was characterized by helplessness, indecisiveness, and clinging behavior. DSM-II (American Psychiatric Association, 1968) relegated passive–dependent personality to "other personality disorders of specified types" and provided no description. In DSM-III (American Psychiatric Association, 1980), three criteria were specified; these pertained to passivity and lack of independence, subordination of one's own needs, and lack of self-confidence.

DSM-III-R (American Psychiatric Association, 1987) gave the disorder its present name and expanded the definition to nine criteria. The essential feature became a "pervasive pattern of dependent and submissive behavior" with five criteria required for a diagnosis (see Table 11.1). Most of the criteria are elaborations of the passivity and subordination included in DSM-III. However, lack of self-confidence was dropped, and several criteria reflecting anxious attachment and fear of loss of an important person were added. In addition, a criterion reflecting sensitivity to criticism was added.

The criteria for dependent personality disorder were critically examined for possible revision for DSM-IV. The purpose of this chapter is to review the key issues addressed in the revision process, as well as current thinking with regard to the criteria and diagnosis of this disorder.

## STATEMENT OF ISSUES

The major issues addressed were as follows:

- To what extent does dependent personality disorder overlap conceptually with other personality disorders?
- To what extent does dependent personality disorder overlap empirically with other disorders?
- How do the individual criteria for dependent personality disorder perform (e.g., sensitivity and specificity)?
- Is dependent personality disorder characterized by single or multiple components?
- Is there gender bias in the application of dependent personality disorder?

TABLE 11.1. DSM-III-R and DSM-IV Diagnostic Criteria for Dependent Personality Disorder

| DSM-III-R criteria | DSM-IV criteria |
| --- | --- |
| A pervasive pattern of dependent and submissive behavior, beginning by early adulthood and present in a variety of contexts, as indicated by at least *five* of the following: | A pervasive and excessive need to be taken care of that leads to submissive and clinging behavior and fears of separation, beginning by early adulthood and present in a variety of contexts, as indicated by five (or more) of the following: |
| (1) is unable to make everyday decisions without an excessive amount of advice or reassurance from others | (1) has difficulty making everyday decisions without an excessive amount of advice and reassurance from others |
| (2) allows others to make most of his or her important decisions, e.g., where to live, what job to take | (2) needs others to assume responsibility for most major areas of his or her life |
| (3) agrees with people even when he or she believes they are wrong, because of fear of being rejected | (3) has difficulty expressing disagreement with others because of fear of loss of support or approval. **Note:** Do not include realistic fears of retribution |
| (4) has difficulty initiating projects or doing things on his or her own | (4) has difficulty initiating projects or doing things on his or her own (because of a lack of self-confidence in judgment or abilities rather than a lack of motivation or energy) |
| (5) volunteers to do things that are unpleasant or demeaning in order to get other people to like him or her | (5) goes to excessive lengths to obtain nurturance and support from others, to the point of volunteering to do things that are unpleasant |
| (6) feels uncomfortable or helpless when alone, or goes to great lengths to avoid being alone | (6) feels uncomfortable or helpless when alone because of exaggerated fears of being unable to care for himself or herself |
| (7) feels devastated or helpless when close relationships end | (7) urgently seeks another relationship as a source of care and support when a close relationship ends |
| (8) is frequently preoccupied with fears of being abandoned | (8) is unrealistically preoccupied with fears of being left to take care of himself or herself |
| (9) is easily hurt by criticism or disapproval | |

*Note.* From APA (1987, p. 354) and APA (1994, pp. 668–669). Copyright 1987 and 1994 by the American Psychiatric Association. Reprinted by permission.

# LITERATURE REVIEW

These issues were examined on the basis of a review of the literature published from January 1980 to May 1990. Forty-seven articles appeared under the direct subject heading "dependent personality disorder," and 38 additional articles were identified by using related descriptive terms. Other information and data were collected from book chapters on the topic, journal articles not abstracted on Medline, and reports of unpublished data.

## Conceptual Overlap

Conceptual overlap of dependent personality disorder features can be found with borderline, avoidant, and histrionic personality disorders.

### Borderline Personality Disorder

Both dependent and borderline personality disorders are characterized by fear of abandonment. However, the behavioral patterns of these two disorders are quite different. Fear of abandonment elicits rage and manipulation in borderline personality disorder; in contrast, it elicits submissive and clinging behavior in dependent personality disorder. Whereas borderline patients have difficulty being alone under any circumstances, for dependent patients the issue is more the need to be attached or to have access to a strong other on whom they can rely for care and support. Borderline and dependent personality disorders can be further distinguished by more general patterns of interpersonal relationships. A key feature of borderline personality disorder is intense and unstable relationships; this is not a characteristic of dependent personality disorder.

### Avoidant Personality Disorder

Both dependent and avoidant personality disorders are characterized by feelings of inadequacy, sensitivity to criticism, and need for reassurance. However, like borderlines, dependents can also be distinguished by their quite distinct behavior patterns. Avoidant personality disorder is based on fear of humiliation and rejection, which results in social timidity and withdrawal. At the heart of dependent personality disorder is an excessive need for attachment, which leads to fears of separation and to submissive and clinging behavior.

### Histrionic Personality Disorder

Both dependent and histrionic personality disorder are characterized by a need for reassurance and approval. In histrionic personality disorder, however, the need is for approval and praise in and of itself, whereas in dependent personality disorder the need is more for reassurance because of doubt about one's judgment and ability. That is, the dependent individual needs to be assured by others that his or her actions are correct.

TABLE 11.2. Percentages of Subjects Diagnosed with Dependent Personality Disorder Receiving Other Specific Axis II Diagnoses

| Study | PRN | SZD | SZT | ATS | BDL | HST | NAR | AVD | OCP | PAG | Sing. |
|---|---|---|---|---|---|---|---|---|---|---|---|
| **DMS-III** | | | | | | | | | | | |
| Pfohl et al. (1986) | | | | | 41 | 29 | | 18 | 6 | 28 | 47 |
| Zanarini et al. (1987) | 7 | | 45 | 30 | 86 | 54 | 22 | 25 | 9 | 25 | 7 |
| Dahl (1986) | | | | | 25 | 25 | | 75 | | | |
| Morey (1988) | 29 | 9 | 26 | 3 | 51 | 29 | 26 | 49 | 9 | 17 | |
| Trull et al. (1987) | | 0 | | | | | | 50 | | | |
| **DSM-III-R** | | | | | | | | | | | |
| Morey (1988) | 29 | 9 | 12 | 3 | 51 | 29 | 26 | 49 | 9 | 17 | |
| Skodol et al. (1988) | 24 | | 30 | 15 | 85 | 30 | 58 | 73 | 30 | 12 | |
| Skodol et al. (1988) | 36 | 3 | 24 | 3 | 79 | 33 | 21 | 70 | 27 | 18 | |

Note. Key to personality disorder abbreviations: PRN, paranoid; SZD, schizoid; SZT, schizotypal; ATS, antisocial; BDL, borderline; HST, histrionic; NAR, narcissistic; AVD, avoidant; OCP, obsessive–compulsive; PAG, passive–aggressive; Sing., percentage with only dependent personality disorder.

## Empirical Overlap

Studies have shown considerable diagnostic overlap of both DSM-III and DSM-III-R dependent personality disorder with other personality disorders, particularly borderline personality disorder (see Table 11.2). Over 50% of patients with dependent personality disorder also had borderline personality disorder in two of four studies using DSM-III criteria and all three studies using DSM-III-R criteria. The second most frequent overlap was with avoidant personality disorder, although there was also frequent overlap with histrionic and schizotypal personality disorders. Relatively few patients met criteria for dependent personality disorder and for no other Axis II disorders. The percentage of personality disorder patients with a single diagnosis of dependent ranged from 7% to 47%, with a median of 20%, in five studies.

## PERFORMANCE OF CRITERIA

Widiger (personal communication) has recently summarized data from five studies on the relationship between specific DSM-III-R criteria and diagnosis of dependent personality disorder. He concluded that criterion 9 ("is easily hurt by criticism or disapproval") performs particularly poorly in all the studies, as it is consistently nonspecific for this diagnosis.

Loranger (personal communication) provided data on criteria performance in a sample of 136 nonpsychotic, nonbipolar patients who were assessed using the Personality Disorder Examination. Criterion 7 ("feels devastated or helpless when a close relationship ends") and criterion 9 ("feelings easily hurt by criticism or disapproval") did particularly poorly in two ways. First, the endorsement rate of each was very high in patients who had no personality disorder. Second, the endorsement rate on each was extremely high (usually over 80%) in almost all personality disorders, including dependent. These two criteria, therefore, were not at all specific to dependent personality disorder. The item with the lowest endorsement rate for dependent personality disorder was criterion 5 ("volunteers to do things that are unpleasant or demeaning in order to get other people to like him or her").

## UNITARY CONCEPT

Whether dependency is characterized by a single or by multiple dimensions has received considerable attention (Hirschfeld, Klerman, Chodoff, et al., 1976; Livesley, Schroeder & Jackson, 1990b; Birchnell, 1988). Interpersonal dependency, as a personality feature, has been investigated by Hirschfeld and colleagues (Hirschfeld, Klerman, Chadoff, et al., 1976; Hirschfeld, Klerman, Gough, et al., 1977). Using a self-report inventory that was tested empirically on both normal and depressed samples, they found that interpersonal dependency contained three components: emotional reliance on an another person, lack of social self-confidence, and assertion of autonomy. Emotional reliance on another person is reflective of intensity and fragility of attachment. Lack of social self-confidence is more reflective of general dependency—that is, social compliance, lack of assertiveness, lack of independent judgment, and a general desire to go along with the group. Thus, it is reflective of one's relationship to other people in general, not just one or two very key people. Assertion of autonomy is the degree to which one claims a complete lack or need for others.

Livesley and colleagues have extended the issues of attachment and dependency to dependent personality disorder (Livesley, Jackson, & Schroeder, 1989; Livesley et al. 1990). They developed a pool of items to assess major dimensions of attachment and dependency, and identified five dimensions of attachment and five of dependency on a conceptual basis. The attachment dimensions included the following (1) fear of loss of an attachment figure, (2) need for affection, (3) need for proximity to the attachment figure, (4) feelings of security based on physical presence of the attachment figure, and (5) strong protest at separation from the attachment figure. The dimensions of dependency were as follows: (1) low self-esteem, (2) need for advice and reassurance, (3) need for constant reassurance and approval, (4) need for care and support, and (5) submissiveness.

Scales assessing the individual dimensions comprising the attachment and dependency constructs were administered to general-population and clinical samples and were analyzed by means of multivariate methods. A principal-components factor analysis yielded two factors that accounted for nearly 72% of the variance and corresponded to attachment and dependency. The correlation between the combined attachment scale and the combined dependency scale was .62. Table 11.3 shows the correspondence of the DSM-III-R criteria for dependent personality disorder with the dimensions of attachment and dependency.

The findings of the studies of Hirschfeld et al. and Livesley et al. are consistent. The emotional reliance on another person component of interpersonal dependency corresponds closely to the concept of attachment. The lack of social self-confidence component of interpersonal dependency corresponds closely to the concept of general dependency. Together, these studies suggest that the two distinguishable dimensions of attachment and general dependency may be components of dependent personality disorder; therefore, diagnostic criteria should assess both.

TABLE 11.3. Correspondence between DSM-III-R Criteria and Dimensions of Dependent Personality Disorder as Proposed by Livesley and Colleagues

| DSM-III-R criteria | Attachment | | | | | Dependency | | | | |
|---|---|---|---|---|---|---|---|---|---|---|
| | Separation protest | Secure base | Proximity seeking | Feared loss | Need for affection | Need for care/support | Low self-esteem | Submissiveness | Need for advice and reassurance | Need for approval |
| (1) is unable to make everyday decisions | | | | | | | | | × | |
| (2) allows others to make important decisions | | | | | | | | × | × | |
| (3) agrees with people out of fear of rejection | | | | | | | | × | | |
| (4) has difficulty initiating things on own | | | | | | | | | × | |
| (5) does things to get others to like him or her | | | | | | | | × | | |
| (6) avoids occasions of being alone | | × | | | | | | | | |
| (7) feels devastated when relationships end | × | | × | | | | | | | |
| (8) is preoccupied with fear of abandonment | | | | × | | | | | | |
| (9) is easily hurt by criticism/ disapproval | | | | | | | | | | |

## Gender Bias

The issue of potential gender bias in diagnosis has been hotly debated in psychiatry, particularly for dependent personality disorder (Brown, 1986; Frances & Widiger, 1987; Gunderson, 1983; Kaplan, 1983; Williams & Spitzer, 1983). Unfortunately, there has been far more rhetoric than research on this issue, with a few exceptions. Widiger and Spitzer (1991) have recently completed a scholarly investigation of the issue, in which they distinguished between sex differences and sex bias in terms of etiology, sampling, diagnosis, assessment procedures, and criteria.

Three studies have reported data relevant to the question of whether the criteria for dependent personality disorder are biased toward diagnosing more women than men. Kass, Spitzer, and Williams (1983) investigated the distribution of DSM-III personality disorders by sex in two large groups of psychiatric patients, using clinicians' diagnoses. They found that dependent personality disorder was diagnosed 2.5 to 4 times more often in women than in men in two large clinical samples with no standard assessment procedures. In contrast, Reich (1987), using standardized instruments (interview and self-report), did not confirm the Kass et al. finding. Instead, Reich found that the percentage of females with dependent personality disorder (using either instrument) mirrored the percentage of females in the clinic.

In another study, Reich, Nduaguba, and Yates (1988) investigated age and sex distribution of DSM-III personality cluster traits, assessed by a self-report measure, in a randomly sampled community population. They did not report findings for dependent personality disorder traits separately. There was a significant difference between males and females only for subjects in the 31–40 age range; in this age group, women had higher scores on all Axis II clusters. Thus, where there were differences between the sexes, these were not specific to dependent personality disorder or even to the "anxious" cluster.

The findings regarding gender bias are far from conclusive. However, when standardized measures are used, women are not more frequently diagnosed with dependent personality disorder than males. This suggests that clinician behavior, rather than the diagnostic criteria, requires more intensive study.

## SIGNIFICANCE OF THE ISSUES FOR DSM-IV

The goal for DSM-IV was to address these issues as carefully and completely as possible, in an attempt to improve the definition of dependent personality disorder.

1. With regard to the conceptual overlap, especially with borderline, avoidant, and histrionic personality disorders, we proposed to include the

conceptual core of dependent personality disorder as a necessary criterion for this disorder. Therefore, an individual with dependent personality disorder must demonstrate a pervasive and excessive need to be taken care of that leads to submissive and clinging behavior and fears of separation.

2. We view dependent personality disorder as composed of both excessive attachment needs and excessive instrumental dependency needs. Criteria assessing these qualities have been included in DSM-IV.

3. Criteria that have been found to perform poorly or to be ambiguous have been modified or deleted.

4. We have examined all the criteria from the vantage of gender bias and have endeavored to make them all free of this. This, of course, may not lead to equal distribution between the sexes, but it will avoid the creation of artifactual differences.

It is our belief that these changes will sharpen the concept and the diagnosis of dependent personality disorder, will reduce overlap with other disorders, and will address sex bias issues.

## CHANGES PROPOSED FOR AND MADE IN DSM-IV

Each criterion section below begins with the DSM-III-R wording, followed by an explication of the intended meaning of the criterion. Next is our proposal for DSM-IV, together with the rationale for the proposed modification. Finally, the criterion as actually published in DSM-IV is given, along with an explanation of any changes from the proposal. The DSM-III-R and DSM-IV criteria are listed in Table 11.1, above. Note that the numbering of the criteria in DSM-IV reflects that in DSM-III-R (for many other personality disorders, this is not the case).

### Essential Feature

The essential feature of dependent personality disorder as proposed for and published in DSM-IV is as follows: "A pervasive and excessive need to be taken care of that leads to submissive and clinging behavior and fears of separation."

### Criterion I

*DSM-III-R*

In DSM-III-R, criterion 1 is as follows: "is unable to make everyday decisions without an excessive amount of advice or reassurance from others." Individuals with dependent personality disorder lack confidence in their own abilities and will wait for others to reassure them. This is in contrast to the "constantly seeks or demands reassurance, approval, or praise" DSM-III-R criterion for histrionic personality disorder (American Psychiatric Association, 1987, p. 349). For the histrionic person, the praise itself is the goal; for the dependent person, having someone else make the decision is the goal.

### Proposed Revision

We proposed this revision of criterion 1: "is unable to make *everyday* decisions without an excessive amount of advice and reassurance from others." The emphasis on "everyday" was intended to distinguish it from criterion 2, which deals with important decisions.

### DSM-IV

In the published version of DSM-IV, the proposed wording of criterion 1 has been altered slightly to readd: "has difficulty making everyday decisions without an excessive amount of advice and reassurance from others." The emphasis on "everyday" has been dropped because of the change in the published wording of criterion 2 (see below).

## Criterion 2

### DSM-III-R

Criterion 2 in DSM-III-R is as follows: "allows others to make most of his or her important decisions, for example, where to live, what job to take." This criterion extends criterion 1 to important decisions. Because the stakes are higher, these individuals will not try to make a decision, even with a great deal of advice and reassurance; rather, they will passively allow others to make these decisions for them. At the heart of this is a lack of confidence in their own judgment.

### Proposed Revision

We suggested this revision of criterion 2: "allows others to make most of his or her *important* decisions, for example, where to live, what job to take." The emphasis on "important" was intended to distinguish it from criterion 1, which deals with everyday decisions.

### DSM-IV

Criterion 2 as published in DSM-IV differs somewhat from our originial proposal: "needs others to assume responsibility for most major areas of his or her life." It was decided that the new wording makes the point about important decisions more forcefully than simply italicizing "important" does.

## Criterion 3

*DSM-III-R*

Criterion 3 in DSM-III-R reads as follows: "agrees with people even when he or she believes they are wrong, because of fear of being rejected." In these individuals, the need for support and nurturance is overpowering. To disagree with others might evoke anger or rejection, which would leave the individuals unable to function.

*Proposed Revision*

We proposed the following revision of criterion 3: "has difficulty expressing disagreement with others because of fear of their anger or loss of support." It is not the rejection per se that motivates the compliance, but rather the consequences of rejection—that is, the loss of care and support. The proposed change was intended to emphasize the fear of anger or loss of support.

*DSM-IV*

Criterion 3 as published in DSM-IV is as follows: "has difficulty expressing disagreement with others because of fear of loss of support or approval. **Note:** Do not include realistic fears of retribution." It was decided that the criterion should distinguish between realistic and unrealistic feared consequences.

## Criterion 4

*DSM-III-R*

In DSM-III-R, criterion 4 is as follows: "has difficulty initiating projects or doing things on his or her own." Because of a lack of confidence in their own abilities, these individuals have difficulty starting anything on their own. This is not necessarily due to a lack of energy or motivation, but rather to a belief that they are not up to the task.

*Proposed Revision*

We proposed this revision of criterion 4: "has difficulty independently initiating projects or doing things on his or her own. This is due to a lack of self-confidence in judgment and/or abilities not to a lack of motivation or energy." The proposed change was meant to emphasize that lack of confidence in judgment and/or abilities is what results in difficulty in independent initiation, rather than the absence of energy or motivation.

*DSM-IV*

The published version of criterion 4 in DSM-IV differs only slightly from the proposed version: "has difficulty initiating projects or doing things on his or her own (because of a lack of self-confidence in judgment or abilities rather than a lack of motivation or energy)."

## Criterion 5

*DSM-III-R*

Criterion 5 in DSM-III-R is as follows: "volunteers to do things that are unpleasant or demeaning in order to get other people to like him or her." The issue here is not a strong need to be liked in and of itself, but rather a need to gain support or nurturance. Also, the individual does not do unpleasant or demeaning tasks because that is what he or she "deserves" or because the individual wishes to induce guilt, as in the case of self-defeating personality. The purpose is to increase the likelihood of obtaining care and nurturance. Performing services for other people may have this effect.

*Proposed Revision*

We suggested the following revision of criterion 5: "goes to excessive lengths to obtain nurturance and support from others, to the point of volunteering to do things that are unpleasant." This change was intended to emphasize the reason for the behavior in order to distinguish it from self-defeating behavior. In self-defeating personality disorder, the motivation for volunteering for unpleasant tasks is to induce guilt or to martyr and/or devalue oneself.

*DSM-IV*

The proposed criterion has been published in DSM-IV without alterations.

## Criterion 6

*DSM-III-R*

Criterion 6 in DSM-III-R reads as follows: "feels uncomfortable or helpless when alone, or goes to great lengths to avoid being alone." Individuals with dependent personality disorder are afraid of being alone because they believe that they will be unable to function when alone. To be alone is to be helpless. These individuals have a strong need for a "secure base" or for proximity to important other(s) on whom they can depend. This is in contrast to individuals with borderline personality disorder, who experience a sense of emptiness and lack of a sense of self, and need others to fill them up and give them an identity. For borderline personality disorder, the fear of being alone is moment-to-moment; for dependent personality disorder, the fear is of not having access to a strong other when advice or reassurance is needed.

## Proposed Revision

We proposed this revision of criterion 6: "feels uncomfortable or helpless when alone because of exaggerated fears of inability to care for himself or herself." The change was intended to emphasize the reason for the feelings of discomfort and helplessness when alone, and to help distinguish this criterion from one of the criteria for borderline personality disorder: "frantic attempts to avoid real or imagined abandonment" (American Psychiatric Association, 1994, p. 654).

## DSM-IV

Again, the proposed criterion appears in DSM-IV without alteration.

## Criterion 7

### DSM-III-R

In DSM-III-R, criterion 7 is as follows: "feels devastated or helpless when close relationships end." This is similar to criterion 6, except that the stakes are higher because a close relationship is involved. The loss of this close relationship leaves the individual with dependent personality disorder unable to function without the help of the important person. This differs from the sense of emptiness, lack of identity, or inner direction experienced by the person with borderline personality disorder who is suffering the loss of an important relationship. Individuals with avoidant personality disorder may also be devastated by the end of a close relationship. They differ from those with dependent personality disorder, however, in their reaction to the end of a relationship: Avoidant individuals are likely to withdraw from relationships, in contrast to dependent individuals, who are likely to quickly replace the lost relationship.

## Proposed Revision

We suggested the following revision of criterion 7: "when close relationships end, undiscriminatingly seeks another relationship to provide nurturance and support." Because of the high endorsement rate of this criterion both in other personality disorders and in other psychiatric disorders, we attempted to make the criterion more specific to dependent personality disorder—in particular, to address the overlap with avoidant personality disorder. In addition, as immediate seeking of another relationship may be a common expression of dependency in males, we felt that this broadening of the criterion might improve the sensitivity of the criteria set to males with abnormal dependency.

## DSM-IV

Criterion 7 as published in DSM-IV is as follows: "urgently seeks another relationship as a source of care and support when a close relationship ends."

## Criterion 8

### DSM-III-R

Criterion 8 in DSM-III-R reads: "is frequently preoccupied with fears of being abandoned." The issue here is the experience of anxiety about being left to take care of oneself without advice, reassurance, and support from an important other person. The individual with dependent personality disorder feels helpless, and the prospect of abandonment fuels fears and anxiety. The issue is not so much the actual abandonment, but rather the prospect of being without help.

### Proposed Revision

We proposed this revision of criterion 8: "is frequently preoccupied with fears of being left to take care of himself or herself." The change was meant to emphasize the fear of being without support and to distinguish this criterion from the fear of abandonment in the borderline.

### DSM-IV

The published version of criterion 8 in DSM-IV differs by only one word from the proposed version: "is unrealistically preoccupied with fears of being left to take care of himself or herself." As in the case of criterion 3, it was decided that the criterion should distinguish between realistic and unrealistic fears.

## Criterion 9

### DSM-III-R

Criterion 9 in DSM-III-R is as follows: "is easily hurt by criticism or disapproval." The dependent individual suffers from low self-confidence and low self-esteem, and therefore criticism or disapproval is particularly devastating. Thus, this individual is likely to be more sensitive to criticism or disapproval.

*Proposed Revision*

We suggested dropping this item in DSM-IV. This symptom is found in other personality disorders and other psychiatric disorders, and is not specific to dependent personality disorder.

*DSM-IV*

In the published version of DSM-IV, the item has been dropped as suggested.

## REFERENCES

Alnaes, R., & Torgersen, S. (1988a). The relationship between DSM-III symptom disorders (Axis I) and personality disorders (Axis II) in an outpatient population. *Acta Psychiatrica Scandinavica, 78,* 485–492.

Alnaes, R., & Torgersen, S. (1988b). DSM-III symptom disorders (Axis I) and personality disorders (Axis II) in an outpatient population. *Acta Psychiatrica Scandinavica, 78,* 348–355.

American Psychiatric Association. (1952). *Diagnostic and statistical manual of mental disorders* (1st ed.). Washington, DC: Mental Hospitals Service.

American Psychiatric Association. (1968). *Diagnostic and statistical manual of mental disorders* (2nd ed.). Washington, DC: Author.

American Psychiatric Association. (1980). *Diagnostic and statistical manual of mental disorders* (3rd ed.). Washington, DC: Author.

American Psychiatric Association. (1987). *Diagnostic and statistical manual of mental disorders* (3rd ed., rev.). Washington, DC: Author.

American Psychiatric Association. (1994). *Diagnostic and statistical manual of mental disorders* (4th ed.). Washington, DC: Author.

Birchnell, J. (1988). Defining dependence. *British Journal of Medical Psychology, 61,* 222–223.

Blashfield, R. K., & Breen, M. J. (1989). Face validity of the DSM-III-R personality disorders. *American Journal of Psychiatry, 146,* 1575–1579.

Brown, L. S. (1986). Gender role analysis: A neglected component of psychological assessment. *Psychotherapy, 23,* 243–248.

Craig, R. J. (1988). A psychometric study of the prevalence of DSM-III personality disorders among treated opiate addicts. *International Journal of the Addictions, 23,* 115–124.

Dahl, A. A. (1986). Some aspects of the DSM-III personality disorders illustrated by a consecutive sample of hospitalized patients. *Acta Psychiatrica Scandinavica, 73*(Suppl. 328), 61–67.

Davidson, J., Miller, R., & Strickland, R. (1985). Neuroticism and personality disorder in depression. *Journal of Affective Disorders, 8,* 177–182.

Fishbain, D. A., Goldberg, M., Meagher, B. R., Steele, R., & Rosomoff, H. (1986). Male and female chronic pain patients categorized by DSM-III psychiatric diagnostic criteria. *Pain, 26,* 181–197.

Frances, A., & Widiger, T. (1987). A critical review of four DSM-III personality disorders: Borderline, avoidant, dependent, and passive–aggressive. In G. Tischler

(Ed.), *Diagnosis and classification in psychiatry* (pp. 269–289). New York: Cambridge University Press.

Greenberg, R. P., & Bornstein, R. F.(1988a). The dependent personality: I. Risk for physical disorders. *Journal of Personality Disorders, 2,* 126–135.

Greenberg, R. P., & Bornstein, R. F. (1988b). The dependent personality: II. Risk for psychological disorders. *Journal of Personality Disorders, 2,* 136–143.

Gunderson, J. (1983). DSM-III diagnosis of personality disorders. In J. Frosch (Ed.), *Current perspectives on personality disorders* (pp. 20–39). Washington, DC: American Psychiatric Press.

Hirschfeld, R. M., Klerman, G. L., Chodoff, P., Korchin, S., & Barrett, J. (1976). Dependency–self-esteem–clinical depression. *Journal of the American Academy of Psychoanalysis, 4,* 373–388.

Hirschfeld, R. M., Klerman, G. L., Gough, H. G., Barrett, J., Korchin, S. J., & Chodoff, P. (1977). A measure of interpersonal dependency. *Journal of Personality Assessment, 41,* 610–618.

Hogg, B., Jackson, H. J., Rudd, R. P., & Edwards, J. (1990). Diagnosing personality disorders in recent-onset schizophrenia. *Journal of Nervous and Mental Disease, 178,* 194–199.

Joffe, R. T., & Regan, J. J. (1988). Personality and depression. *Journal of Psychiatric Research, 22,* 279–286.

Kaplan, M. (1983). A woman's view of DSM-III. *American Psychologist, 38,* 786–792.

Kass, F., Spitzer, R. L., & Williams, J. B. W. (1983). An empirical study of the issue of sex bias in the diagnostic criteria of DSM III Axis II personality disorders. *American Psychologist, 38,* 799–801.

Korenblum, M., Golombek, H., Marton, P., & Stein, B. (1987). The classification of disturbed personality functioning in early adolescence. *Canadian Journal of Psychiatry, 32,* 362–367.

Levine, J., Tischer, P., Antoni, M., Green, C., & Millon, T. (1985). Refining personality assessments by combining MCMI high point profiles and MMPI codes: Part II. MMPI code 27/72. *Journal of Personality Assessment, 49,* 501–507.

Livesley, W. J., Jackson, D. N., & Schroeder, M. L. (1989). *The structure of personality pathology in a general population sample.* Unpublished manuscript.

Livesley, W. J., Reiffer, L. L., Sheldon, A. E., & West, M. (1987). Prototypicality ratings of DSM-III criteria for personality disorders. *Journal of Nervous and Mental Disease, 175,* 395–401.

Livesley, W. J., Schroeder, M. L., & Jackson, D. N. (1990). Dependent personality disorder and attachment problems. *Journal of Personality Disorders, 4,* 232–240.

Malow, R. M., West, J. A., Williams, J. L., & Sutker, P. B. (1989). Personality disorders classification and symptoms in cocaine and opioid addicts. *Journal of Consulting and Clinical Psychology, 57,* 765–767.

Mavissakalian, M., & Hamann, M. S. (1988). Correlates of DSM-III personality disorder in panic disorder and agoraphobia. *Comprehensive Psychiatry, 29,* 535–544.

Mavissakalian, M., Hamann, M. S., & Jones, B. (1990). A comparison of DSM III personality disorders in panic/agoraphobia and obsessive–compulsive disorder. *Comprehensive Psychiatry, 31,* 238–244.

McElroy, R. A. Jr., Davis, R. T., & Blashfield, R. K. (1989). Variations on the family resemblance hypothesis as applied to personality disorders. *Comprehensive Psychiatry, 30,* 449–456.

Mezzich, J. E., Fabrega, H. Jr., & Coffman, G. A. (1987). Multiaxial characterization of depressive patients. *Journal of Nervous and Mental Disease, 175,* 339–346.

Morey, L. C. (1988). Personality disorders in DSM-III and DSM-III-R: Convergence, coverage, and internal consistency. *American Journal of Psychiatry, 145,* 573–577.

Overholser, J. C., Kabakoff, R., & Norman, W. H. (1989). The assessment of personality characteristics in depressed and dependent psychiatric inpatients. *Journal of Personality Assessment, 53,* 40–50.

Pfohl, B., Coryell, W., Zimmerman, M., & Stangl, D. (1986). DSM-III personality disorders: Diagnostic overlap and internal consistency of individual DSM-III criteria. *Comprehensive Psychiatry, 27,* 21–34.

Piersma, H. L. (1987). The MCMI as a measure of DSM-III Axis II, diagnoses: An empirical comparison. *Journal of Clinical Psychology, 43,* 478–483.

Pilkonis, P. A. (1988). Personality prototypes among depressives: Themes of dependency and autonomy. *Journal of Personality Disorders, 2,* 144–152.

Pilkonis, P. A., & Frank, E. (1988). Personality pathology in recurrent depression: Nature, prevalence, and relationship to treatment response. *American Journal of Psychiatry, 145,* 435–441.

Poldrugo, F., & Forti, B. (1988). Personality disorders and alcoholism treatment outcome. *Drug and Alcohol Dependence, 21,* 171–176.

Reich, J. H. (1987). Sex distribution of DSM-III personality disorders in psychiatric outpatients. *American Journal of Psychiatry, 144,* 485–488.

Reich, J. H. (1989). Familiarity of DSM-III dramatic and anxious personality clusters. *Journal of Nervous and Mental Disease, 177,* 96–100.

Reich, J. H. (1990). *Phenomenological overlap of DSM-III avoidant and dependent personality disorders.* Unpublished manuscript.

Reich, J. H., Nduaguba, M., & Yates, W. (1988). Age and sex distribution of DSM III personality cluster traits in a community population. *Comprehensive Psychiatry, 29,* 298–303.

Reich, J. H., Noyes, R. Jr., & Troughton, E. (1987). Dependent personality disorder associated with phobic avoidance in patients with panic disorder. *American Journal of Psychiatry, 144,* 323–326.

Reich, J. H., & Troughton, E. (1988). Comparison of DSM-III personality disorders in recovered depressed and panic disorder patients. *Journal of Nervous and Mental Disease, 176,* 300–304.

Reich, J. H., Yates, W., & Nduaguba, M. (1989). Prevalence of DSM-III personality disorders in the community. *Social Psychiatry and Psychiatric Epidemiology, 24,* 12–16.

Shea, M. T., Glass, D. R., Pilkonis, P. A., Watkins, J., & Docherty, J. P. (1987). Frequency and implications of personality disorders in a sample of depressed outpatients. *Journal of Personality Disorders, 1,* 27–42.

Skodol, A. E., Rosnick, L., Kellman, D., Oldham, J. M., & Hyler, S. E. (1988). Validating structured DSM-III-R personality disorder assessments with longitudinal data. *American Journal of Psychiatry, 145,* 1297–1299.

Smith, T. W., O'Keefe, J. L., & Jenkins, M. (1988). Dependency and self-criticism: Correlates of depression or moderators of the effects of stressful events. *Journal of Personality Disorders, 2,* 160–169.

Spitzer, R. L., Williams, J. B., Kass, F., & Davies, M. (1989). National field trial of the DSM-III-R diagnostic criteria for self-defeating personality disorder. *American Journal of Psychiatry, 146,* 1561–1567.

Stangl, D., Pfohl, B., Zimmerman, M., Bowers, W., & Corenthal, C. (1985). A structured interview for the DSM-III personality disorders: A preliminary report. *Archives of General Psychiatry, 42,* 591–596.

Thompson, L. W., Gallagher, D., & Czirr, R. (1988). Personality disorder and outcome in the treatment of later life depression. *Journal of Geriatric Psychiatry, 21,* 133–153.

Trull, T. J., Widiger, T. A., & Frances, A. (1987). Covariation of criteria sets for avoidant, schizoid, and dependent personality disorders. *American Journal of Psychiatry, 144,* 767–771.

Tyrer, P., Casey, P., & Call, J. (1983). Relationship between neurosis and personality disorder. *British Journal of Psychiatry, 142,* 404–408.

Waldinger, R. J. (1986, June). Assessing borderline personality. *Medical Aspects of Human Sexuality,* pp. 76–88.

Widiger, T. A., & Sanderson, C. (1987). The convergent and discriminant validity of the MCMI as a measure of the DSM-III personality disorders. *Journal of Personality Assessment, 51,* 228–242.

Widiger, T. A., & Spitzer, R. L. (1991). Sex bias in the diagnosis of personality disorders: Conceptual and methodological issues. *Clinical Psychology Review, 11,* 1–22.

Williams, J. B. W., & Spitzer, R. L. (1983). The issue of sex bias in DSM-III [A critique of "A woman's view of DSM-III" by Marcie Kaplan]. *American Psychologist, 38*(7), 793–798.

Yager, J., Landsverk, J., Edelstein, C. K., & Hyler, S. E. (1989). Screening for Axis II personality disorders in women with bulimic eating disorders. *Psychosomatics, 30,* 255–262.

Yates, W. R., Sieleni, B., Reich, J., & Brass, C. (1989). Comorbidity of bulimia nervosa and personality disorder. *Journal of Clinical Psychiatry, 50,* 57–59.

Zanarini, M. C., Frankenburg, F. R., Chauncey, D. L., & Gunderson, J. C. (1987). The Diagnostic Interview for Personality Disorders: Interrater and test–retest reliability. *Comprehensive Psychiatry, 28,* 467–480.

Zimmerman, M., & Coryell, W. (1989). DSM-III personality disorder diagnoses in a nonpatient sample: Demographic correlates and comorbidity. *Archives of General Psychiatry, 46,* 682–689.

# Commentary on Dependent Personality Disorder

W. John Livesley

If one accepts the underlying premises of the DSM system there is little that is controversial about the DSM-IV (American Psychiatric Association, 1994) criteria set for dependent personality disorder. The thorough review of the recent literature on dependency provided by Hirschfeld, Shea, and Weise in Chapter 11 shows that the diagnosis as delineated in DSM-IV has good support from the clinical and research literature. The essential feature of the diagnosis as stated in DSM-IV captures the main components of dependent behavior, and the diagnostic criteria appear to provide a satisfactory representation of the diagnosis. If one does not accept the premises of DSM-IV, however, the diagnosis of dependent personality disorder provides an excellent illustration of the fundamental problems with the DSM approach to the classification of personality disorders.

## THE ESSENTIAL FEATURE

The concept of dependent personality disorder held by clinicians covers a wide variety of behaviors: reliance on others and institutions; need for approval; submissiveness and unassertiveness; need for affection, care, and support; need for advice and reassurance; and a variety of attachment behaviors, including fear of losing attachment figures and difficulty in separating from them (Livesley, Schroeder, & Jackson, 1990). As Hirschfeld and colleagues note, this concept has two main components: dependency behaviors and attachment behaviors. Attachment theory, especially as explicated by Bowlby (1969, 1977), distinguishes between attachment behavior, which consists of "any form of behavior that results in a person attaining or retaining proximity to some other differentiated and preferred individual who is usually conceived as stronger and/or wiser" (Bowlby, 1977, p. 203) and dependency behaviors, which consist of generalized actions designed to elicit assistance, guidance, and approval. Unlike attachment, dependency is not directed toward a specific person, nor are these behaviors concerned with promoting the sense of security that comes from proximity to attachment figures. Empirical studies using multivariate statistical techniques have confirmed the distinction between attachment and dependency (Livesley et al., 1990).

The two component structure of dependent personality disorder was not recognized in DSM-III-R. Pathological attachment was omitted from the definition of the essential feature of the diagnosis which states that the diagnosis involves "a pervasive pattern of dependent and submissive behavior" (American Psychiatric Association, 1987, p. 354). Nevertheless, as Hirschfeld and colleagues point out, the DSM-III-R diagnostic criteria set includes both attachment and dependency items. Modification of the essential feature in DSM-IV to read "a pervasive and excessive need to be taken care of, that leads to submissive and clinging behavior and fears of separation" (American Psychiatric Association, 1994, p. 668) is obviously something of an improvement. By including more than submissiveness and dependency, the diagnosis provides a better representation of the concept of dependent personality held by clinicians. Attachment behaviors are not actually mentioned in the essential feature, which is unfortunate, because attachment theory could have provided a rational basis for constructing the criteria set. This failure illustrates the reluctance of DSM to draw upon well-established theories even when these are well supported by empirical evidence. A consequence is that Axis II lacks coherence and a theoretical rationale (see Jackson & Livesley, Chapter 23).

## DIAGNOSTIC CRITERIA

Although the way the essential feature of the diagnosis is defined in DSM-IV is an improvement, the way this feature is translated into a set of diagnostic criteria is less satisfactory. The criteria set appears to include both dependency and attachment items; thus, we can expect the diagnosis to possess satisfactory content validity. But items written to assess the attachment component do not really capture the essence of attachment as conceptualized by Bowlby. Criteria such as "goes to excessive lengths to obtain nurturance . . . ," "feels . . . helpless when alone . . . ," and " . . . preoccupied with fears of being left . . . " (American Psychiatric Association, 1994, pp. 668–669) do not express the core feature of attachment—namely, the desire to attain and maintain proximity to an attachment figure, because a sense of security is dependent upon this proximity. This leads to a desire for closeness, especially at times of stress or uncertainty; fear of, and protest about, separation; and the ability to cope effectively only when the attachment figure is considered to be available and responsive.

When systematic empirical studies are conducted, the DSM-IV items may well be found to function satisfactorily, because they are sufficiently saturated with attachment content. But the fact that there is doubt raises questions about the content validity of the diagnosis. The problem arises from a fundamental shortcoming of the DSM approach to date: Diagnostic items have been selected by a committee process that has not, as far as we are informed, involved establishing in an explicit and systematic way a consensual definition of the diagnosis to guide the committee when selecting diagnostic items (Livesley & Jackson, 1992). Instead, the committee has relied on the assumption that each member has the same understanding of the meaning of a diagnostic concept—an assumption that is questionable and unnecessary. The failure to define diagnoses is a fundamental flaw in the system; it continues to be repeated with each revision, and it limits the scientific value of the classification.

## THE STRUCTURE OF DEPENDENT PERSONALITY DISORDER

The two-component structure of the diagnosis raises the question of whether dependency and attachment behaviors should be combined into a single diagnostic category or whether they should form two separate diagnostic entities. Ultimately, resolution of this issue will depend in part on whether the single diagnosis obscures important clinical information—that is, whether dependency behaviors and attachment behaviors have sufficiently different etiologies that the two behaviors respond differently to treatment interventions. Meanwhile, Hirschfeld and colleagues have attempted to justify combination into a single category by citing data showing that the two sets of behaviors are highly intercorrelated. The implication is that they have allowed empirical evidence to determine the position adopted for DSM-IV. But there are good grounds for questioning this assumption. An alternative interpretation is that the decision to use a single diagnostic category was determined by the basic philosophical assumptions of Personality Disorders Work Group about the nature of mental disorders, and that this position has influenced the way the data have been interpreted.

DSM-IV, like its predecessors, is based on neo-Kreapelinian assumptions about the nature of mental disorders (Blashfield, 1984; Klerman, 1978). Basic to this philosophical position is the assumption that disorders are discrete entities. The conservative approach adopted for DSM-IV has made it difficult to discard this assumption, despite overwhelming evidence that in the case of personality disorders the simplistic categorical model of DSM is inconsistent with the way personality is organized.

As Hirschfeld and colleagues point out, the two components of dependent personality disorder intercorrelated approximately .60 in one study. On the basis of this intercorrelation, they consider that it is appropriate to include both features in a single category. But this value is not absolute; by selecting items differently, it would be possible to increase or decrease the correlation. In any case, the correlation is significantly less than the reliability of the scales involved, suggesting that the two scales assess distinct but related components of personality. Thus the issue of whether there should be one or two diagnostic constructs is theoretical, not empirical. If one adopts the difficult-to-substantiate position that there are a fixed number of personality disorder diagnoses, each defined by a set of phenotypic features, then it would be appropriate to use a single diagnostic construct to represent the psychopathology of the attachment–dependency domain. If one accepts the empirical evidence that the phenotypic features of personality disorder are best represented by a dimensional model, however, more options are available. The two dimensions could be kept separate at one level of the dimensional structure to permit detailed analysis of possible differences in etiology and treatment outcome, but could be combined into a single higher-order dimension for other purposes. Thus the breadth or narrowness of the diagnostic constructs that are adopted depends on the purpose for which the classification is being used.

Given the decision to retain categorical diagnoses, the definition of dependent personality disorder in DSM-IV is appropriate. But it is perhaps unfortunate that a valuable opportunity has been lost to reconceptualize personality disorders and develop a classification that is more consistent with empirical data.

## REFERENCES

American Psychiatric Association. (1987). *Diagnostic and statistical manual of mental disorders* (3rd ed., rev.). Washington, DC: Author.

American Psychiatric Association. (1994). *Diagnostic and statistical manual of mental disorders* (4th ed.). Washington, DC: Author.

Blashfield, R. K. (1984). *The classification of psychopathology.* New York: Plenum.

Bowlby, J. (1969). *Attachment and loss: Vol. 1, Attachment.* London: Hogarth Press.

Bowlby, J. (1977). The making and breaking of affectional bonds. *British Journal of Psychiatry, 130,* 201–210, 431–431.

Klerman, G. L. (1978). The evolution of a scientific nosology. In J. C. Shershow (Ed.), *Schizophrenia: Science and practice.* Cambridge, MA: Harvard University Press.

Livesley, W. J., & Jackson, D. N. (1992). Guidelines for developing, evaluating, and revising the classification of personality disorders. *Journal of Nervous and Mental Disease, 180,* 609–618.

Livesley, W. J., Schroeder, M. L., & Jackson, D. N. (1990). Dependent personality disorder and attachment problems. *Journal of Personality Disorders, 4,* 232–240.

# CHAPTER 12

# Obsessive–Compulsive Personality Disorder

BRUCE PFOHL
NANCY BLUM

The DSM-III-R (American Psychiatric Association [APA], 1987) criteria for obsessive–compulsive personality disorder represent an attempt to capture a historical concept whose implications and validity are largely unknown. The modern roots of obsessive–compulsive personality disorder go back at least as far as Freud, who described the anal character type. In his classic 1908 paper, Freud outlined the anal character as arising from a defense against anal eroticism. He described such individuals as "orderly, parsimonious and obstinate. . . . Orderly covers the notion of bodily cleanliness, as well as conscientiousness in carrying out small duties and trustworthiness. . . . Parsimony may [include] . . . avarice; and obstinacy can go over into defiance, to which rage and revengefulness are easily joined" (p. 169).

In 1921, Abraham developed this concept further with a rich description of character traits, which has been concisely summarized in a review by Oldham and Frosch (1988):

> Abraham emphasized the compulsive person's pleasure in indexing, classifying, and compiling lists, his tendency to arrange things symmetrically and to divide things with minute exactness, and his ambivalence toward order or cleanliness betrayed by fastidiousness on the surface but disarray or lack of cleanliness underneath. He also noted the compulsive person's pleasure in possession, often resulting in an inability to throw away worn out or worthless objects. The compulsive's penchant to postpone every action is combined with an often unproductive perseverance and preoccupation with preserving correct social appearances.

An earlier version of this chapter was published in the *Journal of Personality Disorders*, 1991, *5*, 363–375. Copyright 1991 by The Guilford Press. Adapted by permission.

Yet, in close personal relationships, the compulsive refuses to accommodate himself to others, expects compliance, has an exaggerated criticism of others, and insists on controlling interactions with others. Finally, Abraham noted the generally morose or surly attitude of the compulsive, reflecting a state of constant tension. (p. 245)

The DSM-I (American Psychiatric Association, 1952) criteria for compulsive personality and the nearly identical DSM-II (American Psychiatric Association, 1968) criteria for obsessive–compulsive personality (abstracted in Table 12.1) emphasized the "orderly" component of this personality type. DSM-III (American Psychiatric Association, 1980) expanded the description with five operational criteria, of which four were required for diagnosis. DSM-III-R made relatively minor changes to the five criteria and added four more, requiring five of nine criteria to make the diagnosis. These criteria (see Table 12.2 for the full DSM-III-R and DSM-IV [American Psychiatric Association, 1994] criteria) capture most of the traits described by Freud and Abraham.

It is interesting to note that despite the fact that almost all diagnostic systems that include personality disorders recognize the existence of this concept, the name of this disorder has undergone repeated revision:

Psychoanalytic:                          Anal character
DSM-I:                                   Compulsive personality
DSM-II:                                  Obsessive–compulsive personality
DSM-III:                                 Compulsive personality disorder
DSM-III-R:                               Obsessive–compulsive personality disorder
*International Classification*
*of Diseases,* ninth revision
(ICD-9):                                 Anankastic personality

## SIGNIFICANT ISSUES

Members of the Personality Disorders Work Group and consultants participating in the DSM-IV revision process raised the following issues: Are criteria congruent with the descriptive literature? Are criteria internally consistent? Are criteria supported by external validators? How is obsessive–compulsive personality disorder related to obsessive–compulsive disorder and other Axis I disorders? Is obsessive–compulsive personality disorder distinct from other personality disorders? Are the structure of the diagnostic criteria and the threshold for diagnosis appropriate? What is the best name for this disorder?

## LITERATURE REVIEW

When the empirical literature on the DSM-III or DSM-III-R criteria for obsessive–compulsive personality disorder and relevant data sets were evalu-

TABLE 12.1. Prototypical Traits for Obsessive–Compulsive Personality Disorder

*DSM-III-R (American Psychiatric Association, 1987) obsessive–compulsive personality disorder*

Perfectionism
Preoccupation with details, rules, order, organization
Insistence that others submit to exactly his or her way of doing things
Excessive devotion to work
Indecisiveness
Overconscientiousness, scrupulousness, and inflexibility (not in DSM-III)
Restricted expression of affection
Lack of generosity (not in DSM-III)
Inability to discard worn out or worthless objects (not in DSM-III)

*DSM-II (American Psychiatric Association, 1968) obsessive–compulsive personality*

Excessive concern with conformity and adherence to standards of conscience
Rigidity, overinhibition, overconscientiousness
Inability to relax easily

*ICD-9 (World Health Organization, 1977) anankastic personality*

Rigidity
Personal insecurity and doubt[a]
Conscientiousness, checking, stubbornness, and caution
Perfectionism and meticulous accuracy
Unwelcome thoughts and impulses (not as severe as in obsessional neurosis)[a]

*Freud's (1908) anal character*

Orderliness: bodily cleanliness, conscientiousness in carrying out small duties, trust-
  worthy
Parsimony: may include greed
Obstinacy: argumentative, perhaps to the point of rage and revengefulness[a]

*Abraham's (1921) anal character*

Pleasure in indexing, compiling lists, and arranging things symmetrically
Superficial fastidiousness masking disarray underneath
Pleasure in possession; inability to throw away worn out or worthless objects
Tendency to postpone every action; unproductive perseverance
Preoccupation with preserving correct social appearance
In close personal relationships, refusal to accommodate others; expectations of
  compliance
Exaggerated criticism of others; insistence on controlling interactions with others [a]
Generally morose or surly attitude

*Lazare et al. (1966, 1970) (from Lazare–Klerman Trait Scale)*

Orderliness
Strong superego
Perseverance
Obstinacy
Rigidity                                                                    *(cont.)*

TABLE 12.1 (cont.)

*Lazare et al. (1966, 1970) (from Lazare–Klerman Trait Scale)*
   Parsimony
   Emotional constriction
   Rejection of others[b]
   Self-doubt[a, b]

*Additions to essential feature suggested by Personality Disorders Work Group advisors*
   Preoccupation with mental and interpersonal control
   Inflexibility of thinking, feeling, and behavior

[a]Traits not represented in DSM-III-R criteria.
[b]Items not consistently supported by factor analysis.

ated, a high threshold for recommending changes in the criteria and a low threshold for suggesting alternatives needing further research were adopted. The former was considered necessary because the varied history of this diagnostic concept and lack of empirical research created an almost irresistible temptation to make changes reflecting the composition of the study committee rather than real progress in knowledge about the disorder. The latter was felt to be necessary because the need for progress in this area mandates that future investigators explore a rich variety of alternatives as well as current criteria, in order to identify weaknesses and potential better ways to represent the diagnosis.

## Are Criteria Congruent with the Descriptive Literature?

Because there is only limited empirical research supporting the DSM-III-R criteria for obsessive–compulsive personality disorder, it is worthwhile to examine whether the criteria at least capture those traits historically associated with this personality type. The traits elucidated by Freud and Abraham have been cited previously and are summarized in Table 12.1. Because several features mentioned in the literature are not represented in DSM-III-R or DSM-IV, some experimental criteria based on these features are proposed at the end of the chapter, in the hope that future research will clarify their relationship with obsessive–compulsive personality disorder.

   Lazare and colleagues were the first to examine psychoanalytic concepts of personality by systematically using factor analysis to determine whether the theoretically derived components truly clustered together (Lazare, Klerman, & Armor, 1966, 1970). They began (Lazare et al., 1966) with a series of traits representing the oral, obsessive, and hysterical personality constructs, and used a 200-item self-report rating scale to operationalize the measurement of the underlying traits. Each trait was assessed by seven true–false items. Table 12.1 summarizes the "obsessional" traits examined in this study. The test (later called the Lazare–Klerman Trait Scale) was given to a series

TABLE 12.2. DSM-III-R and DSM-IV Diagnostic Criteria for Obsessive–Compulsive Personality Disorder

| DSM-III-R criteria | DSM-IV criteria |
|---|---|
| A pervasive pattern of perfectionism and inflexibility, beginning by early adulthood and present in a variety of contexts, as indicated by at least *five* of the following: | A pervasive pattern of preoccupation with orderliness, perfectionism, and mental and interpersonal control, at the expense of flexibility, openness, and efficiency, beginning by early adulthood and present in a variety of contexts, as indicated by four (or more) of the following: |
| (1) perfectionism that interferes with task completion, e.g., inability to complete a project because own overly strict standards are not met | (1) is preoccupied with details, rules, lists, order, organization, or schedules to the extent that the major point of the activity is lost |
| (2) preoccupation with details, rules, lists, order, organization, or schedules to the extent that the major point of the activity is lost | (2) shows perfectionism that interferes with task completion (e.g., is unable to complete a project because his or her own overly strict standards are not met) |
| (3) unreasonable insistence that others submit to exactly his or her way of doing things, **or** unreasonable reluctance to allow others to do things because of the conviction that they will not do them correctly | (3) is excessively devoted to work and productivity to the exclusion of leisure activities and friendships (not accounted for by obvious economic necessity) |
| (4) excessive devotion to work and productivity to the exclusion of leisure activities and friendships (not accounted for by obvious economic necessity) | (4) is overconscientious, scrupulous, and inflexible about matters of morality, ethics, or values (not accounted for by cultural or religious identification) |
| (5) indecisiveness: decision making is either avoided, postponed, or protracted, e.g., the person cannot get assignments done on time because of ruminating about priorities (do not include if indecisiveness is due to excessive need for advice or reassurance from others) | (5) is unable to discard worn-out or worthless objects even when they have no sentimental value |
| (6) overconscientiousness, scrupulousness, and inflexibility about matters of morality, ethics, or values (not accounted for by cultural or religious identification) | (6) is reluctant to delegate tasks or to work with others unless they submit to exactly his or her way of doing things |
| (7) restricted expression of affection | (7) adopts a miserly spending style toward both self and others; money is viewed as something to be hoarded for future catastrophes |

*(cont.)*

TABLE 12.2. (cont.)

| DSM-III-R criteria | DSM-IV criteria |
|---|---|
| (8) lack of generosity in giving time, money, or gifts when no personal gain is likely to result | (8) shows rigidity and stubbornness |
| (9) inability to discard worn-out or worthless objects even when they have no sentimental value | |

*Note.* From APA (1987, p. 356) and APA (1994, pp. 672–673). Copyright 1987 and 1994 by the American Psychiatric Association. Reprinted by permission.

of female psychiatric patients. An obsessional dimension emerged, characterized by orderliness, strong superego, perseverance, obstinacy, rigidity, rejection of others, parsimony, and emotional constriction.

There have been at least two replication studies—one by Lazare et al. (1970) and one by Torgersen and Psychol (1980). Self-doubt (including difficulty in making decisions) was not associated with the obsessional dimension in any of the three studies. Rejection of others was associated with the obsessional dimension in the first study of female patients by Lazare et al. (1966); Torgersen and Psychol (1980) found an association among men but not among women. Rejection of others is defined by such items as "I often tend to express my resentment against a person by having nothing more to do with him," and "I usually keep myself somewhat aloof and hard to approach." This concept is captured by experimental criterion 6 in the list at the end of this chapter.

The Lazare–Klerman Trait Scale assesses obstinacy with such descriptions as "I do not usually back down from my opinions even when others argue with me." This contrasts with the items measuring oral aggression, which did not cluster with the obsessional dimension and which include items such as "I tend to make biting or sarcastic remarks when I criticize other people." There was also little association with the aggression item "I get into a fighting mood when the occasion seems to demand it." At least from the perspective of this self-report inventory, there is little overt evidence for the predisposition of "rage and revengefulness" noted by Freud (1908).

As outlined in Table 12.1, the DSM-III-R criteria set captures almost all the traits historically associated with the character type. Abraham's (1921) descriptions of "exaggerated criticism of others" and "generally morose or surly attitude" are not directly included in DSM-III-R, although the former may be implied by criterion 3, which refers to a conviction that others cannot be trusted to do things correctly. Likewise, Lazare et al.'s trait "rejection of others" is not captured directly. It is interesting that the few traits mentioned in the literature but not represented in DSM-III-R represent more overt expressions of hostility toward or contempt for others with different points of view. The factor-analytic data suggest that such traits may be only weakly associated with the obsessional dimension.

## Are Criteria Internally Consistent?

"Internal consistency" refers to how well the components of a criteria set appear to cluster together in individual patients. The analysis becomes a type of "bootstrap" procedure in which the criteria as a whole are assumed to approximate a real diagnostic entity, and patients are categorized as cases or noncases according to the criteria set taken as a whole. Individual criteria can then be examined according to their frequency among cases ("sensitivity") and rarity among noncases ("specificity"). It is also useful to examine the frequency of the diagnosis among individuals scoring positive on a specific criterion ("positive predictive value"). Such information can be useful for identifying which criteria increase discrimination from other disorders, and which do not discriminate or are not strongly related to the syndrome defined by the remaining criteria.

Only limited data are available for DSM-III-R. Data from four unpublished data sets are discussed here. The Freiman and Widiger (1989) data set is based on a study of 50 hospitalized psychiatric patients who received a structured interview for personality assessment. The Millon and Tringone (1989) data set is based on 584 patients described by clinicians as part of a mail survey. DSM-III-R criteria were paraphrased in this study. The Morey and Heumann (1988) data set is based on a mixed group of 291 patients who received an unstructured clinical interview. The Pfohl and Blum (1990) data set is based on the Structured Interview for DSM-III-R Personality Disorders (SIDP-R; Pfohl, Blum, Zimmerman, & Stangl, 1989) as used with a mixed group of 112 nonpsychotic inpatients, outpatients, and normal controls. Despite a lack of obsessive–compulsive personality disorder cases, the Freiman and Widiger (1989) study still provides useful information about specificity of individual criteria.

The statistics for these four studies are presented in Table 12.3. The two worst-performing criteria in each category are enclosed in parentheses. Results varied across studies, suggesting the need for cautious interpretation. The sensitivity for the nine criteria averaged approximately .50 or better across the three informative studies, with the exception of criteria 8 and 9. Given that these two criteria had very high specificity scores and that only five criteria are required for diagnosis, this may not be a problem.

Criterion 3 — "unreasonable insistence that others submit to exactly his or her way of doing things, or unreasonable reluctance to allow others to do things because of the conviction that they will not do them correctly" — showed low specificity in one study and very low positive predictive value in two of three studies (see Table 12.3). In the Morey and Heumann (1988) study, this criterion was present in 74% of obsessive–compulsive personality disorder cases, 81% of histrionic cases, 77% of narcissistic cases, and 83% of passive–aggressive cases. In our study (Pfohl & Blum, 1990), this criterion was present in 74% of obsessive–compulsive personality disorder cases, 75% of narcissistic personality disorder cases, and 60% of borderline personal-

TABLE 12.3. Internal-Consistency-Based Diagnostic Statistics for DSM-III-R
Obsessive–Compulsive Personality Disorder Criteria

| Study | Freq[b] | Criteria[a] | | | | | | | | |
|---|---|---|---|---|---|---|---|---|---|---|
| | | 1 | 2 | 3 | 4 | 5 | 6 | 7 | 8 | 9 |
| *Sensitivity* | | | | | | | | | | |
| Freiman & Widiger (1989) | 0 | – | – | – | – | – | – | – | – | – |
| Millon & Tringone (1989) | 60 | .47 | .47 | (.27)[c] | .75 | (.17) | .50 | .47 | – | – |
| Morey & Heumann (1988) | 23 | .65 | .78 | .74 | .61 | .74 | .54 | .96 | (.30) | (.22) |
| Pfohl & Blum (1990) | 31 | .87 | .87 | .74 | (.42) | .87 | .58 | .55 | (.29) | .48 |
| *Specificity* | | | | | | | | | | |
| Freiman & Widiger | 0 | .88 | .92 | .78 | .92 | (.56) | .96 | (.64) | .90 | .86 |
| Millon & Tringone | 60 | .87 | .90 | .82 | .81 | (.64) | .85 | (.74) | – | – |
| Morey & Heumann | 23 | .86 | .88 | (.53) | .90 | (.56) | .84 | .71 | .90 | .97 |
| Pfohl & Blum | 31 | .74 | (.62) | .72 | .91 | (.69) | .78 | .74 | .86 | .78 |
| *Positive predictive value* | | | | | | | | | | |
| Freiman & Widiger | 0 | – | – | – | – | – | – | – | – | – |
| Millon & Tringone | 60 | .29 | .36 | (.15) | .31 | (.06) | .28 | .17 | – | – |
| Morey & Heumann | 23 | .29 | .35 | (.12) | .35 | (.13) | .22 | .22 | .21 | .36 |
| Pfohl & Blum | 31 | .56 | .47 | .50 | .65 | .52 | .50 | (.45) | (.45) | (.45) |

[a]Numbers for criteria correspond to those in the DSM-III-R column in Table 12.2.
[b]Frequency of obsessive–compulsive personality disorder diagnosis in each study. Total sample size for each study was $n = 84$ (Freiman & Widiger, 1989), $n = 584$ (Millon & Tringone, 1989), $n = 291$ (Morey & Heumann, 1988), and $n = 112$ (Pfohl & Blum, 1990).
[c]Parentheses indicate the two worst-performing items in each study.

ity disorder cases. Given the lack of consistency across studies, more data
would be desirable.

Criterion 5—"indecisiveness: decision making is either avoided, post-
poned, or protracted . . . "—showed low sensitivity in one of three studies
and low specificity in four out of four studies. The positive predictive value
was very low in two out of three studies. In the Morey and Heumann (1988)
study, this criterion was present in 74% of obsessive–compulsive personality disorder cases, 78% of dependent personality disorder cases, 71% of
avoidant personality disorder cases, and 63% of schizotypal personality disorder cases. In the Pfohl and Blum (1990) study, this criterion was present
in 87% of obsessive–compulsive personality disorder cases, 71% of paranoid personality disorder cases, 64% of dependent personality disorder cases,
62% of avoidant personality disorder cases, and 67% of schizotypal personality disorder cases. Thus, there was fair agreement across studies that this
criterion might be a problem.

The remaining criteria appeared to have acceptable internal consis-

tency statistics, or at least failed to show any consistent evidence of weakness across studies.

## Are the Criteria Supported by External Validators?

Although almost no external validity data are available on DSM-III-R criteria for obsessive–compulsive personality disorder, it should be noted that external validators are the most desirable basis for revising criteria. For
example, if obsessive–compulsive personality disorder were conceptualized
as resulting from a certain parental style, then the criteria should identify
individuals raised in this type of family. If obsessive–compulsive personality disorder were considered adaptive in certain professions (e.g., accoun-
tants), then it might be possible to show higher rates of obsessive–compulsive
personality disorder among these professions. Biological markers might also
be sought, since most clinicians accept that personality is in part genetic.
No data sets of this type were available to guide the process of revising specific
criteria for DSM-IV.

## How Is the Personality Disorder Related to Obsessive–Compulsive Disorder and Other Axis I Disorders?

Although DSM-III-R lists obsessive–compulsive disorder, hypochondriasis,
major depression, and dysthymia as possible complications of obsessive–
compulsive personality disorder, there are few data to support this list. The
data that do exist usually begin with patients with a specific Axis I diagnosis
and examine rates of personality disorder. This design does not allow any
valid estimate about the risk of Axis I disorders in patients with a given personality disorder.

The overlap between obsessive–compulsive personality disorder and obsessive–compulsive disorder deserves special attention, because the similarity in names implies similar or related disorders and may lead to confusion.
Prior to the introduction of DSM-III criteria, Pollak (1979) reviewed studies
that examined the co-occurrence of obsessive–compulsive neurosis and obsessive–compulsive personality disorder (Ingram, 1961; Rosenberg, 1967; Sandler & Hazari, 1960). He summarized: "Clearly there is no necessary
one-to-one relationship between obsessional personality and obsessional neurosis, despite the occasional findings that more obsessive–compulsive neu-
rotics than would be expected by chance show evidence of a premorbid
obsessional personality" (p. 232).

The findings for studies using DSM-III and DSM-III-R criteria are similar. The literature review for DSM-IV focused on studies employing clinical
and structured interviews, because it was not clear that any of the available
self-report personality measures were truly assessing DSM-III or DSM-III-R
criteria for obsessive–compulsive personality disorder. Rasmussen and
Tsuang (1986) studied a series of 44 outpatients with DSM-III obsessive–

compulsive disorder, who were assessed with a clinical interview and check-list. Twenty-four patients (55%) met criteria for DSM-III compulsive perso-nality disorder. There was no control group. The next most common personality diagnosis was histrionic personality disorder (9%). Baer, Jenike, and Ricciardi (1990) used the Structured Interview for DSM-III Personality Disorders (SIDP; Pfohl, Stangl, & Zimmerman, 1982; Stangl, Pfohl, Zimmer-man, & Bowers, 1985) to assess DSM-III personality criteria in a series of 96 patients with obsessive–compulsive disorders. Six (6%) of the patients met criteria for compulsive personality disorder. Forty-four (45%) met criter-ia for other personality diagnoses, with mixed, dependent, and histrionic personality disorders being the most common. The same authors (Janike & Baer, personal communication) have used the SIDP-R (Pfohl et al., 1989) to assess DSM-III-R personality disorder criteria in a series of 59 patients with obsessive–compulsive disorder; 15 (25%) of these cases met the criteria for obsessive–compulsive personality disorder.

In a preliminary report of a collaborative project, Pfohl, Black, and Noyes (1988) compared the rates of obsessive–compulsive personality dis-order in several diagnostic groups studied at the University of Iowa with the SIDP. DSM-III compulsive personality disorder was diagnosed in 22 (19%) of 114 obsessive–compulsive patients, in 5 (6%) of 78 patients with major depression, and in 7 (8%) of 83 patients with panic disorder. Two other per-sonality diagnoses were more common than compulsive personality in the patients with obsessive–compulsive disorder: avoidant personality disorder (22%) and dependent personality disorder (21%). In a smaller series of pa-tients interviewed with the SIDP-R, the criteria for DSM-III-R obsessive–com-pulsive personality disorder were met in 7 (31%) of 22 patients with obsessive–compulsive disorder, 7 (35%) of 20 patients with generalized anxi-ety disorder, 6 (30%) of a mixed group of 20 nonpsychotic inpatients with other diagnoses (most often major depression), and none of the 10 normal controls.

There are even fewer data regarding the association between obses-sive–compulsive personality disorder and other Axis I disorders. The data presented here indicate that obsessive–compulsive personality disorder is not uncommon among patients with affective and anxiety disorders. Although there are references in the literature to various measures of ob-sessional character traits predisposing to depression (Kendell & Discipio, 1970; Matussek & Feil, 1983; Perris, Eisemann, & von Knorring, 1984), other studies failed to find such an association (Hirschfeld, Klerman, Clayton, & Keller, 1983; Hirschfeld et al., 1989).

In summary, available studies suggest that the majority of patients with Axis I obsessive–compulsive disorder do not meet Axis II criteria for obses-sive–compulsive personality disorder. Among patients with obsessive–com-pulsive disorder who do have a personality disorder, several other personality disorders may be just as common as or more common than obsessive–com-pulsive personality disorder. It is not possible to determine at this time whether patients with obsessive–compulsive disorder are more likely to meet criteria for obsessive–compulsive personality disorder than patients with other Axis I diagnoses. The relationship between obsessive–compulsive personality disorder and other Axis I disorders is even less clear.

## Is the Personality Disorder Distinct from Other Personality Disorders?

There have been some inconsistent and surprising overlaps between obsessive–compulsive personality disorder and other Axis II disorders across studies. Table 12.4 presents the rates of other comorbid personality diagnoses, which were unexpectedly high across several studies. Although it might be reasonable to consider that some diagnoses (e.g., paranoid personality disorder) really are associated with many obsessive–compulsive personality disorder traits, others (e.g., borderline personality disorder) are theoretically at the opposite end of the spectrum. The findings may relate to the fact that other personality disorders may have similar behaviors, but for different reasons. For example, unreasonable insistence that others submit to their wishes, indecisiveness, and lack of generosity may all exist in individuals with other personality disorders, although the motivation for these behaviors may differ in ways not easily captured by the criteria. The differences between studies may relate in part to the manner of assessment of criteria. For example, some structured interviews provide specific questions to determine whether the indecisiveness is part of an overall tendency to ponder or part of a need for excessive reassurance from others. Some of the experimental criteria listed at the end of this chapter attempt to make such distinctions. Another approach would be to build such distinctions into the "explications" in the text of the diagnostic manual.

## Are the Structure of the Diagnostic Criteria and the Threshold for Diagnosis Appropriate?

As noted previously, the DSM-III criteria for compulsive personality disorder required four of five criteria to make the diagnosis. The DSM-III-R Personality Disorders Advisory Group chose to expand the description to nine criteria, of which only five were required (see Table 12.2). The nine criteria were thought to provide a better representation of the full domain of traits in the clinical descriptions of obsessive–compulsive personality disorder. The requirement of only five of nine criteria allowed for greater variation among patients in how the personality disorder was expressed. Such a major change in the structure of the criteria would be expected to have some effect on the rate of diagnosis. The data in Table 12.4 suggest that the rate of diagnosing obsessive–compulsive personality disorder was roughly twice as high when DSM-III-R criteria were used as when DSM-III criteria were used.

TABLE 12.4. Percentages of Obsessive–Compulsive Personality Disorder (OCPD) Patients with Selected Comorbid Personality Disorder Diagnoses

| Study | Criteria | Number of OCPD cases | Sample size | Comorbid diagnoses (%) | | | | |
|-------|----------|----------------------|-------------|----------|-----------|------------|-------------|----------|
| | | | | Paranoid | Histrionic | Borderline | Narcissistic | Avoidant |
| Pfohl et al. (1986) | DSM-III | 7 | 131 | 0 | 43 | 29 | 14 | 29 |
| Zanarini (1989) | DSM-III | 17 | 253 | 17 | 39 | 72 | 28 | 50 |
| Morey & Heumann &1988) | DSM-III-R | 23 | 291 | 22 | 13 | 9 | 30 | 56 |
| Skodol (1989) | DSM-III-R | 21 | 97 | 33 | 24 | 86 | 48 | 62 |
| Pfohl & Blum (1990) | DSM-III-R | 31 | 112 | 52 | 36 | 26 | 16 | 52 |
| Pfohl & Blum (1990) | Modified[a] | 19 | 112 | 68 | 37 | 16 | 26 | 47 |

[a]The modified criteria were identical to DSM-III-R criteria, except that criterion 5 was deleted and five of the remaining eight criteria were required for diagnosis.

The best way to clarify the impact of the changes from DSM-III to DSM-III-R would be to apply both criteria sets to the same set of patients. We (Pfohl & Blum, 1990) assessed a mixed group of 72 nonpsychotic inpatients and outpatients with normal intellectual functioning, using the SIDP for DSM-III personality diagnoses and the SIDP-R for DSM-III-R diagnoses. Eleven (15%) patients met DSM-III criteria for compulsive personality disorder, and 20 (27%) met DSM-III-R criteria for obsessive–compulsive personality disorder. Of the 11 patients who met DSM-III criteria, 9 met DSM-III-R criteria. This suggests that the main effect of the last set of changes was to expand the number of patients qualifying for this diagnosis. It is not clear whether this represented an improvement.

As already noted, one problem with the DSM-III-R criteria is the unexpectedly high overlap with other personality disorders. The elimination of criteria with low specificity (i.e., criteria that are frequently present in other personality disorders) represents one approach to decreasing overlap that can be tested with existing data sets. An example of this approach is represented in the bottom row of Table 12.4. When criterion 5 was eliminated and five of the remaining eight criteria were required for diagnosis, the rate of diagnosis in the Pfohl and Blum (1990) data set dropped from 31 (28%) to 19 (17%). The overlap with borderline personality disorder dropped from 26% to 16%, but the overlap with several other personality disorders actually increased. It may be that requiring five of fewer criteria (eight) selects for more severe cases, and that more severe cases may be more likely to score positive on a variety of dimensions.

It is possible that the overlap between diagnoses is not a matter of problematic criteria, but rather reflects the fact that personality traits do vary in individuals in a way that crosses the conceptual boundaries implied by the Axis II diagnoses. If this were true, a series of continuous trait dimensions might capture the true state of nature better than the DSM-III-R categories do. Such a radical departure from this approach to Axis II was considered for DSM-IV by the Personality Disorders Work Group, but rejected (see Widiger & Sanderson, Chapter 22, this volume).

## What Is the Best Name for the Disorder?

Obsessive–compulsive personality disorder cannot be viewed as a necessary or even a common prerequisite to the development of Axis I obsessive–compulsive disorder; nor is it the most common personality diagnosis in patients with obsessive–compulsive disorder. The similarity in names represents a source of confusion to those learning to use and apply the DSM system. Jenike and Baer (personal communication) have expressed the concern that the similarity in names might lead to confusion among clinicians about what treatments are most effective for each disorder.

ICD-9 and ICD-10 use the term "anankastic personality," and DSM-II included the alternative label "anankastic personality" in parentheses. Although the term "anankastic personality disorder" would separate the personality disorder from the Axis I disorder, its adoption would violate the guiding principle of avoiding labels that do not have a descriptively clear meaning in the English language. The Personality Disorders Work Group therefore recommended no change in the name for DSM-IV

## CHANGES MADE IN DSM-IV

Obsessive–compulsive personality disorder represents an attempt to operationalize a concept that has long been part of the psychiatric literature. The criteria possess good content validity with respect to the descriptive literature, including the factor-analytic work of Lazare et al. (1966, 1970). Problems with this disorder include the high degree of overlap with other personality disorders and the lack of empirical studies that might provide external validity for the DSM-III-R criteria. The relationship between Axis I obsessive–compulsive disorder and obsessive–compulsive personality disorder is apparently weak, and it is unfortunate that the similarity in names may lead to confusion.

The DSM-IV diagnostic criteria for obsessive–compulsive personality disorder are listed in Table 12.2. Although there was good reason to conclude that certain improvements were needed, there was some disagreement among advisors and work group members about how much data ought to be accumulated before a change was accepted as a valid improvement. The following changes have been made.

1. There was a consensus that the essential feature of this disorder could be better described as follows: "A pervasive pattern of preoccupation with orderliness, perfectionism, and mental and interpersonal control, at the expense of flexibility, openness, and efficiency."

2. Because criterion 3 as worded in DSM-III-R has failed to discriminate the diagnosis clearly from other disorders, the following change in wording was made to emphasize the unique features of this trait in obsessive–compulsive personality disorder: "is reluctant to delegate tasks or to work with others unless they submit to exactly his or her way of doing things" (this is now DSM-IV criterion 6).

3. Because DSM-III-R criterion 5 ("indecisiveness . . . ") showed poor discrimination in recent studies and weak association with the disorder in factor-analytic studies, it was decided that this criterion should be deleted.

4. DSM-III-R criterion 7 ("restricted expression of affection") has also been deleted because of poor discriminant properties.

5. It was recommended that DSM-III-R criterion 8 be reworded to capture the parsimonious quality of the disorder more effectively. The new criterion reads: "adopts a miserly spending style toward both self and others; money is viewed as something that must be hoarded or cautiously invested to provide for future catastrophes" (this is now DSM-IV criterion 7).

6. Because the rate of diagnosis of this disorder appeared to be much higher in studies using DSM-III-R as compared to DSM-III criteria, it originally seemed reasonable to require five of the eight remaining criteria for diagnosis of this disorder. However, DSM-IV as published requires only four of the eight criteria.

7. A new criterion, "shows rigidity and stubbornness," has been introduced into DSM-IV (it is criterion 8 there) to capture these prototypical features, which were only indirectly represented in DSM-III-R.

## CRITERIA PROPOSED FOR RESEARCH

In addition to the changes described above, the following experimental criteria were formulated to operationalize some concepts described in the literature, in the hope that they may help future researchers:

1. Making the "correct" decision often becomes a time-consuming and complicated process that he or she is loath to entrust to anyone else.

2. Maintains loyalty to a select group of friends or family, yet overt expressions of affection toward these individuals is highly restricted or nonexistent.

3. Periods of rigid adherence to authority are punctuated by great irritation or overt anger when authority figures are perceived as "bending the rules."

4. Argues stubbornly with others who have a different political or

philosophical viewpoint and considers opposing opinion as utterly without merit.

5. Is critical and judgmental of others, for example, prone to make biting and sarcastic remarks.

6. Dispenses with others who fail to accommodate to his or her exacting standards and demands by refusing to have anything more to do with them.

## REFERENCES

Abraham. K. (1921). Contributions to the theory of the anal character. In K. Abraham, *On character and libido development*. New York: Basic Books, 1966.

American Psychiatric Association. (1952). *Diagnostic and statistical manual of mental disorders* (1st ed.). Washington, DC: Mental Hospitals Service.

Amercian Psychiatric Association. (1968). *Diagnostic and statistical manual of mental disorders* (2nd ed.). Washington, DC: Author.

American Psychiatric Association. (1980). *Diagnostic and statistical manual of mental disorders* (3rd ed.). Washington, DC: Author.

American Psychiatric Association. (1987). *Diagnostic and statistical manual of mental disorders* (3rd ed., rev.). Washington, DC: Author.

American Psychiatric Association. (1994). *Diagnostic and statistical manual of mental disorders* (4th ed.). Washington, DC: Author.

Baer, L., Jenike, M. A., & Ricciardi, J. (1990). Standardized assessment of personality disorders in obsessive–compulsive disorder. *Archives of General Psychiatry, 47,* 826–830.

Freiman, K., & Widiger, T. (1989). [Co-occurrence and diagnostic efficiency statistics]. Unpublished raw data.

Freud, S. (1908). Character and anal eroticism. In J. Strachey (Ed. and Trans.), *The standard edition of the complete psychological works of Sigmund Freud* (Vol. 9). London: Hogarth Press, 1959.

Hirschfeld, R. A. M., Klerman, G. L., Clayton, P. J., & Keller, M. B. (1983). Personality and depression. *Archives of General Psychiatry, 40,* 993–998.

Hirschfeld, R. A. M., Klierman, C. L., Lavori, P., Keller, M. B., Grimth, P., & Coryell, W. (1989). Premorbid personality assessments of first onset of major depression. *Archives of General Psychiatry, 46,* 345–350.

Ingram, I. M. (1961). The obsessional personality and obsessional illness. *American Journal of Psychiatry, 1*(17), 1016–1019.

Kendell, R. E., & Discipio, W. J. (1970). Obsessional symptoms and obsessional personality traits in patients with depressive illness. *Psychological Medicine, 1,* 65–72.

Lazare, A., Klerman, G., & Armor, D. J. (1966). Oral, obsessive and hysterical personality patterns. *Archives of General Psychiatry, 14,* 624–630.

Lazare, A., Klerman, G., & Armor, D. J. (1970). Oral, obsessive and hysterical personality patterns: Replication of factor analysis in an independent sample. *Journal of Psychiatric Research, 7,* 275–279.

Matussek, P., & Feil, B. F. (1983). Personality attributes of depressive patients. *Archives of General Psychiatry, 40,* 783–790.

Millon, T., & Tringone, R. (1989). [Co-occurrence and diagnostic efficiency statistics]. Unpublished raw data.

Morey, L., & Heumann, K. (1988). [Co-occurrence and diagnostic efficiency statistics]. Unpublished raw data.

Oldham, J. M., & Frosch, W. A. (1988). Compulsive personality disorder. In R. Michels, J. O. Cavenar, H. K. H. Brodie, A. M. Cooper, S. B. Guze, L. L. Judd, G. L. Klerman, & A. J. Solnit (Eds.), *Psychiatry*. Philadelphia: J. B. Lippincott.

Perris, C., Eisemann, M., & von Knorring, L. (1984). Personality traits in former depressed patients and healthy subjects without past history of depression. *Psychopathology, 17,* 178–186.

Pfohl, B., Black, D., & Noyes, R. Jr. (1988). *Axis I/Axis II comorbidity findings* (Abstract). American Psychiatric Association Annual Meeting, Montreal.

Pfohl, B., & Blum, N. (1990). [Co-occurrence and diagnostic efficiency statistics]. Unpublished raw data.

Pfohl, B., Blum, N., Zimmerman, M., & Stangl, D. (1989). *The Structured Interview for DSM-III-R Personality Disorders (SIDP-R)*. Iowa City: Department of Psychiatry, University of Iowa.

Pfohl, B., Coryell, W., Zimmerman, M., & Stangl, D. (1986). DSM-III personality disorders: Diagnostic overlap and internal consistency of individual DSM-III criteria. *Comprehensive Psychiatry, 27,* 21–34.

Pfohl, B., Stangl, D., & Zimmerman, M. (1982). *The Structured Interview for DSM-III Personality Disorders (SIDP)*. Iowa City: Department of Psychiatry, University of Iowa.

Pollak, J. M. (1979). Obsessive compulsive personality: A review. *Psychological Bulletin, 86,* 225–241.

Pollak, J. M. (1987). Relationship of obsessive–compulsive personality to obsessive–compulsive disorder: A review of the literature. *Journal of Psychology, 121,* 137–148.

Rasmussen, S. A., & Tsuang, M. T. (1986). Clinical characteristics and family history in DSM-III obsessive–compulsive disorder. *American Journal of Psychiatry, 143,* 317–322.

Rosenberg, C. M. (1967). Personality and obsessional neurosis. *British Journal of Psychiatry, 113,* 471–477.

Sandler, J., & Hazari, A. (1960). The "obsessional": On the psychological classification of obsessional character traits and symptoms. *British Journal of Medical Psychology, 33,* 113–122.

Skodol, A. (1989).[Co-occurrence and diagnostic efficiency statistics]. Unpublished raw data.

Stangl, D., Pfohl, B., Zimmerman, M., & Bowers, W. (1985). A structured interview for DSM-III personality disorders. *Archives of General Psychiatry, 42,* 591–596.

Torgersen, S., & Psychol, C. (1980). The oral, obsessive and hysterical personality syndromes: A study of hereditary and environmental factors by means of the twin method. *Archives of General Psychiatry, 37,* 1272–1277.

World Health Organization. (1977). *International classification of diseases* (9th revision). Geneva: Author.

Zanarini, M. (1989). [Co-occurrence and diagnostic efficiency statistics]. Unpublished raw data.

# Commentary on Obsessive–Compulsive Personality Disorder

Jerrold M. Pollak

Obsessive–compulsive personality disorder has a well-established place in the clinical literature, beginning with the observations made by Freud and other classical psychoanalysts about the constellation of so-called "anal character traits" (e.g., Freud, 1908; Jones, 1918). Since that time, clinicians and theorists working within a broadly defined psychodynamic framework (e.g., Mallinger, 1982, 1984; Salzman, 1980) and from a social learning perspective (Millon, 1981) have refined our understanding of the abnormal and normal variants of this personality pattern. Relative to most other personality patterns, obsessive–compulsive personality has also been the subject of considerable empirical investigation, including a number of factor-analytic and experimental studies that have been reviewed previously (Pollak, 1979, 1987a). This research literature is moderately supportive of a clustering of traits that conforms reasonably well to clinical descriptions, including early analytic observations of anal character. Obsessive–compulsive personality is a highly familiar personality construct (Lazare, 1989), and obsessive–compulsive personality disorder is not a controversial psychiatric diagnosis (Widiger & Frances, 1988). As pointed out by Pfohl and Blum in their thoughtful and comprehensive review in Chapter 12, the longevity of the construct of obsessive–compulsive personality disorder is reflected in its inclusion (under various names) in all editions of the *Diagnostic and Statistical Manual of Mental Disorders,* including DSM-IV (American Psychiatric Association, 1994).

Obsessive–compulsive traits are probably widely disseminated in the normal population. This personality type is best understood as falling on a continuum of severity—from an adaptive coping style, particularly suitable for managing the complex demands of modern industrial society (Monroe, 1974; Oldham & Frosch, 1992; Perry & Vaillant, 1989), to exaggerated and maladaptive expressions falling within the neurotic to borderline levels of structural personality organization (Goldstein, 1985). In clinical practice, the point at

which obsessive–compulsive patterns constitute psychopathological deviation is not always clear (Gunderson, 1988; Oldham & Frosch, 1992; Perry
& Vaillant, 1989), and modest heterogeneity in clinical presentation is
common.

## DIAGNOSTIC CRITERIA

The DSM-III-R (American Psychiatric Association, 1987) criteria for obsessive–compulsive personality disorder constitute a clear improvement over
the DSM-III (American Psychiatric Association, 1980) criteria for compulsive personality disorder. First, the DSM-III-R criteria are more faithful to
analytic descriptions and to the findings of empirical research. Second, by
increasing the number of criteria within a polythetic framework, DSM-III-R
reflects an enhanced appreciation of the diversity in clinical presentation
of maladaptive obsessive–compulsive patterns.

A computer search of relevant citations through the latter part of 1993,
conducted for this commentary, identified only a small number of additional
studies on this construct that have been completed since the most recent
review (Pollak, 1987a) and the publication of DSM-III-R. Moreover, the kinds
of studies completed have continued to be of questionable relevance for enhancing the definitional clarity of obsessive–compulsive personality disorder, and specifically for bolstering its external validity. Thus, Pfohl and Blum
are quite correct in stating that insufficient new knowledge has accumulated since the publication of DSM-III-R to justify significant alteration of the
diagnostic criteria in DSM-IV. Specifically, there is insufficient empirical evidence to anchor the criteria to a single dominant or pathognomonic feature or to order the items in terms of importance to diagnosis.

The changes described by Pfohl and Blum in Chapter 12 are in keeping with the intent of DSM-IV to refine the wording of existing diagnostic
criteria for established categories and to eliminate items with a high degree
of overlap with other personality disorder categories, rather than to strive
for significant reconceptualization or redefinition (Hirschfeld, 1993).

Pfohl and Blum note that DSM-III-R criterion 5 ("indecisiveness . . . ")
has been deleted, and that criterion 3 ("unreasonable insistence that others
submit to exactly his or her way of doing things . . . ") has been reworded.
It is a well-established idea among clinicians that problematic decision making is a key feature of the behavioral style of individuals with pathological
obsessive–compulsive patterns (e.g., Rado, 1959). Difficulty with decision making is also a characteristic that continues to be identified in studies of self-
report measures of obsessive–compulsive personality traits (McCann, 1992).
Still, because self-doubt (including explicit difficulty with decision making)
failed to correlate with the obsessive dimension identified in factor analytic
studies and also has been shown to have low specificity, the deletion of this
criterion in DSM-IV is reasonable. At the same time, Pfohl and Blum's ex-

perimental criterion 1 may prove helpful in salvaging this concept in modi-fied form. In its coupling of the arduous nature of decision making with a staunch reluctance to delegate decision making to others, this experimen-tal criterion also appears to acknowledge the counterdependent nature of maladaptive obsessive–compulsive personality, emphasized in psychodynam-ic formulations, in a way that potentially can be reliably assessed.

The experimental criteria are generally sound and deserve serious con-sideration in future discussions of modifications in diagnostic criteria. DSM-IV criterion 7 nicely reflects analytic descriptions of the stingy quality of individuals with obsessive–compulsive personality disorder (Fromm, 1947; Jones, 1918; Reich, 1949). This criterion might be expanded in the future to include a penurious approach to the use of time, as this is included in DSM-III-R criterion 8 and has been emphasized in analytic descriptions (Jones, 1918; Pettit, 1969).

Experimental criterion 2 aptly describes the juxtaposition of loyalty to significant others with compromise in overt display of affection toward these same individuals. This criterion may prove to be useful in differentiating persons with obsessive–compulsive personality disorder, who have intact ca-pacities for dedication and loyalty, from individuals with narcissistic person-ality disorder, who are thought to lack such capacities but who share some behavioral similarities with individuals with obsessive–compulsive personality disorder: hostility; inordinate need for interpersonal control; and a perfec-tionistic, competitive, and driven lifestyle (Akhtar, 1989; Horowitz, 1989).

Experimental criteria 3, 4, and 5 are good operational definitions, as described in analytic writings, of the often-cited proclivities of persons with obsessive–compulsive personality disorder to be highly opinionated and authoritarian and to be excessively critical of the ideas and actions of others (Abraham, 1921). At the same time, experimental criteria 4, 5, and/or 6 may be found to have excessive overlap with a new diagnostic criterion for nar-cissistic personality disorder: "shows arrogant, haughty behaviors or attitudes" (American Psychiatric Association, 1994, p. 661; see Gunderson, Ronning-stam, & Smith, Chapter 9, this volume).

Experimental criterion 6 may also create confusion when considered in relation to experimental criterion 2. More specifically, the individual with an obsessive–compulsive personality disorder is depicted as remaining loy-al to significant others, yet as rejecting anyone failing to conform to his or her expectations (experimental criterion 6).

Experimental criterion 3 addresses well the strong identification with authority and the conformist aspect of obsessive–compulsive personality dis-order. However, neither the DSM-III-R criteria, the DSM-IV criteria, nor the experimental criteria appear to directly address the resistance to authority — typically in a furtive, withholding manner — which historically has also been seen as a key aspect of obsessive–compulsive personality disorder, especial-ly in the writing of psychodynamic clinicians (e.g., Rado, 1959). Reference is made to this feature in the narrative section of the DSM-III-R description of obsessive–compulsive personality disorder, but is not included in the diagnostic criteria section itself. On the other hand, formal inclusion of such a criterion might create undesirable overlap with the new criteria for passive–aggressive (negativistic) personality disorder (see Millon & Radovanov, Chapter 14, this volume).

Similarly, neither the DSM-III-R criteria, the DSM-IV criteria, nor the experimental criteria appear to address adequately the demand sensitivity component of obsessive–compulsive personality disorder, described so well by Mallinger (1982). This involves a negative and sometimes hostile and defiant response to demands or expectations, which are perceived in an exaggerated fashion.

Although, to a significant degree, thresholds for DSM-III-R diagnoses are arbitrary (Widiger, 1992), it was a sound proposal to continue to require five of the remaining eight DSM-III-R criteria after the deletion of criterion 5, because it might decrease the rate of false-positive diagnoses. This would be desirable in light of the unclear boundaries between normal and abnormal obsessive–compulsive personality patterns; the fairly widespread prevalence of obsessive–compulsive traits in the normal population, particularly in men; and the well-documented proclivity of clinicians to overpathologize (Ziskin & Faust, 1988). The requirement of DSM-IV of only four of eight criteria may serve to increase the rate of false-positive diagnoses.

## ESSENTIAL FEATURE

Modifying the essential feature of obsessive–compulsive personality disorder to include a preoccupation with mental and interpersonal control is a positive change that is consistent with the emphasis in recent dynamic thinking on exaggerated mechanisms of intrapersonal and interpersonal control in this disorder (Mallinger, 1984; Salzman, 1980). It is also timely, given recent conceptualizations of personality disorders as enactments of disordered thought–feeling–action patterns in relation to significant others (McLemore & Brokaw, 1987). The emphasis on interpersonal control may also sensitize clinicians to the potential value of more active and interpersonally focused psychotherapeutic methods, both individual and group, in the modification of maladaptive obsessive–compulsive personality patterns (Gunderson, 1988; Perry & Vaillant, 1989; Salzman, 1980).

Repositioning the concept of in flexibility so that it is described as a consequence of maladaptive obsessive–compulsive traits, rather than as part of the essential feature of the disorder per se, is also a welcome change. Inflexibility is a rather vague and general concept that can be said to characterize all maladaptive personality patterns to varying degrees.

## RELATIONSHIP OF OBSESSIVE–COMPULSIVE DISORDER TO OBSESSIVE–COMPULSIVE PERSONALITY DISORDER

Traditional psychodynamic teaching has maintained that obsessive–compulsive personality is the primary, if not exclusive, predisposing maladaptive personality pattern in the development of obsessive–compulsive disorder. Dynamic thinking has also held that these two psychiatric entities should be conceptualized as falling on a continuum of severity and as sharing common dynamics and etiology (e.g., Salzman, 1980). In contrast to this venerable opinion, empirical studies as reviewed by Baer and Jenike (1992) indicate that obsessive–compulsive disorder and obsessive–compulsive personality disorder are distinct disorders. Obsessive–compulsive disorder is associated with significant Axis II comorbidity; most studies have reported that more than 50% of individuals with obsessive–compulsive disorder met DSM-III criteria for one or more personality disorders. Pfohl and Blum note in Chapter 12, however, that the majority of individuals with obsessive–compulsive disorder do not have obsessive–compulsive personality disorder. Also, most individuals with obsessive–compulsive personality disorder never develop obsessive–compulsive disorder (Pollak, 1987b).

Moreover, in studies applying DSM-III personality disorder criteria, compulsive personality disorder was not more frequently associated with obsessive–compulsive disorder than were other personality disorder diagnoses. It may also be the case that obsessive–compulsive disorder predisposes to personality pathology, including obsessive–compulsive traits, rather than developing in response to maladaptive obsessive–compulsive personality patterns (Stein, Hollander, & Skodol, 1993).

It remains unknown, however, whether consistent use of DSM-III-R or DSM-IV criteria (which are more in accord with psychodynamic conceptualizations) will show that the prevalence of obsessive–compulsive personality disorder in obsessive–compulsive disorder is higher than previously reported (Baer & Jenike, 1992), or whether obsessive–compulsive personality disorder shows modestly higher rates of comorbidity than other personality disorders with obsessive–compulsive disorder.

## OVERLAP IN TERMINOLOGY

In any case, these two psychiatric conditions have far less in common that the striking similarity in their names would suggest. Indeed, the overlap in terminology used to describe them is likely to increase the probability of confusion in diagnosis, especially among inexperienced clinicians. However, in the absence of viable alternative terms, that would more readily distinguish these two disorders, the overlapping terminology will, as pointed out by Pfohl and Blum, have to remain for now.

It was prudent for DSM-IV to include more explicit clarification regarding differential diagnosis than was included in DSM-III-R. More specifically, DSM-IV indicates that obsessive–compulsive disorder involves obsessions and compulsions absent in obsessive–compulsive personality disorders and that the two disorders are considered distinct diagnoses despite the similarity in their names.

## CONCLUSIONS

Finally, although this is not addressed by Pfohl and Blum in Chapter 12, the DSM-III-R description of impairment associated with obsessive–compulsive personality disorder—that is, "This disorder frequently is quite incapacitating, particularly in its effect on occupational functioning" (American Psychiatric Association, 1987, p. 355)—has been called into question by empirical data suggesting that obsessive–compulsive personality disorder is associated with less functional impairment than most other personality disorders (Nakao et al., 1992). DSM-IV now states: "Obsessive–compulsive personality traits in moderation may be especially adaptive, particularly in situations that reward high performance. Only when these traits are inflexible, maladaptive, and persisting and cause significant functional impairment or subjective distress do they constitute Obsessive–Compulsive Personality Disorder" (American Psychiatric Association, 1994, p. 672).

## REFERENCES

Abraham, K. (1921). Contributions to the theory of the anal character. In K. Abrahams, *Selected papers on psychoanalysis.* London: Hogarth Press, 1927.

Akhtar, S. (1989). Narcissistic personality disorder: Descriptive features and differential diagnosis. *Psychiatric Clinics of North America, 12,* 505–529.

American Psychiatric Association. (1980). *Diagnostic and statistical manual of mental disorders* (3rd ed.). Washington, DC: Author.

American Psychiatric Association. (1987). *Diagnostic and statistical manual of mental disorders* (3rd ed., rev.). Washington, DC: Author.

American Psychiatric Association. (1994). *Diagnostic and statistical manual of mental disorders* (4th ed.). Washington, DC: Author.

Baer, L., & Jenike, M. A. (1992). Personality disorders in obsessive–compulsive disorder. *Psychiatric Clinics of North America, 15,* 805–812.

Freud, S. (1908). Character and anal eroticism. In E. Jones (Ed.), *Sigmund Freud: Collected papers* (Vol. 2). London: Hogarth Press, 1925.

Fromm, E. (1947). *Man for himself.* New York: Rinehart.

Goldstein, W. N. (1985). Obsessive–compulsive behavior, DSM-III and a psychodynamic classification of psychopathology. *American Journal of Psychotherapy, 46,* 346–359.

Gunderson, J. (1988). Personality disorders. In A. M. Nicholi (Ed.), *The new Harvard guide to modern psychiatry.* Cambridge, MA: Harvard University Press.

Hirschfeld, R. M. A. (1993). Personality disorders: Definition and diagnosis. *Journal of Personality Disorders, 7*(Suppl.), 9–17.

Horowitz, M. J. (1989). Clinical phenomenology of narcissistic pathology. *Psychiatric Clinics of North America, 12,* 531–539.

Jones, E. (1918). Anal character traits. In E. Jones, *Papers on psychoanalysis.* London: Balliere, Tindall & Cox, 1938.

Lazare, A. (1989). Personality. In A. Lazare (Ed.), *Outpatient psychiatry.* Baltimore: Williams & Wilkins.

Mallinger, A. E. (1982). Demand-sensitive obsessionals. *Journal of the American Academy of Psychoanalysis, 10,* 407–426.

Mallinger, A. E. (1984). The obsessive's myth of control. *Journal of the American Academy of Psychoanalysis, 12,* 147–165.

McCann, J. T. (1992). A comparison of two measures for obsessive–compulsive personality disorder. *Journal of Personality Disorders, 6,* 18–23.

McLemore, C. W., & Brokaw, D. W. (1987). Personality disorders as dysfunctional interpersonal behavior. *Journal of Personality Disorders, 1,* 270–285.

Millon, T. (1981). *Disorders of personality: DSM-III, Axis II.* New York: Wiley.

Monroe, R. R. (1974). Obsessive behavior: Integration of psychoanalytic and other approaches. In S. Arieti (Ed.), *American handbook of psychiatry* (Vol. 2). New York: Basic Books.

Nakao, K., Gunderson, J. G., Phillips, K. A., Tanaka, N., Yorifugi, K., Takaishi, J., & Nishimura, T. (1992). Functional impairment in personality disorders. *Journal of Personality Disorders, 6,* 24–33.

Oldham, J. M., & Frosch, W. A. (1992). Compulsive personality disorder. In R. Michels (Ed.), *Psychiatry* (rev. ed.). Philadelphia: J. B. Lippincott.

Perry, J. C., & Vaillant, G. E. (1989). Personality disorders. In H. I. Kaplan & B. J. Sadock (Eds.), *Comprehensive textbook of psychiatry* (5th ed, Vol. 2). Baltimore: Williams & Wilkins.

Pettit, T. F. (1969). Anality and time. *Journal of Consulting and Clinical Psychology, 33,* 170–174.

Pollak, J. M. (1979). Obsessive–compulsive personality: A review. *Psychological Bulletin, 86,* 225–241.

Pollak, J. (1987a). Obsessive–compulsive personality: Theoretical and clinical perspectives and recent research findings. *Journal of Personality Disorders, 1,* 248–262.

Pollak, J. (1987b). Relationship of obsessive–compulsive personality to obsessive–compulsive disorder: A review of the literature. *Journal of Psychology, 121,* 137–148.

Rado, S. (1959). Obsessive behavior. In S. Arieti (Ed.), *American handbook of psychiatry* (Vol. 1). New York: Basic Books, 1974.

Reich, W. (1949). *Character analysis* (3rd ed.) (V. R. Carafagno, Trans.). New York: Farrar, Straus.

Salzman, L. (1980). *Treatment of the obsessive personality.* New York: Jason Aronson.

Stein, D. J., Hollander, E., & Skodol, A. E. (1993). Anxiety disorders and personality disorders. *Journal of Personality Disorders, 7,* 87–104.

Widiger, T. A. (1992). Categorical vs. dimensional classification: Implications from and for research. *Journal of Personality Disorders, 6,* 287–300.

Widiger, T. A., & Frances, A. J. (1988). Personality disorders. In J. A. Talbott, R. E. Hales, & S. C. Yudofsky (Eds.) *Textbook of psychiatry.* Washington, DC: American Psychiatric Press.

Ziskin, J., & Faust, D. (1988). *Coping with psychiatric and psychological testimony* (Vol. 1). Marina del Rey, CA: Law and Psychology Press.

# PART III

# APPENDED AND DELETED DIAGNOSES

# CHAPTER 13

# Depressive Personality Disorder

KATHARINE A. PHILLIPS
ROBERT M. A. HIRSCHFELD
M. TRACIE SHEA
JOHN G. GUNDERSON

Depressive personality has a long and rich history, dating back to at least the time of Emil Kraepelin (1921). Under such rubrics as "depressive character," "melancholic temperament," and "subaffective dysthymia," it has been described by clinical theorists from diverse perspectives and has been used by clinicians for years (Phillips, Gunderson, Hirschfeld, & Smith, 1990). Despite its clinical tradition and its formal recognition in European psychiatry by the ninth revision of the *International Classification of Diseases* (ICD-9; World Health Organization, 1978), depressive personality disorder remains a controversial concept. It was considered for inclusion in DSM-IV (American Psychiatric Association [APA], 1994) for these reasons: (1) This disorder's historical tradition is substantial; (2) its omission has been criticized by authors from notably diverse theoretical perspectives (Kernberg, 1987; Akiskal, 1989; A. T. Beck, personal communication, 1990); (3) empirical evidence in its support is accumulating; and (4) certain Axis I and II disorders may be biogenetically linked, suggesting that depressive personality disorder might represent a trait-like, temperamental variant of Axis I mood disorders.

Although Kraepelin (1921) clearly described a depressive temperament the concept may actually have originated millennia ago, in the descriptions by Hippocrates and Aristotle of a "black gall," or melancholic, personality type. Although this temperament was postulated to predispose individuals to more severe melancholic episodes, it was not considered to be entirely

An earlier version of this chapter was published in the *Journal of Personality Disorders*, 1993, 7, 30–42. Copyright 1991 by The Guilford Press. Adapted by permission.

pathological. In fact, Aristotle suggested that all those who excelled in philosophy, politics, poetry, or arts are melancholics (Smith 1908–1931, p. 953). Kraepelin and several other German phenomenologists (Kretschmer, 1925; Tellenbach, 1980) subsequently described a depressive temperament, which they believed was pathological and "characterized by a permanent gloomy emotional stress in all the experiences of life" (Kraepelin, 1921, p. 118). Like Hippocrates and Aristotle, they postulated that this personality type was a milder, trait-like variant—or substrate—of major mood disorder that predisposed individuals to more severe depressive or manic episodes. It was, in other words, considered a subaffective "rudiment" from which more florid manic or depressive episodes "rise like mountain peaks from a structurally similar plain" (Slater & Roth, 1969; pp. 191–192). Kraepelin believed these individuals to be predominantly gloomy, despondent, and despairing, as well as serious, burdened, guilt-ridden, self-reproaching, self-denying, and lacking in self-confidence. He considered this personality type to be inherited, to be expressed early in life, and to persist throughout life, either as the temperament alone or as the "point of departure" for more florid major depressive or manic episodes.

Kurt Schneider (1923) also described a depressive personality, which he called "depressive psychopathy." Like Kraepelin, he considered these individuals to be gloomy, pessimistic, serious, and incapable of enjoyment or relaxation; he also saw them as quiet, skeptical, worrying, duty-bound, and self-doubting. Unlike Kraepelin, Schneider believed depressive personality to be linked to normal personality and other personality disorders, but not to major mood disorder.

Several psychoanalysts (Berliner, 1966; Kahn, 1975; Arieti & Bemporad, 1980; Simons, 1986) have also described an enduring depressive personality, which they believe to derive from disturbed early object relations rather than an abnormal constitution. Laughlin (1967) and subsequently Kernberg (1987), like the German phenomenologists, have proposed that these individuals are overly serious, somber, burdened, responsible, conscientious, and highly critical of themselves and others, and have attributed these characteristics to an excessively severe superego. However, Kernberg has posited that they do not necessarily express their criticism of others and that they may inhibit the expression of angry or aggressive thoughts and feelings. Laughlin, in fact, suggested that this inhibition of aggression can be so extreme that such persons may appear overly polite, agreeable, compliant, passive, and even subservient. Finally, unlike the German phenomenologists, Laughlin and Kernberg have posited the importance of overdependence on the love, support, and acceptance of others, although these traits may be masked by a counterdependence designed to protect against rejection. Kernberg, like Kraepelin, has suggested that this personality type may predispose an individual to depressive episodes, which tend to occur when the individual's overly high standards or dependency needs are not met.

Although cognitive and behavioral theorists have not described a depres-

sive personality per se, some of their work on enduring, depressogenic beliefs may have relevance to this disorder. For example, Beck (1967) and Alloy, Abramson, Metalsky, and Hartlage (1988) believe that persons prone to
major depression have chronically distorted negative cognitions, which predispose them to the development of more severe depressive episodes. However,
these theories focus primarily on the premorbid features of major depression, rather than on a depressive personality type that may or may not predispose individuals to depressive episodes.

Depressive personality disorder had no clear equivalent in DSM-I (American Psychiatric Association, 1952), but in DSM-II (American Psychiatric Association, 1968) it appears to have been subsumed by the heterogeneous
diagnosis of depressive neurosis. The subsequent placement of depressive
neurosis on Axis I in DSM-III (American Psychiatric Association, 1980) as
dysthymic disorder, rather than on Axis II as depressive personality disorder, was controversial (Akiskal, 1983; Goldstein & Anthony, 1988). It has been
argued that dysthymia is an overly broad category that includes both mild
affective disorders and trait-like temperamental or characterological depressive personality traits, and that the latter should be teased out from dysthymia
and placed on Axis II (Goldstein & Anthony, 1988; Cooper & Michels, 1981).
However, it has also been acknowledged that questions about this putative
disorder remain, many of which are addressed in this chapter.

## SIGNIFICANT ISSUES

The issues addressed by the DSM-IV Personality Disorders Work Group and
covered in this chapter are as follows:

1. What diagnostic instruments have been developed, and how do the
   individual criteria for depressive personality disorder perform?
2. To what extent can depressive personality disorder be distinguished
   conceptually from other personality disorders and Axis I mood disorders?
3. To what extent can depressive personality disorder be distinguished
   empirically from other personality disorders and Axis I mood disorders?
4. Is depressive personality disorder a "normal" type of temperament
   rather than a personality disorder?

Despite depressive personality's long and rich historical tradition, it has
only recently received empirical attention. Thus, there are many unanswered
questions about this disorder, many of which focus on nosological issues.
In particular, it has been suggested that depressive personality may be a
redundant concept, overlapping excessively with other personality
disorders—in particular, self-defeating, dependent, obsessive–compulsive,

and avoidant personality disorders. Others question whether depressive personality might overlap significantly with Axis I mood disorders, such as dysthymia; a related concern is that patients with chronic mood disorder might be misdiagnosed with a personality disorder and consequently might receive inadequate somatic treatment (although a personality disorder diagnosis should not rule out the use of medication). Another question is whether depressive personality refers to a relatively "normal" type of temperament, rather than a personality disorder with associated distress and impairment. For all of these reasons, the depressive personality remains a controversial entity in need of further empirical study.

## LITERATURE REVIEW

A Medline search of the psychiatric literature using such index terms as "dysthymia" and the combined terms "depression" and "personality" generated approximately 50 references. Historical references on depressive personality were also reviewed, and additional sources were obtained from their bibliographies. Ten researchers and advisors with an interest in depressive personality disorder (both advocates and individuals with a neutral stance) identified relevant historical or empirical sources, provided feedback on the disorder's descriptive features, and commented on its possible inclusion in DSM-IV. Finally, empirical work in progress was identified and included in the review.

### Diagnostic Instruments and Criteria Performance

Akiskal's (1989) recent modifications of his 1983 criteria for depressive personality (subaffective dysthymia), which were based on Schneider's (1923) description, are as follows:

> Indeterminate early onset (<21 years)
> Habitually long sleeper (>9 hours of sleep)
> Psychomotor inertia, which is typically worse in the morning
> At least five of the following traits:
>
> 1. Gloomy, pessimistic, humorless, or incapable of fun
> 2. Quiet, passive, and indecisive
> 3. Skeptical, hypercritical, or complaining
> 4. Brooding and given to worry
> 5. Conscientious or self-disciplining
> 6. Self-critical, self-reproaching, and self-derogatory
> 7. Preoccupied with inadequacy, failure, and negative events, to the point of morbid enjoyment of one's failures. (p. 223)

Several studies to date have shown that good interrater reliability can be achieved both for the number of depressive personality traits present

($r$ = .86) and for presence or absence of the diagnosis (kappa = .82; Klein, 1990; Klein, Clark, Dansky, & Margolis, 1988). Another study, using Schneider's description of depressive personality disorder (Standage, 1979), similarly found a high interrater reliability (kappa = .75) for the disorder's presence or absence. Akiskal's criteria also have acceptable internal consistency (alpha = .61 [Klein, 1990]; alpha = .73 [Klein & Miller 1993]) comparable to that of other DSM-III-R (American Psychiatric Association, 1987) personality disorders (Morey, 1988). In Klein's research, the one item that did not correlate highly with the others was conscientiousness.

Because assessment of Akiskal's and Schneider's criteria was not based on a structured interview, such an interview—the Diagnostic Interview for Depressive Personality Disorder—was recently developed (Gunderson, Phillips, Triebwasser, & Hirschfeld, 1994). This interview, which originally included all 32 putative depressive personality disorder traits mentioned in the literature, has good interrater reliability both for most individual traits and for the overall diagnosis (kappa = .62). Internal consistency is also high (alpha = .93). Hypochondriasis and conscientiousness, however, did not correlate highly with other items, and they have therefore been eliminated from the revised version of the instrument. On the basis of interviews with patients and normal controls, a cutoff score for the diagnosis that yields an acceptable sensitivity (89%) and specificity (83%) was determined. Factor analysis of the diagnostic interview, using the DSM-IV Mood Disorders Field Trial version of the Diagnostic Interview for Depressive Personality Disorder on a sample of 491 subjects, produced the following factors: negativistic, introverted/tense, passive/unassertive, and self-denying. Importantly, with few exceptions, depressive personality disorder traits as assessed by the interview do not appear to correlate significantly with Axis I depressive symptoms, as independently assessed with the 24-item Hamilton Rating Scale for Depression or the Structured Clinical Interview for DSM-III-R.

Klein (1990), using Akiskal's criteria, reported on the test–retest stability of the depressive personality disorder diagnosis over a 6 month interval; the number of depressive personality disorder traits rated as present in the initial and follow up evaluations correlated .43 ($p$ < .001). In addition, there was a 71% concordance on the presence or absence of the diagnosis (kappa = .41). Gunderson et al. reported a test–retest reliability on the Diagnostic Interview for Depressive Personality of .41 (kappa) after a follow-up interval of more than one year and with different raters at baseline and follow-up (Gunderson et al., 1994).

## Conceptual Distinction from Other Disorders

It has been suggested that depressive personality disorder may overlap conceptually with self-defeating (Kernberg, 1984), dependent (Kernberg, 1984), obsessive–compulsive (Schneider, 1923), and avoidant (Standage, 1986) personality disorders. Some of the conceptual similarities and differences between depressive personality disorder and other personality disorders, and between depressive personality disorder and dysthymia, are discussed below.

### Self-Defeating Personality Disorder

Kernberg (1987) has suggested that depressive and self-defeating personality disorders are closely related constructs, as reflected by his use of the term "depressive–masochistic personality." However, Simons (1986) has noted that patients with self-defeating personality disorder unconsciously torture and blackmail others, provoking retaliation, so that their "inner struggle is externalized and then acted out with the external world" (p. 594). In contrast, individuals with depressive personality disorder internalize their conflict, which leads to self-torture and self-defeat in the absence of provoked retaliation from others. Whereas individuals with self-defeating personality disorder actively reject opportunities for pleasure and have a negative reaction when positive events occur, those with depressive personality disorder simply find it difficult to get any enjoyment or pleasure out of such opportunities and events.

### Dependent Personality Disorder

Unlike the German phenomenologists, several psychoanalysts feature dependency in their description of depressive personality disorder (Kernberg, 1987; Kahn, 1975). Kernberg, however, believes that although these individuals are overly dependent on the approval of others, they are not overtly clinging and often appear counterdependent (Kernberg, 1990). As such, they tend to reject others before they can be rejected, to avoid feeling disappointed and frustrated when their dependency needs are not met.

### Obsessive–Compulsive Personality Disorder

Although "conscientious," "duty-bound," and "self-disciplining"—traits resembling obsessive–compulsive personality disorder—have been proposed to characterize depressive personality disorder (Schneider, 1923; Tellenbach, 1961; Laughlin, 1967; Kernberg, 1987; Akiskal, 1989; Simons, 1986), preliminary empirical evidence does not support the inclusion of these traits in the depressive personality disorder construct (Klein et al., 1988; Phillips et al., 1994). These disorders also differ conceptually in that individuals with obsessive–compulsive personality disorder are more constricted in their expression of affection and not necessarily persistently gloomy; they also adopt a controlling interpersonal style, whereas those with depressive personality disorder are often passive and unassertive (Kernberg, 1990).

### Avoidant Personality Disorder

Although it has been proposed that depressive personality disorder, like avoidant personality disorder, is characterized by shyness and introversion

(Schneider, 1923; Akiskal, 1989; Simons, 1986), individuals with depressive personality disorder are less reluctant to enter into relationships, and hence have more and better relationships with others (Kernberg, 1984). According to Kernberg, persons with depressive personality disorder have an enormous sense of personal responsibility and therefore attempt to relate well to others, which may result in good surface relations at the cost of tension and doubts about whether they deserve others' love and friendship (Kernberg, 1984). In addition, individuals with avoidant personality disorder are not necessarily chronically gloomy and unhappy.

## Borderline Personality Disorder

In borderline personality disorder, mood is unstable and perturbed by outbursts of anger, whereas anger tends to be unexpressed in depressive personality disorder. Relationships in borderline personality disorder are also often unstable, with alternation between extremes of idealized expectations and the perception of bitter betrayals, whereas in depressive personality disorder relationships are more stable and more consistently involve unexpressed negative thoughts about others (Kernberg, 1984). The severe identity disturbance marked by vacillation and extreme "badness" seen in borderline personality disorder is not characteristic of the stable low self-esteem seen in depressive personality disorder. Individuals with depressive personality disorder tend toward behavioral constriction and constraint, unlike the impulsiveness of those with borderline personality disorder (Kernberg, 1990).

## Passive–Aggressive Personality Disorder

The negativism of passive–aggressive personality disorder is often directed toward authority figures and expressed in response to demands. In contrast, individuals with depressive personality disorder have often been suggested to be compliant and particularly anxious to please authority figures (Laughlin, 1967). In addition, individuals with passive–aggressive personality disorder are not necessarily persistently gloomy and dysphoric.

The recent reconceptualization of passive–aggressive personality disorder, and the parenthetical addition of "negativistic" to its name (see Chapter 14), create possible overlap with depressive personality disorder because both now share the features of pessimism and criticism of others. The criticism expressed by those with passive–aggressive (negativistic) personality disorder, however, is preferentially directed at authority figures, whereas that expressed in depressive personality disorder is not. In addition, individuals with depressive personality disorder may be more likely to inhibit expression of critical, hostile, or aggressive thoughts or feelings, and to feel guilty and blame themselves rather than others. Moreover, their mood is generally gloomy and unhappy, rather than sullen, irritable, and angry.

*Dysthymia*

It has also been suggested that depressive personality disorder may overlap excessively with Axis I mood disorders—in particular, the primary, early-onset type of dysthymia (Kocsis, 1991). However, by definition, dysthymia is a mild, chronic form of mood disorder, not a personality disorder. Some more specific theoretical differences between depressive personality disorder and dysthymia include the following:

1. Depressive personality disorder by definition has an early onset (beginning by early adulthood), whereas dysthymia can begin at any age.
2. Depressive personality disorder is chronic and persistent, whereas dysthymia can remit.
3. Depressive personality disorder is characterized primarily by personality traits rather than symptoms.
4. Many depressive personality disorders traits are cognitive, intrapsychic, and interpersonal, in contrast to dysthymia's symptoms, which are largely somatic.

## Empirical Distinction from Other Disorders

Several researchers have investigated the overlap between depressive personality disorder and other psychiatric disorders—in particular, personality and mood disorders. In the earliest study, Standage (1986), using Schneider's concept of the depressive personality, reported on four patients with depressive personality disorder. One patient had a diagnosis of avoidant personality disorder, one had avoidant traits, and two had a diagnosis of mixed personality disorder.

In a study of 177 outpatients, Klein (1990) assessed overlap with DSM-III schizotypal and borderline personality disorders and mood disorders. Patients were assessed at baseline and 6 months later with an expanded version of the Schedule for Affective Disorders and Schizophrenia, the Family History Research Diagnostic Criteria interview, and Akiskal's criteria for depressive personality disorder. A significantly greater proportion of those patients with depressive personality disorder than of those without the disorder received a diagnosis of schizotypal personality disorder (23% vs. 7%), but the two groups did not differ significantly on rates of borderline personality disorder.

In a study of 54 subjects (Phillips et al., 1994), both depressive personality disorder and a full range of DSM-III-R Axis II disorders were assessed independently, using Gunderson et al.'s (1994) Diagnostic Interview for Depressive Personality Disorder and the Diagnostic Interview for Personality Disorders—Revised. Minimal to moderate overlap was found between depressive personality disorder and any particular Axis II disorder. Only 13% of subjects with depressive personality disorder also met criteria for a Cluster A disorder, with none meeting criteria for schizotypal personality disorder. Nineteen percent met criteria for at least one Cluster B disorder, with only 10% meeting criteria for borderline personality disorder. The overlap was highest with the "anxious cluster" disorders, with 48% of subjects with depressive personality disorder also meeting criteria for at least one Cluster C disorder: 29% met criteria for avoidant, 10% for dependent, 10% for passive–aggressive, and 13% for obsessive–compulsive personality disorder. Only 13% of subjects with depressive personality disorder also met criteria for self-defeating personality disorder. Thus, it appears that depressive personality disorder does not overlap significantly with—and is not completely subsumed by—any specific DSM-III-R Axis II disorder.

Regarding the overlap with Axis I dysthymia, Klein found that significantly more patients with than without depressive personality disorder also met criteria for DSM-III dysthymia, but the two disorders appeared to be distinct: In a clinical sample, only 30% met criteria for both depressive personality and dysthymia (kappa = .22; Klein, 1990), and in a nonclinical sample, only 19% met criteria for both depressive personality disorder and dysthymia (kappa = .25; Klein & Miller, 1993). Similarly, Phillips et al. (1992) found that in a clinical sample in which depressive personality disorder and dysthymia were blindly assessed, only 35% of subjects with depressive personality disorder also met criteria for DSM-III-R dysthymia, and only 16% met criteria for the primary early-onset type of dysthymia. Thus, depressive personality disorder and dysthymia appear to be distinct constructs.

Regarding the possible relationship of depressive personality disorder to other Axis I mood disorders, Klein et al. (1988) found that patients with depressive personality disorder had more severe depression and significantly more family members with bipolar disorder or hospitalization for mood disorder than patients without depressive personality disorder had. They had less severe depression and fewer relatives with unipolar depression than patients with dysthymia. Klein et al. (1988) also found a similar familial relationship between depressive personality disorder and major mood disorder in another study, in which depressive personality disorder was more common in offspring of patients hospitalized for major depression than in offspring of normal controls or patients hospitalized for medical disorders. Similarly, Wetzel, Cloninger, Hong, and Reich (1980) found that depressive personality traits were more likely than other traits to occur in relatives of patients with major depression. On the basis of these findings, Klein (1990) and Klein and Miller (1993) have concluded that although depressive personality disorder appears to be distinct from dysthymia, it may nonetheless be related to major mood disorder and dysthymia; it appears to be a less symptomatic, more trait-like variant of mood disorder than is dysthymia. This "spectrum relationship" posited for depressive personality disorder and major mood disorder is similar to that documented for schizotypal personality disorder and schizophrenia (Baron, Gruen, Asnis, & Kane, 1983; Gunderson & Siever, 1985).

Akiskal's work similarly suggests that depressive personality disorder can be differentiated from dysthymia. Yerevanian and Akiskal (1979) prospectively studied 150 outpatients with "characterological depression"—a mild, chronic depressive illness of early insidious onset that is similar to DSM's early-onset dysthymia. They found that early-onset dysthymia consisted of two subtypes—"depressive personality" and "character-spectrum disorder" (Akiskal et al., 1980; Akiskal, 1983). Patients with depressive personality (or "subaffective dysthymia") shared features with a unipolar depressed control group: shortened rapid-eye-movement (REM) latency; family history of unipolar or bipolar mood disorder; relatively normal developmental history; good social outcome; more frequent superimposed and melancholic major depressive episodes; and good response to antidepressant medications, lithium, and social skills training. In contrast, character-spectrum disorder (a heterogeneous mix of personality disorders—primarily histrionic and antisocial—with secondary dysphorias) was characterized by normal REM latency; family history of alcoholism and sociopathy, but not mood disorder; childhood parental loss, separation, or divorce; poor social outcome; nonmelancholic major depressive episodes; poor response to antidepressant medication; and polysubstance and alcohol abuse.

Hauri and Sateia (1984) replicated Akiskal's REM latency findings. Rhimer (1990) subsequently found that patients with depressive personality, but not character-spectrum disorder, had abnormal results on the dexamethasone suppression test and responded to sleep deprivation. Akiskal (1989) has concluded, like Klein, that depressive personality is a variant of classic mood disorder that is chronic, subsyndromal, and trait-like (rather than episodic, symptomatic, and state-like), all of which warrant its classification as a personality disorder. He has also concluded that, like major mood disorder, depressive personality disorder can improve with antidepressant medication, underscoring the fact that a personality disorder diagnosis should not rule out the use of medication. Finally, Akiskal (1989) believes that depressive personality disorder is a subset of early-onset dysthymia and that it differs from other forms of dysthymia, such as the late-onset type and the character-spectrum subtype of early-onset dysthymia.

The work cited above suggests that depressive personality disorder may be distinct from existing mood and personality disorders, and that it may be a trait-like, personality variant of Axis I mood disorders. Although, like all psychiatric disorders, it has some overlap with other diagnostic categories, that overlap appears to be incomplete. Further research is needed to confirm these findings, however.

## Is Depressive Personality Disorder a "Normal" Type of Temperament?

Several proponents of the depressive personality suggest that it may constitute a type of temperament—a relatively "normal," constitutionally based personality type—rather than a personality disorder with associated distress and impairment. Indeed, Tellenbach's "typus melancholicus," in particular, may be closer to a relatively normal temperament type that predisposes to major depressive episodes than to a personality disorder. However, preliminary data, based on the Global Adjustment Scale, indicate that depressive personality disorder may be associated with significant impairment in functioning (Klein & Miller, 1992), suggesting that it is a clinically significant entity. This question—temperament variant versus disorder—needs to be further addressed by future research.

This question also has implications for Kraepelin's (and subsequently, Akiskal's) other proposed temperament types—hyperthymic, cyclothymic, and irritable (Kraepelin, 1921; Akiskal, 1989). Do these personality types constitute disorders, with associated distress and impairment? Or are they relatively normal, nonpathological constitutional traits that may exist on a spectrum with, and perhaps predispose individuals to, the Axis I mood disorders?

## PLACEMENT IN DSM-IV

A major question faced by the Personality Disorders Work Group was whether depressive personality disorder should be included in DSM-IV. In support of its inclusion were its long historical tradition, advocacy by expert clinicians from diverse theoretical perspectives, and some empirical evidence. However, more data were and still are needed, especially data confirming its distinctiveness from other diagnoses (notably dysthymia and near-neighbor personality disorders).

The work group considered several options for the diagnosis: inclusion on Axis II; listing in the appendix of proposed diagnoses requiring further study; and omission from DSM-IV altogether. In light of the strong historical tradition and preliminary empirical evidence, the work group recommended inclusion in the appendix of proposed diagnoses; the disorder accordingly appears in Appendix B of the published DSM-IV (American Psychiatric Association, 1994). This action reflects the work group's belief that certain Axis II disorders may be on a spectrum with certain Axis I disorders—in other words, that certain personality disorders may be early-onset, enduring, trait-like variants of the more episodic and severely symptomatic Axis I disorders, and may share similar family history, treatment response, and perhaps etiology. Such a link has been demonstrated for schizophrenia and schizotypal personality disorder, and may also exist for Axis I mood disorders and depressive personality disorder, as suggested by Akiskal's and Klein's research. Some groups have expressed the concern that if depressive personality disorder is actually a type of dysthymia but is placed on Axis II, their patients may not receive adequate somatic treatment; however, this concern reflects the false assumption that personality disorders are devoid of biological underpinnings and should not be treated with medication. In fact, as suggested by the spectrum concept, certain personality disorders, including depressive personality disorder, are likely to be at least partly biological in origin and may warrant such treatment. Nonetheless, the work group had some concerns about including this disorder as a full-fledged member of Axis II in DSM-IV. First, delineation from other Axis II disorders and from dysthymia requires further confirmation. Second, the question of whether this personality type constitutes a personality disorder or a variant of normal personality needs to be addressed further. For these reasons, it was decided that depressive personality disorder should be included in an appendix as described above.

An alternative would have been to combine depressive personality disorder and Axis I dysthymia, as has occurred in ICD-10. Although depressive personality disorder was a separate disorder (a type of affective personality disorder) in ICD-9, it is subsumed under dysthymia in ICD-10 — a category that includes both affective symptoms (such as insomnia and poor concentration) and some of the personality traits characteristic of depressive personality disorder (pessimism, brooding, and feelings of inadequacy) (World Health Organization, 1978, 1992). Similarly, an alternative criterion B in Appendix B broadens the DSM-IV criteria for dysthymia to include several depressive personality disorder characteristics, such as pessimism, brooding, and feelings of inadequacy. However, at this time, empirical support for combining these disorders is limited; indeed, what evidence is available suggests that they are distinct but related disorders.

## DSM-IV CRITERIA FOR DEPRESSIVE PERSONALITY DISORDER

The research criteria for depressive personality disorder in DSM-IV represent characteristics commonly described in the clinical and empirical literature; these criteria are listed in Table 13.1, and the rationale for each is discussed briefly below. Because the symptoms of a major depressive episode may produce some of these features, it is important to ascertain that the features do not occur exclusively during major depressive episodes, as the exclusionary criterion in the DSM-IV list (criterion B) indicates. That is, they should not be symptoms (state-like), but rather an individual's personality characteristics (trait-like). Thus, they should be pervasive, of late adolescent or early adult onset, and persistent and stable rather than short-lived and episodic. They should also cause significant distress and/or impairment in functioning.

Criterion 1 in the DSM-IV list is as follows: "usual mood is characterized by dejection, gloominess, cheerlessness, joylessness, unhappiness." The rationale for this criterion is reasonably self-evident: The predominant mood of individuals with depressive personality disorder is dysphoric — in particular, gloomy and unhappy. Although the mood may fluctuate, it is fairly persistently negative and somber (Kraepelin, 1921; Schneider, 1923; Laughlin,

TABLE 13.1. DSM-IV Research Criteria for Depressive Personality Disorder

A. A pervasive pattern of depressive cognitions and behaviors beginning by early adulthood and present in a variety of contexts, as indicated by five (or more) of the following:
   (1) usual mood is dominated by dejection, gloominess, cheerlessness, joylessness, unhappiness
   (2) self-concept centers around beliefs of inadequacy, worthlessness, and low self-esteem
   (3) is critical, blaming, and derogatory toward self
   (4) is brooding and given to worry
   (5) is negativistic, critical, and judgmental toward others
   (6) is pessimistic
   (7) is prone to feeling guilty or remorseful

B. Does not occur exclusively during Major Depressive Episodes and is not better accounted for by Dysthymic Disorder.

*Note.* From APA (1994, p. 733). Copyright 1994 by the American Psychiatric Association. Reprinted by permission.

1967; Akiskal, 1989; Simons, 1986). These individuals are often overly serious, lack a sense of humor, and feel they do not deserve to have fun or be happy (Laughlin, 1967; Kernberg, 1990).

Criterion 2 is as follows: "self-concept centers around beliefs of inadequacy, worthlessness, and low self-esteem." This criterion is included because individuals with depressive personality disorder feel inferior and tend to doubt and undervalue their self-worth and abilities (Kraepelin, 1921; Schneider, 1923; Berliner, 1966; Kahn, 1975; Akiskal, 1989; Simons, 1986; Arieti & Bemporad, 1980).

Criterion 3 reads: "is critical, blaming, and derogatory toward self." The rationale for this criterion is that individuals with depressive personality disorder are harsh in their self-judgments, tending to be self-critical and disparaging of their accomplishments, performance, and conduct (Kraepelin, 1921; Tellenbach, 1961; Berliner, 1966; Laughlin, 1967; Kahn, 1975; Arieti & Bemporad, 1980; Simons, 1986; Akiskal, 1989).

Criterion 4, "is brooding and given to worry," is included in the DSM-IV list because individuals with depressive personality disorder tend to ruminate about and persistently dwell on negative and unhappy thoughts (Schneider, 1923; Laughlin, 1967; Simons, 1986; Akiskal, 1989). Similarly, criterion 5, "is negativistic, critical, and judgmental toward others," is included because individuals with depressive personality disorder tend to judge others as harshly as they judge themselves. They tend to see and expect the worst in others and focus on others' failings rather than on their positive attributes (Berliner, 1966; Kernberg, 1987; Akiskal, 1989; Simons 1986). Criterion 6, "is pessimistic," is included because individuals with depressive personality disorder tend to have negative expectations for the future, see life as futile, and anticipate the worst (Schneider, 1923; Laughlin, 1967; Akiskal, 1989; Simons, 1986).

Finally criterion 7 reads: "is prone to feeling guilty or remorseful." This criterion is included because individuals with depressive personality disorder have a tendency to feel remorseful about their behavior and excessively blame themselves for their failings (Kraepelin, 1921; Schneider, 1923; Tellenbach, 1961; Laughlin, 1967; Kahn, 1975; Berliner, 1966; Kernberg, 1987).

Other criteria, proposed by some clinicians and researchers, may in the future be added to those listed in Table 13.1 if they are supported by data from ongoing studies of depressive personality.

- "is quiet, introverted, passive, and unassertive" (Schneider, 1923; Berliner, 1966; Laughlin, 1967; Akiskal, 1989; Simons, 1986).
- The following may be added to criterion 5: "although such thoughts are often difficult to express and often kept to themselves" (Laughlin, 1967; Kernberg, 1987; Berliner, 1966; Kahn, 1975).

The empirical attention that depressive personality disorder is currently receiving reflects its rich historical and clinical tradition. Ongoing studies should resolve some of the controversies that surround it—whether it is a personality disorder or a "normal" type of temperament, whether it is distinct from existing mood and personality disorders or related to Axis I mood disorders, and how it may best be treated. Such data should also usefully inform this disorder's definition, conceptualization, and placement in future editions of DSM.

## REFERENCES

Akiskal, H. S., Rosenthal, T. L., Haykal, R. F., Lemmi, H., Rosenthal, R. H., & Scott-Straus, A. (1980). Characterological depressions: Clinical and sleep EEG findings separating "subaffective dysthymia" from "character spectrum disorder." *Archives of General Psychiatry, 37,* 777–783.

Akiskal, H. S. (1983). Dysthymic disorder: Psychopathology of proposed chronic depressive subtypes. *American Journal of Psychiatry, 140,* 11–20.

Akiskal, H. S. (1989). Validating affective personality types. In L. Robins & J. Barrett (Eds.), *The validity of psychiatric diagnosis.* New York: Raven Press.

Alloy, L. B., Abramson, L. Y., Metalsky, G. I., & Hartlage, S. (1988). The hopelessness theory of depression: Attributional aspects. *British Journal of Clinical Psychology, 27,* 5–21.

American Psychiatric Association. (1952). *Diagnostic and statistical manual of mental disorders* (1st ed.). Washington, DC: Mental Hospitals Service.

American Psychiatric Association. (1968). *Diagnostic and statistical manual of mental disorders* (2nd ed.). Washington, DC: Author.

American Psychiatric Association. (1980). *Diagnostic and statistical manual of mental disorders* (3rd ed.). Washington, DC: Author.

American Psychiatric Association. (1987). *Diagnostic and statistical manual of mental disorders* (3rd ed., rev.). Washington, DC: Author.

American Psychiatric Association. (1994). *Diagnostic and statistical manual of mental disorders* (4th ed.). Washington, DC: Author.

Arieti, S., & Bemporad, J. R. (1980). The psychological organization of depression. *American Journal of Psychiatry, 137,* 1360–1365.

Baron, M., Gruen, R., Asnis, L., & Kane, J. (1983). Familial relatedness of schizophrenia and schizotypal states. *American Journal of Psychiatry, 140,* 1437–1442.

Beck, A. T. (1967). *Depression: Causes and treatment.* Philadelphia: University of Pennsylvania Press.

Berliner, B. (1966). Psychodynamics of the depressive character. *Psychoanalysis Forum, 1,* 244–251.

Cooper, A. M., & Michels, R. (1981). Book review: American Psychiatric Association: *Diagnostic and statistical manual of mental disorders,* 3rd ed. *American Journal of Psychiatry, 138,* 128–129.

Goldstein, W. N., & Anthony, R. N. (1988). The diagnosis of depression and the DSMs. *American Journal of Psychotherapy, 42,* 180–196.

Gunderson, J. G., Phillips, K. A., Triebwasser, J. T., & Hirschfeld, R. M. A. (1994). Diagnostic Interview for Depressive Personality. *American Journal of Psychiatry, 151,* 1300–1304.

Gunderson, J. G., & Siever, L. (1985). Relatedness of schizotypal to schizophrenic disorders. *Schizophrenia Bulletin, 11,* 532–537.

Hauri, P., & Sateia, M. J. (1984). REM sleep in dysthymic disorders. *Sleep Research, 13,* 119.

Hirschfeld, R. M. A., Shea, M. T., & Phillips, K. A. (1992). Depressive personality disorder in DSM-IV. In *1992 CME syllabus and proceedings summary: American Psychiatric Association 145th Annual Meeting, Washington, D.C.* Washington, DC: American Psychiatric Association.

Kahn, E. (1975). The depressive character. *Folia Psychiatrica Neurologica Japonica, 29,* 291–303.

Kernberg, O. (1984). *Severe personality disorders: Psychotherapeutic strategies.* New Haven, CT: Yale University Press.

Kernberg, O. (1987). Clinical dimensions of masochism. In R. A. Glick & D. I. Meyers (Eds.), *Masochism: Current and psychotherapeutic contributions.* Hillsdale, NJ: Analytic Press.

Kernberg, O. (1990, May 16). *Differential diagnosis of the depressive–masochistic personality disorder.* Paper presented at the 143rd Annual Meeting of the American Psychiatric Association, New York.

Klein, D. N. (1990). Depressive personality: Reliability, validity, and relation to dysthymia. *Journal of Abnormal Psychology, 99,* 412–421.

Klein, D. N., Clark, D. C., Dansky, L., & Margolis, F. T. (1988). Dysthymia in the offspring of parents with primary unipolar affective disorder. *Journal of Abnormal Psychology, 97,* 265–274.

Kocsis, J. H. (1991). Resolved: Depressive personality is a useful construct that should be included in DSM-IV. In *1991 CME syllabus and proceedings summary: American Psychiatric Association 144th Annual Meeting, New Orleans.* Washington, DC: American Psychiatric Association.

Kraepelin, E. (1921). *Manic–depressive insanity and paranoia.* (R. M. Barclay, Trans.; G. M. Robertson, Ed.). Edinburgh: E, & S, Livingstone.

Kretschmer, E. (1925). *Physique and character* (W. J. H. Sprott, Trans.). New York: Harcourt, Brace.

Laughlin, H. P. (1967). *The neuroses.* Stoneham, MA: Butterworths.

Morey, L. C. (1988). The categorical representation of personality disorder: A cluster analysis of DSM-III-R personality features. *Journal of Abnormal Psychology, 97,* 314–321.

Phillips, K. A., Gunderson, J. G., Hirschfeld, R. M. A., & Smith, L. E. (1990). A review of the depressive personality. *American Journal of Psychiatry, 147,* 830–837.

Phillips, K. A., Gunderson, J. G., Kimball, C. R., Triebwasser, J., & Faedda, G. (1992). An empirical study of depressive personality. In *1992 CME syllabus and proceedings summary: American Psychiatric Association 145th Annual Meeting, Washington, D.C.* Washington, DC: American Psychiatric Association.

Rhimer, Z. (1990). Dysthymia: A clinician's perspective. In S. W. Burton & H. S. Akiskal (Eds.), *Dysthymic disorder.* London: Gaskell/Royal College of Psychiatrists.

Schneider, K. (1923). *Clinical psychopathology.* (M. W. Hamilton, Trans.). London: Grune & Stratton, 1959.

Simons, R. C. (1986). Psychoanalytic contributions to psychiatric nosology: Forms of masochistic behavior. *Journal of the American Psychoanalytic Association, 35,* 583–608.

Slater, E., & Roth, M. (1969). *Clinical psychiatry* (3rd ed.). Baltimore: Williams & Wilkins.

Smith, J. A., & Ross, W. D. (Eds.). (1908–1931). *The works of Aristotle.* Oxford: Clarendon Press.

Standage, K. F. (1979). The use of Schneider's typology for the diagnosis of personality disorders: An examination of reliability. *British Journal of Psychiatry, 135,* 238–242.

Standage, K. (1986). A clinical and psychometric investigation comparing Schneider's and the DSM-III typologies of personality disorders. *Comprehensive Psychiatry, 27,* 35–45.

Tellenbach, H. (1980). *Melancholy: History of the problem, endogeneity, typology, pathogenesis, clinical considerations* (E. Eng, Trans.). Pittsburgh: Duquesne University Press.

Wetzel, R. D., Cloninger, C. R., Hong, B., & Reich, T. (1980). Personality as a subclinical expression of the affective disorders. *Comprehensive Psychiatry, 21,* 197–205.

World Health Organization. (1978). *International classification of diseases* (9th revision). Geneva: Author.

World Health Organization. (1992). *The ICD-10 classification of mental and behavioural disorders: Diagnostic criteria for research.* Geneva: Author.

Yerevanian, B. I., & Akiskal, H. S. (1979). "Neurotic," characterological, and dysthymic depressions. *Psychiatric Clinics of North America, 2,* 595–617.

# Commentary on Depressive Personality Disorder: A False Start

PETER MCLEAN
SHEILA WOODY

When mental disorders are recognized, information on prevalence and the discovery of both mechanisms and effective treatments need not be far behind. Such has been the case, for example, with panic disorder. However, premature or inaccurate identification of a disorder can sponsor confusion. Phillips, Hirschfeld, Shea, and Gunderson have noted in Chapter 13 that limited recognition has been granted to depressive personality disorder in DSM-IV (American Psychiatric Association, 1994) by identifying it as a proposed diagnostic category needing further study. Two nosological issues are important in considering the merits of depressive personality disorder: categorical versus dimensional classification, and Axis I versus Axis II classification of the phenomenon of chronic, low-grade depressed mood. This commentary provides a critical appraisal of the diagnostic concept of depressive personality disorder through an examination of these nosological issues, and reviews the DSM-IV criteria. We conclude that the phenomenon of chronic depressed mood may best be conceptualized in a state–trait format, in which the state is characterized by major depression and the trait by chronic, low-grade depressed mood (dysthymia).

## RATIONALE FOR INCLUSION IN DSM-IV

Phillips et al. cite several reasons why depressive personality disorder was considered for inclusion in DSM-IV—historical descriptions and putative biogenetic influence. They start by noting the substantial historical tradition, in which writers over the ages have described a depressive character or temperament. Such accounts are difficult to interpret, because descriptions frequently fail to distinguish between observed and inferred data (Chodoff, 1973), with the result that symptoms and explanations are both presented as evidence for depressive personality disorder or depressive personality. Depressive personality disorder has never, up to now, been included in the DSM; Phillips et al. feel that this exclusion has been controversial and that sufficient empirical evidence is now available to justify its inclusion, at least in the "for further study" appendix. Regardless of whether chronic depression is an Axis I or II disorder, or whether this phenomenon is best described dimensionally rather than categorically, the measurement goals of validity and reliability still apply. A focus on these empirical goals will identify knowledge deficiencies and guide future studies.

Phillips et al. also suggest a possible biogenetic linkage between depressive personality disorder and Axis I mood disorders. This suggestion appears gratuitous, however, since unequivocal evidence of biogenetic influence is lacking, and since such evidence would not be conceptually decisive in making a case for depressive personality disorder. Klein, Clark, Dansky, and Margolis (1988) found that the offspring of unipolar depressed patients exhibited higher rates of affective disorder, major depression, and dysthymia relative to controls, but environmental influences were not taken into account. When the relative genetic and environmental contributions to individual differences in depressive symptoms have been studied more closely, heritability has been shown to be less influential than family rearing and unique life experiences (Gatz, Pederson, Plomin, Nesselroade, & McClearn, 1992).

## CHRONIC DEPRESSION:
## PERSONALITY VERSUS MOOD DISORDER

In reviewing the evidence that chronic depression represents a personality rather than a mood disorder, Phillips et al. state the issues as follows: What diagnostic instruments have been developed to assess depressive personality disorder, and how do they perform? Can depressive personality disorder be both conceptually and empirically distinguished from Axis I mood disorders and other personality disorders? Finally, is depressive personality a "normal" type of temperament rather than a personality disorder? We review these issues in turn.

### Diagnostic Instruments

Good interrater reliabilities for presence or absence of disorder (kappa = .68–.80) have been reported by Standage (1979) and both Klein et al. (1988) and Klein (1990), using Akiskal's (1983) criteria. Both Akiskal and Standage derived their criteria from Schneider's (1923) description of depressive personality disorder. Moderate test–retest stability for depressive personality disorder classification has been reported by Klein (1990) over a 6-month interval (kappa = .41). This is similar to Prusoff, Merikangas, and Weissman's (1988) finding for test–retest stability of depressive personality over a 3- to 6-year follow-up (kappa = .45). Interestingly, the test–retest reliability for major depressive episode over the same period was twice as high (kappa = .80). Gunderson, Phillips, and Triebwasser (1992) have taken diagnosis of depressive personality disorder a step further in the development of a structured interview for depressive personality disorder.

As we see, most of the evidence in support of depressive personality disorder derives from demonstrations of interrater reliability. Test–retest reliability has been variable and has been reported as lower for depressive personality disorder than for major depression (Prusoff et al., 1988). This is problematic, since depressive personality disorder by definition is a stable construct, whereas major depressive episode is a fluctuating phenomenon. The diagnostic criteria for depressive personality disorder have varied somewhat among investigators, and now DSM-IV has made significant changes in the criteria. Although there are no data available on diagnostic reliability for the DSM-IV research criteria, there is little reason to worry that the proposed criteria will prove less reliable than other criteria. The challenge will be to increase test–retest reliability and to establish validity.

## Conceptual and Empirical Distinction from Other Disorders

In Chapter 13, Phillips et al. reiterate their earlier position (Phillips, Gunderson, Hirschfeld, & Smith, 1990)—namely, that there is a need to clarify the relationship between depressive personality disorder and both Axis I depressive disorders and Axis II personality disorders. However, little progress appears to have been made. In terms of Axis II disorders, part of the problem is that these disorders suffer from overlap and inconsistency in diagnostic criteria. Such inconsistency seems unavoidable when incompatible theoretical orientations form the basis for Axis II disorder descriptions. Phillips et al., for example, cite phenomenologists, psychoanalysts, and a cognitive theorist in support for the construct of depressive personality disorder. Descriptors for inclusion–exclusion are variable, reflecting the poor conceptual distinction among disorders. Empirical evidence for distinction between depressive personality disorder and Axis II disorders is also equivocal. Klein (1990) and Standage (1986) both report high rates of comorbidity among Axis II disorders and depressive personality, indicating a moderate degree of shared variance. In a recent study using structured interviews to assess both depressive personality disorder and Axis II disorders, Phillips, Gunderson, Kimball, Treibwasser, and Faedda (1992) report a range of overlap between depressive personality disorder and Axis II disorders from 13% (Cluster A) to 48% (Cluster C), but they conclude that the overlap is not significant.

The major challenge to depressive personality disorder is to demonstrate

how it differs from dysthymia. Phillips et al. distinguish depressive personality disorder from dysthymia theoretically, on the basis of age of onset,
course, and modality of symptom expression. Depressive personality disorder, consistent with its being called a personality disorder, is thought to have
a late adolescent or early adult onset. However, according to DSM-III-R
(American Psychiatric Association, 1987), dysthymia usually begins in childhood, adolescence, or early adulthood. The course of depressive personality disorder is regarded as persistent and stable, whereas DSM-III-R describes
the course of dysthymia as chronic and allows for no more than 2 months'
freedom from symptoms in any 2-year period (for adults). These are thin
distinctions. Finally, criteria for diagnosis of dysthymia are based on somatic and affective symptoms, whereas Phillips et al. point out that depressive
personality disorder traits involve some cognitive, intrapsychic, and interpersonal traits, in addition to somatic and affective symptoms. Does this mean
that dysthymia is devoid of cognitive, intrapsychic, and interpersonal traits
of depression? Can somatic, cognitive, affective, intrapsychic, and interpersonal symptoms of dysthymia and depressive personality disorder be reliably distinguished? Furthermore, DSM-IV alternative criterion B for dysthymic
disorder (American Psychiatric Association, 1994, p. 718) includes interpersonal, behavior and cognitive symptoms, in addition to the standard somatic and affective symptoms, thus making dysthymic disorder (alternative
criterion B) and depressive personality disorder virtually redundant. A number of empirical studies have shown overlap between depressive personality disorder and dysthymia diagnoses (Akiskal et al., 1980; Klein, 1990; Phillips
et al., 1992), and there is broad agreement that these two constructs are in-
adequately separated. It is noteworthy that in the move from the 9th to 10th
revisions of the *International Classification of Diseases* (World Health Organization, 1978, 1992), depressive personality has been combined with dysthymia.

## Depressive Personality: "Normal" Type of Temperament or Personality Disorder?

In the classification of cognitive, emotional, and behavioral expression of
mental functioning, there has been enduring controversy over the merits
of categorical as opposed to dimensional approaches (Kendall, 1975; Lorr,
1986). In categorical classification systems, discontinuity and qualitative
differences are assumed, whereas in dimensional classification systems, distinctions between people are assumed to be quantitative and normally distributed on a linear continuum (Moras & Barlow, 1992). Phillips et al.
recognize the possibility that depressive personality disorder may represent
a more intense form of "normal" temperament, but have opted for an Axis
II categorical representation in which depressive personality disorder is related to, but distinct from, dysthymia. DSM-IV has required a more rigorous
standard of evidence and documentation than its predecessors (Frances,

Widiger, & Pincus, 1989)—an empirical process that leads inevitably to a dimensional consideration of psychopathology (Barlow, 1992). Within the dimensional model, broader issues of chronic, low-grade depression become easier to evaluate, because more contextual information is available when a dimensional system is used. These broader issues include the relationship between chronic mild depression and the constructs of affective instability, temporal stability of personality structure, behavioral and cognitive manifestations of depressed mood, and appropriate thresholds along the normal–abnormal continuum.

Phillips et al. acknowledge the possibility that depressive personality disorder may represent the pathological end of a depressive temperament dimension, and call for further research to address this possibility. Consideration of depressive personality disorder as a variant of normal temperament is incomplete, however, without reference to the major work on temperament within the personality research literature. What is the relationship between depressive personality and (1) the neurotocism factor of the "Big Five" dimensions of personality (Goldberg, 1980); (2) Eysencks's (1986) neuroticism factor, which identifies nine subordinate trait terms (anxious, depressed, emotional, tense, moody, shy, irrational, low self-esteem, guilt feelings); or (3) the dimension of negative affect identified by Watson and Clark (1984)? Researchers of widely diverging theoretical persuasions almost universally accept neuroticism as one of the basic dimensions of personality (John, 1990). Given the relatively high overlap between depressive personality disorder and Cluster C diagnoses (Phillips et al., 1992), it is unclear whether or not the construct of depressive personality disorder (or indeed dysthymia) is simply a clinical representation of neuroticism.

## DSM-IV PROPOSED CRITERIA
## FOR DEPRESSIVE PERSONALITY DISORDER

Phillips and her colleagues describe the criteria for depressive personality disorder that have been included in DSM-IV Appendix B. These criteria are similar to Akiskal's (1983) criteria for depressive personality. Specifically, Akiskal's requirements for psychomotor inertia and excessive sleep have been dropped, and the requirements of significant distress and/or impairment of functioning as the result of symptoms have been added. Moreover, depressive personality disorder must not occur exclusively during episodes of major depression. Finally, the list of seven traits (five required by Akiskal) has been modified. The trait "conscientious or self-disciplining" has been omitted, and there are new trait descriptors involving cognitive (e.g., beliefs), intrapsychic, and interpersonal (e.g., critical attitude toward others) domains. As in Akiskal's list, at least five of the seven traits must be positive for diagnostic determination. These refinements to Akiskal's (1983) criteria, particularly the requirements for occurrence at times other than major depressive episodes and for evidence of distress and/or impairment in functioning, should improve performance in reliability checks. However, there is no reason to expect better separation from dysthymia than has been achieved previously. Again, it is noteworthy that DSM-IV alternative criterion B for dysthymic disorder (American Psychiatric Association, 1994, p. 718), compared to DSM-IV criteria for dysthmic disorder (p. 349), almost eclipses the new criterion for depressive personality disorder. It remains likely that the DSM-III-R dysthymia criteria, with emphasis on somatic symptoms, and the DSM-IV criteria for depressive personality disorder, with emphasis on trait-like symptoms reflecting cognitive, affective, and intrapsychic phenomenon, are assessing different facets of the same thing—dysthymia.

## OUTSTANDING ISSUES

Three outstanding issues raised by this review of Phillips et al.'s chapter have led us to the conclusion that the concept of depressive personality disorder represents a false start. First, the concept of depressive personality disorder has been developed in isolation from the large and rich empirical literature in personality. Nosological arguments aside, the constructs of chronic problems hypothesized to be related to personality need to be developed in the context of the wide empirical literature on personality. Neuroticism consistently emerges in personality research as a basic dimension of personality. How does the temperament dimension of depressive personality differ? A number of investigators (e.g., Costa & McCrae, 1990; Wiggins & Pincus, 1992) have demonstrated that the five-factor model of personality envelops both normal and abnormal dimensions of personality, leaving open the possibility that depressive personality disorder may represent the abnormal expression of a normal personality dimension. Furthermore, depressive symptoms have been shown to predict future psychiatric disorders over a period of up to 16 years in a continuous, graded-risk fashion, presumably because they represent a normal personality dimension of vulnerability akin to neuroticism (Zonderman, Herbst, Schmidt, Costa, & McCrae, 1993).

Second, there is a serious need for longitudinal data on affective variation in both general-population and clinical samples. Little information is available on the frequency, duration, intensity, and quality of affective variation and dysregulation within nonclinical samples over the course of a day, week, or month. It is apparent that affective instability is the issue, and that single "snapshots" to assess symptoms or traits against disorder criteria may not be the best method of informing us about depressive personality and its relationship to neuroticism. Longitudinal data involving cognitive, behavioral, affective, and symptomatic expressions of the key descriptors of depressive personality, dysthymia, and neuroticism would be most useful. Recent efforts are promising: the "longitudinal, expert, all data" (LEAD) standard (Spitzer, 1983; Pilkonis, Heape, Ruddy, & Serrao, 1991) to develop validity consensus, and the use of prototypical exemplars to assess behavioral manifestations of personality (Livesley & Schroeder, 1990). These and similar methods should be applied to any proposed Axis II construct.

Finally, the questionable distinction between depressive personality disorder and dysthymia remains problematic. We suggest that a state–trait configuration, with major depressive episode representing the state and dysthymia representing the trait, would be an alternate way of viewing the relationship between episodic and characterological expression of depression. In this case, dysthymia represents the pathological end of the normal dimension of depressive personality or neuroticism. We believe that such a classification would generate a more productive line of inquiry than would modifying the DSM-IV research criteria for depressive personality disorder.

## REFERENCES

Akiskal, H. S. (1983). Dysthymic disorder: Psychopathology of proposed chronic depressive subtypes. *American Journal of Psychiatry, 140,* 11–20.

Akiskal, H. S., Rosenthal, T. L., Haykal, R. F., Lemmi, H., Rosenthal, R. H., & Scott-Straus, A. (1980). Characterological depression: Clinical and sleep EEG findings separating "subaffective dysthymia" from "character spectrum disorder." *Archives of General Psychiatry, 37,* 777–783.

American Psychiatric Association. (1987). *Diagnostic and statistical manual of mental disorders* (3rd ed., rev.). Washington, DC: Author.

American Psychiatric Association. (1994). *Diagnostic and statistical manual of mental disorders* (4th ed.). Washington, DC: Author.

Barlow, D. H. (1992). Diagnosis, DSM-IV, and dimensional approaches. In A. Ehlers, W. Fiegenbaum, I. Florin, & J. Margraf (Eds.), *Perspectives and promises of clinical psychology* (pp. 13–21). New York: Plenum Press.

Chodoff, P. (1973). The depressive personality: A critical review. *International Journal of Psychiatry, 11*(2), 196–217.

Costa, P. T., & McCrae, R. R. (1990). Personality disorders and the five-factor model of personality. *Journal of Personality Disorders, 4*(4), 362–371.

Eysenck, H. J. (1986). Models and paradigms in personality research. In A. Angleitner, A. Furnham, & G. Van Heck (Eds.), *Personality psychology in Europe: Vol. 2. Current trends and controversies* (pp. 213–232). Lisse, The Netherlands: Swets & Zeitlinger.

Frances, A., Widiger, T., & Pincus, A. (1989). The development of DSM-IV. *Archives of General Psychiatry, 46,* 373–375.

Gatz, M., Pederson, N. W., Plomin, R., Nesselroade, J. R., & McClearn, G. E. (1992). Importance of shared genes and shared environments for symptoms of depression in older adults. *Journal of Abnormal Psychology, 101,* 701–708.

Goldberg, L. R. (1980). *Some ruminations about the structure of individual differences: Developing a common lexicon for the major characteristics of human personality.* Paper presented at the annual convention of the Western Psychological Association, Honolulu.

Gunderson, J. G., Phillips, K. A., & Triebwasser, J. T. (1992). Diagnostic Interview for Depressive Personality Disorder. In *1992 CME syllabus and proceedings sum-*

*mary: American Psychiatric Association 145th Annual Meeting, Washington, D.C.* Washington, DC: American Psychiatric Association.

John, O. P. (1990). The search for basic dimensions of personality. In P. McReynolds, J. C. Rosen, & G. J. Chelune (Eds.), *Advances in psychological assessment* (pp. 1–37). New York: Plenum Press.

Kendall, R. E. (1975). *The role of diagnosis in psychiatry.* Oxford, England: Blackwell Scientific.

Klein, D. N. (1990). Depressive personality: Reliability, validity, and relation to dysthymia. *Journal of Abnormal Psychology, 99,* 412–421.

Klein, D. N., Clark, D. C., Dansky, L., & Margolis, E. T. (1988). Dysthymia and the offspring of parents with primary unipolar affective disorder. *Journal of Abnormal Psychology, 97,* 265–274.

Livesley, W. J., & Schroeder, M. L. (1990). Dimensions of personality disorder: The DSM-III-R Cluster A diagnoses. *Journal of Nervous and Mental Disease, 178*(10), 627–635.

Lorr, M. (1986). Classifying psychotics: Dimensional and categorical approaches. In T. Millon & G. L. Klerman (Eds.), *Contemporary directions in psychopathology: Toward the DSM-IV* (pp. 331–345). New York: Guilford Press.

Moras, K., & Barlow, D. H. (1992). Dimensional approaches to diagnosis and the problem of anxiety and depression. In A. Ehlers, W. Fiegenbaum, I. Florin, & J. Margraf (Eds.), *Perspectives and promises of clinical psychology* (pp. 23–37). New York: Plenum Press.

Phillips, K. A., Gunderson, J. G., Hirschfeld, R. M. A., & Smith, L. E. (1990). A review of the depressive personality. *American Journal of Psychiatry, 147,* 830–837.

Phillips, K. A., Gunderson, J. G., Kimball, C. R., Triebwasser, J,. & Faedda, G. (1992). An empirical study of depressive personality. In *1992 CME syllabus and proceedings summary: American Psychiatric Association 145th Annual Meeting, Washington, D.C.* Washington, DC: American Psychiatric Assocation.

Pilkonis, P. A., Heape, C. L., Ruddy, J., & Serrao, P. (1991). Validity in the diagnosis of personality disorders: The use of the LEAD standard. *Psychological Assessment: A Journal of Consulting and Clinical Psychology, 3*(1), 46–54.

Prusoff, B., Merikangas, K., & Weissman, M. (1988). Lifetime prevalence and age of onset of psychiatric disorders: Recall 4 years later. *Psychiatry Research, 22,* 107–117.

Schneider, K. (1923). *Clinical psychopathology* (M. W. Hamilton, Trans.). London: Grune & Stratton, 1959.

Spitzer, R. L. (1983). Psychiatric diagnosis: Are clinicians still necessary? *Comprehensive Psychiatry, 24,* 399–411.

Standage, K. (1979). The use of Schneider's typology for the diagnosis of personality disorders: An examination of reliability. *British Journal of Psychiatry, 135,* 238–242.

Standage, K. (1986). A clinical and psychometric investigation comparing Schneider's and the DSM-III typologies of personality disorders. *Comprehensive Psychiatry, 27,* 35–45.

Watson, D., & Clark, L. A. (1984). Negative affectivity: The disposition to experience aversive emotional states. *Psychological Bulletin, 96,* 465–490.

Wiggins, J. S., & Pincus, A. L. (1992). Personality: Structure and assessment. *Annual Review of Psychology, 43,* 473–504.

World Health Organization. (1978). *International classification of diseases* (9th revision). Geneva: Author.

World Health Organization. (1992). *The ICD-10 classification of mental and behavioral disorders: Diagnostic criteria for research.* Geneva: Author.

Zonderman, A. B., Herbst, J. H., Schmidt, C. Jr., Costa, P. T. Jr., & McCrae, R. R. (1993). Depressive symptoms as a nonspecific, graded risk for psychiatric diagnoses. *Journal of Abnormal Psychology, 102*(4), 544–552.

# CHAPTER 14

# Passive–Aggressive (Negativistic) Personality Disorder

THEODORE MILLON
JELENA RADOVANOV

With the exception of the two new "appended" personality disorders in DSM-III-R (American Psychiatric Association [APA], 1987), passive–aggressive personality disorder was one of two or three of DSM-III's (American Psychiatric Association, 1980) original group of Axis II disorders that elicited considerable discussion at Personality Disorders Work Group meetings and within the post-DSM-III critical literature. As noted below, questions were raised concerning the very legitimacy of passive–aggressive as a personality disorder, and several group members and consultants wondered whether an expansion of its rather narrow range of diagnostic criteria to that of a more broadbased "negativistic personality disorder" would enhance its viability in this regard (Frances & Widiger, 1987; Millon, 1981).

The descriptive features that characterize the disorder have been portrayed in considerable detail by numerous distinguished clinicians for close to a century under a variety of designations. Its most recent revival, termed the "passive–aggressive personality trait disturbance" in DSM-I (American Psychiatric Association, 1952), represented the manner in which the disorder was expressed in the armed forces during World War II. However, numerous early theorists portrayed diversely labeled "dispositions" and "characters" whose features included those of passive–aggressive personality disorder, but parallel more closely the broadly formulated outline for the newly reconceptualized passive–aggressive (negativistic) personality disorder.

Six major etiological perspectives have emerged in regarded to the pas-

An earlier version of this chapter was published in the *Journal of Personality Disorders*, 1993, 7, 78–85. Copyright 1993 by The Guilford Press. Adapted by permission.

sive–aggressive personality: the psychoanalytical/dynamic, behavioral, cognitive, interpersonal, social learning, and biological models.

Stricker and Gold (1988) describe the psychodynamic approach as focusing on the infantile and childhood experiences, in order to build an understanding of the developmental history of the individual's maladaptive behaviors and current dysfunction. They emphasize the adequacy of the individual's ego functions, inter- and intrapsychic conflict, and level of psychosexual development, as well as the cohesiveness and consistency of the individual's sense of self. According to their continuum approach to the personality disorders (measured by the severity of dysfunction in the above-mentioned areas), Sticker and Gold consider passive–aggressive personality to fall in the midrange of personality disorders, between neurotic and psychotic.

Karl Abraham (1924) refined Freud's psychosexual stages by breaking the oral stage down into distinct biting and sucking stages (Millon, 1981). Abraham claimed that an individual could become fixated at either stage. Widiger, Frances, Spitzer, and Williams (1988) have described the passive–aggressive individual as being fixated in Abraham's oral-biting stage and thus exhibiting an "oral-sadistic" character. The features of this character include a combination of envy, hostility, jealousy, and ambivalence toward others. Basing his observations on Abraham's concept, Menninger (1940) portrayed these personalities as "inclined to blame the world for everything unpleasant that happens to them ... [to be] cantankerous, contemptuous, petulant—inclined to find everything wrong ... [to be] emotionally soured [and] perpetually discontented" (p. 394). Reich (1933) described a personality in which the individual is prone to complaining, obstruction of the goals of others, followed by overwhelming unconscious guilt (Kernberg, 1984). Reich referred to the passive–aggressive approach of such individuals as an "infantile spite reaction" (Millon, 1981).

Within the behavioral school, the argument about personality and traits is waged most heavily. There is clear division as to what constitutes personality (Turner & Turkat, 1988). Perry and Flannery (1982) view passive–aggressive behavior as a maladaptive "expression of anger in social interactions." According to McCann (1988), these individuals either have failed to learn appropriate assertive behaviors, experience inhibition of assertive reactions because of excessive anxiety, or anticipate punishment for assertive behavior.

Cognitive theorists examine the individual's belief system and thought schemas to uncover the basis for the personality disorder. According to Murray (1988), the cognitive approach views personality as a complex information-processing system, in which the individual receives information from the environment and assigns meaning to this input. Murray suggests that each personality has a "core rubric" consisting of beliefs about the self and life in general, and conclusions based on these beliefs. A core rubric for the passive–aggressive personality might contain the following assumptions: (1) I am misunderstood and unappreciated; (2) Life is treacherous and full of people who will take advantage of you; (3) Therefore, it is better not to put yourself out for people because you will end up getting hurt.

Beck and colleagues' (Beck, Freeman, & Associates, 1990) cognitive theory on the passive–aggressive personality is very similar to the core rubrics described by Murray. Beck et al. state that the individual's affective response stems from his or her uncontrolled automatic thoughts. These thoughts in turn arise from basic assumptions about the world and self that each person carries. A passive–aggressive individual may feel depressed because he or she thinks that "no one ever gives me credit for the things I do." This thought may arise from a more unconscious assumption that "things always go wrong" or from an assumption that "people should always show me respect if they like me." According to the cognitive approach, the behavioral, interpersonal, and affective components of the personality disorder result from unrealistic or faulty cognitions.

According to the interpersonal perspective, personality disorders reflect a pathological pattern of interpersonal relationships (Endler & Edwards, 1988; Widiger & Frances, 1985). Wiggins (1982) and Kiesler (1986) propose that personality should be conceived as falling along an interpersonal circumplex with two defining dimensions: affiliation (agreeable vs. quarrelsome) and power (dominant vs. submissive). Kiesler describes the passive–aggressive as being individual "lazy–submissive" and "quarrelsome and aloof" in his or her relationships with others.

Social learning theory classifies personality along three dimensions: self–other, pain–pleasure, and active–passive (Millon, 1990). According to Millon, the passive–aggressive individual is best described as "active–ambivalent," meaning that the individual is conflicted between self-gratification and the need to please others. The active dimension arises from the individual's active attempts to manipulate his or her environment in order to achieve maximum gratification. According to McCann (1988), this personality pattern results from contradictory parental attitudes during childhood. As a child, the individual receives mixed messages from the environment, and learns that the world is unpredictable and that he or she must remain wary. The individual longs for affection, but feels that affection is given erratically and may be withdrawn unexpectedly.

The psychobiological approach to personality is a very old model, dating back at least to the time of Hippocrates. Several biological theories include physiological and genetic factors in their descriptions of the personality makeup of the passive–aggressive individual. Kraepelin (1913), Bleuler (1924), Aschaffenburg (1922), Hellpach (1920), and Schneider (1923) all speculated on the constitutional contributions to personality and described individuals who today would probably be diagnosed as passive–aggressives (McCann, 1988; Millon, 1981). For example, Kraepelin (1913) wrote about individuals with constitutions that incline them to "take all things hard and feel the unpleasantness in every occurrence," as well as to "show an extraordinary fluctuating emotional equilibrium . . . often in an unpleasant way." Bleuler (1924) spoke of these personalities as being "irritable of mood," and Aschaffenburg (1922) described them as "dissatisfied personalities who go through life as if they were perpetually wounded." Hellpach (1920) depicted them as "fussy people of sour disposition," and Schneider (1923), referring to them as "ill-tempered depressives," characterized them as nagging, spiteful, and malicious, tending to be "doggedly pessimistic and rejoice when things go wrong."

Siever and Davis (1991) have proposed a model of personality that incorporates biological factors such as cognitive and perceptual organization, impulsivity and aggression controls, and anxiety and inhibition physiological control. McCann (1988) and Klar, Siever, and Coccaro (1988) speculate that there may exist biochemical factors that predispose an individual toward being more moody or irritable. Millon (1981) reported that a large number of "difficult to manage" infants become passive–aggressives as adults, indicating that some early-onset factor (perhaps genetic or constitutional) may be involved in this personality disorder.

## STATEMENT OF ISSUES

From the literature (both past and recent), as well as Personality Disorders Work Group discussions and consultants' missives, there appeared to be five main issues or questions that needed to be answered for DSM-IV (American Psychiatric Association, 1994).

1. Should the prototypical traits selected to represent the DSM-III-R passive–aggressive category's essential feature be modified to include aspects of a more broadly conceived negativistic personality disorder?

2. Despite its problematic character, do prevalence data for DSM-III or DSM-III-R passive–aggressive personality disorder give evidence that a broadened concept of this personality disorder would achieve an adequate prevalence level or diagnostic usage?

3. Can DSM-III or DSM-III-R passive–aggressive personality disorder be differentiated from personality disorders with which it has important traits in common?

4. On the basis of the DSM-III and DSM-III-R formulations, do the clinical features of passive–aggressive personality disorder demonstrate acceptable levels of diagnostic reliability, internal consistency, and external validity?

5. Can DSM-III-R passive–aggressive personality disorder be expanded to comprise a more full-range personality disorder on the basis of the historic clinical literature, which suggests additional and diverse trait criteria?

## SIGNIFICANCE OF THE ISSUES

"Passive–aggressive personality disorder" was first introduced into the nomenclature in a U.S. War Department technical bulletin in 1945, to describe military personnel who expressed their opposition to authority figures in an indirect, "subverting" manner, rather than openly and directly. The term was carried over into both the U.S. Joint Armed Services and Standard Veterans Administration classification systems shortly thereafter, and included as part of DSM-I in 1952. Although recognized in that manual as but one of several subtypes of aggressive expression, it has not been accepted internationally (e.g., it has never been included in the *International Classification of Diseases*); it was reluctantly included in both DSM-II (American Psychiatric Association, 1968) and DSM-III (American Psychiatric Association, 1980) because of its narrow scope as a personality disorder, and DSM-III included the stipulation that its diagnosis not be made in conjunction with any other personality disorder (the only personality disorder restricted in this manner); it has achieved minimal clinical usage (a meager case history or theoretical literature); and it has prompted a very small body of empirical studies. In several critical reviews of the DSM system (Kernberg, 1984; Zimmerman, 1988), passive–aggressive personality disorder has been noted as among those DSM-III-R categories least supportable for inclusion in DSM-IV (see, in particular, Blashfield, Sprock, & Fuller, 1990).

Although the form of expression (indirect or passive hostility) is undoubtedly a feature of this personality style, it is usually but one of several covariant features—a number of which were well described in the pre-World War II literature where oppositional and negativistic expression included cognitive, interpersonal, self-image-related, and affective, as well as behavioral, characteristics.

The main issue, confronted by the Personality Disorders Work Group therefore, was whether a more comprehensive formulation—that of "negativistic personality disorder," inclusive of multiple criterion domains (a defining feature of any personality disorder)—would achieve greater acceptance by the profession, prove to be more clinically useful, and stimulate greater empirical research than its more narrowly focused DSM-III-R passive–aggressive forerunner.

## LITERATURE REVIEW

Dialogue Information Services provided Medline and other less medically oriented computer searches of the 1978–1990 literature, and were guided by terms such as "passive–aggressive personality," "oppositional behavior," "negativism," "aggression," and the like. References prior to that period were also drawn upon, owing to the fact that the disorder has forerunners in the clinical literature going back to the 1920s. The literature specific to the label "passive–aggressive personality disorder," however, is quite sparse. Empirical studies associated with DSM-III and DSM-III-R formulations do include passive–aggressive personality disorder, but rarely as a primary focus; where it is found, it is included, for the most part, simply as a member of the Axis II group. A total of 17 articles and chapters were located that contained more than just a passing reference to the designation.

Comments from advisors and consultants also were not extensive. A coordinated body of diagnostic criteria and comorbidity data for all the personality disorders, including the passive–aggressive personality disorder, was supplied by numerous investigators (Blashfield, 1988; Dahl, 1986; First & Spitzer, 1989; Freiman & Widiger, 1989; Millon & Tringone, 1989; Morey & Heumann, 1988; Pfohl & Blum, 1990; Skodol, 1989; Zanarini, 1989).

## Traits Selected for the Essential Feature

As briefly noted in prior pages, clinical theorists of an earlier period Kraepelin, Abraham, Bleuler, Schneider) described "character types" similar to passive–aggressive personality disorder that predated the official World War II designation; their conceptions, however, encompassed a wider range of clinical features than the singular element of resistance to external demands. More contemporary researchers seeking to identify a core or essential set of features have found a similar, but again, a wider range of elements to typify and be central to the construct. Small, Small, Alig, and Moore (1970) found those categorized as having passive–aggressive personality disorder to be notable for the "stormy nature of their personal relationships." Whitman, Trosman, and Koenig (1954) observed earlier that among the distinctive features of this personality disorder was the "conflict between . . . dependency needs and guilt feelings," resulting in "pseudoaggression" and "fears of external retaliation." Although Livesley, Reiffer, Sheldon, and West (1987) reported that "resistance to demands of adequate performance" was central to the disorder, they also found features such as stubbornness and procrastination. To Kiesler (1986), the core element of the passive–aggressive construct is the combination of quarrelsomeness and submissiveness. Work group members and advisors suggested additional characterizing features, such as "sullen affect and deliberate rudeness," "resentfully argumentative and irritable," and "feelings of victimization." Given the work group's desire to broaden the characterization of this disorder, the following phrase was proposed as the essential feature description of negativistic personality disorder in its September 1991 deliberations: "A pervasive patter of argumentativeness, oppositional behavior, and negative and defeatist attitudes." In DSM-IV as published (American Psychiatric Association, 1994), the essential feature of passive–aggressive (negativistic) personality disorder is described as follows: "A pervasive pattern of negativistic attitudes and passive resistance to demands for adequate performance" (p. 734).

## Data Pertaining to Prevalence Level and Diagnostic Usage

A truly representative epidemiological study has yet to be carried out on the DSM personality disorders (Weissman, 1990). Nevertheless, as summarized in a series of studies reported to the work group, passive–aggressive personality disorder prevalences ranged from .00 to .52 (Widiger, 1991). This lack of consensus may reflect a lack of uniform standards and methodologies (inclusion of "second" and "third" diagnoses, etc.). In studies with larger numbers of subjects, the clinical usage rate ranges from .02 to .08. In those cases in which a secondary, co-occurrent personality disorder was assigned, the frequency of passive–aggressive personality disorder secondary diagnosis was roughly 10% (Millon & Tringone, 1989). Despite questions concerning its adequacy as conceived in DSM-III and DSM-III-R, clinicians appear to use the diagnosis. It would appear reasonable, therefore, to assume that a more comprehensive formulation, such as that for the newly reconceptualized passive–aggressive (negativistic) personality disorder, would prove at least equally useful and discriminating.

## Differentiation from Other Personality Disorders

Diagnostic overlap statistics do not indicate an unusual pattern of comorbidities for DSM-III or DSM-III-R passive–aggressive personality disorder—a fact that may reflect the DSM-III proscription for codiagnosing this disorder. At best, there is a weak indication of a correspondence between passive–aggressive and borderline personality disorders (perhaps reflecting the shared ambivalence about many matters in these disorders), as well as a more unexpected covariance with narcissistic personality disorder (Morey & Heumann, 1988). Among the studies with larger $n$'s (Millon & Tringone, 1989), there are minor correspondences between passive–aggressive personality disorder and self-defeating and sadistic personality disorders, suggesting that the passive–aggressive personality disorder "dynamic" is composed of both timorous and hostile qualities. With the advent of the broadened construct and the more diverse set of traits of passive–aggressive (negativistic) personality disorder, both the disorder's prevalence and its pattern of comorbidity may shift. This is one of the reasons why the work group decided that the new construct should be placed in DSM-IV's Appendix B rather than in the manual's main text (see below).

## Clinical Features: Diagnostic Reliability, Internal Consistency, and External Validity

Rather poor reliability statistics have been found for passive–aggressive personality disorder. Kappas for the DSM-III criteria set were especially unimpressive. This reflected, in part, the fact that the disorder was characterized by essentially one trait; in general, reliability figures are usually poor for constructs composed of a small item pool. As of this writing, the work group has not been able to develop reliability statistics on either DSM-III-R passive–aggressive personality disorder or the broadened DSM-IV passive–aggressive (negativistic) personality disorder; the self-report DSM-II Passive–Aggressive Personality Disorder Scale, associated with the DSM-III-R formulation and aspects of the negativistic pattern, does show an improvement over its pre-DSM-III version (Millon, 1987). Perhaps this signifies that a more comprehensive set for this disorder's criteria will lead to improved reliability.

Large unpublished studies carried out by work group members and consultants (e.g., Freiman & Widiger, 1989; Millon & Tringone, 1989; Morey & Heumann, 1988) have furnished data (sensitivity, specificity, positive and negative predictive value, and phi coefficients) on each of the DSM-III-R passive–aggressive personality disorder criteria. (Additional studies concerning the expanded criteria for DSM-IV underway, but incomplete.) A brief review of the DSM-III-R data is in order. In general, the various studies show somewhat similar results, although the magnitude of validity numbers was appreciably higher in some projects than in others. These data indicate relatively weak discriminability among passive–aggressive personality disorder criteria; they overlapped appreciably with antisocial and somewhat less with narcissistic criteria scores. Strong criteria overlap was seen in some studies with paranoid personality disorder and (where included) with DSM-III-R sadistic personality disorder. Finally, the internal consistency statistics for passive–aggressive personality disorder may be spuriously high. This may reflect the fact that many DSM-III-R passive–aggressive criteria say the same thing, or something close to the same thing; for example, criterion 1 ("procrastination . . . ") and criterion 3 ("seems to work deliberately slowly . . . ") may be indistinguishable. So, too, may criterion 2 ("becomes sulky . . . when asked to do something he or she does not want to do"), criterion 4 ("protests . . . that others make unreasonable demands on him or her") and criterion 7 "resents useful suggestions from others . . . ").

## Can Passive–Aggressive Personality Disorder Be Expanded to Comprise a More Full-Range Disorder?

A major "issue" raised by several Personality Disorders Work Group consultants related to whether passive–aggressive personality disorder is a "true" personality disorder, or whether it is merely a single trait—essentially that of a defense mechanism whose presence is based on a psychodynamic inference (Perry & Flannery, 1982). Indeed, some consultants and group members wondered whether it should exist at all as a personality disorder in DSM-IV. It has never achieved acceptance in Europe, as noted earlier. Moreover, perhaps the scarcity of literature on the disorder indicates a lack of both clinical and research interest; if so, some asked, should it be deleted from the Axis II list (Blashfield, Sprock, & Fuller, 1990)?

On the other hand, might these "difficulties" have arisen from the manner in which the disorder has previously been formulated, both before and after DSM-III? Viewed differently, might there not be a more valid and clinically useful diagnostic entity here (more in line with what Kraepelin, Abraham, Bleuler, Schneider, and Menninger described) than that which World War II military psychiatrists fashioned in highly restrictive terms? And if the work group were to enlarge the scope of this diagnostic entity's "criteria" to include a multiple-domain set of character traits, might not both clinical usage and research literature grow?

Although the DSM-III-R criterion set was improved over that of DSM-III, many group members and consultants felt that it might be further enhanced if a wider range of trait domains were tapped than currently, such as several of the following, derived from a number of diverse sources (e.g., Kraepelin, Schneider, Reich, Horney, Millon, Cameron, Shapiro, et al.):

Frequently irritable and erratically moody
A tendency to report being easily frustrated and angry
Discontented self-image, as expressed in feeling misunderstood and unappreciated by others
Characteristically pessimistic, disgruntled, and disillusioned with life
Interpersonal ambivalence, as seen in a struggle between acting dependently acquiescent and being assertively independent
The use of unpredictable and sulking behaviors to provoke discomfort in others
Sullen discontent and perennial complaining
Anguished and discontented with themselves, but never satisfied with others either

Dissatisfaction with the passive–aggressive designation itself has been raised, both in the literature and in work group deliberations. To explore a more broadened, "civilian", and neutral nomenclature for this disorder, a number of authors have suggested alternative designations. We quote from one review of these alternatives (Frances & Widiger, 1987):

1. "Passive–aggressive personality disorder" emphasizes the ambivalent coexistence of dependence and oppositionalism, but it has the problems of etiological connotation and previous misuse in military settings.

2. "Oppositional personality disorder" provides continuity with the section on childhood disorders and is interpersonally descriptive, but has an excessively narrow connotation that captures only the interpersonal aspect of the syndrome.

3. "Negativistic personality disorder" is appealingly broad and clearly descriptive and it captures both interpersonal and intrapsychic aspects of behavior, but [it] is a new term without tradition. . . . This term does suggest less about underlying dynamics than the term "passive–aggressive," and opens a broader scope for the introduction of new and appropriate criteria. (p. 284)

## CHANGES PROPOSED FOR AND MADE IN DSM-IV

It was the view of the Personality Disorders Work Group that there were grounds for maintaining the key criteria from DSM-III-R. However, many of these are highly specific and essentially redundant, and it was felt that they should be collapsed into a few general trait descriptors. On the other hand, the scope of the DSM-III-R criteria appears narrowly restricted to the label's origins in military settings. A decision was made to enlarge the scope to encompass nondynamic behavioral, cognitive, and affective features that the historic clinical literature indicates often coexist in syndromal form with the passive–aggressive element.

Two options were discussed. The first and more conservative stance would be to retain, but refine, the DSM-III-R criteria for passive–aggressive personality disorder. The second option, the one favored by the work group, was to introduce a new category to replace or supplement passive–aggressive personality disorder. This new personality disorder would encompass a broader range of oppositional trait features, in line with the clinical literature, and would be placed in an Appendix so as to permit clinicians and researchers to evaluate its utility and efficiency. The passive–aggressive element would continue as one significant component. However, the new designation would permit the introduction of new criteria of a more cognitive and affective character—clinical features that may coexist in syndromal form with the core passive–aggressive behaviors, but accord better with the established pre-World War II literature.

The following criteria comprised the list initially developed by the work group and its advisors and consultants:

1. passively resists fulfilling routine social and occupational tasks (e.g., behaviorally procrastinates, is inefficient)
2. complains of being victimized, misunderstood, and unappreciated by those with whom he or she lives and works
3. is sullen, irritable, and argumentative, especially in reaction to the wishes or expectations of others, and communicates a pervasive mix of angry and pessimistic attitudes toward numerous and diverse events (e.g., cynically notes the potentially troublesome aspects of situations that are going well)
4. unreasonably criticizes and scorns authority
5. expresses envy and resentment toward those apparently more fortunate
6. claims to be luckless, ill-starred, and jinxed in life; personal discontent is more a matter of whining and grumbling than of feeling forlorn or despairing
7. alternates between hostile assertions of personal autonomy and independence, and acting contrite and dependent

TABLE 14.1. DSM-III-R Diagnostic Criteria for Passive–Aggressive Personality Disorder, and DSM-IV Research Criteria for Passive–Aggressive (Negativistic) Personality Disorder

| DSM-III-R criteria | DSM-IV criteria |
|---|---|
| A pervasive pattern of passive resistance to demands for adequate social and occupational performance, beginning by early adulthood and present in a variety of contexts, as indicated by at least *five* of the following: | A. A pervasive pattern of negativistic attitudes and passive resistance to demands for adequate performance, beginning by early adulthood and present in a variety of contexts, as indicated by four (or more) of the following: |
| (1) procrastinates, i.e., puts off things that need to be done so that deadlines are not met | (1) passively resists fulfilling routine social and occupational tasks |
| (2) becomes sulky, irritable, or argumentative when asked to do something he or she does not want to do | (2) complains of being misunderstood and unappreciated by others |
| (3) seems to work deliberately slowly or to do a bad job on tasks that he or she really does not want to do | (3) is sullen and argumentative |
| (4) protests, without justification, that others make unreasonable demands on him or her | (4) unreasonably criticizes and scorns authority |
| (5) avoids obligations by claiming to have "forgotten" | (5) expresses envy and resentment toward those apparently more fortunate |
| (6) believes that he or she is doing a much better job than others think he or she is doing | (6) voices exaggerated and persistent complaints of personal misfortune |
| (7) resents useful suggestions from others concerning how he or she could be more productive | (7) alternates between hostile defiance and contrition |
| (8) obstructs the efforts of others by failing to do his or her share of the work | |
| (9) unreasonably criticizes or scorns people in positions of authority | |
| | B. Does not occur exclusively during Major Depressive Episodes and is not better accounted for by Dysthymic Disorder. |

*Note.* From APA (1987, pp. 357–358) and APA (1994, pp. 734–735). Copyright 1987 and 1994 by the American Psychiatric Association. Reprinted by permission.

The work group originally felt that such a reformulation might accord better with the designation of "negativistic personality disorder," which would also provide a behaviorally less overt and indirectly expressed adult variant of the child/adolescent oppositional defiant disorder. In DSM-IV as published, however, the old nomenclature was not abolished. The reformulated disorder is now referred to as "passive–aggressive personality disorder (negativistic personality)"; it has been called "passive–aggressive (negativistic) personality disorder" here for the sake of brevity.

In other respects, however, the work group's second option has been implemented in the published manual more or less as it was proposed. Table 14.1 presents the DSM-IV research criteria for passive–aggressive (negativistic) personality disorder (with the DSM-III-R criteria for passive–aggressive personality disorder alongside for purposes of comparison); it can be seen that the published criteria are briefer than the proposed ones but do not differ from them in any important way. Furthermore, as suggested by the work group, the new disorder has been placed in DSM-IV's Appendix B to indicate that it awaits further study. The features of the disorder are described in greater detail in the accompanying text in Appendix B (American Psychiatric Association, 1994, pp. 733–734).

## REFERENCES

Abraham, K. (1924). The influence of oral eroticism on character formation. In K. Abraham, *Selected papers on psychoanalysis.* London: Hogarth Press, 1927.

American Psychiatric Association. (1952). *Diagnostic and statistical manual of mental disorders* (1st ed.). Washington, DC: Mental Hospitals Service.

American Psychiatric Association. (1968). *Diagnostic and statistical manual of mental disorders* (2nd ed.). Washington, DC: Author.

American Psychiatric Association. (1980). *Diagnostic and statistical manual of mental disorders* (3rd ed.). Washington, DC: Author.

American Psychiatric Association. (1987). *Diagnostic and statistical manual of mental disorders* (3rd ed., rev.). Washington, DC: Author.

American Psychiatric Association. (1994). *Diagnostic and statistical manual of mental disorders* (4th ed.). Washington, DC: Author.

Aschaffenburg, G. (1922). Constitutional psychopathies. In *Handbook of medical practice* (Vol. 4). Leipzig: Barth.

Beck, A. T., Freeman, A., & Associates. (1990). *Cognitive therapy of personality disorders.* New York: Guilford Press.

Blashfield, R. (1988). [Similarity matrix for personality disorders]. Unpublished raw data.

Blashfield, R., Sprock, J., & Fuller, A. (1990). Suggested guidelines for including/excluding categories in the DSM-IV. *Comprehensive Psychiatry, 31,* 15–19.

Bleuler, E. (1924). *Textbook of psychiatry* (A. A. Brill, Trans.). New York: MacMillan.

Dahl, A. A. (1986). Some aspects of the DSM-III personality disorders illustrated by a consecutive sample of hospitalized patients. *Acta Psychiatrica Scandinavica, 73*(Suppl. 328), 61–67.

Endler, N. S., & Edwards, J.M. (1988). Personality disorders from an interactional perspective. *Journal of Personality Disorders, 2,* 326–333.

First, M., & Spitzer, R. (1989). [Diagnostic efficiency statistics]. Unpublished raw data.

Frances, A., & Widiger, T. (1987). A critical review of four DSM-III personality disorders. In G. Tischer (Ed.), *Diagnosis and classification in psychiatry.* New York: Cambridge University Press.

Freiman, K., & Widiger, T. (1989). [Co-occurrence and diagnostic efficiency statistics]. Unpublished raw data.

Hellpach, W. (1920). Amphithymia. *Zeitschrift fuer die Gesamte Neurologice und Psychiatrie, 52,* 136–152.

Kernberg, O. F. (1984). *Severe personality disorders: Psychotherapeutic strategies.* New Haven, CT: Yale University Press.

Kiesler, D. J. (1986). The 1982 interpersonal circle: An analysis of DSM-III personality disorder. In T. Millon, & G. L, Klerman (Eds.), *Contemporary directions in psychopathology: Toward the DSM-IV.* New York: Guilford Press.

Klar, H., Siever, L. J., & Coccaro, E. (1988). Psychobiologic approaches to personality and its disorders: An overview. *Journal of Personality Disorders, 2,* 334–341.

Kraepelin, E. (1913). *Psychiatrie: Ein Lehrbuch* (8th ed., Vol. 3). Leipzig: Barth.

Livesley, W. J., Reiffer, L. I., Sheldon, A. E., & West, M. (1987). Prototypicality ratings of DSM-III criteria for personality disorders. *Journal of Nervous and Mental Disease, 175,* 395–401.

McCann, J. T. (1988). Passive–aggressive personality disorder: A review. *Journal of Personality Disorders, 2,* 170–179.

Menninger, K. (1940). Character disorders. In J. E. Brown (Ed.), *The psychodynamics of abnormal behavior.* New York: McGraw-Hill.

Millon, T. (1981). *Disorders of personality: DSM-III, Axis II.* New York: Wiley–Interscience.

Millon, T. (1987). *Millon Clinical Multiaxial Inventory-II Manual (MCMI-II).* Minneapolis: National Computer Systems.

Millon, T. (1990). *Toward a new personology: An evolutionary model.* New York: Wiley.

Millon, T., & Tringone, R. (1989). [Co-occurrence and diagnostic efficiency statistics]. Unpublished raw data.

Morey, L., & Heumann, K. (1988). [Co-occurrence and diagnostic efficiency statistics]. Unpublished raw data.

Murray, E. J. (1988). Personality disorders: A cognitive view. *Journal of Personality Disorders, 2,* 37–43.

Perry, J. C., & Flannery, R. B. (1982). Passive–aggressive personality disorder: Treatment implications of a clinical typology. *Journal of Nervous and Mental Disease, 170,* 164–173.

Pfohl, B., & Blum, N. (1990). [Internal consistency statistics for the DSM-III-R personality disorder criteria]. Unpublished raw data.

Reich, W. (1933). *Charakter analyse.* Leipzig: Sexpol Verlag.

Schneider, K. (1923). *Psychopathic personalities.* London: Cassell, 1950.

Siever, L. J., & Davis, K. L. (1991). A psychobiological perspective on the personality disorders. *American Journal of Psychiatry, 148,* 1647–1658.

Skodol, A. (1989). [Co-occurrence and diagnostic efficiency statistics]. Unpublished raw data.

Small, I. F., Small, J. G., Alig, V. B., & Moore, D. F. (1970). Passive–aggressive personality disorder: A search for a syndrome. *American Journal of Psychiatry, 126,* 97–107.

Stricker, G., & Gold, J. R. (1988). A psychodynamic approach to the personality disorders. *Journal of Personality Disorders, 2,* 350–359.

Turner, S. M., & Turkat, I. D. (1988). Behavior therapy and the personality disorders. *Journal of Personality Disorders, 2,* 342–349.

Weissman, N. M. (1990). *The epidemiology of personality disorder: A 1990 update.* Paper presented at the Conference on the Personality Disorders, Williamsburg, VA.

Whitman, R. M., Trosman, H., & Koenig, R. (1954). Clinical assessment of passive–aggressive personality. *Archives of Neurology and Psychiatry, 72,* 540–549.

Widiger, T. A. (1991). DSM-IV reviews of the personality disorders: Introduction to special series. *Journal of Personality Disorders, 5,* 136–148.

Widiger, T. A., & Frances, A. (1985). The DSM-III personality disorders: Perspectives from psychology. *Archives of General Psychiatry, 42,* 615–623.

Widiger, T. A., Frances, A., Spitzer, R. L., & Williams, J. B. W. (1988). The DSM-III-R personality disorders: An overview. *American Journal of Psychiatry, 145,* 786–795.

Wiggins, J. S. (1982). Circumplex models of interpersonal behavior in clinical psychology. In P. C. Kendall & J. N. Butcher (Eds.), *Handbook of research methods in clinical psychology.* New York: Plenum Press.

Zanarini, M. (1989). [Co-occurrence and diagnostic efficiency statistics]. Unpublished raw data.

Zimmerman, M. (1988). Why are we rushing to publish DSM-IV? *Archives of General Psychiatry, 45,* 1135–1138.

# Commentary on Passive–Aggressive (Negativistic) Personality Disorder

ELIZABETH BAERG

In their chapter, Millon and Radovanov review the issues that have led to the reconceptualization of DSM-III-R's (American Psychiatric Association, 1987) passive–aggressive personality disorder as the more global passive–aggressive (negativistic) personality disorder, which addresses a broader spectrum of oppositional expression, in DSM-IV (American Psychiatric Association, 1994). They believe that the changes made in DSM-IV will more accurately reflect clinical reality and stimulate research interest. This commentary reviews some problems associated with the DSM-III-R passive–aggressive personality disorder diagnosis, and suggests that these problems remain unresolved by subsuming the construct under a new diagnostic category. In addition to a discussion about diagnostic continuity between adult and childhood disorders, potential problems with the discriminant validity of passive–aggressive (negativistic) personality disorder are addressed.

The rich historical tradition of the passive–aggressive construct suggests that it may provide important clinical information, but there are still many questions about its contribution to current understanding of personality problems. Like the other categories of personality disorder, DSM-III-R passive–aggressive personality disorder was found to intercorrelate with all other Axis II diagnoses when both dimensional and categorical, and both interview and self-report, assessment instruments were used (Widiger et al., 1990). Unlike the other diagnostic categories, this commonly co-occurring diagnosis did not show a specific pattern of intercorrelations. This finding has led the authors to suggest that passive–aggressive behavior may be better understood as a situational response than as a specific personality style or trait. They refer to the experience of powerlessness, which may commonly provoke a predictable set of behaviors during a psychiatric hospitalization. It is also possible that some modified form of the construct may be identified as a behavioral dimension of personality pathology (Schroeder & Livesley, 1991).

Both DSM-III-R passive–aggressive and DSM-IV passive–aggressive (negativistic) personality disorders assume a motivational component that is central to the construct definition. Specific behavioral responses can be readily identified, but the motive is difficult to operationalize. This problem will continue to plague the DSM-IV disorder, which operationalizes the motive using complex criteria such as "alternates between hostile defiance and contrition" (American Psychiatric Association, 1994, p. 735).

As with its precursor, poor discriminant validity between diagnostic measures of passive aggressive (negativistic) personality disorder and other personality disorders can be expected. In particular, this reformulated personality disorder shares many criteria with the new depressive personality disorder. Attempts to differentiate the two have addressed the quality of unhappy mood and the underlying motivation of the shared negativistic, critical, and pessimistic criteria. Phillips, Hirschfeld, Shea, and Gunderson (Chapter 13, this volume) describe persons with depressive personality disorder as compliant and anxious to please authorities, and thereby as being "negativistic, critical, and judgmental toward others" (American Psychiatric Association, 1994, p. 733) in a more inhibited manner than patients with passive–aggressive (negativistic) personality disorder, who express these qualities through passive resistance. Differentiation between the two disorders on the basis of quality of mood is equally subtle. Phillips et al. suggest in Chapter 13 that patients with passive–aggressive (negativistic) personality disorder will not necessarily be persistently gloomy and dysphoric, although the criteria (e.g., "is sullen . . . ," "expresses envy and resentment . . . ," "voices exaggerated . . . complaints of personal misfortune"; (American Psychiatric Association, 1994, p. 735) contribute to face validity that could easily include unhappiness.

Millon and Radovanov suggest in Chapter 14 that passive–aggressive (negativistic) personality disorder describes a less overt adult variant of the child and adolescent oppositional defiant disorder. Although it is worthwhile to consider the continuum of childhood disorders such as oppositional defiant disorder with passive–aggressive (negativistic) personality disorder in adults, these data are not yet available. There has been a considerable evolution of the concept of oppositional defiant disorder over the years. Rey (1993) notes that the disorder now describes "a pattern of angry, aggressive, negativistic comportment" rather than the previous "opposition to authority figures." He suggests that the inclusion of an angry and physically aggressive construct, which is supported by factor-analytic studies, makes the as-yet-unsubstantiated link between passive–aggressive personality disorder and oppositional defiant disorder even less likely to be established. If oppositional defiant disorder lies on a physically aggressive dimension with conduct disorder, an analysis of child-to-adult continuity will need to examine the more closely related antisocial personality disorder.

In this commentary, I have taken the position that the solution to the conceptual and psychometric problems of the passive–aggressive construct does not lie in simply reformulating the construct. The new passive–aggressive (negativistic) personality disorder, although it addresses a broader spectrum of behavior, will probably continue to exhibit the problems of its precursor and add little new information to our understanding of personality pathology.

## ACKNOWLEDGMENT

I wish to thank Marsha Schroeder, PhD, for her helpful comments.

## REFERENCES

American Psychiatric Association. (1987). *Diagnostic and statistical manual of mental disorders* (3rd ed., rev.). Washington, DC: Author.

American Psychiatric Association. (1994). *Diagnostic and statistical manual of mental disorders* (4th ed.). Washington, DC: Author.

Rey, J. M. (1993). Oppositional defiant disorder. *American Journal of Psychiatry, 150,* 1769–1778.

Schroeder, M., & Livesley, W. J. (1991). An evaluation of DSM-III-R personality disorders. *Acta Psychiatrica Scandinavica, 84,* 512–519.

Widiger, T. A., Frances, A. J., Harris, M., Jacobsberg, L. B., Fyer, M., & Manning, D. (1990). Comorbidity among Axis II disorders. In J. M. Oldham (Ed.), *Personality disorders: New perspectives on diagnostic validity.* Washington, DC: American Psychiatric Press.

CHAPTER 15

# Sadistic Personality Disorder

SUSAN J. FIESTER
MARTHA GAY

"Sadism" is a term originally used by Krafft-Ebing (1898) to describe the desire to inflict pain upon the sexual object. He also coined the term "masochism" for the desire to have pain inflicted by the sexual object. Freud (1905, 1915, & 1924) further elaborated the concept as an element of male aggressiveness, or a desire to subjugate contained in the biological underpinnings of male sexuality. Freud described two aspects of sadism—one characterized by an active or violent attitude toward the sexual object, and the other characterized by sexual satisfaction that is completely conditional on the humiliation and maltreatment of the sexual object (sexual sadism).

As a concept, sadism has continued to be more prominent in the psychoanalytic literature than within other theoretical frameworks. Numerous other psychoanalysts subsequently expanded and modified Freud's hypotheses, but they basically adhered to the original concepts of the interrelationship of sadism and masochism and the instinctual basis of both (Brenner, 1959; Eissler, 1958; Gero, 1962; Reik, 1941).

As the object relations school of psychoanalysis developed, the concept of sadism shifted from a focus on its instinctual basis to a focus on environmental and interpersonal factors. From this perspective, sadomasochism was conceptualized as a type of object relationship that defends against frank object loss (Avery, 1977; Bieber, 1966; Fromm, 1973; Nydes, 1963; Parker, 1973). The dynamics of sadomasochism are felt to be centered around the struggle to intimidate a potentially deserting partner into believing that the loss of the object will cause him or her significant pain. With the development of self psychology, there was a further evolution of the concept of sadism, based in the dynamics of narcissistic personality disturbance (Kohut,

An earlier version of this chapter was published in the *Journal of Personality Disorders*, 1991, 5, 376–385. Copyright 1991 by The Guilford Press. Adapted by permission.

1971, 1972). Within this framework, the development of the "self" concept is adversely affected by inadequate empathic responses (mirroring) on the part of the mother, leading to a failure to idealize this "selfobject" and failure to form an adequate ego ideal. This results in a failure of internal regulation of self-esteem, which leads to dependence on external objects for a sense of wholeness.

In addition to the existence of several different theoretical frameworks for the concept of sadism, there has also been considerable controversy about which developmental stage is involved in the development of sadistic defenses or personality styles. Some have emphasized Oedipal problems, whereas others have emphasized pre-Oedipal problems or the predominance of developmental periods (e.g., the phallic) as being key. Still others have implicated several different developmental stages as being involved.

Another theoretical controversy centers around whether sadism is a unitary phenomenon or whether more generalized sadistic behavior and sexual sadism are distinct entities, as originally posited by Freud. Several studies (Breslow, 1987; Gosselin & Wilson, 1980; Spengler, 1977) have indicated that sexual sadomasochists generally limit sadistic and masochistic behavior to the sexual domain and rarely engage in more general sadistic behaviors with their partners. There have been no studies to date of personality styles among sexual sadists. However, one study of spouse abusers found three distinctive "personality types" among this violence-prone population (Hamberger & Hastings, 1988).

## HISTORY OF SADISTIC PERSONALITY DISORDER

During the development of DSM-III-R (American Psychiatric Association, 1987), sadistic personality disorder was suggested for inclusion by several psychiatrists who felt that there was a clinical need for a category to describe persons (usually seen in forensic settings) who demonstrated a long-standing maladaptive pattern of cruel, demeaning, and aggressive behavior toward others, but whose personality disturbance did not fit any other DSM-III-R diagnosis. They saw this disorder as distinct from the other personality disorders, including antisocial personality disorder. As a result of discussions with the Advisory Committee on Personality Disorders, eight criteria were subsequently developed along with an exclusion criterion. These criteria were subsequently approved for inclusion in Appendix A of DSM-III-R, entitled "Proposed Diagnostic Categories Needing Further Study." There was substantial controversy about this diagnostic category. The major controversies surrounding the disorder are outlined here, followed by a critical review and summary of data on prevalence, sex bias, comorbidity, differential diagnosis, clinical phenomenology, treatment, and course and prognosis relevant to resolving these controversies.

# SIGNIFICANT ISSUES

The major issues confronted by the Personality Disorders Work Group in debating whether or not to include sadistic personality disorder in DSM-IV. (American Psychiatric Association, 1994) were as follows:

1. What is the prevalence of sadistic personality disorder, and does the diagnostic category have clinical utility?

2. What phenomena (background, functioning, prognosis) are associated with sadistic personality disorder?

3. Is sadistic personality disorder a discrete entity distinguishable from other existing personality disorder diagnoses, or is there significant overlap of this disorder with other Axis II categories?

4. Do the sadistic personality disorder diagnosis and criteria have good performance characteristics (internal consistency)?

5. Does the sadistic personality disorder diagnostic category have good reliability, and is it supported by external validators?

6. Are there problems in applying the sadistic personality disorder criteria? For example, is a high degree of inference required to determine the presence or absence of criteria?

7. Is there sex bias in diagnositc criteria set for the sadistic personality disorder or in the application of the criteria?

8. Will the inclusion of sadistic personality disorder potentially result in harmful consequences for any particular populations?

9. Do data addressing these questions support the continued inclusion of sadistic personality disorder in the diagnostic nomenclature?

# LITERATURE REVIEW

The literature reviewed for sadistic personality disorder covered published articles, chapters, and books on sadism or sadistic personality disorder. Other than for conceptual, theoretical, or historical purposes, all sources that did not involve empirical data were excluded (e.g., case studies). The sources of data were identified through a computer search of English-language journal articles published from 1960 to 1991. Information was also solicited from researchers who had data sets with relevant data on sadistic personality disorder, including unpublished articles and reports. Finally, input was solicited from a wide range of advisors with varied theoretical, clinical, and research backgrounds.

## Prevalence and Clinical Utility

Several studies have examined the prevalence of sadistic personality disorder. Gay (1989) reported on a sample of 235 adults accused of child abuse referred by the juvenile court system for psychiatric evaluation of fitness to be custodial parents. Twelve (5%) met criteria for a diagnosis of sadistic personality disorder. Freiman and Widiger (1989), in a study using the Personality Interview Questionnaire-II, found that 18% of a sample of 50 inpatients (primarily male) in a public psychiatric hospital were diagnosed as having sadistic personality disorder. Millon and Tringone (1989), in a study using an outpatient sample from a wide variety of settings, found that 3% met criteria for sadistic personality disorder. We and our colleagues (Spitzer, Fiester, Gay, & Pfohl, 1991) in a survey that approximately 2.5% of all cases evaluated by forensic psychiatrists over the previous year met criteria for sadistic personality disorder. One recent study using the Personality Disorders Examination found a high prevalence rate (33%) in a group of 21 sex offenders (pedophiles and rapists), most of whom were in prison (Berger, 1991). Thus, three of five studies found a relatively low prevalence (2.5%–5%) of the disorder, and two other studies found much higher prevalence rates (18%–33%). It should be noted that the highest prevalence was in a very specialized forensic population, where the disorder might be expected to be much more prevalent than in the general population.

Several factors may account in part for the low prevalence rates. Discussions with consultants and advisors (particularly those in the forensic field) generally indicated that it may at times be difficult to determine the presence of sadistic personality disorder criteria, as a person must admit to a wide variety of socially unacceptable behaviors—for instance, cruel and aggressive behavior, lying, and frightening and intimidating others. In addition, the disorder may be relatively rare in general-practice settings, as individuals with sadistic personality disorder do not often voluntarily seek treatment.

Regarding the utility of this diagnostic category, only 19% of psychiatrists in our survey (Spitzer et al., 1991) indicated that the diagnosis was "not useful for any particular purpose." Respondents felt that the diagnosis was useful for the following purposes: 75% "for describing the individual's pattern of behavior; 64% "for predicting the individual's likely future pattern of behavior; 61% "for use in providing the court with information that will be relevant in sentencing"; 55% "for making treatment or management decisions, and 51% "for evaluating a parent's fitness for custody" (p. 877). Only 11% noted "for use as a psychiatric defense in mitigating responsibility for a crime" (p. 877). Thus, a majority of the respondents who had at some time evaluated individuals with the diagnosis of sadistic personality disorder believed that it has value in both clinical and forensic settings.

## Phenomenological Studies

There are few descriptive data except for those from a study by Gay (1989, in press; Gay & Fiester, 1991) and from our survey (Spitzer et al., 1991). In the Gay (1989) study, 75% of the subjects with sadistic personality disorder had a history of physical abuse during childhood; 42% reported a history of significant emotional abuse; 16% had experienced early childhood sexual abuse; and 8% reported a history of significant neglect. There was also a very high frequency of loss of parental figure by death during childhood or adolescence (25%) or significant childhood losses (75%). We (Spitzer et al., 1991) also found a high prevalence of childhood abuse and loss (90% emotional abuse, 76% physical abuse, 52% multiple losses, and 41% sexual abuse).

Gay (1989) found that subjects with sadistic personality disorder were surprisingly high-functioning, with 66% having steady employment and few having other legal problems. In addition, they tended to have intense, long-lasting attachments to their chosen partners, which were extremely difficult to break. Subjects with sadistic personality disorder also demonstrated considerable remorse and sadness about the separations and losses precipitated by their violence. The range of their abusive behaviors included verbally demeaning the other, making threats to kill the victim, and actually beating and killing. Abuse of the spouse in addition to the children was frequent (75%), as was abuse toward others outside the immediate family.

Gay also found that there was a very poor prognosis in most cases of sadistic personality disorder, with children being returned to their homes in only two cases (17%) where there had been no recurrence of the child abuse. In both these cases, the person was provided with in-house modeling of appropriate parenting skills. Gay also found that persons with sadistic personality disorder were reluctant to acknowledge their problems and therefore reluctant to seek or receive any type of treatment unless it was remanded by the justice system. She felt that persons with sadistic personality disorder often saw their behaviors as ego-syntonic and consistent with culturally accepted sexist patriarchal values.

## Comorbidity

Several studies have examined the overlap of sadistic personality disorder with other personality disorders. Freiman and Widiger (1989) found the highest overlap with narcissistic (56%), paranoid (44%), and antisocial (44%) personality disorders, and also a moderate amount of overlap with schizotypal, borderline, histrionic, and passive–aggressive personality disorders (33% in each case). Millon and Tringone (1989) used three different means of diagnosing personality disorders (clinical diagnosis, diagnostic checklist, the Millon Clinical Multiaxial Inventory); they found that the greatest overlap of sadistic personality disorder was with antisocial (17–30%), passive–aggressive (15–60%), and narcissistic (8–42%) personality disorders. A small degree of overlap was found with borderline and paranoid personality disorders. Interestingly, some overlap was also found with self-defeating personality disorder (2–15%).

We (Spitzer et al., 1991) found that 37–47% of cases of sadistic personality disorder also met criteria for narcissistic personality disorder, and

67–75% met criteria for antisocial personality disorder. Gay (1989) found a small amount of overlap in her study, with 8% receiving an additional diagnosis of narcissistic personality disorder and 8% receiving a diagnosis of antisocial personality disorder. Finally, Berger (1991) found sadistic personality disorder to be comorbid with avoidant (43%), borderline (29%), antisocial (24%), and paranoid (24%) personality disorders. He found no overlap with self-defeating personality disorder.

Two other studies used different approaches to address the problem of overlap of sadistic personality disorder with other Axis II disorders. In our survey (Spitzer et al., 1991), 76% of the respondents thought it useful to note both sadistic and antisocial personality disorder diagnoses, primarily because sadistic personality disorder indicated specific features that were usually not present in antisocial personality disorder alone. Blashfield and Breen (1989) supplied clinicians with case histories and asked them to give DSM-III-R diagnoses for the cases. Seventy-three percent of the clinicians attributed a sadistic personality disorder diagnosis to the sadistic personality disorder cases. The other most frequent diagnoses given to the sadistic personality disorder cases were antisocial (11%) and paranoid (6%) personality disorders.

Regarding the overlap of sadistic personality disorder with Axis I disorders, Gay (1989, in press) found that 16% met criteria for alcohol dependence. One-third had a prior history of mixed substance abuse, and 8% met criteria for current substance abuse. No other comorbid Axis I disorders were present. In the Spitzer et al. (1991) survey, 27% of cases with sadistic personality disorder also had comorbid major depressive disorder or dysthymia, and 61% had comorbid psychoactive substance abuse or dependence.

The high comorbidity of sadistic personality disorder with narcissistic and antisocial personality disorder as well as with several other personality disorders across a number of studies has raised concern that sadistic personality disorder may not be a distinct entity. It should be noted, however, that the mere presence of overlap or comorbidity does not necessarily imply that the disorder is not distinct from other personality disorders or that it is not a valid category.

## Performance Characteristics

Three studies have examined the performance characteristics of the individual DSM-III-R criteria for sadistic personality disorder (Blashfield & Breen, 1989; Freiman & Widiger, 1989; Millon & Tringone, 1989). Overall, the criterion with the highest correlation (phi coefficient) with the presence–absence of the disorder was criterion 6 (pertaining to intimidation). Criteria with extremely low phi values were 3 (pertaining to harsh treatment or discipline) and 7 (pertaining to restriction of others' autonomy). There were moderately high positive predictive power and high negative predictive power for nearly all of the criteria. High sensitivity was found for criterion 1 (pertain-

ing to living physical cruelty or violence), criterion 4 (pertaining to amusement or pleasure in others' suffering), criterion 5 (pertaining to lying for
the purpose of inflicting harm or pain), and criterion 6. Fairly high sensitivity was found for nearly all criteria in all three studies except for criterion
3, which had very poor sensitivity.

We (Spitzer et al., 1991) reported that the sensitivity of individual criteria
ranged from .65 to .94; the highest sensitivity was for criteria 1, 2, 4, and
6, and the lowest for criterion 5. Specificities ranged from .93 to .99.

In summary, criteria 3 and 7 appeared to have the poorest face validity.
Criteria 1 and criterion 4 appeared to perform well. Overall, the studies
found consistently good performance for nearly all the criteria, with remark-
ably high specificity and generally high sensitivity.

## Reliability and External Validity

Only one study examined test–retest or interrater reliability for sadistic personality disorder. Freiman and Widiger (1989), using master's-level clinical
psychologists for ratings, found a high interrater reliability (85%) for sadistic personality disorder.

To date, no studies have examined external validators such as biochemical variables, response to treatment, course of illness, or family history.

## Problems in Applying the Criteria

No studies were located that examined difficulties in determining the
presence or absence of particular sadistic personality disorder criteria. The
criteria as stated in DSM-III-R are fairly clear and behaviorally based. Several criteria appear to require some degree of inference to determine their
presence, However. For example, criterion 5 requires determining the motivation for lying; criterion 3 requires a judgment about what constitutes "unusually harsh" discipline, and criterion 4 requires a determination of the
subject's affective state in relation to the suffering of others (amusement or
pleasure).

## Sex Bias

Several studies examined differences in the prevalence of sadistic personality disorder in men and women. Gay (1989) found a high ration of males
to females (67% males vs. 33% females). Freiman and Widiger (1989) found
that 100% of the cases of sadistic personality disorder in their study population (which was 70% male) were male. In our survey (Spitzer et al., 1991),
98% of the cases of sadistic personality disorder were male. Thus, empirical
data are consistent with the theoretical literature and clinical case reports,
which have suggested that sadistic behavior is much more common among
men than among women.

Only one study (Sprock, Blashfield, & Smith, 1990) examined issues related to differential assignment of the sadistic personality disorder diagnosis to males versus females. In their study 49 undergraduate students (primarily female), who were not familiar with the DSM-III-R, were presented with stimuli consisting of 142 DSM-III-R criteria for the 11 personality disorders in the main body of the manual, plus self-defeating and sadistic personality disorders. It is not clear whether the raters were asked to evaluate whether the personality characteristics described as "primarily male" represented a normal male or not. Exclusion criteria were not presented, nor was the essential feature for each disorder listed. The stimuli were presented in random order, and subjects were asked to sort the cards along a dimension of gender from features most characteristic of males to those most characteristic of females. Sadistic personality disorder was seen as most typical of males, followed by antisocial and schizoid personality disorders. All criteria associated with sadistic personality disorder were rated in a direction consistent with their overall mean. Male and female raters did not differ in their mean ratings for the diagnosis or for individual symptoms.

The symptoms seen as most strongly associated with male or female gender stereotypes were examined, and an attempt was made to construct a prototypical male and a prototypical female personality disorder. In the case of the prototypical male disorder, the prototype depicted a sadistic man, who was cruel, angry, and aggressive, thus suggesting that sadistic personality disorder is strongly linked to stereotypical male behaviors. All of the symptoms from the male stereotype came from sadistic personality disorder except for one, which came from borderline personality disorder. Since the masculine personality disorder prototype is close to the stereotypical role for males in society, this raises concern about the potential for labeling typical men as having a personality disorder.

## Other Controversies

Critics of the sadistic personality disorder category felt that it was created as a "companion" personality disorder category to justify the inclusion of self-defeating personality disorder by having a comparable sex-role-stereotyped category that applied primarily to men rather than women. It was suspected that this might neutralize criticism regarding self-defeating personality disorder. However, the stimulus for the development of the disorder arose primarily from the clinical observations of forensic psychiatrists, who felt that the DSM system lacked a category to describe sadistic persons.

Another concern involved the potential use of sadistic personality disorder to mitigate responsibility for violent crime. There was a feeling that "diminished responsibility" or "not guilty by reason of insanity" defenses might be used in the defense of a spouse abuser or a person engaging in other violent behavior. In the Spitzer et al. (1991) survey, although 11% of the survey respondents felt that the diagnosis of sadistic personality disorder might be used as a psychiatric defense in mitigating responsibility for a crime, only 1% were familiar with instances in which it had been misused. Other forensic experts who responded to inquiries about the use of the sadistic personality disorder diagnosis as a defense strategy reported that in their experience, this occurred very infrequently. However, this low frequency of use may simply reflect the fact that the diagnosis, not being an "official" personality disorder in DSM-III-R, has been infrequently used.

Seventy-six percent of the respondents in the Spitzer et al. (1991) survey believed that if sadistic personality disorder were to become an "official" personality disorder diagnosis, it would have significant potential for being misused (in either forensic or clinical settings) for mitigating criminal responsibility in spouse or child abuse cases. As one eloquent respondent in this survey noted, "The medicalization of evil deeds becomes an avenue of excuses" (p. 877). However, concern about misuse of a diagnostic category within the judicial system should not necessarily lead to exclusion of that category from the diagnostic nomenclature if it is indeed a useful category. Many diagnoses carry the potential for misuse in forensic settings. It is in part the responsibility of the judicial system to develop guidelines and procedures for appropriate use of psychiatric evaluation and testimony within its domain. As an example, Oregon has passed a statute that disallows a personality disorder as the basis for an insanity defense, thus limiting the potential abuse of personality disorder diagnoses in the legal arena.

Still another concern involved the possible stigmatization of a patient labeled with sadistic personality disorder. One respondent to the survey (Spitzer et al., 1991) felt that patients labeled as having sadistic personality disorder might be abused by correctional or police officers. Finally, a label of sadistic personality disorder in a treatment setting might beget a "blame the perpetrator" attitude, which could interfere with effective treatment.


## CONCLUSIONS AND ACTION TAKEN IN DSM IV

There have been relatively few studies of sadistic personality disorder, with little systematic data collection. Unfortunately, the few studies that have been carried out have significant limitations, involving use of small samples from highly selected populations and other methodological flaws. In a few cases, sadistic personality disorder has been included in the data sets from larger studies examining all the personality disorders. However, in most studies of this type it has generally not been included, in part because of its status as an "unofficial" personality disorder in DSM-III-R.

From the existing data, sadistic personality disorder would appear to be relatively uncommon (2–5%), although it may have a higher prevalence in special forensic populations. There was significant comorbidity with antisocial, narcissistic, and a number of other personality disorders, thus raising questions about the distinctiveness of the disorder. There was a high male–female ratio (approximately 5:1) for the diagnosis, and the disorder was stongly associated with sex-role-stereotyped masculine behavior.

Phenomenologically, there appeared to be a very high prevalence of childhood physical, sexual, and emotional abuse, and of parental death and other significant losses, in the history of subjects with sadistic personality disorder. Whether this might be etiologically related to the disorder was not clear. There have been no studies to lend external validation to the diagnostic category. There was generally very high specificity for the DSM-II-R criteria, as well as excellent sensitivity. The criteria are behaviorally based and do not appear to be particularly ambiguous, although several criteria do require some degree of inference in determining their presence or absence.

Although many psychiatrists felt that the category has utility, a large number were also concerned about potential misuse of this personality disorder category in forensic or clinical settings. However, there are few actual data on abuse or misuse of this diagnosis in clinical or legal settings.

It is surprising that the inclusion of this category in DSM-III-R Appendix A led to little new research. Clearly, more research is needed to determine whether this really is a useful and valid diagnosis, distinct from other personality disorders. A better understanding of the phenomenology and etiology of the disorder (e.g., childhood antecedents and subsequent intrapsychic dynamics) might allow for the development of effective interventions for persons with sadistic personality disorder who are willing and/or able to be engaged in treatment. To make an analogy, research on individuals with antisocial personality disorder who have previously been felt to have a poor prognosis has resulted in identification of a subgroup of patients who are able to form a therapeutic alliance and who benefit from psychotherapy (Woody, McLellan, Luborsky, & O'Brien, 1985).

Identification of subgroups of persons with sadistic personality disorder who could be successfully treated with various interventions (such as the child abusers with sadistic personality disorder who were provided in-home modeling to help change their abusive behaviors; Gay, 1989) could provide one approach toward addressing a widespread societal problem of domestic violence. Thus, this category could have importance in identifying individuals who cause distress and suffering in others and whose behavior may have a significant legal and economic impact.

Despite these considerations, the Personality Disorders Work Group concluded that the current evidence did not support elevating this disorder to the status of an official DSM-IV personality disorder. Nor was it considered appropriate to retain the diagnosis in Appendix B, the DSM-IV equivalent of DSM-III-R Appendix A. (See Widiger, Chapter 17, for further discussion.)

# REFERENCES

American Psychiatric Association. (1987). *Diagnostic and statistical manual of mental disorders data]*. (3rd ed., rev.). Washington, DC: Author.

American Psychiatric Association. (1994). *Diagnostic and statistical manual of mental disorders* (4th ed.). Washington, DC: Author.

Avery, N. (1977). Sadomasochism: A defense against object loss. *Psychoanalytic Review, 64*, 101–109.

Berger, P. (1991). [Unpublished raw data].

Bieber, L. (1966). Sadism and masochism. In S. Arieti, (Ed.), *American handbook of psychiatry* (Vol. 3). New York: Basic Books.

Blashfield, R. K., & Breen, M. J. (1989). Face validity of the DSM-III-R personality disorders. *American Journal of Psychiatry, 146*, 1575–1579.

Brenner, C. (1959). The masochistic character: Genesis and treatment. *Journal of the American Psychoanalytic Association, 7*, 197–226.

Breslow, N. (1987). Locus of control, desirability of control, and sadomasochism. *Psychological Reports, 61*, 995–1001.

Eissler, K. (1958). Notes on the problem of technique in the psychoanalytic treatment of adolescents: With some remarks on perversions. *Psychoanalytic Study of the Child, 13*.

Freiman, K., & Widiger, T. (1989). [Co-occurrence and diagnostic efficiency statistics]. Unpublished raw data.

Freud, S. (1905). Three essays on the theory of sexuality. In J. Strachey (Ed. and Trans.), *The standard edition of the complete psychological works of Sigmund Freud* (Vol. 7). London: Hogarth Press, 1953.

Freud, S. (1915) Instincts and their vicissitudes. In J. Strachey (Ed. and Trans.), *The standard edition of the complete psychological works of Sigmund Freud* (Vol. 14). London: Hogarth Press, 1957.

Freud, S. (1924). The economic problem of masochism. In J. Strachey (Ed. and Trans.), *The standard edition of the complete psychological works of Sigmund Freud* (Vol. 19). London: Hogarth Press, 1961.

Fromm, E. (1973). *The anatomy of human destructiveness*. New York: Holt, Rinehart & Winston.

Gay, M. (1989, May). Personality disorders among child abusers. In R. L. Spitzer (Chair), *Psychiatric diagnosis, victimization and women*. Symposium presented at the 142nd Annual Meeting of the American Psychiatric Association, San Francisco.

Gay, M. (in press). Sadistic personality disorder in a child-abusing population. *Child Abuse and Neglect*.

Gay, M., & Fiester, S. (1991). Sadistic personality disorder. In R. Michels (Ed.), *Psychiatry* (rev. ed., Vol. 1). Philadelphia: J. B. Lippincott.

Gero, G. (1962). Sadism, masochism, and aggression: Their role in symptom formation. *Psychoanalytic Quarterly, 31*, 31–42.

Gosselin, C., & Wilson, G. (1980). *Sexual variations*. New York: Simon & Schuster.

Hamberger, L. K., & Hastings, J. (1988). Characteristics of male spouse abusers consistent with personality disorders. *Hospital and Community Psychiatry, 39*, 763–770.

Kohut, H. (1971). *The analysis of the self*. New York: International Universities Press.

Kohut, H. (1972). Thoughts on narcissism and narcissistic rage. *Psychoanalytic Study of the Child, 27*, 360–400.

Krafft-Ebing, R. (1898). *Psychopathia sexualis* (10th ed.). Stuttgart: Enke.

Millon, T., & Tringone, R. (1989). [Co-occurrence and diagnostic efficacy statistics]. Unpublished raw data.

Nydes, J. (1963). The magical experience of the masturbation fantasy. *American Journal of Psychotherapy, 4,* 303–310.

Parker, S. (1973). *The joy of suffering.* New York: Jason Aronson.

Reik, T. (1941). *Masochism in modern man.* New York: Farrar, Straus.

Spengler, A. (1977). Manifest sadomasochism of males: Results of an empirical study. *Archives of Sexual Behaviour, 6,* 6.

Spitzer, R. L., Fiester, S., Gay, M., & Pfohl, B. (1991). Is sadistic personality disorder a valid diagnosis?: The results of a survey of forensic psychiatrists. *American Journal of Psychiatry, 148,* 875–879.

Sprock, J., Blashfield, R. K., & Smith, B. (1990). Gender weighting of DSM-III-R personality disorder criteria. *American Journal of Psychiatry, 147,* 586–590.

Woody, G. E., McLellan, A. T., Luborsky, L., & O'Brien, C. P. (1985). Sociopathy and psychotherapy outcome. *Archives of General Psychiatry, 42,* 1081–1086.

# CHAPTER 16

# Self-Defeating Personality Disorder

SUSAN J. FIESTER

"Masochistic personality disorder" was first proposed as a category for DSM-III-R (American Psychiatric Association [APA], 1987) in 1983, on the basis of its presumed clinical utility and of precedent within the psychoanalytic, psychiatric, and psychological literature (Kass, Spitzer, Williams, & Widiger, 1989). Clinical experience, a review of the literature, and data from a clinical population were subsequently used to develop 10 criteria. These criteria were modified by the Advisory Committee on Personality Disorders and were subsequently pilot-tested by Kass, MacKinnon, and Spitzer (1986). The proposed category was later discussed at a 1984 meeting of the Advisory Committee on Personality Disorders of the Work Group to Revise DSM-III. Two items were dropped, because one was not felt to be central to the construct and the other was felt to reflect a paraphilia, sexual masochism. A draft version of masochistic personality disorder consisting of nine criteria was developed and published in October 1985 (Work Group to Revise DSM-III, 1985). Another, larger pilot study was carried out by Kass (1987), using the revised criteria.

Concerns were subsequently raised by the APA Committee on Women about potential problems with the diagnosis (e.g., sex bias, association with the psychoanalytic concept of masochism, potential misuse of the disorder in the context of victimization and abuse, and others discussed in depth in later sections of this chapter). In 1985 another meeting of the Advisory Committee on Personality Disorders was held, and these issues were further discussed. As a result, the category was renamed "self-defeating personality disorder" to avoid association with psychoanalytic concepts of female masochism. The criteria were further revised in light of the above-mentioned

An earlier version of this chapter was published in the *Journal of Personality Disorders*, 1991, 5, 194–209. Copyright 1991 by The Guilford Press. Adapted by permission.

criticisms; three criteria were eliminated, five revised, and two added (Work Group to Revise DSM-III, 1986).

A discussion of the rationale for these revisions is provided by Kass et al. (1989). The committee's aim was to emphasize that the category describes psychopathology rather than normative, culturally prescribed behaviors and to emphasize that the diagnosis should only be applied when the pattern of self-defeating behaviors is long-standing (present since early adulthood) and occurs in a variety of contexts. Finally, criteria were added in an attempt to exclude the diagnosis if the behaviors occur only in the context of, or only in response to, an abusive situation, or if the behaviors only occur when the individual is depressed. After further discussion, the APA Board of Trustees initially approved including self-defeating personality disorder in the main body of DSM-III-R; however, the board later decided to place it instead in Appendix A, "Proposed Diagnostic Categories Needing Further Study."

Since the publication of DSM-III-R, the controversy and heated debate about the category have continued, with much opposition to its inclusion being expressed (Caplan, 1985, 1987; Kaplan, 1983; Rosewater, 1987; Walker, 1987; Widiger & Frances, 1989). The major controversies surrounding this disorder are outlined here, followed by a critical review and summary of research data relevant to these questions and controversies.

## SIGNIFICANT ISSUES

The following issues appearing in the literature, and/or growing from discussions among the Personality Disorders Work Group members/advisors, were addressed by the work group in debating whether or not to include self-defeating personality disorders in DSM-IV (American Psychiatric Association, 1994):

1. What is the prevalence of self-defeating personality disorder?

2. Is self-defeating personality disorder a discrete entity that can be reliably distinguished from existing Axis II diagnoses, or is there significant overlap with other personality disorders (comorbidity)?

3. Do the diagnosis and criteria set have good reliability, internal consistency, and validity? And does the diagnosis have clinical utility?

4. Are there problems in applying the criteria? For example, is a high degree of inference required to determine the presence or absence of criteria?

5. Is there sex bias in the diagnostic criteria or in the application of the criteria?

6. Has the inclusion of the diagnosis resulted in harmful consequences for women, and/or might it result in harmful consequences in the future?

7. Is self-defeating personality disorder more appropriately conceived of as a disorder on the affective spectrum than as a personality disorder?

8. Do data addressing these questions support the continued inclusion of self-defeating personality disorder in the diagnostic nomenclature?

# LITERATURE REVIEW

The literature review covered articles published from 1960 to 1991, chapters, or books on masochism and masochistic or self-defeating personality
disorder. Other than for conceptual, theoretical, or historical purposes, all
sources that did not involve empirical data were excluded (e.g., case studies).
Empirical studies cited were included if they used the original criteria or
the final revised criteria listed in DSM-III-R. Studies using the earlier criteria were included because of the paucity of studies on the disorder and the
importance of reviewing all empirical data that were in any way relevant
to determining the fate of self-defeating personality disorder. Further information was solicited from researchers who had data sets relating to the diagnosis and unpublished reports. Input was also solicited from a wide range
of advisors with varied theoretical, clinical, and research backgrounds.

## Prevalence

Several studies have shown a high prevalence of self-defeating personality
disorder in samples of psychiatric patients. Reich (1987) examined 82 randomly selected intakes to a university outpatient clinic and 40 normal volunteers, using a version of the Personality Disorder Questionnaire (PDQ) that
included the originally proposed masochistic personality disorder criteria.
Patients with organic disorders, schizophrenia, mania, or psychosis were excluded from the patient population, and subjects with depressive and psychotic disorders were excluded from the normal population. Reich (1987),
using a cutoff score of six or more criteria, found a prevalence for masochistic
personality disorder of 18.3% in outpatients and 5% in normal subjects.
There was no significant difference between the prevalence in the patient
group as compared to the normal controls, thus raising the question of
whether the criteria might not actually be tapping relatively common personality traits as opposed to frank disorder.

The Reich (1987) study has several methodological limitations. First, the
study used the criteria for the original masochistic personality disorder
category, which differ significantly from those of the DSM-III-R self-defeating
personality disorder category. Exclusion criteria for the patient group did
not include depression, but persons were excluded from the normal control group if they carried a diagnosis of depression. Thus, the patient group,
but not the normal controls, might have received a diagnosis of masochistic
personality disorder even in the presence of depression—a problem that
was later addressed in the revision of the masochistic personality disorder
criteria by adding an exclusion clause. Reich did note that data based on
structured interviews administered to the outpatient group indicated that
the masochistic symptoms occurred at times when the subjects were not clinically depressed and at periods when they were not in situations of psychological or physical abuse. It should also be noted that self-report inventories

of personality disorders may show a tendency toward overdiagnosis (Hyler, Skodol, Kellman, Oldham, & Rosnick, 1990).

A study by Kass et al. (1986) involved 59 patients (64% female, 88% white; mean age = 35 years) in a university psychiatric outpatient clinic. Fifteen psychiatrists were asked to determine the presence or absence of the 10 original masochistic criteria in three to five patients selected from a list of all their patients. Using their own personal criteria, the therapists also rated the severity of masochistic personality disorder on a 4-point scale. Fourteen percent of the sample were diagnosed as having masochistic personality disorder. Kass et al. (1986) did not mention how many of the subjects had a given threshold number of formal masochistic personality disorder criteria. Of all the personality disorders, only borderline personality disorder was diagnosed more frequently (19%). A second study was carried out by Kass (1987), using 367 patients (61% female) from the private practices of a variety of therapists. The 9 criteria for masochistic personality initially proposed for DSM-III-R in the October 1985 draft were interspersed randomly among 13 other randomly chosen personality disorder criteria. Clinicians were asked to rate each trait as present, absent, or unknown. Twenty-two percent of the patients were rated as having six criteria present; 13% had seven or more criteria present; 9% had eight or more present; and 3% had all nine present.

The two Kass studies are obviously limited in that the population samples were middle-class, were primarily white, and were drawn from private practices in a major metropolitan area. In addition, in the Kass (1987) study, patients could have been included even if they had been in treatment for only 1 month. Although the average time in treatment for the sample was 16 months, therapists may not have known whether patients only briefly in treatment had histories of being in, or were currently in, abusive situations. The study also involved a "retrospective" rating by clinicians as opposed to a direct interview. Clinicians were, however, blind to the real purpose of the study. Other problems with the Kass et al. (1986) study have been elaborated by Caplan (1985); these include lack of guidelines for selecting patients and lack of data about how many masochistic patients were selected by each psychiatrist.

In a study reported by Spitzer, Williams, Kass, and Davies (1989), 5,000 psychiatrists were sent a questionnaire about the personality disorder diagnostic criteria being considered for DSM-III-R at the time of the study. Thirty-two criteria were listed, including criteria for borderline, dependent, and self-defeating personality disorders, and seven criteria from other personality disorders listed in random order. Subjects chose the first patient they had treated who came to mind whom they knew well who had a personality disorder. They then indicated which of the criteria applied to the case. They also specified a primary DSM-III (American Psychiatric Association, 1980) personality disorder diagnosis for the case. Spitzer et al. (1989) found a prevalence rate for self-defeating personality disorder of 42% for females and 28% for males. However, this cannot be considered a true prevalence: Spitzer et al. felt that those surveyed may have noticed that a third of the criteria involved self-defeating behavior, and clinicians may have thus preferentially chosen a patient with self-defeating personality disorder.

In the same article, Spitzer et al. (1989) reported on a multisite study of the reliability of the Structured Clinical Interview for DSM-III-R, Axis II (SCID-II) in 85 inpatients/outpatients who had at least one personality disorder diagnosis; this study found a prevalence of self-defeating personality disorder of 7% (as compared to 9% for borderline personality disorder). Interviewers were clinicians with varied training and a broad range of experience levels. Freiman and Widiger (1989), using master's-level clinical psychologists to administer the Personality Interview Questionnaire-II, studied 50 patients in a public hospital setting and found a prevalence rate of 8%. Skodol, Rosnick, Kellman, Oldham, and Hyler (1988) found prevalence rates of 21% using the Personality Disorder Examination (PDE) and 37% using the SCID-II, in a sample of 97 subjects. Millon and Tringone (1989) found 27 cases of self-defeating personality disorder among 584 subjects (5%) using clinician diagnoses, (6%) using a diagnostic checklist, and (5%) using the Millon Clinical Multiaxial Inventory (MCMI). Comparable data were reported by Pfohl (1990).

In summary, several studies found a surprisingly high prevalence of self-defeating personality disorder (14–22%, with two outlying studies with rates of 37% and 42%). In one study the disorder was diagnosed more frequently than any other personality disorder except borderline. Several other studies found much lower prevalence rates (5–8%). It should be noted that many of these studies were carried out with limited and relatively homogeneous samples; few studies used a semistructured interview; and nearly all the studies had major methodological flaws. It is not clear whether the higher or lower prevalence rates would hold up in more methodologically sound studies using larger and more heterogeneous samples.

## Distinctiveness from Other Disorders

Regarding clinician's perceptions of need for the self-defeating personality disorder category, Spitzer et al. (1989) conducted a survey of 2,000 psychiatrists with a special interest in personality disorders. Half of the respondents (620) felt that there was a need for self-defeating personality disorder in DSM-III-R, and half did not. However, if there was a differential return rate—that is, if those psychiatrists who felt that self-defeating personality disorder was a needed category were either more or less apt to return the questionnaire than those who did not feel it was needed—this could have led to a significant bias in the data. There was no relationship between endorsement of the diagnosis and the psychiatrists' gender, type of clinical practice, or years of experience.

Several studies addressed the issue of whether masochistic personality disorder (as originally defined) is distinct from the other personality disorders. Fuller (1986) used 10 case descriptions of patients with masochistic personality disorder, including prototypical and nonprototypical cases. Ten clinicians using the DSM-III criteria could not consistently assign any personality disorder diagnosis to even the nonprototypical "masochism" case descriptions. However, another group of 10 clinicians who applied DSM-III-R criteria to the same case histories could reliably identify the prototypical "masochism" cases as cases of masochistic personality disorder.

In a second study (Fuller & Blashfield, 1989), 150 mental health professionals were asked in one condition to use DSM-III personality disorder categories to diagnose 15 case descriptions that included prototypical and nonprototypicL borderline, passive–aggressive, antisocial, dependent, and masochistic personality disorders. They did not assign diagnoses with high rates of agreement for any other personality disorder diagnosis to the prototypical "masochism" cases when they were asked to use DSM-III Axis II diagnoses, and masochistic personality disorder was not a possible diagnosis. For the three prototypical "masochism" cases, the diagnoses most commonly given were mixed personality disorder or personality disorder not otherwise specified (NOS). Dependent personality disorder was the diagnosis given most commonly (58%) for one nonprototypical case, and avoidant was the one given most commonly (36%) for the other nonprototypical case.

When clinicians were asked to assign DSM-III-R diagnoses to the cases in another condition, they most commonly assigned masochistic personality disorder to each of the prototypical cases (regardless of the sex of the case), whereas the nonprototypical cases most commonly received dependent, avoidant, or NOS diagnoses. The results did not support the idea that the "masochism" cases described could be subsumed under the already existing DSM-III personality disorder diagnoses. It should be noted that it is always possible to generate cases for which a proposed diagnosis will specifically apply; however, for this study, most cases were generated from the literature.

Examining comorbidity, Spitzer et al. (1989) found that self-defeating personality disorder was the sole diagnosis in only 3.8% of cases. In 6% of the cases it was comorbid with dependent, in 5% with borderline, and in 22% with both personality disorders. Thus, there was considerable overlap with other personality disorder categories. A principal-components factor analysis resulted in three factors that did not match the domains of the three personality disorders studied. Three self-defeating personality disorder criteria were contained with the "borderline" factor, and four dependent personality disorder criteria were contained in the "self-defeating" factor; these findings suggest further problems with the concept of self-defeating personality disorder as a separate construct.

Several other studies have addressed the issue of the degree of overlap or comorbidity of masochistic/self-defeating personality disorder with the other personality disorders (Table 16.1). A study by Freiman and Widiger (1989) of 50 subjects, only 4 of whom were diagnosed as having self-defeating

## TABLE 16.1. Comorbidity Percentages

| Study | Number of self-defeating cases | Comorbid diagnoses (%) | | | | | | | | | | | |
|---|---|---|---|---|---|---|---|---|---|---|---|---|---|
| | | PRN | SZD | SZT | ATS | BDL | HST | NAR | AVD | DPD | OCP | PAG | SAD |
| Freiman & Widiger (1989) | 4 | 50 | 50 | 50 | 75 | 100 | 25 | 100 | 100 | 75 | 0 | 25 | 0 |
| Skodol et al. (1988) | | | | | | | | | | | | | |
| PDE | 20 | 30 | 0 | 40 | 20 | 90 | 30 | 50 | 55 | 65 | 55 | 10 | 0 |
| SCID-II | 36 | 43 | 9 | 23 | 11 | 86 | 29 | 26 | 57 | 51 | 23 | 17 | — |
| Millon & Tringone (1989) | | | | | | | | | | | | | |
| Clinical diagnosis[a] | 27 | 0 | 0 | 0 | 0 | 19 | 7 | 0 | 19 | 41 | 4 | 7 | 4 |
| Diagnostic checklist[b] | 31 | 0 | 3 | 0 | 0 | 32 | 3 | 0 | 19 | 74 | 3 | 3 | 0 |
| MCMI[c] | 40 | 0 | '' | 0 | 0 | 20 | 15 | 0 | 55 | 43 | 0 | 35 | 3 |
| Reich (1987) | | | | | | | | | | | | | |
| PDQ | 17 | 12 | 12 | 65 | 12 | 71 | 35 | 0 | 53 | 76 | 59 | 6 | — |
| MCMI | 17 | 0 | 53 | 12 | 6 | 35 | 6 | 0 | 59 | 82 | 6 | 53 | — |
| SIDP | 15 | 0 | 0 | 20 | 7 | 53 | 53 | 7 | 33 | 73 | 27 | 0 | — |
| Blashfield & Breen (1989) | — | 1 | 3 | 0 | 1 | 3 | 1 | 2 | 2 | 3 | 3 | 5 | 2 |
| Spitzer et al. (1989)[d] | — | — | — | — | — | 3 | — | — | 6 | 6 | — | — | — |

Note. Key to personality disorder abbreviations: PRN, paranoid; SZD, schizoid; SZI, schizotypal; ATS, antisocial; BDL, borderline; HSI, histrionic; NAR, narcissistic; AVD, avoidant; DPD, dependent; OCP, obsessive–compulsive; PAG, passive–aggressive; SAD, sadistic.
[a]No cases received a diagnosis of self-defeating personality disorder only.
[b]13% of cases received a diagnosis of self-defeating personality disorder only.
[c]5% of cases received a diagnosis of self-defeating personality disorder only.
[d]8% of cases received a diagnosis of self-defeating personality disorder only; 22% were comorbid with both dependent and borderline personality disorders.

personality disorder, showed that there was a significant overlap between this disorder and other personality disorders.

The greatest overlap occurred with borderline, avoidant, antisocial, and dependent personality disorders. Skodol et al. (1988), using the PDE and the SCID-II, also found a significant overlap with other personality disorders; the greatest overlap occurred with borderline, avoidant, and dependent personality disorders. For the PDE alone, there was also high overlap with narcissistic and obsessive–compulsive personality disorders.

Millon and Tringone (1989) used three different methods of diagnosing personality disorders (clinical diagnosis, a diagnostic checklist, and the MCMI) and examined comorbidity among all the personality disorders. For all three methods of diagnosis, they found the highest overlap of self-defeating personality disorder with dependent, avoidant, and borderline personality disorders. There was also a high degree of overlap with passive–aggressive personality disorder for the MCMI.

Reich (1987) used the PDQ, the MCMI, and the Structured Inteview for DSM-III Personality Disorders (SIDP) as diagnostic instruments and found the greatest overlap (greater than 50% on two of the three instruments) with dependent, avoidant, and borderline personality disorders. Finally, Blashfield and Breen (1989) supplied clinicians with case histories and asked them to make DSM-III-R diagnoses. Seventy-one percent of the clinicians gave a diagnosis of self-defeating personality disorder when presented with a case containing the self-defeating personality disorder criteria. Only very infrequently were self-defeating personality disorder cases assigned other personality disorder diagnoses.

The Reich (1987) study was the only one that examined overlap of masochistic/self-defeating personality disorder with Axis I disorders. Reich found that 15 of 17 patients with masochistic personality disorder had Axis I disorders: 53% had major depressive disorder; 7% had minor depression; 7% had schizoaffective disorder, depressive type; 7% had panic disorder; 20% had a phobia; 13% had obsessive–compulsive disorder; 13% had generalized anxiety disorder; 13% had alcohol abuse; and 7% had drug abuse.

These studies had numerous methodological problems some of which are noted above (including small sample sizes). One strength in several studies was the use of more than one instrument (self-report and semistructured interviews) to assess personality disorder.

In summary, these studies have provided mixed data—some supporting the concept of the self-defeating personality disorder as a distinct entity (Blashfield & Breen, 1989; Fuller, 1986; Fuller & Blashfield, 1989) and others suggesting significant overlap with several other personality disorders (Freiman & Widiger, 1989; Millon & Tringone, 1989; Reich, 1987; Skodol et al., 1988; Spitzer et al., 1989). Interestingly, the studies using case histories that were diagnosed by clinicians tended to suggest the distinctiveness of self-defeating personality disorder, whereas the studies using various instruments to diagnose actual subjects tended to show significant overlap and to argue against the distinctiveness of the diagnosis. Across all studies and all instruments, to greatest comorbidity for masochistic/self-defeating personality disorder was found with borderline, avoidant, and dependent personality disorders. Almost no overlap was found with sadistic personality disorder, and very little was found with antisocial, paranoid, schizoid, schizotypal, and narcissistic personality disorders. However, it should be noted that overlap or comorbidity does not necessarily imply that a disorder is not distinct from other personality disorder categories, nor that it is not a valid category.

## Reliability, Internal Consistency, and Validity

Two studies examined the test–retest or interrater reliability for self-defeating personality disorder. Spitzer et al. (1989), in the SCID-II reliability study, reported test–retest reliability to be only .33—one of the lowest values reported for any personality disorder. Freiman and Widiger (1989) reported interrater reliability to be .49; again, this was one of the lowest for any personality diagnosis.

Few studies have addressed the question of the validity of self-defeating personality disorder, and most of these have addressed only the descriptive validity. Three studies examined the internal consistency of the criteria for masochistic personality disorder. Kass (1987) found only moderate correlations between each masochistic personality disorder criterion and the mean of the other eight masochistic criteria (mean = .35; range = .27 to .40). Kass et al. (1986) found slightly higher correlations (mean = .44; range = .24 to .64). Correlations of each masochistic personality disorder criterion with the 13 nonmasochistic personality disorder criteria ranged from .07 to .29. For six of the nine criteria, correlations with other masochistic criteria were significantly higher than correlations with the mean score for the presence or absence of the 13 nonmasochistic traits. Thus, Kass et al. showed fairly good internal consistency for masochistic personality disorder criteria, with moderate intercorrelations.

The Kass et al. (1986) study also found that the earlier masochistic personality disorder criteria had good internal consistency and showed a moderate degree of intercorrelation. Two traits showed higher correlations with other personality disorders than with the clinicians' own rating of masochistic personality: "Prides self on being ethically or morally superior to others" showed higher correlations with paranoid, narcissistic, dependent, compulsive, and passive–aggressive disorders; and "sexually excited by fantasies of humiliations" showed higher correlations with borderline and avoidant personality disorders.

Eight of the ten "masochism" traits had a substantially higher correlation with the clinicians' ratings of masochistic personality than with each of the existing Axis II personality disorders. In addition, the correlation between the total number of items rated present for each subject and the clinicians' global masochistic personality ratings was .76, suggesting that these eight criteria describe a category consistent with clinicians' concepts of masochism. Unfortunately, the same clinicians rated masochism and masochistic personality disorder, and they may not have been blind to the purpose of the study. This could possibly have contributed to factitiously high internal consistency ratings, and it constitutes a significant methodological flaw limiting the conclusions that can be drawn.

Spitzer et al. (1989) found moderate to high internal consistencies for each of the criteria sets (borderline, dependent, and self-defeating), with a Cronbach's alpha of .70 for self-defeating personality disorder. However, intercorrelations among the criteria sets, were also relatively high when corrected for attenuation, were also relatively high, indicating a relative lack of independence, particularly between dependent and self-defeating personality disorders. In a further survey (Spitzer et al., 1989), each of 222 psychiatrists provided information about two patients they knew well — one with self-defeating personality disorder, and a "control" with any other DSM-III personality disorder. Although the self-defeating personality disorder criteria were significantly more common in patients with the disorder, all eight criteria were relatively common in the control patients (present in 29–51% of cases).

Few data are available on the external validation of self-defeating personality disorder by clinical description, delineation from other disorders, biochemical parameters, response to treatment, course of illness, and family history (genetic factors). Reich (1987) found that patients with self-defeating personality disorder did not differ from outpatients without self-defeating personality disorder on demographic factors such as gender, age, marital status, or education. Reich (1990) did, however, find a higher prevalence of self-defeating personality disorder in first-degree relatives of patients with self-defeating personality disorder; these are the only validity data to date that involve family history. Pfohl (1990) reported a significantly greater frequency of childhood sexual abuse in persons with self-defeating personality disorder than in individuals with the other personality disorders (with the exception of borderline). There has been no research on course, response to treatment, outcome, or biological factors. Thus, there are no research data to support the utility of this category in informing decisions regarding clinical management or choice of treatment, or in predicting treatment outcome. However, it should be kept in mind that adequate external validation studies have been carried out for only a few of the personality disorders.

## Problems in Applying Criteria

One criticism frequently leveled at the personality disorders is that determining the presence or absence of some criteria involves a high degree of inference. Several of the DSM-III-R self-defeating personality disorder criteria (American Psychiatric Association, 1987, pp. 373–374) appear to require a high degree of inference in determining their presence or absence — for example, criterion 8: ("engages in excessive self-sacrifice that is unsolicited by the intended recipients of the sacrifice"). Different clinicians and researchers may have very different perceptions of thresholds for "excessive" self-sacrifice. In addition, in a society that tends to encourage self-sacrificial behavior on the part of women as one aspect of the stereotyped feminine role, it is not clear how the diagnostician would determine what constitutes "excessive" self-sacrifice. Would the threshold for such self-sacrifice differ for men and women, given that the normative behaviours for the masculine versus feminine sex roles differ? Likewise, it may be difficult to determine whether the self-sacrifice is solicited or unsolicited by the intended recipient. Although self-sacrifice may not be explicitly encouraged, more subtle communication of such an expectation could be present.

A high degree of inference is also required in order to determine whether the person is uninterested in or "rejects people who consistently treat him or her well" (criterion 7). What constitutes being "treated well" may differ by gender, social class, ethnic or cultural group, and/or race. Finally, for "chooses people and situations that lead to disappointment, failure, or mistreatment even when better options are clearly available" (criterion 1), it is unclear how the diagnostician would adequately judge whether "better options are clearly available." For example, a patient of low socioeconomic level who lives in an environment and culture of poverty, substance abuse, violence, and general deprivation may well be involved with people or situations leading to disappointment, failure, or mistreatment. Given certain external conditions or limitations, it may be quite unclear whether other "better options" are in fact available and are realistic options for the person. Unfortunately, no studies have been carried out to determine whether the degree of inference required poses an actual problem in making the diagnosis of self-defeating personality disorder—for example, whether clinicians differ markedly in their assessments.

## Sex Bias

The issue of sex bias is a complex one and is discussed in depth in several papers (Kaplan, 1983; Kass, Spitzer, & Williams, 1983; Williams & Spitzer, 1983). Sprock, Blashfield, and Smith (1990) point out that apparent sex differences in the frequency of assigning a particular diagnosis can result from the following: (1) inherent gender bias in the diagnostic criteria—that is, bias within the criteria themselves that reflect sex-role stereotypes (societal prescriptions about which types of behavior are healthy vs. pathological for males vs. females); (2) gender bias in the way clinicians apply the criteria; (3) real differences in the prevalence of the disorders in males and females as a reflection of different susceptibilities to the disorder, based on psychological, biological, genetic, social, and/or environmental factors; or (4) any combination of these three factors. So, although there appear to be gender differences in the diagnosis of personality disorders other than self-defeating personality disorder—with females being more often diagnosed with histrionic and dependent personality disorders, and males being more frequently diagnosed as having antisocial, schizoid, passive–aggressive, and paranoid personality disorders—it is not clear why this is the case. Furthermore, the occurrence of a disorder in women versus men may have different implications.

Several studies have addressed the issue of differences in the frequencies of diagnosis of self-defeating personality disorder in men and women. In the Kass et al. (1986) study, six of the patients diagnosed as having masochistic personality disorder were female (75%) and two were male (25%). The correlation of the mean of the 10 masochistic traits (absent vs. present) with the sex of the eight patients (male vs. female) was not statistically significant; however, the small $m$ in both Kass studies limits the conclusions that can be drawn from the data. In the Kass (1987) study, for five of the nine masochistic personality disorder criteria, there was a higher than expected female-to-male ratio. Interestingly, no association was found between social class and the presence of masochistic criteria, except for one criterion. The Spitzer et al. (1989) study, as noted in the section on prevalence, found a 1.5:1 female–male ratio (42% vs. 28%) for the self-defeating personality disorder diagnosis.

Spitzer et al. (1989) reported from a separate survey that when clinicians provided information about two patients they knew well—one with self-defeating personality disorder, and one with any other DSM-III personality disorder—62% of the self-defeating personality disorder patients versus 55% of the other personality disorder patients were female. In the study by Reich (1987), 58% of the outpatient masochistic subjects were women, which was not significantly different from the percentage of women in the outpatient population as a whole. Reich (1987) also examined sex differences in the prevalence of individual criteria and found a significantly higher prevalence in females of two criteria ("sacrifices own needs for the needs of others" and "taken advantage of and not complaining," which is no longer a criterion); however, the overall $F$ was not significant.

In the first part of their survey of self-defeating personality disorder, Spitzer et al. (1989) regressed the 204 patients diagnosed as having self-defeating personality disorder on the eight diagnostic criteria, using sex as a covariate. No item showed a significant interaction with sex. Of particular interest was the trend for criterion 1 ("chooses people and situations . . . ") to be associated with the diagnosis for females, whereas criterion 2 ("rejects or renders ineffective the attempts of others to help him or her") tended to be associated with the diagnosis for males.

Additional studies have examined potential bias in the assignment of the self-defeating personality disorder diagnosis, using ratings of case histories rather than diagnosis of actual subjects. Fuller and Blashfield (1989) selected 15 case histories to present to clinicians. Five case histories had been shown in previous studies to be prototypes of other personality disorder diagnoses, while five were nonprototypical personality disorder diagnoses. Five cases represented masochistic personality disorder, with three of these being prototypical cases. Three groups participated (150 psychiatrists, 150 psychologist clinicians, and 150 clinicians of various training). In all cases thought to be prototypes (except for one masochistic personality disorder case), more than 70% of clinicians assigned the proper diagnosis. Reversing the sex of the cases did not affect the DSM-III-R Axis II diagnoses for either the prototypical or the nonprototypical cases. Even when the investigators examined the impact of the sex of the clinician performing the ratings, no significant differences were found, except for one case in which the female clinicians were more likely to diagnose the case as masochistic personality disorder when the case was written to describe a female, and male clinicians were more likely to use the masochistic personality disorder diagnosis when the case was written to describe a male. Thus, the authors concluded that their data did not support a hypothesis of sex bias.

In another study (Sprock et al., 1990), 49 undergraduate students in an introductory psychology course who were unfamiliar with the DSM-III-R were presented with 142 cards, each containing one of the criteria for the DSM-III-R personality disorders (including self-defeating and sadistic) in random order. They were instructed to sort the cards along a dimension of gender, from features most characteristic of males to those most characteristic of females. Dependent personality disorder was seen as the most characteristic of females, followed by histrionic and avoidant personality disorders. Sadistic personality disorder was seen as most typical of males, followed by antisocial and schizoid personality disorders. Self-defeating, obsessive–compulsive, paranoid, and schizotypal personality disorders fell near the mean. Males and females did not differ in mean ratings for diagnoses or for individual symptoms. Although subjects did associate criteria used to define DSM-III-R personality disorder with societally stereotyped gender roles, self-defeating personality disorder was not found to be particularly related to gender; this finding suggests that the current criteria do not reflect stereotyped female sex role behaviors, but are equally applicable to males and females.

In summary, the available empirical data suggest that self-defeating personality disorder is diagnosed overall somewhat more frequently in women than in men, and that some individual self-defeating personality disorder criteria are rated as present more frequently in women than in men. Experimental studies have not found a sex bias in the application of the diagnosis for either male or female clinicians. Furthermore, one prototype study (Sprock et al., 1990) found that the prototypical personality disorder for the female gender was closest to dependent, not self-defeating personality disorder. The question of whether there are real differences in the prevalence of self-defeating personality disorder in females versus males awaits further research.

Another concern involves the potential diagnosis of self-defeating personality disorder in women who are merely exhibiting behaviors that conform to the societal expectations for the female sex role. Walker (1987) points out that some behaviors fitting certain self-defeating personality disorder criteria may actually be adaptive (e.g., in terms of enhancing a woman's desirability for marriage and motherhood, or of enhancing the probability of survival in a violent encounter); thus, it seems the possible that of normal women in traditional roles could be characterized as having personality disorders. Although Sprock et al.'s (1990) research found the feminine personality disorder prototype to be close to the stereotypical role of a normal female in society, this would seem to be more of a concern for dependent personality disorder than for self-defeating personality disorder, because the feminine personality disorder prototype was of a dependent female rather than a self-defeating one. In addition, Reich (1987) found that only 5% of his "normal" sample received a diagnosis of self-defeating personality disorder. If there were a real potential for the diagnosis to be applied to women who are merely exhibiting behavior that conforms to the expected female sex role, then one would expect a far greater rate of self-defeating personality disorder in the general population than 5%, which represented only two cases in Reich's study. Furthermore, the sex of these two cases was not even specified. In addition, a body of psychological research suggests that various types of self-defeating behaviors are relatively common in the general population (Baumeister & Scher, 1988; Curtis, 1989).

## Possible Misapplications of the Diagnosis: "Blaming the Victim" and Misuse in Abuse Situations

Critics of self-defeating personality disorder suggested that the inclusion of the diagnosis in DSM-III-R would have widespread negative effects in many arenas for women (Caplan, 1985, 1987; Kaplan, 1983; Rosewater, 1987; Walker, 1987; Widiger & Frances, 1989). One concern was with the potential misapplication of the diagnosis in the forensic setting. For example, in a case where a woman is being prosecuted for harming a physically abusive spouse, a diagnosis of self-defeating personality disorder could possibly be used by the prosecution to "blame" the woman for remaining in the abusive relationship and turn attention away from the use of a legitimate psychiatric diagnosis in the defense—for example, post-traumatic stress disorder ("battered woman syndrome"). Furthermore, the diagnosis might be used in cases where parental "fitness" is an issue, leading to women being deprived of custody of their children. Concern has also been expressed regarding the potential harmful effects in treatment settings, where therapists might conclude that women are responsible for their predicaments (i.e., "blame the victims") and assume a negative therapeutic stance that would undermine the therapeutic effort and result in a negative outcome. Alternatively, self-defeating personality disorder may have utility in conceptualizing specific treatment approaches, as in the Berglas (1985, 1988) subtypes of those who fear success, those who pursue victory through defeat, and those who derive secondary gain through sadomasochistic relationships.

No research or clinical reports were located that addressed the issue of actual harm occurring to women in clinical, forensic, or other settings as a result of the use of the diagnosis. In addition, no anecdotal information was obtained from the various consultants and forensic experts regarding specific instances of misuse or abuse of the disorder in forensic settings, although there are reports in the literature that suggest the potential for misuse (Snell, Rosenwald, & Robey, 1964). A broader survey or another form of data collection might be helpful in determining whether this is a realistic concern.

Another major concern has involved potential inappropriate application of the diagnosis to women in abusive situations. Critics have feared that the behaviors included as diagnostic criteria in DSM-III-R may be characteristic of women who are physically, sexually, and/or psychologically abused, and that this could lead to misdiagnosis of a personality disorder in persons who have "chronic" post-traumatic stress disorder as a result of prior victimization. Critics of the diagnosis feel that many self-defeating behaviors represent accommodation or response to various types of physical and/or psychological victimization, and that the behaviors decrease in frequency or disappear if the abuse is eliminated. Frances (1980) has also noted that it is often difficult in cross-sectional evaluation to determine the extent to which current behaviors represent enduring, lifelong patterns or are primarily a function of the patient's current clinical state and/or role expectations. In order to deal with this initial criticism, the DSM-III-R Advisory Committee on Personality Disorders added an exclusion criterion stating that the diagnosis can not be made when the behaviors occur exclusively in response to or in anticipation of being physically, sexually, or psychologically abused. However, as Walker (1987) notes, interviewers or therapists may frequently neglect to assess the history of or current presence of abuse. Even when they do inquire, abuse may often not be acknowledged by the victims.

The problem is further complicated by the fact that some women may have suppressed knowledge of earlier abuse, and recall of the abuse experiences may occur only during treatment (Herman & Schatzow, 1987). Herman and Schatzow found a relationship between the severity and duration of the abuse and the degree to which memory of the abuse had been repressed, thus suggesting that those women most severely affected by the impact of previous abuse are those least likely to recall and/or report the abuse during a diagnostic assessment.

## Relationship to the Affective Disorders Spectrum

Another controversy has centered around the proposition that self-defeating personality disorder is really a disorder on the affective spectrum, not a personality disorder. There is a clinical and theoretical tradition supporting the concept of a depressive–masochistic personality. This is perhaps best described by Kernberg (1984), who also briefly reviews the origin of the concept in the writings of early psychoanalysts (Kraepelin, Schneider, Fenichel, and others). Akiskal (1983) similarly proposes a character spectrum disorder as a chronic depressive subtype, based on his research on dysthymic disorder. Furthermore, many of the criterion features of self-defeating personality disorder are present in patients who suffer from depression — for example, guilty responses to positive events, rejecting opportunities for pleasure, failing to accomplish tasks, and rejecting others who treat him or her well. Thus, in some cases it may be difficult to tease apart whether the self-defeating behaviors are reflecting maladaptive personality traits or are manifestations of current or more long-standing depressive illness.

Examination of the self-defeating personality disorder criteria also indicates some overlap with traits described in the literature as being characteristic of the "depressive personality." However, there is little overlap with the criteria for depressive personality disorder that have been included in Appendix B pf DSM-IV (see Phillips, Hirschfeld, Shea, & Gunderson, Chapter 13, this volume). Of interest in relation to this problem are data from the Reich (1987) study, which showed a high level of comorbidity of Axis I diagnoses in patients with masochistic personality disorder (53% had major depression and 7% minor depression) before the exclusion criterion for depression was added.

In summary, it appears that there is confusion regarding the nature of the relationship of self-defeating personality disorder to the affective disorders. However, it does not appear that the disorder can satisfactorily be subsumed under the category of depressive personality disorder, at least as this category is defined in DSM-IV Appendix B.

## CONCLUSIONS AND ACTION TAKEN IN DSM-IV

Since the inclusion of self-defeating personality disorder in Appendix A of DSM-III-R, several studies have been carried out to investigate prevalence, internal consistency of the criteria set, the clinical utility of the disorder, validity, overlap with other personality disorder, and potential sex bias in the criteria and their clinical application. Although there has been progress in the attempt to elucidate the nature of self-defeating personality disorder, the small body of research that has been carried out over the past several years has significant limitations, as previously noted. Data from existing studies have shown a relatively high prevalence; a fairly high female–male sex ratio; good internal consistency; significant overlap with several other personality disorders (particularly borderline, dependent, and avoidant personality disorders); some possible inherent sex bias in the criteria; an apparent lack of sex bias in the application of the criteria by clinicians; and lack of differentiation of patients with self-defeating personality disorder from patients with other disorders in terms of demographic factors other than gender. Few data were available with which to address the issue of external validity (e.g., associated features, impairment, complications, predisposing factors, family history, and biological markers), except for one study showing increased prevalence of the disorder in relatives of probands with self-defeating personality disorder, and another showing an increased frequency of childhood sexual abuse in person with the disorder. There are no formal data on the potential harmful effects of use of the diagnosis in clinical, forensic, or other settings. There is little or no information about whether the diagnosis implies something about the course of illness or prognosis, or helps inform decisions regarding treatment, as no studies of course, prognosis, or treatment outcome have been carried out. In addition, many critics expressed significant concerns about the potential negative consequences of including the disorder in DSM-IV.

In summary, although there is a historical tradition and some support for the clinical utility of self-defeating personality disorder, the Personality Disorders Work Group felt that data were lacking to support its inclusion in DSM-IV, either in the body of the manual or in Appendix B. In the absence of such supportive data, the DSM-IV committee decided that self-defeating personality disorder, should be omitted from the classification. (See Widiger, Chapter 17, for further discussion).

## REFERENCES

Akiskal, H. (1983). Dysthymic disorder: Psychopathology of proposed chronic depressive subtypes. *American Journal of Psychiatry, 140,* 11–20.

American Psychiatric Association. (1980). *Diagnostic and statistical manual of mental disorders* (3rd ed.). Washington, DC: Author.

American Psychiatric Association. (1987). *Diagnostic and statistical manual of mental disorders* (3rd ed., rev.). Washington, DC: Author.

American Psychiatric Association. (1994). *Diagnostic and statistical manual of mental disorders* (4th ed.). Washington, DC: Author.

Baumeister, R. F., & Scher, S. J. (1988). Self-defeating behavior patterns among normal individuals: Review and analysis of common self-destructive tendencies. *Psychological Bulletin, 104,* 3–22.

Berglas, S. (1985). Self-handicapping and self-handicappers: A cognitive/attributional model of interpersonal self protective behaviour. *Perspectives in Personality, 1,* 235–270.

Berglas, S. (1988, August). *Toward treatment matching for patients suffering a self-defeating personality disorder: Anticipatory negative therapeutic reactions.* Paper presented at the 96th Annual Meeting of the American Psychological Association, Atlanta.

Blashfield, R. K., & Breen, M. J. (1989). Face validity of the DSM-III-R personality disorders. *American Journal of Psychiatry, 146,* 1575–1579.

Caplan, P. J. (1985). *The myth of women's masochism.* New York: Dutton.

Caplan, P. J. (1987). The Psychiatric Association's failure to meet its own standards: The dangers of the self-defeating personality disorder category. *Journal of Personality Disorders, 1,* 178–182.

Curtis, R. (Ed.). (1989). *Self-defeating behaviors: Experimental research, clinical impressions, and practical implications.* New York: Plenum Press.

Frances, A. (1980). The DSM-III personality disorder section: A commentary. *American Journal of Psychiatry, 137,* 1050–1054.

Freiman, K., & Widiger, T. (1989). [Co-occurrence and diagnostic efficiency statistics]. Unpublished raw data.

Fuller, A. K. (1986). Masochistic personality disorder: A diagnosis under consideration. *Jefferson Journal of Psychiatry, 4,* 7–21.

Fuller, A. K., & Blashfield, R. K. (1989). Masochistic personality disorder: A prototype analysis of diagnosis and sex bias. *Journal of Nervous and Mental Disease, 177,* 168–172.

Herman, J., & Schatzow, E. (1987). Recovery and verification of memories of childhood. *Psychoanalytic Psychology, 4,* 1–14.

Hyler, S., Skodol, A., Kellman, D., Oldham, J., & Rosnick, L. (1990). Validity of the Personality Diagnostic Questionnaire Revised: Comparison with two structured interviews. *American Journal of Psychiatry, 147,* 1043–1048.

Kaplan, M. (1983). A woman's view of DSM-III. *American Psychologist, 38,* 786–792.

Kass, F. (1987). Self-defeating personality disorder: An empirical study. *Journal of Personality Disorders, 1,* 168–173.

Kass, F., Mackinnon, R. A., & Spitzer, R. L. (1986). Masochistic personality: An empirical study. *American Journal of Psychiatry, 143,* 216–218.

Kass, F., Spitzer, R. L., & Williams, J. B. W. (1983). An empirical study of the issue of sex bias in the diagnostic criteria of DSM III Axis II personality disorders. *American Psychologist, 38,* 799–801.

Kass, F., Spitzer, R. L., Williams, J. B. W., & Widiger, T. A. (1989). Self-defeating personality disorder and DSM-III-R: Development of the diagnostic criteria. *American Psychologist, 146,* 1022–1026.

Kernberg, O. (1984). *Severe personality disorders.* New Haven, CT: Yale University Press.

Millon, T., & Tringone, R. (1989). [Co-occurrence and diagnostic efficacy statistics]. Unpublished raw data.

Pfohl, B. (1990, November). *Discussion.* Paper presented at the NIMH Conference on Personality Disorders, Williamsburg, VA.

Reich, J. (1987). Prevalence of DSM-III-R self-defeating (masochistic) personality disorder in normal and outpatient populations. *Journal of Nervous and Mental Disease, 175,* 52–54.

Reich, J. (in press). Familiality of self-defeating personality disorder. *Journal of Nervous and Mental Disease.*

Rosewater, L. B. (1987). A critical analysis of the proposed self-defeating personality disorder. *Journal Personality Disorders, 1,* 190–195.

Skodol, A., Rosnick, L., Kellman, D., Oldham, J., & Hyler, S. (1988). Validating structured DSM-III-R personality disorder assessment with longitudinal data. *American Journal of Psychiatry, 145,* 1297–1299.

Snell, J., Rosenwald, R., & Robey, A. (1964). The wife-beater's wife. *Archives of General Psychiatry, 11,* 107–112.

Spitzer, R. L., Williams, J. B. W., Kass, F., & Davies, M. (1989). National field trial of the diagnostic criteria for self-defeating personality disorder. *American Journal of Psychiatry, 146,* 1561–1567.

Sprock, J., Blashfield, R. K., & Smith, B. (1990). Gender weighting of DSM-III-R personality disorder criteria. *American Journal of Psychiatry, 147,* 586–590.

Walker, L. (1987). Inadequacies of the masochistic personality disorder diagnosis for women. *Journal of Personality Disorders, 1,* 183–189.

Widiger, T. A., & Frances, A. J. (1989). Controversies concerning the self-defeating personality disorder. In R. Curtis (Ed.), *Self-defeating behaviours: Experimental research, clinical impressions, and practical implications.* New York: Plenum Press.

Williams, J. B. W., & Spitzer, R. L. (1983). The issue of sex bias in DSM-III. *American Psychologist, 38,* 793–798.

Work Group to Revise DSM-III. (1985, October). *DSM-III-R in development.* Washington, DC: American Psychiatric Association.

Work Group to Revise DSM-III. (1986, August). *DSM-III-R in development* (2nd draft). Washington, DC: American Psychiatric Association.

# CHAPTER 17

# Deletion of Self-Defeating and Sadistic Personality Disorders

THOMAS A. WIDIGER

The self-defeating and sadistic personality disorders were included within Appendix A of DSM-III-R, "Proposed Diagnostic Categories Needing Further Study" (American Psychiatric Association [APA], 1987, p. 367). This appendix also contained the late luteal phase dysphoric disorder. The DSM-III-R decisions regarding the self-defeating personality disorder and the late luteal phase dysphoric disorder generated the most controversy in the revision process for DSM-IV. The DSM-IV Personality Disorders Work Group decided to delete the self-defeating and sadistic personality disorders entirely from the manual (Task Force on DSM-IV, 1993; American Psychiatric Association, 1994). It is the purpose of this chapter to present and discuss these decisions.

## SELF-DEFEATING PERSONALITY DISORDER

A masochistic personality disorder diagnosis was included in DSM-III (American Psychiatric Association, 1980). It was grouped with the examples of "atypical, mixed, or other personality disorder" (American Psychiatric Association, 1980, p. 329), along with the impulsive and immature personality disorders (the category was renamed "personality disorder not otherwise specified" [NOS] in DSM-III-R; American Psychiatric Association, 1987, p. 358). Masochistic personality traits, described as "the need to be disappointed or humiliated" (American Psychiatric Association, 1980, p. 274), were also discussed within the differential diagnosis section on sexual masochism.

The diagnosis had been considered for an official code number in DSM-III. Why it did not become an officially recognized personality disorder is "not entirely clear" (Kass, Spitzer, Williams, & Widiger, 1989, p. 1023). Its inclusion was said to be opposed by some who felt that it would overlap too much with the Axis I diagnosis of dysthymia (Widiger & Frances, 1989): Both disorders would be describing a chronically pessimistic, depressed, gloomy, self-destructive, and self-defeating behavior pattern. Kass et al. (1989), however, recalled that it was rejected simply because it was proposed "only shortly before the manual went to press" (p. 1023), and "at the time it seemed as though a descriptive approach to defining the category would be impossible, since the psychoanalytic literature on the disorder focused primarily on psychodynamic rather than descriptive features" (p. 1023).

Frances (1980), a member of the DSM-III Advisory Committee on Personality Disorders, presented his objections to this decision in his early commentary on Axis II of DSM-III. He noted the inconsistency of the DSM-III Task Force decisions to provide a characterological variant of schizophrenia within Axis II (i.e., schizotypal personality disorder), and yet to subsume characterological variants of mood disorders—particularly DSM-II cyclothymic personality disorder (American Psychiatric Association, 1968) and *International Classification of Diseases*, ninth revision (ICD-9), affective personality disorder (which included a depressive type; World Health Organization, 1978)—within the mood disorder diagnoses of cyclothymia and dysthymia. "The inclusion of dysthymic disorder (chronic depressive disorder or depressive neurosis) is a . . . controversial and worrisome decision" (Frances, 1980, p. 1052). The dysthymia diagnosis cuts a broad swath across a large and heterogeneous population. It includes persons with "psychological conflicts that make them pessimistic, self-defeating, and unhappy" (Frances, 1980, p. 1052). Frances suggested that the diagnosis of dysthymia should have been confined to persons with vegetative symptoms: "Nonvegetative chronic depression should have appeared separately under one or another title (I would have preferred depressive or masochistic personality) in the personality disorders section" (p. 1052). Objections to the failure to include a masochistic–depressive personality disorder among the officially recognized personality disorders within DSM-III was subsequently reiterated by various prominent and influential clinicians and researchers (e.g., Asch, 1986; Frances & Cooper, 1981; Gunderson, 1983; Kernberg, 1984; Simons, 1987a).

Spitzer, as chair of the Work Group to Revise DSM-III, responded to these criticisms by developing (in collaboration with Kass and MacKinnon) a criteria set for a masochistic personality disorder. Their proposal, however, placed considerably more emphasis upon the masochistic than upon the depressive aspects of the behavior patterns described by Frances (1980), Kernberg (1984), and others. A pilot test of the criteria set indicated good internal consistency and correlation with clinicians' diagnoses of masochistic personality disorder (Kass, MacKinnon, & Spitzer, 1986). A proposal to provide this diagnosis with an official code number in DSM-III-R was then approved by the DSM-III-R Advisory Committee on Personality Disorders in 1984, and nine criteria were developed and published in the initial draft of DSM-III-R (Work Group to Revise DSM-III, 1985).

The decision to emphasize masochism was helpful in differentiating the proposed personality disorder from the mood disorder of dysthymia, but the emphasis upon masochism also generated considerable opposition and controversy, with formal objections by the APA's Committee on Women and the American Psychological Association's Program on Women (Kass et al., 1989). The major concerns were that the diagnosis would resurrect and provide credibility to an archaic analytic hypothesis that persons (particularly women) unconsciously associate pain with pleasure (Caplan, 1984), and that the diagnosis would often be used to blame victims of abuse for their victimization (Walker, 1984). Victims of abuse may often appear to be submissive, compliant, and resigned for their own self-protection (Browne, 1993); once they are removed and protected from the abuse, their behavior may change (Walker, 1984).

These concerns were understandable. The theoretical orientation of the early proponents for the diagnosis was largely psychoanalytic (e.g., Asch, 1986; Frances & Cooper, 1981; Gunderson, 1983; Kernberg, 1984; Simons, 1987a), and the initial efforts to formulate and pilot the diagnosis were uninformed by the literature and research on victimization (Holden, 1986). A meeting was held on November 18, 1985, to discuss and address the concerns. Attending the meeting were advisory committee members and advisors, as well as opponents of the proposal. It was decided at this meeting to rename the diagnosis "self-defeating personality disorder" to dissociate it from the early theories of masochism; to revise the criteria set to further minimize the likelihood that normal persons (particularly women) would be given the diagnosis; and to provide a special exclusion criterion that the symptoms not occur only in response to or in anticipation of being physically, sexually, or psychologically abused.

The controversy, however, did not subside. The proposal continued to generate vituperative commentaries in local and national news media, protest demonstrations, and threats of legal action (Coalition against Misdiagnosis, 1986; Rosewater, 1986). The APA Board of Trustees appointed an ad hoc committee to review the efforts made by the Work Group to Revise DSM-III, paying particular attention to self-defeating personality disorder and other controversial proposals. On December 3, 1985, the committee recommended that self-defeating personality disorder be included within an appendix to DSM-III-R; on December 7, 1985, the APA Board of Trustees recommended that it be included in the body of the manual; but in June 1986, the board reversed this decision and recommended placing self-defeating personality disorder within an appendix (Kass et al., 1989).

A revision of the criteria set appeared in an appendix to the second draft of DSM-III-R (Work Group to Revise DSM-III, 1986). The appendix at this time was designated for "new categories added to DSM-III-R that are controversial" (Work Group, 1986, p. VIII:1). The name and description of this appendix did not suggest that it was for diagnoses not being given official recognition. In fact, one of the members of this appendix, periluteal phase dysphoric disorder (changed to "late luteal phase dysphoric disorder" in DSM-

III-R and "premenstrual dysphoric disorder" in DSM-IV), was given its own code number and listed within the class of "other disorders associated with physiologic functions" (along with eating and sleep disorders). Self-defeating personality disorder was given the code number of a personality disorder NOS (301.89). However, in the final version of DSM-III-R this appendix was titled "Proposed Diagnostic Categories Needing Further Study" (American Psychiatric Association, 1987, p. 367), and its stated rationale was "to facilitate further systematic clinical study and research" (American Psychiatric Association, 1987, p. 367).

The interpretation and understanding of this appendix have themselves been controversial. The diagnoses within the appendix were said to lack official recognition or approval because they were not included among the officially recognized diagnoses and were not given their own unique code numbers (Widiger, Frances, Spitzer, & Williams, 1988). However, they were included within the manual of officially recognized disorders; they were given a set of criteria for their diagnosis; a code number that could be used for their diagnosis was provided (e.g., 301.89 for self-defeating personality disorder); and a description of their predisposing factors, complications, prevalence, family history, and associated features was also provided. It is difficult to argue that the APA did not consider self-defeating personality disorder to exist—or that the APA was not providing a significant degree of recognition and approval—when it provided a set of diagnostic criteria, gave a code number for diagnosis, and indicated the prevalence, predisposing factors, and family history of self-defeating personality disorder. The provision within DSM-III-R Appendix A did at least provide a quasi-official recognition.

The inclusion of self-defeating personality disorder within DSM-III-R generated considerable controversy. The second issue of the *Journal of Personality Disorders* devoted a special section to the diagnosis (Widiger, 1987), including papers representing the opposing perspectives (i.e., Caplan, 1987; Kass, 1987; Liebowitz, 1987; Rosewater, 1987; Shainess, 1987; Simons, 1987b; Walker, 1987). Many commentaries and reviews have appeared since then. Some have provided a compelling rationale for the diagnosis (e.g., Cooper, 1993), whereas others have provided compelling critiques of its validity and concerns regarding its potential misapplication (e.g., Herman, 1988). A variety of empirical studies on self-defeating personality disorder were also published, but few were directly relevant to the central issues, benefits, and/or concerns regarding the diagnosis.

Spitzer, Williams, Kass, and Davies (1989) did document that many clinicians did indeed support its inclusion. Fifty-one percent of 620 psychiatrists who had noted an interest in personality disorders in APA's *Biographical Directory* indicated that they had seen patients with a pattern of self-defeating behavior; that none of the DSM-III personality disorders were adequate for describing and understanding this behavior; and that they felt there was a need for the diagnosis in DSM-III-R. On the other hand, the survey was conducted in early 1986, and the respondents may not have been sufficiently

aware of the specific issues regarding the diagnosis. One could also interpret the results as indicating an absence of consensus, because 49% of the
respondents indicated no need for the diagnosis. On still another hand, it
would be unusual for any new proposed diagnosis to have widespread
familiarity and support.

Many studies reported significant prevalence rates, but these studies also
indicated substantial overlap and co-occurrence with existing personality disorder diagnoses, particularly the dependent, avoidant, and borderline personality disorders (Fiester, 1991; Reich, 1987; Spitzer et al., 1989). It was never
demonstrated that the diagnosis was describing a behavior pattern that was
not adequately represented by existing diagnoses. The rationale for its inclusion was that "many clinicians believe that no other personality disorder
is adequate to describe this particular pattern of personality disturbance in
which the individual is drawn to situations or relationships in which he or
she will suffer; undermines pleasurable experiences; and prevents others
from helping him or her" (Work Group to Revise DSM-III, 1986, p. IX:43).
There were anecdotal/case history data to support this contention (e.g., Cooper, 1993; Widiger, 1988), but there was no systematic research. For example,
it was not at all clear that the 711 cases of self-defeating personality disorder
reported in Spitzer et al. (1989), the 48 cases in Kass (1987), or the 17 cases
of masochistic personality disorder (as originally defined) in Reich (1987)
involved persons for whom self-defeating personality traits were important
in treatment or in understanding their pathology. Simply meeting the criteria
for the diagnosis, particularly in the context of co-occurring Axis I and Axis
II disorders, would not demonstrate that the diagnosis would have any utility or relevance to understanding the person's predominant issues, problems,
needs, or conflicts. These studies indicated substantial prevalence for the
*diagnosis,* not for the *disorder.*

Most studies reported that more females than males were given the diagnosis (Kass, 1987; Kass et al., 1986; Reich, 1987; Spitzer et al., 1989), but
this is consistent with the theoretical and clinical expectations for the disorder (Widiger & Frances, 1989; Widiger & Spitzer, 1991). Sprock, Blashfield,
and Smith (1990) reported no significant sex-typing within the criteria set,
suggesting that it did not reflect stereotypically feminine sex-role behavior.
Fuller and Blashfield (1989) found that clinicians were just as likely to diagnose males with self-defeating personality disorder as females when provided with descriptions of males with self-defeating symptomatology.

No studies addressed the central issues regarding the diagnosis, such
as the concern that female victims of abuse would be overdiagnosed with
self-defeating personality disorder. There is justification for this concern.
A historical illustration is provided by Snell, Rosenwald, and Robey (1964),
who explained the occurrence of 12 husbands charged with assault and battery as "filling masochistic needs of the wife and . . . necessary for the wife's
(and the couple's) equilibrium" (p. 110). DSM-III-R provided the exclusion
criterion that the behaviors used to make the diagnosis of self-defeating per-

sonality disorder were not to "occur exclusively in response to, or in anticipation of, being physically, sexually, or psychologically abused" (American
Psychiatric Association, 1987, p. 374). However, none of the popular self-
report inventories for the assessment of the DSM-III-R personality disorders
(e.g., the Millon Clinical Multiaxial Inventory-II [Millon, 1987] and the Personality Diagnostic Questionnaire—Revised [Hyler & Rieder, 1987]) provide
any questions to assess for this exclusion criterion; yet data regarding the
prevalence and family history of self-defeating personality disorder have at
times been based on such inventories (e.g., Reich, 1987, 1989). No mention
of the exclusion criterion is even made in some of the DSM-III-R personality disorder semistructured interviews that include self-defeating personality disorder (e.g., Loranger, 1988).

Complicating this issue is the likelihood that some proportion of wom-
en who are being victimized may indeed have self-defeating personality traits.
For example, Snyder and Fruchtman (1981) identified four distinct patterns
of abuse in a sample of 119 persons from a shelter for battered women. At
least one pattern was consistent with the presence of a personality disorder.
These women had experienced extensive violence within their families of
origin. All of them reported substantial parental neglect and abuse on at
least a monthly basis. Snyder and Fruchtman (1981) concluded that these
women "have grown to expect violence and accept it as part of their lives"
(pp. 883–884). Nearly half of them reported abuse in adulthood by persons
other than a current boyfriend; 27% had been abused by their spouses pri-
or to marriage; and they were much more likely than other battered women
to reject the intervention of the shelter in order to return to their assailants
(i.e., 60% left the shelter).

A history of victimization in childhood can result in chronic, enduring,
and pervasive attitudes of self-blame, pessimism, and self-denigration that
will be consistent with self-defeating personality disorder (Baumeister &
Scher, 1988; Browne, 1993; Curtis, 1989; Herman, 1992). Walker's (1984)
learned helplessness model for adult victimization (which results in part from
a history of childhood victimization) is itself consistent with self-defeating
personality disorder (Widiger & Frances, 1989). These persons may not be
seeking pain and suffering (or unconsciously associating pain or suffering
with pleasure), but they can develop an ego-syntonic acceptance of abuse,
or a belief (identity) that they are persons for whom victimization is an expected, natural, and accepted occurrence. Such persons are likely to be revic-
timized. On the other hand, these persons are likely to represent only a
minority of battered women (Strube, 1988). In the study by Snyder and
Fruchtman (1981), the women who appeared to have accepted victimization
constituted only 9% of the total sample of 119 battered women, indicating
the importance of being cautious in diagnosing self-defeating personality
disorder in battered women and in generalizing from such cases to other
victims of abuse.

What the DSM-IV Personality Disorders Work Group needed were empirical studies on the relevance and role of the self-defeating personality disorder diagnosis in victims of abuse. No such studies were known or made available to the work group (Fiester, 1991; Chapter 18). The research on self-defeating personality disorder often failed to consider the occurrence and influence of victimization on the diagnosis (e.g., Reich, 1987; Spitzer et al., 1989), and the research on victimization failed to assess adequately for the occurrence and influence of self-defeating personality traits (e.g., Rosewater, 1987; Walker, 1984).

The self-defeating personality disorder diagnosis continued to be controversial throughout the development of DSM-IV. The debate often generated more heat than light (e.g., Caplan, 1991). Some participants appeared to be more interested in the preservation and even escalation of the controversy than in its resolution. After several meetings, the work group reached an initial consensus that self-defeating personality disorder should not be given its own code number in DSM-IV and at best would be included in an appendix (Fiester, 1991; Task Force on DSM-IV, 1991; Frances et al., 1991). Some members of the work group favored its deletion from the manual, and some favored retaining it within an appendix, but none were without some ambivalence regarding their recommendation.

The final decision was to delete the diagnosis entirely from DSM-IV (American Psychiatric Association, 1994). The balance was perhaps tipped in part by the occurrence of a court case in which the self-defeating personality disorder diagnosis was apparently being used in the defense of a prominent psychiatrist who was being sued by a female resident for an alleged discrimination. It was unlikely that the diagnosis would be influential in the outcome of this case, but the case did provide an immediate and vivid illustration of the potential influence and potential misuse of the diagnosis. The inclusion within an appendix would appear to provide a credibility to the diagnosis that may not yet be warranted. Potential misuse does not negate or belie the validity of a diagnosis (Fiester, 1991), but the validity of self-defeating personality disorder is itself questionable. A diagnosis that has the potential for harm against a particular segment of the population should be held to an especially high standard of validation before it is given any official credibility.

It is possible, however, that the DSM-IV Personality Disorders Work Group and the DSM-IV Task Force succumbed to the political pressure to delete the diagnosis (Walker, 1989). The deletion of the diagnosis will be a disservice to persons, including women, for whom maladaptive self-defeating traits represent a central and significant problem in their lives. However, its presence in DSM-III-R and in the *DSM-IV Sourcebook* (Widiger, Frances, Pincus, Davis, & First, 1991) should be sufficient encouragement to the proponents of the diagnosis to pursue the documentation of its validity and clinical utility (Pincus, Frances, Davis, First, & Widiger, 1992). In addition, the presence of depressive personality disorder in Appendix B of DSM-IV (Task Force, 1993; American Psychiatric Association, 1994) will represent many of the self-defeating traits (e.g., pessimism and self-blame) that were included in the original proposals by Frances (1980), Frances and Cooper (1981), and Kernberg (1984), without the excess baggage provided by the construct of masochism.

## SADISTIC PERSONALITY DISORDER

The initial impetus for the sadistic personality disorder was provided by a forensic psychiatrist, Martha Gay. Gay worked (and continues to work) with perpetrators and victims of abuse. She noticed in the 1985 draft of DSM-III-R (Work Group to Revise DSM-III, 1985) the presence of a diagnosis that would apply to the adult victims of abuse (i.e., masochistic personality disorder), but no diagnosis that would apply well to the perpetrators of the abuse. She suggested that many of these perpetrators have sadistic personality traits.

Spitzer was responsive to this suggestion and noted the proposal in the November 18, 1985, meeting of proponents, opponents, and other persons concerned with the DSM-III-R masochistic personality disorder proposal. Spitzer cited the existence of the sadistic personality disorder proposal in response to an argument that DSM-III-R would be labeling victims of abuse as having a mental disorder, but not the perpetrators. His rejoinder was subsequently characterized as an effort at a "horse trade," or offering sadistic personality disorder in exchange for the withdrawal of the opposition to masochistic personality disorder (Leo, 1985). Perceptions and memories of meetings, particularly ones in which there has been heated debate, are often inconsistent and inaccurate. In my opinion, the characterization of the proposal as an effort at a horse trade was quite inaccurate and misleading (Widiger et al., 1988).

Sadistic personality disorder appeared in the second draft of DSM-III-R (Work Group to Revise DSM-III, 1986). The rationale provided for its inclusion was as follows: "Although systematic studies of this category are lacking, it was added to DSM-III-R because many clinicians who evaluate individuals (primarily men) who abuse spouses or children believe there is a need for identifying this particular pattern of personality disturbance" (Work Group to Revise DSM-III, 1986, p. IX:43). Sadistic personality disorder was included within the appendix for "new controversial categories" (Work Group to Revise DSM-III, 1986, p. VIII:1). The rationale at this time for the appendix was to highlight the importance of being especially careful and cautious in the use of the diagnoses contained therein: "These categories may have a high potential for misapplication; therefore, these diagnoses should be given only after an especially careful differential diagnostic evaluation and when the diagnostic criteria are clearly met" (Work Group to Revise DSM-III, 1986, p. VIII:1). One might question whether the same admonition should not apply to the diagnosis of any and all mental disor-

ders. In any case, as noted earlier in the discussion of self-defeating personality disorder, the final decision was for this appendix to be called "Proposed Diagnostic Categories Needing Further Study" (American Psychiatric
Association, 1987, p. 367), and for its rationale to be "to facilitate further
systematic clinical study and research" (American Psychiatric Association,
1987, p. 367). Sadistic personality disorder was not given its own unique code
number (it was provided with the personality disorder NOS code number
of 301.90). In other words, presentation within DSM-III-R Appendix A was
intended to encourage research on particular diagnoses that were not yet
being given official approval or recognition (rather than to emphasize especially careful diagnosis of disorders having a high potential for misuse).

Some, however, have questioned the rationale of providing diagnoses
within the DSM primarily for the purpose of stimulating the research needed to determine whether they should be given official approval. "Including
an unproven experimental diagnostic category in DSM-IV may confer upon
that category an approval which it does not yet merit" (Pincus et al., 1992,
p. 114). Pincus et al. (1992) cited in particular the DSM-III-R sadistic personality disorder: "Research should drive DSM and not the other way around"
(p. 114). The DSM attempts to wear many and often conflicting hats (Frances,
Pincus, Widiger, Davis, & First, 1990). A manual that provides the list of officially recognized disorders to guide clinical, treatment, insurance, disability, forensic, and other important social and clinical decisions will complicate
and confuse these decisions if it also considers its purpose to include guiding the future direction of research. It will not always be clear which diagnoses have been approved for clinical practice and which have not. A manual
with the purpose of generating and guiding future research would probably be quite different from DSM-III-R and DSM-IV, and would perhaps be
more appropriately the domain of a research agency (e.g., the National Institute of Mental Health) that could develop a manual of new diagnoses, conditions, and constructs in need of additional or special research. The
"proposed diagnostic categories" appendix to any edition of the DSM should
at least be confined to those proposals that the respective work group and
task force believe will be approved in the next edition.

The inclusion of sadistic personality disorder in Appendix A of DSM-
III-R was not particularly successful in generating research. This may,
however, reflect in part the limited amount of time that had transpired since
its appearance (Zimmerman, 1988) and in part the infrequency of research
focused on any specific personality disorder other than the borderline,
schizotypal, and antisocial disorders (Blashfield, 1993). In any case, the only
published studies on sadistic personality disorder were those conducted by
the original proponents of the diagnosis (i.e., Gay, in press; Spitzer, Fiester,
Gay, & Pfohl, 1991). Most of the prevalence and comorbidity findings reported by Fiester and Gay (1991) were obtained simply by the presence of the
sadistic personality disorder criteria set within DSM-III-R semistructured interviews, the findings from which were made available to the Personality Dis-

orders Work Group (Widiger, 1991). These prevalence rates could have been obtained by any set of proposed personality disorder diagnostic criteria. Even something as farcical or satirical as the "delusional dominating personality disorder" proposed by Pantony and Caplan (1991) will obtain a prevalence rate.

The study by Gay (1989, in press), however, does provide credible support for the diagnosis. Gay found that 5% of 235 consecutive adults accused of child abuse met the DSM-III-R criteria for sadistic personality disorder, which required that the sadistic behavior not be confined to just one person. Of these 12 males, 9 abused both their wives and their children. Most importantly, 10 of these 12 persons apparently failed to meet the DSM-III-R criteria for any other personality disorder (only 1 was given a diagnosis of antisocial personality disorder). Only half had any past or current Axis I disorder, and this was confined in each case to a substance-related disorder, which would not negate or conflict with a diagnosis of sadistic personality disorder. None were considered to have a sexually sadistic paraphilia. In addition, these 12 persons had a history that would be consistent with the development of maladaptive personality traits. For example, 9 of the 12 reported a history of substantial physical abuse as a child (2 also reported sexual abuse).

The findings of the study by Spitzer et al. (1991), however, were mixed. Spitzer et al. conducted the survey to document the statement that "many clinicians who evaluate individuals . . . who abuse spouses or children believe there is a need for identifying this particular pattern of personality disturbance" (Work Group to Revise DSM-III, 1986, p. IX:43). Spitzer et al. sent a questionnaire in July 1989 to all of the 1,390 members of the American Academy of Psychiatry and the Law. Usable responses were provided by 279 respondents (i.e., 20%). When asked whether they had "ever personally evaluated, in a forensic setting, an individual who demonstrated a pervasive pattern of cruel, demeaning, and aggressive behavior that meets the [DSM-III-R] criteria for sadistic personality disorder [provided] above" (p. 876), 52% ($n$ = 141) answered yes. They further indicated that they had personally evaluated, on average, six such individuals (or 4% of their total evaluations per year). Seventy-five percent of the persons who met the DSM-III-R sadistic criteria were also said to meet the DSM-III-R criteria for antisocial personality disorder, but 73% of their psychiatrists indicated that it would still be useful to provide both diagnoses. The diagnosis of sadistic personality disorder would provide unique and special emphasis on aggressive personality traits (Widiger et al., 1988).

Psychiatrists' opinions regarding the inclusion of sadistic personality disorder in DSM-IV, however, were less encouraging. A majority of the respondents (66%) believed that the diagnosis had considerable potential for misuse, particularly in the mitigation of criminal responsibility in cases of child or spouse abuse. Only 11% of the respondents believed that it would be "very useful and should be included" (Spitzer et al. 1991, p. 877); 29% believed that it was of "no or limited value and likely to be abused" (p. 877); and 16% indicated that it was "perhaps useful, but [there were] inadequate data to justify its inclusion" (p. 877). In other words, only 11% supported its inclusion, and 45% clearly opposed it. These results are inconsistent with the original impression that "many" forensic psychiatrists believe there is a need for its inclusion, unless one interprets 11% as being "many" and ignore the 45% who clearly opposed its inclusion. It should be noted that the remaining 44% indicated that the diagnosis could be useful "but should only be included in DSM-IV if there is any research or clinical data demonstrating its utility (validity) as a diagnosis that is distinct from other personality disorders" (p. 877). The only such data were provided by Gay (1989, in press) and Spitzer et al. (1991). Gay's findings are encouraging but need to be replicated (e.g., a sample of 12 sadistic personality disorder subjects is minimal, and the finding that only 2 of them met the DSM-III-R criteria for another personality disorder should be replicated). In other words, one could interpret the Spitzer et al. survey as indicating that 89% of forensic psychiatrists actually opposed the inclusion of the diagnosis.

The DSM-IV Personality Disorders Work Group not only recommended that sadistic personality disorder not be elevated to the body of the manual, but also that it be deleted entirely from the manual. The rationale for retaining it within an appendix was "the hope that its continued presence will stimulate future research that will help in deciding its ultimate fate" (Fiester & Gay, 1991, p. 384). However, as indicated above, it was decided that this would not be a sufficient rationale for the inclusion of sadistic personality disorder within the manual. Provision within an appendix, it was felt, would provide a credibility and quasi-official recognition that is not yet warranted. There are likely to be sadistically aggressive and domineering persons who are not adequately characterized by the antisocial personality disorder diagnosis (Gay & Fiester, 1991; Widiger et al., 1988), but before the diagnosis is given any official credibility, there should be more systematic research.

## CONCLUSIONS

Self-defeating personality disorder was the personality diagnosis that created the most controversy in the preparation of both DSM-III-R and DSM-IV. It will now be of interest whether self-defeating and sadistic personality disorders disappear from the clinical and research literature, or whether there is sufficient motivation and support to generate the necessary research for their consideration in DSM-V. What the authors of DSM-V will need to reach a fully informed decision will be objective and dispassionate research that is focused directly on the key issues, such as the clinical utility (benefits and harm) and validity of a diagnosis of self-defeating personality disorder to victims of abuse and of sadistic personality disorder to perpetrators of abuse. In addition, it will also be useful to further clarify the purpose (and to assess the effect) of diagnoses included in a DSM appendix for further study.

## REFERENCES

American Psychiatric Association. (1968). *Diagnostic and statistical manual of mental disorders* (2nd ed.). Washington, DC: Author.

American Psychiatric Association. (1980). *Diagnostic and statistical manual of mental disorders* (3rd ed.). Washington, DC: Author.

American Psychiatric Association. (1987). *Diagnostic and statistical manual of mental disorders* (3rd ed., rev.). Washington, DC: Author.

American Psychiatric Association. (1994). *Diangostic and statistical manual of mental disorders* (4th ed.). Washington, DC: Author.

Asch, S. S. (1986). The masochistic personality. In R. Michels (Ed.), *Psychiatry* (Vol. 1, pp. 1–9). Philadelphia: J. B. Lippincott.

Baumeister, R. F., & Scher, S. J. (1988). Self-defeating behavior patterns among normal individuals: Review and analysis of common self-destructive tendencies. *Psychological Bulletin, 104,* 3–22.

Blashfield, R. K. (1993, September). *Growth of the personality disorder literature from 1975 to 1991.* Poster presented at the 3rd International Congress on the Disorders of Personality, Cambridge, MA.

Browne, A. (1993). Violence against women by male partners. *American Psychologist, 48,* 1077–1087.

Caplan, P. J. (1984). The myth of women's masochism. *American Psychologist, 39,* 130–139.

Caplan, P. J. (1987). The Psychiatric Association's failure to meet its own standards: The dangers of self-defeating personality disorder as a category. *Journal of Personality Disorders, 1,* 178–182.

Caplan, P. J. (1991). How do they decide who is normal? The bizarre, but true, tale of the DSM process. *Canadian Psychology, 32,* 162–170.

Coalition against Misdiagnosis. (1986). *Information packet: The DSM-III-R diagnoses.* Seattle, WA: Author.

Cooper, A. M. (1993). Psychotherapeutic approaches to masochism. *Journal of Psychotherapy Practice and Research, 2,* 1–13.

Curtis, R. C. (Ed.). (1989). *Self-defeating behaviors: Experimental research, clinical impressions, and practical implications.* New York: Plenum Press.

Fiester, S. J. (1991). Self-defeating personality disorder: A review of data and recommendations for DSM-IV. *Journal of Personality Disorders, 5,* 194–209.

Fiester, S. J., & Gay, M. (1991). Sadistic personality disorder: A review of data and recommendations for DSM-IV. *Journal of Personality Disorders, 5,* 376–385.

Frances, A. J. (1980). The DSM-III personality disorders section: A commentary. *American Journal of Psychiatry, 137,* 1050–1054.

Frances, A. J., & Cooper, A. M. (1981). Descriptive and dynamic psychiatry: A perspective on DSM-III. *American Journal of Psychiatry, 138,* 1198–1202.

Frances, A. J., Pincus, H. A., Widiger, T. A., Davis, W. W., & First, M. B. (1990). DSM-IV: Work in progress. *American Journal of Psychiatry, 147,* 1439–1448.

Frances, A. J., Widiger, T. A., First, M. B., Pincus, H. A., Tilly, S. M., Miele, G. M., & Davis, W. W. (1991). DSM-IV: Toward a more empirical diagnostic system. *Canadian Psychology, 32,* 171–173.

Fuller, A. K., & Blashfield, R. K. (1989). Masochistic personality disorder: A prototype analysis of diagnosis and sex bias. *Journal of Nervous and Mental Disease, 177,* 168–172.

Gay, M. (1989, May). Personality disorders among child abusers. In R. L. Spitzer (Chair),

*Psychiatric diagnosis, victimization and women.* Symposium conducted at the 142nd Annual Meeting of the American Psychiatric Association, San Francisco.

Gay, M. (in press). Sadistic personality disorder in a child-abusing population. *Child Abuse and Neglect.*

Gay, M., & Fiester, S. J. (1991). Sadistic personality disorder. In R. Michels (Ed.), *Psychiatry* (rev. ed., Vol. 1, pp. 1–13). Philadelphia: J. B. Lippincott.

Gunderson, J. G. (1983). DSM-III diagnosis of personality disorders. In J. Frosch (Ed.), *Current perspectives on personality disorders* (pp. 20–39). Washington, DC: American Psychiatric Press.

Herman, J. (1988). *Self-defeating personality disorder and sadistic personality disorder: A conceptual critique and review of recent research.* Unpublished manuscript.

Herman, J. (1992). *Trauma and recovery.* New York: Basic Books.

Holden, C. (1986). Proposed new psychiatric diagnoses raise charges of gender bias. *Science, 231,* 327–328.

Hyler, S. E., & Rieder, R. (1987). *The Personality Diagnostic Questionnaire — Revised.* New York: New York State Psychiatric Institute.

Kass, F. (1987). Self-defeating personality disorder: An empirical study. *Journal of Personality Disorders, 1,* 168–173.

Kass, F., MacKinnon, R. A., & Spitzer, R. L. (1986). Masochistic personality disorder: An empirical study. *American Journal of Psychiatry, 143,* 216–218.

Kass, F., Spitzer, R. L., Williams, J. B. W., & Widiger, T. A. (1989). Self-defeating personality disorder and DSM-III-R: Development of the diagnostic criteria. *American Journal of Psychiatry, 146,* 1022–1026.

Kernberg, O. F. (1984). *Severe personality disorders* (pp. 77–94). New Haven, CT: Yale University Press.

Leo, J. (1985, December 2). Battling over masochism: Psychiatrists and feminists debate "self-defeating" behavior. *Time,* p. 76,

Liebowitz, M. R. (1987). Commentary on the criteria for self-defeating personality disorder. *Journal of Personality Disorders, 1,* 196–199.

Loranger, A. W. (1988). *Personality Disorders Examination (PDE) manual.* Yonkers, NY: DV Communications.

Millon, T. (1987). *Millon Clinical Multiaxial Inventory-II Manual (MCMI-II).* Minneapolis, MN: National Computer Systems.

Pantony, K., & Caplan, P. J. (1991). Delusional dominating personality disorder: A modest proposal for identifying some consequences of rigid masculine socialization. *Canadian Psychology, 32,* 120–133.

Pincus, H. A., Frances, A. J., Davis, W. W., First, M. B., & Widiger, T. A. (1992). DSM-IV and new diagnostic categories: Holding the line on proliferation. *American Journal of Psychiatry, 149,* 112–117.

Reich, J. H. (1987). Prevalence of DSM-III-R self-defeating (masochistic) personality disorder in normal and outpatient populations. *Journal of Nervous and Mental Disease, 175,* 52–54.

Reich, J. H. (1989). Familiality of DSM-III self-defeating personality disorder. *Journal of Nervous and Mental Disease, 178,* 597–598.

Rosewater, L. B. (1986, August). The DSM-III-R: Ethical and legal implications for feminist therapists. In R. Garfinkel (Chair), *Politics of diagnosis: Feminist psychology and the DSM-III-R.* Symposium conducted at the 94th Annual Meeting of the American Psychological Association, Washington, DC.

Rosewater, L. B. (1987). A critical analysis of the proposed self-defeating personality disorder. *Journal of Personality Disorders, 1,* 190–195.

Shainess, N. (1987). Masochism—or self-defeating personality? *Journal of Personality Disorders, 1,* 174–177.

Simons, R. C. (1987a). Applicability of DSM-III to psychiatric education. In G. T. Tischler (Ed.), *Diagnosis and classification in psychiatry: A critical appraisal of DSM-III* (pp. 510–529). New York: Cambridge University Press.

Simons, R. C. (1987b). Self-defeating and sadistic personality disorders: Needed additions to the diagnostic nomenclature. *Journal of Personality Disorders, 1,* 161–167.

Snell, J., Rosenwald, R., & Robey, A. (1964). The wife-beater's wife: A study of family interaction. *Archives of General Psychiatry, 11,* 107–112.

Snyder, D., & Fruchtman, L. (1981). Differential patterns of wife abuse: A data-based typology. *Journal of Consulting and Clinical Psychology, 49,* 878–885.

Spitzer, R. L., Fiester, S. J., Gay, M., & Pfohl, B. (1991). Results of a survey of forensic psychiatrists on the validity of the sadistic personality disorder diagnosis. *American Journal of Psychiatry, 148,* 875–879.

Spitzer, R. L., Williams, J. B. W., Kass, F., & Davies, M. (1989). National field trial of the DSM-III-R diagnostic criteria for self-defeating personality disorder. *American Journal of Psychiatry, 146,* 1561–1567.

Sprock, J., Blashfield, R. K., & Smith, B. (1990). Gender weighting of DSM-III-R personality disorder criteria. *American Journal of Psychiatry, 147,* 586–590.

Strube, M. J. (1988). The decision to leave an abusive relationship: Empirical evidence and theoretical issues. *Psychological Bulletin, 104,* 236–250.

Task Force on DSM-IV. (1991). *DSM-IV options book: Work in progress.* Washington, DC: American Psychiatric Association.

Task Force on DSM-IV. (1993). *DSM-IV draft criteria.* Washington, DC: American Psychiatric Association.

Walker, L. E. A. (1984). *The battered woman syndrome.* New York: Springer.

Walker, L. E. A. (1987). Inadequacies of the masochistic personality disorder diagnosis for women. *Journal of Personality Disorders, 1,* 183–189.

Walker, L. E. A. (1989). Psychology and violence against women. *American Psychologist, 44,* 695–702.

Widiger, T. A. (1987). The self-defeating personality disorder: Introduction. *Journal of Personality Disorders, 1,* 157–160.

Widiger, T. A. (1988). Treating self-defeating personality disorders. *Hospital and Community Psychiatry, 39,* 819–821.

Widiger, T. A. (1991). DSM-IV reviews of the personality disorders: Introduction to special series. *Journal of Personality Disorders, 5,* 122–134.

Widiger, T. A., & Frances, A. J. (1989). Controversies concerning the self-defeating personality disorder. In R. C. Curtis (Ed.), *Self-defeating behaviors: Experimental research, clinical impressions, and practical implications* (pp. 289–309). New York: Plenum Press.

Widiger, T. A., Frances, A. J., Pincus, H. A., Davis, W. W., & First, M. B. (1991). Toward an empirical classification for the DSM-IV. *Journal of Abnormal Psychology, 100,* 280–288.

Widiger, T. A., Frances, A. J., Spitzer, R. L., & Williams, J. B. W. (1988). The DSM-III-R personality disorders: An overview. *American Journal of Psychiatry, 145,* 786–795.

Widiger, T. A., & Spitzer, R. L. (1991). Sex bias in the diagnosis of personality disorders: Conceptual and methodological issues. *Clinical Psychology Review, 11,* 1–22.

Work Group to Revise DSM-III. (1985). *DSM-III-R in development*. Washington, DC: American Psychiatric Association.

Work Group to Revise DSM-III. (1986). *DSM-III-R in development* (2nd draft). Washington, DC: American Psychiatric Association.

World Health Organization. (1978). *International classification of diseases* (9th revision). Geneva: Author.

Zimmerman, M. (1988). Why are we rushing to publish DSM-IV? *Archives of General Psychiatry, 45*, 1135–1138.

# PART IV

# BASIC ISSUES AND ALTERNATIVE PERSPECTIVES

# CHAPTER 18

# On the Importance of Theory to a Taxonomy of Personality Disorders

ROGER DAVIS
THEODORE MILLON

How can we best conceptualize and organize the clinical data that comprise personality disorders? Not only are these data complex, but they can be approached from a variety of frames of reference. Behaviorally, they can be conceived and grouped as complex response patterns to environmental stimuli. Biophysically, they can be approached and analyzed as sequences of complex neural and chemical activity. Intrapsychically, they can be inferred and categorized as networks of entrenched unconscious processes that bind anxiety and conflict. Quite evidently, the complexity and intricacy of personological phenomena make it difficult not only to establish clear-cut relationships among phenomena, but also to find simple ways in which these phenomena can be classified or grouped. Should we artificially narrow our perspective to one data level to obtain at least a coherency of view? Or should we trudge ahead with formulations that bridge domains, but threaten to crumble by virtue of their complexity and potentially low internal consistency?

Because of such intrinsic complexity, psychologists are still seeking a completely satisfying approach to personality and its nexus with psychopathology. Despite many prolonged and brilliant ruminations, the current state of psychopathological nosology resembles Ptolemy's astronomy of over 2,000 years ago: Our diagnostic categories describe, but they do not really explain. Like so many crystalline spheres, each lies in its own orbit, for the most part uncoordinated with the others. We do not know why this universe takes its ostensive form. There is no law of gravity that undergirds and binds our psychopathological cosmos together. In fact, the word "cosmos" implies an intrinsic unity, a laudable ideal, which is not appropriate in its usage: Our "star charts," our DSMs, remain aggregations of taxons, not true taxonomies. Their reliability, but dubious validity, lend our field the illusion of science but not its substance.

Perhaps the most radical option is simply to dispense with taxonomies altogether. Of course, that is impossible. Both clinically and scientifically, a taxonomy serves certain functional ends. Clinically, it provides a means of organizing pathological phenomena—the signs and symptoms or manifestations of mental disorder. By abstracting across persons, a taxonomy formalizes certain clinical commonalities and relieves the clinician of the burden of conceptualizing each patient *sui generis,* as an entity so existentially unique that it has never been seen before nor ever will be again. For psychopathology to be practiced at all, there cannot be as many groups as individuals. Even if the formal categories that constitute a taxonomy are but convenient fictions of dubious reality, some groups are better than no groups at all.

On a deeper, scientific level, knowledge about nature depends crucially on the representations of nature encoded in a classification system. Only mystics presumably possess the ability to transcend the gulf between subject and object in a mutual absorption of mind and nature. Indeed, the very lure of mystical knowledge is that it is unmediated. Mysticism promises a direct mode of seeing—one that possesses an "absolute" quality difficult to argue with. Were such knowledge possible and readily available, science itself would be unnecessary. Mind and nature would be perfectly coordinated, without any need of intermediate representations and nomological linkages. In this sense, perhaps the most existentially disappointing aspect of religion is that there is more than one: The mystics have gone to the mountain and come back with different tales.

Despite such disappointments, taxonomists of personology can learn much from the mystics, both as a point of contrast and as a point of departure. By making the comparison we at least know what our goals are. In short, we want what the mystics have (or say they have): We want a clear vision; we want freedom from confusion. Our greatest dream is one of almost mystical insight, wherein our representational blinders are removed and the inner essences of reality are revealed—for the purposes of this chapter, the substantive structural and functional variables that comprise personology and its nexus with psychopathology.

Scientifically, however, the actual mystical experience leaves something to be desired. Usually it resists representation, perhaps actively so, proving ultimately too numinous and ineffable to articulate. Science, of course, cannot afford the luxury of being numinous and ineffable. Science depends on self-conscious knowledge. What is numinous to the mystic is vague to the scientist. Whereas mystics comprehend nature in its totality as a radically open system of seamless unity, scientists must create artificially closed relational systems. We are wedded to representational systems, including taxonomies—so wedded, in fact, that the abandonment of all representational schemas would be an abandonment of knowledge itself. In the best of all possible worlds, of course, we would have both the experience of true seeing and a representational system by which to articulate it; such is the holy grail of a taxonomy of personality disorders. And only such a taxonomy "should be viewed as having objective existence in nature" (Hempel, 1965, p. 146), as carving nature at its joints or affording a sense of communion that goes beyond intervening variables and construct systems — the only true validity, that which comes from an intuition of nature as it is. A scientist born thinking within such a taxonomy might never become conscious of the representational aspect; the taxonomy would be completely transparent. Whether such a taxonomy exists or whether it must remain an ideal that all actual taxonomies will fall short of to various degrees, only just such a taxonomy will prove ultimately scientifically satisfying for the personality disorders, and ultimately satisfying to the researchers and clinicians who must work inside it.

The examination of intentions that has formed the theme of this introduction to our chapter is be continued throughout. What is interesting is how assumptions about what the world is like inform how the world is investigated and what qualifies as worthy of being designated as truth. We argue that only a theoretical approach is prepared to reveal the "essential entities" called personality disorders that have "objective existence" in nature. In one way or another, our discussion returns to the issue of the "comorbidity" of the personality "disorders." Much of the recent research and commentary addressed to the problems of Axis II concerns comorbidity, so an investigation of the assumptions underlying this area of contention is potentially illuminating. The prevailing view is that comorbidity is a great evil, as if any at all were too much. This view is backed up by empirical research showing that many patients are diagnosed with four or more personality disorders. More troublesome is the fact that, since we lack the direct knowledge of the mystics, we cannot be sure whether this enigmatic state of affairs is an intrinsic feature of the personological domain itself or whether it is a by-product of intervening variables.

## CONCEPTUAL OPENNESS VERSUS CONCEPTUAL SPECIFICITY

### Theoretical and Empirical Approaches to Personality Syndromes

How should personological phenomena be investigated? Should we remain close to the assumptions and constructs of common sense, refining our measures until we can advance with sure-footed precision? Or should we seek conceptual innovations that will partition the personological realm in ways that are more theoretically and clinically fruitful? One option would be to anchor personological phenomena directly in the empirical world of observables in a one-to-one fashion, tying each attribute to only one indicator. Each

attribute would then be its own mode of measurement, possessing no information beyond that contained in the procedure itself; this is akin to what
have been called "operational definitions" (Bridgeman, 1927).

The virtue of operational definitions lies in their precision, but their
vice lies in their scope. Ultimate empirical precision can only be achieved
if every defining feature that distinguishes a taxon is anchored to a single
observable in the real world—that is, a different datum for every difference
observed between personality syndromes. This goal is simply not feasible
or desirable: The subject domain of personology is inherently more weakly
organized than that of the so-called "hard" sciences. As one moves from physics and chemistry into biological and psychological arenas, unidirectional
causal pathways give way to feedback and feedforward processes, which in
turn give rise to emergent levels of description that are more inferential than
the physical substrates underlying them. Intrapsychic formulations, for example, require that the clinician transcend the level of the merely observable. Owing to their abstract and hypothetical character, these indeterminate
and intervening concepts are known as "open concepts" (Pap, 1953).

The polar distinction between operational definitions and open concepts represents in part an epistemological continuum from conceptual specificity to conceptual openness—a continuum from those who prefer to employ
data derived from empirical/practical contexts to those who prefer to draw
their ideas from more causal/theoretical sources (Millon, 1987). Each end
of this polarity embraces a compromise between scope and precision. The
virtue of each hides its vices. The advantage of operationism is obvious: Personality syndromes and the attributes of which they are composed are rend-
ered unambiguous. Diagnostic identifications are directly translatable into
measurement procedures, maximizing precision. However, the direct map-
ping of attributes to the measurement procedures required ignores the
biases inherent in any one procedure, so that operationism is fatally deficient in scope.

The advantage of open concepts is likewise obvious: Open concepts acknowledge the desirability of multiple measurement procedures and encourage their users to move freely in more abstract and inferential realms.
Each open concept can be embedded in a theoretical matrix or network from
which its meaning is derived through its relations with other open concepts,
with only indirect reference to explicit observables. The disadvantage is that
open concepts may become so circuitous in their references that they become tautological and completely decoupled from the empirical realm. No
doubt clarity gets muddled in statements such as this: "In the borderline individual the mechanisms of the ego disintegrate when libidinous energies
overwhelm superego introjections." In such formulations, the "scope" of a
theory overwhelms the testability of its empirical linkages, rendering precision zero.

Obviously, every scientific model is a simplification of nature and thus
involves some compromise between scope and precision. We are not yet mys-

tics at the beginning of a science: Unlike the individual born thinking in a taxonomy that carves nature at its joints, we are acutely conscious that the relations among our naive representations are not those intrinsic to the subject domain itself. No one today would seriously put the humoral theory of Hippocrates forward as a model of personality syndromes. Instead, such formulations resemble the more or less unrefined and often self-contradictory knowledge of common sense, rather than the well-criticized and well-corroborated knowledge of science. But, as disputable as common sense is, it is nevertheless the point of departure for scientific knowledge (Pepper, 1942) and a source of common-sense taxonomies. Hempel (1965) framed this progression in terms of stages:

> The development of a scientific discipline may often be said to proceed from an initial "natural history" stage . . . to more and more theoretical stages, in which increasing emphasis is placed upon the attainment of comprehensive theoretical accounts of the empirical subject matter under investigation. The vocabulary required in the early stages of this development will be largely observational: It will be chosen so as to permit the description of those aspects of the subject matter which are ascertainable fairly directly by observation. The shift toward systematization is marked by the introduction of new, "theoretical" terms, which refer to various theoretically postulated entities, their characteristics, and the processes in which they are involved; all these are more or less removed from the level of directly observable things and events.
>
> These terms have a distinct meaning and function only in the context of the corresponding theory. (pp. 139–140)

What is it that distinguishes these two broad approaches at the level of the individual? What is it that each individual scientist does to execute his or her approach? Evidently, the theoretical approach is driven primarily by taking perspective on sense-near representations in order to discover underlying theoretical/casual relations from which a more coherent, internally corroborating system of constructs might be established. New constructs are generated, "more or less removed from the level of directly observable things and events." Some old ones are discarded, while others have their meaning sharpened or transformed as the system of relations is made more explicit. A process of reflection seems essential. Such representations are referred to here as "theoretical constructs," to reinforce their abstract origins in the mind of a reflective scientist.

The empirical approach, by contrast, is inherently suspicious of theory and tends to keep close to sense-near representations. As such, the vocabulary of empiricism remains "largely observational," in Hempel's terms. As an ideal type, empirical preoccupations tend toward the progressive refinement of methods of observing of pre-existing constructs, rather than the generation of new ones; they tend toward ever greater agreement of one observer with another (interrater reliability), an observer with himself or herself (reliability over occasions), and greater purity of observation (internal consistency).

Few scientists today are naive empiricists. However, as noted by Kukla (1989), "no science embraced empiricism more wholeheartedly than psychology." Moreover, some of the assumptions underlying empiricism are insidious and difficult to escape from, even when one ostensibly believes in the utility of theory. Foremost among criticisms is that the empiricism of common sense, naive realism, believes that the world it takes in is the world as it is. Common-sensical empiricism literally believes that its constructs are the world. There is no reason to leave the security of immediate perception. Ultimately, this agenda rests on the assumption that theory-neutral data exist—that is, that one can know the world without transforming it. In the world view of radical empiricism, there are no mediating mental constructs to foul things up. If only this were so, then every act of observation would be an act of knowledge. Each small fact would present us with an objectivity to be plucked from the world like fruit, collected as a hobby, or catalogued like microscope slides. Because naive empiricism remains unconscious of the potentially deceiving role of mental constructs, it believes itself to be carving nature at its joints just as it is. Naive empiricism, then, is really a false mysticism that breaches the gulf between subject and object by denying that any such gulf exists; it is a naive realism, believing that what you see is what you get.

## What Has Cognitive Value to Empiricism?

Does naive realism inform thinking about personality disorders? Yes, mainly in the way of what is believed to possess cognitive value in terms of making personological discriminations. Pepper (1942) casts the discussion as follows:

> The standing criticism to which rough data are subjected is that they are not pure observations, but are loaded with interpretation. . . . A datum, as its derivation indicates, is supposed to be something given, and purely given, entirely free from interpretation. The search for multiplicative corroboration is the effort on the part of a datum to confirm its claim to purity.
>
> Refined data [therefore] consist of pointer readings and correlations among pointer readings.
>
> Where data are concerned, the aim is to attain cognitive items so clear and distinct and simple that disagreement about them among men can scarcely arise. That is what has driven multiplicative refinement to pointer readings, and what gives these data such great reliability. No special skill is needed to note what mark on a dial a black needle rests upon. Anyone with a pair of eyes and a most elementary capacity for following instructions can take a pointer reading. The most brilliant scientist and his most stupid student both easily agree about the reading. Everybody who can look at it can see for himself where the pointer comes. That excessive naivete, and just that, is what makes the evidence so credible and refined. (pp. 51–53)

How do personality psychologists seek out "items so clear and distinct . . . that disagreement can hardly arise"? As in the hard sciences, these are concerned with signal and noise, though in a statistical rather than a physical sense. One of these techniques is aggregation (e.g. Epstein, 1979), based on Abraham Lincoln's old proverb: "It is true that you may fool all of the people some of the time; you can even fool some of the people all the time; but you can't fool all of the people all the time." From Lincoln's proverb we can extract various forms of reliability—namely, reliability over subjects and over occasions. More importantly, we can extract perhaps the principlal touchstone of empiricism: that with enough pure observations, the essence of personality will be revealed. By sampling randomly among possible observational units, potential biases distribute themselves equally, so that only signal (what is common to the units) is additive. The emphasis on aggregation reaches its highest point in meta-analytic studies, where the results of numerous studies are pooled in order to permit investigators to better estimate the "true" correlations and effect sizes. Efforts to "confirm [the] claim to purity" of a datum have lead to the creation of and preference for tests of high internal consistency: A scale should be a pure pointer reading, measuring only its intended construct and nothing but the construct.

## The Empirical View of Error

More than anything else, the obsession with error and with what is deemed as error gives insight into the empirical mindset. If the kind of seeing, the empirical methodologies, are not at fault, then the problem must be the degree of seeing—a problem that the empiricist seeks to mitigate through aggregation. Like any scientist, the empiricist wants to see personality syndromes clearly. Unlike theorists, however, who can take perspective on the naive category system and the system of relations that common sense has furnished as a means of refining common sense, naive empiricists have only their pointer readings to preoccupy them in their search for what is really real. Accordingly, they favor the discrete and atomistic. Scales that are factorially complex—those that operationalize a diagnostic type, for example—are inherently suspected of impurity, of confounding two or more essential entities.

The search for pure pointer readings turns especially ugly when the pointer readings have high internal consistency, but are nevertheless intercorrelated. Correlated pointer readings are inherently ambiguous. Does $A$ cause $B$, does $B$ cause $A$, or are both $A$ and $B$ the product of some third entity? A confusion of levels often ensues. Let us assume for the moment that a narcissism scale is factor-analyzed and two factors are extracted, called "egocentricity" and "dominance"; now we have a higher-order concept, narcissism, and two lower-order extracts. Do egocentricity and dominance drive narcissism, so that narcissism is a convenient fiction, a label applied to people who are egocentric and dominant? Or does narcissism simply express itself through egocentricity and dominance? This confusion leads to a taxonomic quandary. If lower-order traits drive higher-order concepts, then a taxonomy of personality disorders should be articulated at the trait level. The traits are what are really real. However, if the higher-order constructs simply express themselves through lower-order traits, then the taxonomy should be articulated at this more molar level.

When the number of traits expands to 20 or so, the intercorrelations involved in the resulting $20 \times 20$ correlation matrix are almost impossible to make sense of. How is one to escape from this confusion? One option is simply to eliminate the intercorrelations, ideally with a factor analysis. Ambiguities are suppressed and the desire for precision is satisfied through the extraction of orthogonal or independent dimensions. The variance unaccounted for by the factor model is deemed to be error variance or variance attributable to measurement error, and the converse is also thought to be true: The variance accounted for is personologically relevant information. One has only to name the resulting factors to feel that something of great value has been discovered. Taken to an extreme, this view demands that every entity in its purview, whether dimensional or categorical, must be independent of every other entity at the same level of abstraction to be "really real." In dimensional terms, existence equals orthogonality. In categorical terms, existence equals discreteness. Comorbidity is error.

If empiricism is sustained by assumptions that are scientifically untenable, one might expect that it would suffer the fate of old generals and just fade away. What other forces might be responsible for its pervasiveness? An empirical approach to personality disorders gets a big boost from the disease or medical model. The disease model furnishes the intercorrelational paranoia of naive empiricism with a paradigm that validates this very paranoia. Naive empiricism demands independent or discrete entities, and the disease model backs it up with its emphasis on discrete underlying causes. Naive empiricism tends to stay close to common sense, to the world of physical, observable, concrete objects. Likewise, the disease model posits real and independent material entities creating and sustaining an insidious disease process as underlying mental disorders.

However, personality disorders are not "foreign" entities or lesions that intrude insidiously within the person to undermine healthy functioning. The archaic notion that all mental disorders represent external intrusions or internal disease processes is an offshoot of prescientific ideas, such as the notion that demons or spirits "possess" or cast spells on a person. The role of infectious agents has reawakened this archaic view. This conception also appeals to the less sophisticated clinician, for it enables him or her to believe that the insidious intruder can be identified, hunted down, and destroyed. Indeed, the very language in which clinically interesting personality patterns are discussed has been appropriated from the disease model and involves "medical jargon highly prejudicial to the issue" (Carson, 1993, p. 98). Usage of the terms "diagnosis," "disorder," and "comorbidity" is most unfortunate,

invoking images of some underlying, unitary disease process and perpetu-
ating the misconception that health and disease exist as a dichotomy rather
than as a continuum. One cannot be both infected and uninfected at the
same time. The result is that Axis II is being discussed in the terminology
of Axis I.

Unfortunately, there is no alternative vocabulary through which to discuss personality patterns of clinical interest in a manner appropriate to the
intrinsic nature of the personality domain. The term "personality syndrome"
is only slightly better than "personality disorder," and the term "personality
pathology" is worse. Personality is inherently more fluid and dimensionalized than the dichotomies imposed on it by the disease model, representing
a tightly knit organization of attitudes, habits, and emotions that shades
progressively from normality to abnormality. No sharp line divides normal
from pathological behavior. Not only is personality so complex that certain
areas of psychological functioning operate normally while others do not,
but environmental circumstances change in such a way that behaviors and
strategies that prove adaptive at one time fail to do so at another.

Moreover, there is a sense in which the "diagnosis" of personality pathology is irrelevant to any particular case. The adoption of the multiaxial model,
recognizing the embeddedness of classical psychiatric problems in the personological–psychosocial interaction, is a genuine structural advance in the
conception of psychopathological behavior — one far superior to a horizontal cacophony that represents psychiatric, personological, and psychosocial
problems as all existing on the same plane. In the multiaxial model, personality disorders have been given a contextual role. This acknowledges that
the significance of the Axis I symptoms varies as a function of the interaction between Axis II and Axis IV — that is, between the patient's inherent
dispositions and his or her psychosocial environment. Even if the individual does not receive an Axis II diagnosis, the nature of this interaction is still
relevant to the treatment of the case, since the Axis I symptoms must be understood contextually rather than on their own terms. Thus the model has
been structurally composed to favor the explanation of the symptoms or
presenting complaints.

## CONCEPTUAL ASPIRATION: MONOTAXONIC
## AND POLYTAXONIC EMPIRICAL APPROACHES
## TO A TAXONOMY OF PERSONALITY DISORDERS

What other forces might modulate the connection among theory, empiricism, and taxonomy? In what is here called the "monotaxonic" approach,
a smaller piece of the larger pie becomes the object of theoretical speculation or empirical investigation. As its name suggests, this orientation is concerned with what goes on within a single taxonomic unit of analysis, whether
this is a categorical, dimensional, prototypical, or circumplical segment.

Whatever the unit of analysis, its core feature is that it does not attempt to bring order to the entire personality milieu, but rather limits its aspirations to some more circumscribed area of interest. At the opposite extreme is what is here called the "polytaxonic" approach, which seeks to impose some structural edifice upon the entire personological domain. This orientation seeks to explicate latent entities, through either a deductive theoretical approach or a multivariate mathematical approach (such as cluster analysis or factor analysis). Whatever the taxonomic unit of analysis, its core feature is its intention to parse the entire personological domain.

Crossing these two polarities — the first concerning a disposition to take perspective on observations in order to create a coherent theoretical framework versus a disposition to remain close to pre-existing categories or dimensions and refine one's observations; the second concerning a disposition to parse a portion of the personological totality versus a disposition to be concerned with the totality itself — leads to a four-category metataxonomy of approaches to the personality disorders. The derived categories are best viewed as prototypes. That is, just as there is a natural heterogeneity among clinical features of personality, such that not all patients exhibit identical features, there is also a heterogeneity among approaches to the personological domain. Many, but not all, approaches or methodologies can easily be placed within this framework. The monotaxonic and polytaxonic empirical approaches are now discussed; the monotaxonic and polytaxonic theoretical orientations are considered later in ths chapter.

## The Descriptive Monotaxonic Empirical Approach

Prototypically, the descriptive monotaxonic empirical approach tends to focus on a single diagnostic category. As with any empirical approaches to taxonomy, the direction of the argument is from measure to reality. Accordingly, what is learned is learned through exploring the structure of the measures or instruments themselves, rather than through generating new concepts by some process of theoretical refinement. Typically, single or multiple measures are decomposed psychometrically into their constituent elements — again, often through factor analysis.

Obviously, since this approach demands an isomorphism between instrument and reality, it is at its weakest when it employs only a single scale or procedure. The biases that accompany the scale tend to distort the necessary isomorphism and compromise the interpretation of results. Increasingly self-conscious of their heritage, studies of this kind employ multiple measures in the analysis, as a means of extending the aggregation principle to the scale level. Just as the biases inherent in any one item fail to accumulate in a large representative sample of items, the biases inherent in any one scale presumably fail to accumulate when aggregated. Thus whatever components are extracted are components not merely of a single intervening variable, but of reality itself. Again, the direction of the argument is from intervening variable to the nature of the personality variable of interest.

The inherently decompositional methodology of this top-down empiricism tends to get this approach associated with reductionism, and to multiply the number of essential personological features without limit. Nowhere is this better seen than in the history of trait psychology, where the sheer number of traits ultimately casts doubt on the "reality" of any one trait. Apparently, our belief that a particular classification system "carves nature" can sustain shorter lists of categories or dimensions better than longer or interminable lists. With a shorter list, there is the feeling that the boundaries of a domain are known; as the list length increases, the model becomes more unsatisfying, until a feeling that there is no constraint on the number of units of analysis sets in.

## The Descriptive Polytaxonic Empirical Approach

Prototypically, like its cousin above, the descriptive polytaxonic empirical approach is driven by the refinement of sense-near representations. Taxonomically, however, it is concerned not with a smaller piece of the larger pie, but with deriving the entire set of categories or dimensions of the personality domain. Like any empirical approach to taxonomy, it depends crucially on an isomorphism between reality and sense-near representations. That is, the direction of the argument is from these representations to reality, or, in psychological terms, from reliability to validity. What is learned is learned by gathering many diverse measures and subjecting these to a multivariate analysis, which seeks to distill their commonalities or clusters. Typically, the process of theoretical reflection and refinement is not engaged, and few constructs beyond those named by measures entering the data analyses are generated. Whereas the monotaxonic approach may be thought of as working from the top down, moving in the direction of greater specificity as larger units are distilled into smaller ones, this approach works from the bottom up, moving in the direction of greater commonality, combining smaller units into those of greater bandwidth.

The five-factor model of personality is perhaps the epitome of the descriptive polytaxonic empirical approach. Use of sense-near representations is ensured through the lexical hypothesis, which assumes that "most of the socially relevant and interpersonally salient personality characteristics have become encoded in the natural language" (John, 1990, p. 67). According to Digman (1990), the five-factor model has been replicated across multiple data sources, in children and adults, and in several different languages. The factor-analytic method lends the empiricist a way of dealing with the intercorrelations that are so confusing at a sense-near level through the method of factor rotation, the explicit purpose of which is to render the factors more interpretable. Although rotations that yield intercorrelated factors are possible, an orthogonal rotation is by far the most popular; it suppresses the ambiguous intercorrelations out of existence, thus creating a model of laudable scope, if somewhat illusionary precision. Discreteness is quantified as the angle between dimensions, and dimensions that are completely discrete or orthogonal are preferred.

Because of its ability to rotate factors and present completely discrete dimensions as results, factor analysis offers a means of rehabilitating trait psychology. Recall that the top-down or monotaxonic approach tends to multiply the number of units of analysis without limit. Factor analysis restores the short list, recalling George Miller's "seven plus or minus two" — the number of elements in any group or series that human cognition seems to prefer.

## Professional Language versus Common Language

An interesting issue that has recently emerged concerns the tenability of the lexical hypothesis itself for clinical domains of personality. Whereas dimensions of normal personality may be encoded as low-inference representations in the language, those of the clinical or professional language are by definition not so encoded. An argument for the sufficiency of the five-factor model with respect to personality disorders is in fact an argument that the professional language contains nothing that is incremental to the superficialities of the normal lexicon. Otherwise the five-factor model could only be characterized as insufficient rather than sufficient for clinical work. Is the clinical language nothing more than a recapitulation or a pretentious elaboration of the popular judgment — just new wine in normal bottles? If so, then the conclusion that must be drawn is that the thinking of the last hundred years or so is completely redundant with respect to the judgments of normal persons as encoded in the common language.

Fortunately, professional languages differ from the common language, however, because they serve a different purpose. As Hempel (1965) noted, the early stages of the development of a science are characterized by descriptive and observational vocabulary — for example, that contained in the English-language dictionaries culled by the original investigators in the lexical tradition, Allport and Odbert (1936). The clinical language, however, reflects the contributions of various historical schools and their theoreticians, according to the latent structures and processes each believed to be operative. This suggests the possibility that the professional language might also be explored empirically, but with the object of clarifying the essential dimensions of personality disorders through an analysis of the professional vocabulary of psychopathology. Differences between the resulting structures could potentially bear on the validity of the lexical hypothesis, since information surplus to that contained within the five-factor model must be considered unique to the professional language.

Livesley, Jackson, and Schroeder (1989, 1992) attempted to determine whether the underlying trait patterns implicit in the professional language would arrange themselves in a pattern similar to that of the DSM-III (American Psychiatric Association, 1980). These investigators constructed 100 scales according to a content analysis of the professional literature, and subjected these scales to an oblique rather than an orthogonal rotation, resulting in 15 factors and accounting for 75% of the variance of the original 100 scales. Recall the inverse relationship between scope and precision. If the role of error variance is neglected, at this factoring level one-quarter of the information specific to the professional language as contained in the original scales was lost. Schroeder, Wormworth, and Livesley (1992, 1994) reported a four-factor solution of the Dimension Assessment of Personality Pathology-Basic Questionnaire (DAPP-BQ) developed to provide a shorter representation of these 100 scales. This solution accounted for 67% of the total variance. These authors also performed a canonical correlation using the five-factor model as operationalized with the Neuroticism, Extraversion, Openness Personality Inventory (NEO-PI) (Costa & McCrae, 1985) to predict DAPP-BQ scales. A strong but imperfect relationship was found.

The existence of linkages between the common-language five-factor model and the Livesley et al. professional-language model should be comforting both to common-language speakers and to psychopathologists and theorists. First, it indicates that those traits encoded in the common language, however coarse, are not so devoid of information of intrinsic personological importance that their usage is completely unjustified — certainly a situation that would surprise common-language speakers if it were indeed the case. Second, it indicates that theorists and others who have made terminological contributions to the professional language have not become so self-bootstrapped that their innovations float completely untethered to more common-sensical notions. There is partial overlap between these two universes of discourse, as there should be.

## THEORETICAL APPROACHES TO PERSONALITY DISORDERS

Assuming that one's temperament is oriented more toward theoretical explanation than toward empirical description — in other words, that one's propensity runs more toward reflecting on the near-sense representations and propositions of common sense as a means of refining them — how might one go about one's labors? Are there different kinds of theoretical approaches? If so, what are the potential benefits of each for producing a taxonomy of personality disorders? Is a synthesis possible, such that the strengths of each might be combined in a coherent framework? How does each regard the comorbidity or codiagnosis of personality disorders?

Two kinds of theory must be distinguished. Again, the distinction is one concerning the scope of inquiry — whether a single or a few diagnostic categories are addressed (here referred to as a "monotaxonic" orientation) or whether the entire domain of personality pathology is parsed in its entirety (here referred to as a "polytaxonic" orientation). The former orientation is primarily concerned with a single taxonomic unit of analysis, whether this is a categorical, dimensional, or circumplical segment or a DSM hierarchical cluster; its core feature is that it does not attempt to bring order to the entire personality milieu, but limits its aspirations.

## The Explanatory Monotaxonic Theoretical Orientation

The within-category theoretical orientation is probably what comes to mind when most people think about theory or testing a theory. Because it is limited in scope, it is primarily concerned with the essential elements that eventuate in and sustain a particular kind of personality pattern. In its most impressive longitudinal incarnation, models for personality pathology produced by this approach may be explicated through diagrams and flow charts that detail the developmental history of the disorder, complete with the inputs of various factors that predispose individuals to or immunize them against the disorder along the way. Alternately, it may develop as a stage model, with pathology representing the regression to earlier stages of development (as in the oral character, the anal character, etc.).

Although this approach potentially leads to gains in precision, it tends to be somewhat deficient in scope. Since the intention is to understand the origins of pathology, it accepts whatever categories are given it and then it accounts for the developmental origin of these pathologies. Moreover, there is a tendency to parse the particular personality pattern in terms of a single-area clinical domain, whether this is behavioral, phenomenological, intrapsychic, or biophysical. The classical view of narcissism, for example, contends that it is the result of developmental arrests or regressions to earlier periods of fixation. An important elaborator of the narcissism construct is Kohut (1971). Kohut does not challenge the content as such, but rather the sequence of libidinal maturation, which he believed has its own developmental line and sequence of continuity into adulthood. That is, it does not fade away by becoming transformed into object libido, as contended by classical theorists, but unfolds into its own set of mature narcissistic processes and structures. Pathology occurs as a consequence of failures to integrate one of the two major spheres of self-maturation, the "grandiose self" and the "idealized parent imago." If an individual is disillusioned, is rejected, or experiences cold and unempathic care at the earliest stages of self-development, serious pathology (e.g., psychotic or borderline states) will occur. Trauma or disappointment at a later phase will have somewhat different repercussions, depending on whether the difficulty centers on the development of the grandiose self or on the parental imago.

What is notable is that Kohut's is a developmental theory of self and not a personality characterization. Indeed, it is difficult for developmental models to give rise to the kind of taxonomies of scope that are needed for the DSM (see Millon & Davis, 1995, however). Thus, although the explanatory monotaxonic theoretical approach may illuminate the developmental origins of personality pathology (though almost certainly with some bias as to domains of content), this approach works best when it is not held to account for why certain individuals have been segregated into a particular pattern of disorders in the first place. It needs to be given its pathology to begin with; it is nongenerative with respect to categories of personality disorder.

Theories that bridge multiple clinical domains are far fewer, perhaps because any attempt to do so seeks the assimilation of elements that to some extent intrinsically resist unification—otherwise, they could hardly be thought of as existing as domains at all. Accordingly, these models also tend to be reductionistic, in the sense that while all of these domains are domains of an integrated organism, only one area is focused on at a time. Relevant manifestations of pathology from other areas tend to be reduced to operations in that one. Often this kind of reductionism is passive rather than active, in that other domains are passively ignored. As a result, the same diagnostic term, anchored exclusively to one domain, may acquire diverse connotations. Of course, organismic domains have been with us much longer than relatively well-developed taxonomies such as the DSM's.

## The Explanatory Polytaxonic Theoretical Orientation

The monotaxonic theoretical orientation seeks to explain the origins of personality pathology, but typically it must be given its raw material (the disorder of interest) first, and work backward from there. Can a complete science rest on such a foundation? Is it enough merely to accept some external consensus concerning which constellations of traits or disorders are problematic? Whereas the periodic table is the unique province of chemistry, the problematic behaviors that are to be carved up into diagnostic categories are often given to psychopathologists by parties whose standards are extrinsic to psychopathology as a science. The polytaxonic approach, however, asks that categories of personality pathology account for themselves, by persistently inquiring: "Why these categories rather than others?"

Philosophers of science agree that the system of kinds undergirding any domain of inquiry must itself be answerable to the question that forms the very point of departure for the scientific enterprise: Why does nature take this particular form rather than some other? Accordingly, one cannot merely accept any list of kinds or dimensions as given, even if it has been arrived at by committee consensus. Instead, a taxonomic scheme must be justified, and to be justified scientifically, it must be justified theoretically. Taxonomy and theory, then, are intimately linked. Quine (1977) makes a parallel case:

> . . . one's sense of similarity or one's system of kinds develops and changes . . . as one matures. . . . And at length standards of similarity set in which are geared to theoretical science. The development is away from the immediate, subjective, animal sense of similarity to the remoter objectivity of a similarity deter-

> mined by scientific hypotheses . . . and constructs. Things are similar in the later
> or theoretical sense to the degree that they are . . . revealed by science. (p. 171)

Is such a taxonomy possible? The stakes are nothing less than whether personology is to possess its own intrinsic taxonomy or to remain a pseudoscience that provides a service to the larger society, establishing diagnostic
standards according to extrinsic standards. Perhaps we live in a more en-
lightened age, but was it not so long ago that Sullivan (1947) proposed the
"homosexual personality"? Or that the "masochistic personality" came under fire as being prejudicial against women? Although the DSM was deliberately and appropriately formulated atheoretically in order not to alienate
special-interest groups among psychological consumers, ultimately we will
require some way of culling the wheat from the chaff that depends on scientific necessity rather than decision by committee.

The deductive approach generates a true taxonomy to replace the primitive aggregation of taxons that preceded it. This generative power is what
Hempel (1965) meant by the "systematic import" of a scientific classification.
Meehl (1978) has noted that theoretical systems comprise related assertions,
shared terms, and coordinated propositions that provide fertile grounds for
deducing and deriving new empirical and clinical observations. What is elaborated and refined in theory, then, is understanding: an ability to see relations more clearly, to conceptualize categories more accurately, and to create
greater overall coherence in a subject—that is, to integrate its elements in
a more logical, consistent, and intelligible fashion. Pretheoretical taxonomic boundaries that were set according to clinical intuition and empirical study
can now be affirmed and refined according to their constitution along underlying polarities. These polarities lend the model a holistic, cohesive structure that facilitates the comparison and contrast of groups along fundamental
axes, thus sharpening the meanings of the taxonomic constructs derived.

## Manifest and Latent Similarity

In Hempel's (1965) terms, all natural classifications are classifications, but
not all classifications are natural. Not all classification systems carve nature
at its joints, affording the kind of "true seeing" discussed previously. In fact,
an infinite number of classification systems, whether dimensional or categorical, could be proposed for the personality disorders. In this sense, the
purpose of deductive theory is to cull from an infinite number of ways of
grouping clinical phenomena only those that have the potential to "carve
nature"—that is, those that have systematic import with respect to further
hypotheses, and ultimately for methods of therapy and intervention. Hempel (1965) distinguished these two kinds of classifications:

> . . . distinctions between "natural" and "artificial" classifications may well be ex-
> plicated as referring to the difference between classifications that are natural

and those that are not: in a classification of the former kind, those characteristics of the elements which serve as criteria of membership in a given class are associated, universally or with high probability, with more or less extensive clusters of other characteristics. . . . [A] classification of this sort should be viewed as somehow having objective existence in nature, as "carving nature at the joints," in contradistinction to "artificial" classifications, in which the defining characteristics have few explanatory or predictive connections with other traits . . . (pp. 146–147)

What happens, however, when the two are confounded—that is, when more theoretically grounded taxons that carve nature exist side by side in a taxonomy with those based on superficial appearances. As noted, the difference between natural and artificial classification turns on the distinction between manifest or empirical and latent or theoretical levels of similarity. Table 18.1 represents possible agreement and disagreement between manifest and latent levels of similarity for two individuals.

As indicated by the table, for a universe of two patients' presentations, four possibilities exist. Beginning with the first one, we see that two empirically similar presentations may in fact be similar. In this case, what appears to be is indeed the case. Second, two empirically similar presentations may in fact be different. In this case, appearances are deceiving: Two taxons are indicated, but the empirical similarity of the presentations makes them difficult to tease apart. Third, two presentations that appear different may in fact be similar. In this case, again, appearances are deceiving: This time, the empirical difference makes the latent level of similarity (i.e., membership is the same category) difficult to see. Fourth, two presentations that appear different may in fact be different. In this case, different empirical presentations legitimately indicated different category membership. Table 18.1 resembles other tables used to present the logic of diagnostic efficiency statistics, positive and negative predictive power, sensitivity, and specificity (e.g., Baldessarini, Finklestein, & Arana, 1983). Whereas these represent the diagnostic dilemma associated with imperfect predictors in ignorance of the "true" state of nature for a single subject, Table 18.1 represents the nosological dilemma, whereby a classification system must be established on the

TABLE 18.1. Matches and Mismatches for Latent and Manifest Levels of Similarity

| Similar at manifest level? | Similar at latent level? | |
|---|---|---|
| | Yes | No |
| Yes | I. Things that appear similar are in fact similar. | II. Things that appear similar are in fact different. (Nosologically problematic) |
| No | III. Things that appear different are in fact similar. (Nosologically problematic) | IV. Things that appear different are in fact different. |

basis of imperfect attributes, in ignorance of the "true" system that carves natures at its joints. Nosologically, the possibilities represented in quadrants II and III present tremendous difficulties for a classification of personality disorders. Focus on superficial patterns of covariation alone will lead in the second quadrant to the institution of one taxon where two or even many more may be needed, and in the third quadrant to the institution of two (or perhaps many more) where only one in fact exists. But this is the "bet" of empiricism: that things that look alike are alike, and conversely, that things that look different are different — in other words, that there are no cases of mismatched latent and manifest similarity. Such empiricism may be said to have a "horizontal" world view. We might refer to this as the "nature–number" dilemma of empirical taxonomy, in that on the basis of empirical observation alone, it is impossible to fix nonarbitrarily either the nature or the number of the taxons of a classification system. Unless we ask, "Why these particular categories rather than others?", both the nature and number of taxons in a classification system are free to vary — fixed only by virtue of our naive category systems, our preconceptions of natural science, our animal sense of similarity, and, of course, standards extrinsic to our science.

As Quine (1977) noted in his discussion of natural kinds, once the basis on which a system of kinds is founded is explicated, our attachment to a taxonomy loosens in favor of the underlying principles. After all, it was these very underlying principles that allowed the deduction of the taxonomy in the first place. Those who are familiar with the deductive personological taxonomy developed by Millon know, for example, that both the narcissistic and antisocial personalities are independent types, in that both are oriented toward the self. What distinguishes them is primarily their orientation toward their ecologic milieual. Thus, the narcissistic personality is a passive–independent type, and the antisocial personality is an active–independent type. Similarly, the dependent personality is a passive–dependent type; what distinguishes the dependent from the narcissistic personality is primarily an orientation toward others versus an orientation toward self. Nevertheless, both narcissists and antisocials, and narcissists and dependents, share important characteristics.

In the deductive schema explicated by Millon (1981, 1990), the dependent, narcissistic, and antisocial types are deduced from underlying theoretical principles. Far from being orthogonal, then, measures that dimensionalize these types will be correlated because they reflect an intrinsic relationship predicted by the underlying principles. In fact, it is difficult to see how any set of categories that purports to lay claim to scientific necessity through a deductive framework might be dimensionalized and still remain orthogonal, since the deduced types will share common elements, whereas orthogonality is by definition the absence of a relationship. The very generativity of a personological model that claims deductive scientific necessity is then encoded in the intercorrelations of measures of its derived categories. Accordingly, the task of personological science is to account for these intercorrelations, not to suppress them methodologically as is done through factor analysis. Thus the antisocial is very often narcissistic, and the narcissist is also often quite dependent.

Nor must these intercorrelations be confined to the personological domain. As noted, the multiaxial model has been structurally composed to require the explanation of the Axis I symptoms in the context of Axis II personality patterns. Explanation can only occur if some predictions are made. In other words, multiaxial explanation requires that the Axis I disorders not be distributed randomly with respect to Axis II, since if they were distributed randomly, they would again be independent or orthogonal. If a theoretical model of personology is at all worth its salt, it should make some predictions about the way in which various personality styles are psychiatrically dysfunctional—or, in disease terms, make some predictions about Axis I–Axis II comorbidity. Thus the generativity of a personological model with regard to Axis I symptoms will again be encoded in the intercorrelations of measures of Axis I disorders and Axis II personality patterns, which are often discussed as spectrum disorders when these intercorrelations are brought into the foreground.

Far from being a nuisance, then, correlations between diagnostic measures are highly desirable, if these correlations are expected clinically and can be explained theoretically. Significant correlations (dimensional framework) or dual diagnoses (categorical framework) between narcissistic and antisocial personality disorders, for example, should be expected. In fact, the absence of any such correlation should cause us to question the validity of the diagnostic system.

The disadvantage of this approach is that it requires a high degree of clinical and theoretical sophistication. Numerous questions must be answered at theoretical and statistical levels. Are the underlying principles from which the personological taxonomy derived cogent? Do they in fact allow us to understand clinical phenomena? Do they give a complete representation of the subject domain? Do they help explain why each personological type is dysfunctional in some ways and not others? What degree of intercorrelation between the intervening variables that dimensionalize the theory-generated diagnostic types is desirable?

Given these complications and an empirical disposition, perhaps it is more pragmatic in the short run to work with statistically independent gauges extracted through a particular multivariate methodology based on superficial similarities, such as the five-factor model. However, pragmatic virtues are not necessarily scientific, and only a theoretical approach can ultimately form a firm foundation for a science of clinical personology—one that explains rather than merely describes; one that explicates and gives logic to syndromal relationships, rather than forcing them apart to meet archaic and undesirable goals.

# REFERENCES

Allport, G. W., & Odbert, H. S. (1936). Trait-names: A psycho-lexical study. *Psychological Monographs, 47*(No. 211).

American Psychiatric Assocation. (1980). *Diagnostic and statistical manual of mental disorders* (3rd ed.). Washington, DC: Author.

Baldessarini, R., Finklestein, S., & Arana, G. (1983). The predictive power of diagnostic tests and the effect of prevalence of illness. *Archives of General Psychiatry, 40,* 569–573.

Bridgeman, P. W. (1927). *The logic of modern physics.* New York: Macmillan.

Carson, R. C. (1993). Can the Big Five help salvage the DSM? *Psyhological Inquiry, 4,* 98–99.

Costa, P. T., & McCrae, R. R. (1985). *The NEO Personality Inventory manual.* Odessa, FL: Psychological Assessment Resources.

Digman, J. M. (1990). Personality structure: Emergence of the five-factor model. *Annual Review of Psychology, 41,* 417–440.

Epstein, S. (1979). The stability of behavior: I. On predicting most of the people most of the time. *Journal of Personality and Social Psychology, 37,* 1097–1126.

Hempel, C. G. (1965). *Aspects of scientific explanation and other essays in the philosophy of science.* New York: Free Press.

John, O. P. (1990). The "Big Five" factor taxonomy: Dimensions of personality in the natural language and in questionnaires. In L. A. Pervin (Ed.), *Handbook of personality: Theory and research.* New York: Guilford Press.

Kohut, H. (1971). *The analysis fo the self.* New York: International Universities Press.

Kukla, A. (1989). Non-empirical issues in psychology. *American Psychologist, 44,* 785–794.

Livesley, W. J., Jackson, D. N., & Schroeder, M. L. (1989). A study of the factorial structure of personality pathology. *Journal of Personality Disorders, 3,* 292–306.

Livesley, W. J., Jackson, D. N., & Schroeder, M. L. (1992). Factorial structure of traits delineating personality disorders in clinical and general population samples. *Journal of Abnormal Psychology, 101,* 432–440.

Meehl, P. E. (1978). Theoretical risks and tabular asteriks: Sir Karl, Sir Ronald, and the slow progress of soft psychology. *Journal of Consulting and Clinical Psychology, 46,* 806–834.

Millon, T. (1981). *Disorders of personality: DSM-III, Axis II.* New York: Wiley–Interscience.

Millon, T. (1987). On the nature of taxonomy in psychopathology. In C. G. Last & M. Hersen (Eds.), *Issues in diagnostic research.* New York: Plenum Press.

Millon, T. (1990). *Toward a new personology.* New York: Wiley.

Millon, T., & Davis, R. (1995). *Disorders of personality: DSM-IV, Axis II and beyond.* New York: Wiley–Interscience.

Pap, A. (1953). Reduction-sentences and open concepts. *Methods, 5,* 3–30.

Pepper, S. C. (1942). *World hypotheses: A study in evidence.* Berkeley: University of California Press.

Quine, W. V. O. (1977). Natural kinds. In S. P. Schwartz (Ed.), *Naming, necessity, and natural groups.* Ithaca, NY: Cornell University Press.

Schroeder, M. L., Wormworth, J. A., & Livesley, W. J. (1992). Dimensions of personality disorder and their relationship to the Big Five dimensions of personality. *Psychological Assessment, 4,* 47–53.

Schroeder, M. L., Wormworth, J. A., & Livesley. (1994). Dimensions of personality disorder and the five-factor model of personality. In P. T. Costa, Jr., & T. A. Widiger (Eds.), *Personality disorders and the five-factor model for personality.* Washington, DC: American Psychological Association.

Sullivan, H. S. (1947). *Conceptions of modern psychiatry.* New York: Norton.

# CHAPTER 19

# Interrelationships among Categories of Personality Disorders

## M. TRACIE SHEA

The specification of explicit criteria for personality disorders, first introduced in DSM-III (American Psychiatric Association, 1980), has resulted in a substantial increase in empirical investigations. Despite the increase in research, however, surprisingly little is known about the validity of the 11 DSM-III-R (American Psychiatric Association, 1987) specific personality disorder categories and criteria sets. One aspect of such validity is descriptive; that is, do the categories and criteria correspond to clinical reality? Support for descriptive validity would be demonstrated by distinctness (i.e., little overlap) among the disorders, and by similarity of cases within the same diagnosis (homogeneity). Unfortunately, most of the research to date has demonstrated substantial overlap among the personality disorders, as well as heterogeneity within individual disorders (Clark, 1992). A consistent finding is that the majority of individuals with a personality disorder diagnosis receive more than one such diagnosis, and the average number of personality disorder diagnoses per patient has been reported to be as high as 4.6 (Skodol, Rosnick, Kellman, Oldham, & Hyler, 1988). These findings suggest that the 11 DSM-III-R criteria sets do not represent distinct disorders, and thus that the multiple diagnoses received by patients do not represent "comorbid" disorders.

Particularly high rates of overlap have been found among certain pairs and groupings of personality disorders (Oldham et al., 1992). Narcissistic personality disorder was found by these investigators to have high rates of overlap with antisocial, histrionic, and passive–aggressive personality disorders. Borderline and histrionic personality disorders also had high rates of overlap, as did avoidant and schizotypal disorders, and avoidant and dependent disorders. Although overlap occurred most frequently within the same Axis II clusters (i.e., the "dramatic, erratic" and "anxious, fearful" clusters), overlap also occurred among personality disorders in different clusters (e.g., avoidant and schizotypal).

Reducing overlap was a major goal in considering revisions of the personality disorder criteria for DSM-IV (Gunderson, in press; Widiger, 1991a). This effort included analyses of multiple data sets to determine co-occurrence rates and patterns among the disorders. The sensitivity and specificity of each of the criteria were also examined to determine their contribution to the overlap (Widiger, 1991a). It is likely that the modifications of the personality disorder criteria made in DSM-IV (American Psychiatric Association, 1994), based in large part on findings from these analyses, will result in reduced overlap among the disorders and increased homogeneity within disorders. However, it is also likely that overlap and lack of distinctness among the personality disorder categories will remain problematic until more profound changes are made in the DSM system.

The goal of this chapter is to consider features of the DSM classification system that contribute to the lack of clarity regarding boundaries and the excessive rate of overlap among the personality disorders. Different aspects of the system are considered, including the method of classification (categorical) used, as well as the content (i.e., the specific disorders and features of the criteria sets).

## CATEGORICAL SYSTEM

The DSM classification system for personality disorders, like that for the Axis I disorders, is a categorical one, based on the medical model/disease-oriented approach to diagnosis. By definition, this approach assumes that a disorder is present or absent, according to the presence or absence of specified criteria. It has become increasingly clear that this classification approach is not well suited for the domain of personality (e.g., Grove & Tellegen, 1991; Livesley, 1991; Widiger, 1991b). Whereas categorical systems depend upon clear boundaries, most personality features appear to be continuously distributed, without clear separation of abnormality from normality. In addition, the features defined by the various categories are not mutually exclusive; patients can and do show features of more than one disorder. Thus, the boundaries among the categories and between abnormality and normality are inherently indistinct.

Given the limitations of the DSM categorical system, alternative methods of classification have been proposed as more appropriate for the personality disorders. Many in the field have argued for dimensional models, although the choice among the many existing dimensional models is controversial (Widiger, 1991b; Widiger and Frances, 1994; see Widiger & Sanderson, Chapter 22, this volume). Others have noted that the personality disorders are better suited for a prototype-based system of categorization, in which categories are defined by the best (prototypical) examples of the concept, and other cases form a continuum of resemblance (Livesley, 1985).

The DSM-IV Personality Disorders Work Group recognized the limits of the categorical system, but adopted a conservative strategy for change, thus retaining the system. This decision was based on the fact that although a more scientific means of classifying personality disorders is likely to evolve, the current diversity of alternative models, and the absence of definitive data and consensus, argue against more radical changes at this time (Gunderson, in press). Identification of classification models that are better suited to the domain of personality disorders, however, is a critical direction for personality disorder research.

## FEATURES OF THE CRITERIA SETS

In addition to the limitations of a categorical system for personality disorders, certain features of the Axis II criteria sets are likely to contribute to the problems of unreliability, overlap, and heterogeneity within disorders (Shea, 1992). These include (1) lack of clarity regarding the definition and number of constructs covered by the criteria; (2) differences among criteria in level of inference; (3) overlapping criteria; and (4) differences among criteria in terms of explicit statements about motivation.

### Definition and Number of Constructs Covered

Each of the Axis II disorders is defined by a list of typically seven to nine criteria. What constructs are covered by the criteria for each of the disorders is not clear, however, as these are not defined (Livesley, 1987). Conceptually, it appears that the Axis II disorders vary in terms of the number of underlying constructs. For example, two separable dimensions underlying dependent personality disorder have been identified: attachment-related behaviors (need for and proximity to a secure base), and dependency (need for instrumental help) (Livesley, Schroeder, & Jackson, 1990). Although these dimensions are not explicitly defined in the criteria set for this disorder, the set appears to cover both of these constructs. The criteria for paranoid personality disorder appear (at least at a conceptual level) to be more unidimensional, capturing different manifestations of distrust or suspiciousness. Borderline personality disorder appears to consist of more constructs. One study has suggested three relatively distinct subsets of criteria within the DSM-III borderline criteria: an identity cluster (chronic feelings of emptiness or boredom, identity disturbance, and intolerance of being alone); an affect cluster (intense inappropriate anger, instability of affect, and unstable interpersonal relationships); and an impulse cluster (self-damaging acts and impulsive behaviors) (Hurt et al., 1990).

Furthermore, the different constructs or components of the personality disorders are represented by varying numbers of criteria. The polythetic system used for diagnosis (i.e., diagnosis is made if a minimum number of criteria from the criteria set are present), together with varying numbers of criteria assessing varying numbers of constructs, is likely to increase the heterogeneity of subjects with the same personality disorder diagnosis. For example, it is possible for an individual to meet DSM-III criteria for borderline personality disorder without exhibiting any of the traits in one of the three clusters identified by Hurt et al. (e.g., identity disturbance and affective instability may be present without impulsivity). Clearly, this could be an important source of heterogeneity among individuals diagnosed with borderline personality disorder. To take dependent personality disorder as another example, patients can meet criteria predominantly on the basis of attachment behaviors, or, in contrast, primarily on the basis of dependency behaviors.

## Level of Inference of Criteria

The criteria sets for the Axis I disorders capture signs and symptoms of each disorder, and are thus relatively concrete (e.g., delusions, hallucinations, loss of appetite, insomnia, etc.). The domain of personality, in contrast, involves more complex patterns of behaviors, attitudes, and feelings (i.e., traits). In an attempt to improve reliability, however, there has been an attempt in Axis II, similar to that in Axis I, to develop criteria that are as explicit and behaviorally concrete as possible. As a result, the criteria sets are variable in terms of level of inference, with some describing trait constructs and others representing more concrete manifestations of underlying constructs or traits. Criteria defining constructs naturally require more inference than those involving specific behaviors. DSM-IV criteria at the construct level include, for example, "shows perfectionism . . . " (obsessive–compulsive personality disorder; American Psychiatric Association, p. 672), and "has a grandiose sense of self-importance . . . " (narcissistic personality disorder; American Psychiatric Association, 1994, p. 661). In contrast, some of the criteria for paranoid personality disorder are examples of more concrete manifestations of an underlying construct (suspiciousness), such as "is preoccupied with unjustified doubts about the loyalty . . . of [others]," "reads hidden demeaning or threatening meanings into benign remarks or events," and so on (American Psychiatric Association, 1994, p. 637). Some of the criteria sets include a combination of constructs and manifestations of constructs. For example, the narcissistic criterion "has a grandiose sense of self-importance . . . " is followed by illustrative examples of the construct "(e.g., exaggerates achievements and talents, expects to be recognized as superior . . . )" (American Psychiatric Association, 1994, p. 661). Other criteria for this disorder appear to be manifestations of this same construct, such as "believes that he or she is 'special' and unique . . . " and "is preoccupied with fantasies of unlimited success, power, brilliance, beauty, or ideal love" (American Psychiatric Association, 1994, p. 661).

## Overlapping Criteria

Particularly in DSM-III-R, a number of criteria are either similar or identical across different disorders. For example, "has no close friends or confidants (or only one) other than first degree relatives" is a DSM-III-R criterion for schizoid, schizotypal, and avoidant personality disorders (American Psychiatric Association, 1987, p. 340, 342, 353). Examples of similar criteria include "constantly seeks or demands reassurance, approval, or praise" (histrionic; American Psychiatric Association, 1987, p. 349) and "requires constant attention and admiration . . . " (narcissistic; American Psychiatric Association, 1987, p. 352), as well as "frantic efforts to avoid real or imagined abandonment . . . " (borderline; American Psychiatric Association, 1987, p. 348) and "is frequently preoccupied with fears of being abandoned" (dependent; American Psychiatric Association, 1987, p. 353). Responses to the same interview questions will thus result in a positive score for criteria in different disorders. Findings have suggested that co-occurrence rates tend to be highest for those disorders with overlap in their criteria (Oldham et al., 1992).

## Motivation and Meaning of Behavior

The frequent absence in DSM-III-R of explicitness in terms of motivation for the behaviors or behavioral patterns is one reason for artificial overlap. This is particularly important for those criteria that consist of behavioral manifestations of the construct. Benjamin (1993) has noted that the motivation for behaviors that appear to be similar may be quite different for different disorders. Anger, for example, tends to be precipitated by perceptions of abandonment for an individual with borderline personality disorder, whereas criticism or humiliation would be the more likely precipitant for an individual with narcissistic personality disorder. Another example might be absence of close friends, which is a result of an intense fear of rejection for the avoidant, in contrast to a lack of desire for the schizoid. Without statements regarding motivation, such distinctions cannot be made.

In the study by Oldham and colleagues (1992), co-occurrence rates for the same sample of patients were evaluated through the use of two different structured interviews, differing in format. One was the Structured Clinical Interview for DSM-III-R, Axis II (SCID-II; Spitzer, Williams, & Gibbon, 1987), which organizes questions by disorder, and the other was the Personality Disorder Examination (PDE; Loranger, Susman, Oldham, & Russakoff, 1985), in which questions are organized by area of functioning, rather than by disorder. It is interesting that the PDE resulted in higher rates of significant co-occurrence among specific pairs of disorders than the SCID-II. The authors speculate that a reason for this finding is the format of the 1985 version of the PDE, which makes it more difficult for the clinician to weigh the meaning and importance of answers to individual questions because they are not keyed to specific disorders in the interview. (This problem has been partially addressed in later versions of the PDE.) The findings suggest that even when the criteria are not explicit with regard to motivation or meaning of behavior, if questions are asked in the context of a specific disorder, the interviewer may be better able to make judgments about the relevance of the behavior for the disorder in question.

The DSM-IV personality disorder criteria are generally more explicit with regard to motivation than the DSM-III-R criteria. These changes have been made in an attempt to reduce artificial overlap. For example, the schizotypal criterion of excessive social anxiety now reads: "excessive social anxiety that does not diminish with familiarity and tends to be associated with paranoid fears rather than negative judgments about self" (American Psychiatric Association, 1994, p. 645). For avoidant personality disorder, the criterion for social isolation has been revised as follows: "avoids occupational activities that involve significant interpersonal contact, because of fears of criticism, disapproval, or rejection" (American Psychiatric Association, 1994, p. 664). The dependent criterion "feels uncomfortable or helpless when alone" now includes " . . . because of exaggerated fears of being unable to care for himself or herself" (American Psychiatric Association, 1994, p. 668).

## DISCUSSION

Although it is likely that the changes in the personality disorder criteria introduced in DSM-IV will reduce the overlap among diagnoses, it is also likely (and important) that work toward an improved system of classification for personality pathology will continue. A promising direction in this regard is represented by the "dimensional" approach — that is, identifying the basic dimensions that underlie the personality disorders.

There are a number of dimensional models of personality, and conversion to a dimensional approach to personality disorders in the DSM system has frequently been recommended. Widiger (1991b) has summarized the advantages of using a dimensional approach, has noted the empirical support for this approach, and has described the existing dimensional models (see also Widiger & Frances, 1994; Widiger & Sanderson, Chapter 22). These models include the five-factor model, consisting of neuroticism, extraversion, openness, agreeableness, and conscientiousness (Costa & McCrae, 1992); Eysenck's three dimensions of neuroticism, extraversion, and psychoticism (Eysenck, 1987); the four dimensions proposed by Siever and Davis (1991) as underlying the Axis I and Axis II disorders (cognitive disorganization, affective instability, impulsivity, and anxiety); Cloninger's (1987) three dimensions of harm avoidance, novelty seeking, and reward dependence; the interpersonal circumplex dimensions of affiliation and power (Kiesler, 1986;

Benjamin, 1993); and the three-dimensional model of negative emotionality, positive emotionality, and constraint (Tellegen, 1985).

All of the dimensional models attempt to identify the basic components that underlie the domain of personality (and personality disorders), and assume a continuum between normality and abnormality for most dimensions. This assumption has empirical support in the frequent finding of similar factor structures in normal and abnormal samples (e.g., Livesley & Schroeder, 1990, 1991; Livesley, Jackson, & Schroeder, 1992), and in distributions of personality disorder scores, which tend to be continuous rather than dichotomous (Zimmerman & Coryell, 1990).

Livesley has taken a somewhat different approach, directed toward clarification and systematic identification of the components (or dimensions) underlying each of the individual personality disorders. Emphasizing the absence of precise definitions in the DSM system, and the need to define the traits that comprise each diagnosis, he has focused on construct validation (Livesley, 1987; Livesley, Jackson, & Schroeder, 1989). A multistage process has been used to identify and define the traits of each diagnosis, including (1) content analysis of the clinical literature; (2) use of clinician judgments to identify highly prototypical features of each diagnosis; (3) definition of the components of each diagnosis in terms of explicit behavioral dimensions; (4) development of a self-report measure to assess the dimensions; and (5) empirical investigation of the structural relationships between dimensions delineating each diagnosis.

Results have identified some factors that are unique to specific personality disorders, and some that are shared among disorders. Interpersonal exploitation, for example, appears as a prominent feature in factors of antisocial, borderline, histrionic, and narcissistic personality disorders. An example of a unique factor is one identified for borderline personality disorder, reflecting instability or disorganization (i.e., diffuse self-concept, unstable moods, unstable interpersonal relationships, attachment problems) (Livesley & Schroeder, 1991). The authors suggest that the unique factor (labeled "borderline pathology") might be considered the core feature of borderline personality disorder, whereas the other factors that emerged for this disorder (interpersonal exploitation and self-harm) might be considered associated features, since they are shared with other diagnoses (Livesley & Schroeder, 1991).

This work illustrates the usefulness of combining clinical theory and psychometric analyses to clarify and test the validity of the personality disorder classification system. It is also of interest that the relationship between the dimensional measures of the identified personality disorder features and the dimensions of the five-factor model has been investigated, with findings supporting substantial similarity between the five factors and many of the personality disorder scales (Schroeder, Wormworth, & Livesley, 1992).

As the dimensions or traits underlying the personality disorders continue to be clarified, it will be possible to investigate empirically the organization of these traits, and to refine or revise the existing categories on the basis of demonstrated empirical relationships. In a sense, this would be testing the validity of the personality disorders as syndromes—that is, as consisting of groups of traits that are functionally related. For example, the presence of dependent traits (need for instrumental help) might result in excessive attachment needs and behaviors as a way of obtaining the help needed. Or conversely, strong attachment needs could lead to a failure to develop instrumental skills and confidence in such skills, and thus to the development of dependent traits and behaviors. In either case, there would be a functional relationship between these dimensions, and the presence of one would be associated with an increased likelihood of the presence of the other. A functional relationship in a causal sense would not necessarily need to be present among all dimensions, however, as the combination of certain dimensions (occurring for nonrelated reasons) might result in a particular pattern of pathology, and thus a syndrome. For example, the presence of impulsivity together with identity disturbance might lead to a pattern of self-destructive behavior (i.e., a "borderline syndrome"), whereas the combination of impulsivity with lack of conscience or guilt could lead to a pattern of irresponsible or exploitative behavior (i.e., an "antisocial syndrome"). Empirical validation of the groupings of personality dimensions defined by the Axis II disorders could be determined by investigating the most frequent patterns of co-occurrence of the dimensions. This could be done by using cluster analyses of scores on the established dimensions to determine the most common groupings or types (see Blashfield & McElory, Chapter 20, and Jackson & Livesley, Chapter 23, this volume). Also, the frequency of co-occurrence of various pairs of dimensions (dichotomized by defining a cutoff score) could be determined by calculating odds ratios. Development of a more empirically based typology, combined with a classification system that allows gradations of membership (such as a prototype-based system), should result in a more valid and clinically suitable classification of personality disorders.

In summary, the limitations of the DSM classification of personality disorders have become clearer as research in this area has advanced (largely as a result of the introduction of DSM-III). In particular, limitations include the use of an all-or-none categorical system, lack of clarity and definitions of the underlying constructs, and lack of an empirical base demonstrating validity of the disorders. Continuing research should provide a more solid basis for addressing these limitations, and an improved classification system of the personality disorders for DSM-V.

## REFERENCES

American Psychiatric Association. (1980). *Diagnostic and statistical manual of mental disorders* (3rd ed.). Washington, DC: Author.

American Psychiatric Association. (1987). *Diagnostic and statistical manual of mental disorders* (3rd ed., rev.). Washington, DC: Author.

American Psychiatric Association. (1994). *Diagnostic and statistical manual of mental disorders* (4th ed.). Washington, DC: Author.

Benjamin, L. S. (1993). *Interpersonal diagnosis and treatment of personality disorders*. New York: Guilford Press.

Clark, L. A. (1002). Resolving taxonomic issues in personality disorders: The value of larger scale analyses of symptom data. *Journal of Personality Disorders, 6*(4), 360–376.

Cloninger, C. R. (1987). A systematic method for clinical description and classification of personality variants. *Archives of General Psychiatry, 44,* 573–588.

Costa, P. T., & McCrae, R. R. (1992). The five-factor model of personality and its relevance to personality disorders. *Journal of Personality Disorders, 6,* 343–359.

Eysenck, H. (1987). The definition of personality disorders and the criteria appropriate for their description. *Journal of Personality Disorders, 1,* 211–219.

Grove, W. M., & Tellegen, A. (1991). Problems in the classification of personality disorders. *Journal of Personality Disorders, 5,* 31–41.

Gunderson, J. (in press). Introduction to personality disorders. In T. A. Widiger, A. J. Frances, H. A. Pincus, M. B. First, R. Ross, & W. Davis (Eds.), *DSM-IV source book* (Vol. 2). Washington, DC: American Psychiatric Press.

Hurt, S. W., Clarkin, J. F., Widiger, T. A., Fyer, M. R., Sullivan, T., Stone, M. H., & Frances, A. (1990). Evaluation of DSM-III decision rules for case detection using joint conditional probability structures. *Journal of Personality Disorders, 4,* 121–130.

Kiesler, D. (1986). The 1982 interpersonal circle: An analysis of DSM-III personality disorders. In T. Millon & G. L. Klerman (Eds.), *Contemporary directions in psychopathology.* New York: Guilford Press.

Livesley, W. J. (1985). The classification of personality disorders: The choice of category concept. *Canadian Journal of Psychiatry, 30,* 353–358.

Livesley, W. J. (1987). A systematic approach to the delineation of personality disorders. *American Journal of Psychiatry, 144,* 772–777.

Livesley, W. J. (1991). Classifying personality disorders: Ideal types, prototypes or dimensions? *Journal of Personality Disorders, 5,* 52–59.

Livesley, W. J., Jackson, D. N., & Schroeder, M. L. (1989). A study of the factorial structure of personality pathology. *Journal of Personality Disorders, 3*(4), 292–306.

Livesley, W. J., Jackson, D. N., & Schroeder, M. L. (1992). Factorial structure of traits delineating personality disorders in clinical and general population samples. *Journal of Abnormal Psychology, 101,* 432–440.

Livesley, W. J., & Schroeder, M. L. (1990). Dimensions of personality disorder: The DSM-III-R Cluster A diagnoses. *Journal of Nervous and Mental Disease, 178,* 627–635.

Livesley, W. J., & Schroeder, M. L. (1991). Dimensions of personality disorder: The DSM-III-R Cluster B diagnoses. *Journal of Nervous and Mental Disease, 179,* 320–328.

Livesley, W. J., Schroeder, M. L., & Jackson, D. N. (1990). Dependent personality disorder and attachment problems. *Journal of Personality Disorders, 4,* 131–140.

Loranger, A. W., Susman, V. L., Oldham, J. M., & Russakoff, M. (1985). *Personality Disorder Examination (PDE): A structured interview for DSM-III-R personality disorders.* White Plains, NY: New York Hospital–Cornell University Medical Center, Westchester Division.

Oldham, J. M., Skodol, A. E., Kellman, H. D., Hyeler, S. E., Rosnick, L., & Davies, M.

(1992). Diagnosis of DSM-III-R personality disorders by two structured interviews: Patterns of comorbidity. *American Journal of Psychiatry, 149* (2), 213–220.

Schroeder, M. L., Wormworth, J. A., & Livesley, W. J. (1992). Dimensions of personality disorder and their relationships to the Big Five dimensions of personality. *Psychological Assessment, 4,* 47–53.

Shea, M. T. (1992). Some characteristics of the Axis II criteria sets and their implications for assessment of personality disorders. *Journal of Personality Disorders, 6*(4), 377–381.

Siever, L. J., & Davis, K. L. (1991). A psychobiological perspective on the personality disorders. *American Journal of Psychiatry, 148,* 1647–1658.

Skodol, A. E., Rosnick, L., Kellman, D., Oldham, J., & Hyler, S. (1988). Validating structured DSM-III-R personality disorder assessment with longitudinal data. *American Journal of Psychiatry, 145,* 1297–1299.

Spitzer, R. L., Williams, J. B. W., & Gibbon, M. (1987). *Structured Clinical Interview for DSM-III-R personality disorders (SCID-II).* New York: New York State Psychiatric Institute, Department of Biometrics Research.

Tellegen, A. (1985). Structure of mood and personality and their relevance to assessing anxiety, with an emphasis on self-report. In A. H. Tuma & J. D. Maser (Eds.), *Anxiety and the anxiety disorders.* Hillsdale, NJ: Erlbaum.

Widiger, T. A. (1991a). DSM-IV reviews of the personality disorders: Introduction to special series. *Journal of Personality Disorders, 5*(2), 122–134.

Widiger, T. A. (1991b). Personality disorder dimensional models proposed for DSM-IV. *Journal of Personality Disorders, 5,* 386–398.

Widiger, T. A., & Frances, A. J. (1994). Towards a dimensional model for the personality disorders. In P. Costa & T. A. Widiger (Eds.), *Personality disorders and the five-factor model of personality.* Washington, DC: American Psychological Association.

Zimmerman, M., & Coryell, W. (1990). DSM-III personality disorder dimensions. *Journal of Nervous and Mental Diseases, 178,* 686–692.

CHAPTER 20

# Confusions in the Terminology Used for Classificatory Models

ROGER K. BLASHFIELD
ROSS A. MCELROY

With the publication of DSM-III (American Psychiatric Association, 1980) and the decision to place the personality disorders on a separate axis, interest in the classification of personality disorders has increased markedly (Blashfield & McElroy, 1989). One topic attracting attention has been that of the various possible models utilized in classifying these disorders. Among these are a dimensional model, based on descriptive research on normal personality traits; a categorical model, which is the implicit model underlying the classification of personality disorders in DSM-III, DSM-III-R (American Psychiatric Association, 1987), and DSM-IV (American Psychiatric Association, 1994); and a hierarchical model, which suggests that some personality disorders, (e.g., borderline and schizotypal) are more severe and hence should receive higher diagnostic priority.

The discussions of these various models have often involved confusion in terminology. More specifically, we argue that the terms "dimensional" and "categorical," and the terms "cluster" and "hierarchy," have multiple meanings. These meanings have often been confused in the existing literature.

## "DIMENSIONAL" AND "CATEGORICAL"

Most discussions of classificatory models in the last two decades have emphasized a choice between dimensional and categorical models. For instance, a 1991 issue of the *Journal of Personality Disorders* contained six invited papers that analyzed the classification of personality disorders. Four of these six papers (Grove & Tellegen, 1991; Gunderson, Links, & Reich, 1991; Livesley, 1991; Wiggins & Schwartz, 1991) discussed dimensional models as contrasted with categorical models.

To understand how the concepts of a "dimensional" model and a "categorical" model can be used in confusing ways, consider the following example. Suppose that the number of diagnostic criteria for the personality disorders met by a patient is a function of two dimensions: neuroticism and extraversion (Eysenck, 1947, 1953). The first of these dimensions, "neuroticism," is related to the degree of subjective distress that a patient experiences. This dimension has also been referred to as "negative affectivity" (Tellegen, 1985; Watson, Clark, & Tellegen, 1988). Patients with borderline personality disorder will presumably be high on this dimension, whereas patients with narcissistic and antisocial personality disorders will be low. The second dimension, "extraversion" (also called "positive affectivity"), refers to the level of social activity of the patient. Low scores on this dimension are usually considered indicative of introversion, a concept often associated with personality disorders such as avoidant and schizoid. Histrionic individuals, by contrast, will be high on this dimension (i.e., will be extraverted). Notice that what is being presented is a two-dimensional model about the structure of the personality disorders. This model is asserting that personality disorder symptoms can be explained by the two dimensions of neuroticism and extraversion.

Suppose that we administer a test estimating the two dimensions (Clark, 1991; Eysenck & Eysenck, 1975) to a group of patients with personality disorders. Suppose also that we plot the resulting data in the two-dimensional space defined by neuroticism and extraversion. The results might appear as shown in Figure 20.1, in which the data points occur with about equal frequency in different sectors of the space. Results like these are consistent with a dimensional model, because the best way to differentiate patients in Figure 20.1 is in terms of their scores on the two dimensions.

Suppose, however, that when the patient data are plotted, Figure 20.2 results. In this figure, there is a swarm or "cluster" of data points in the upper right-hand corner (i.e., extraverted/distressed patients, or borderline patients); another swarm in the upper left-hand corner (i.e., extraverted/nondistressed patients, or narcissistic patients); and a third swarm in the lower right-hand corner (i.e., introverted/distressed patients, or avoidant and dependent patients). These results are consistent with a categorical model. Knowing the cluster to which a patient belongs are informative, in addition to knowing the patient's score on the two dimensions.

In the language of multivariate statistics, the concepts of "dimensional" and "categorical" represent structural models of the data. That is, the dimensional model in Figure 20.1 suggests that the personality disorder data can be accounted for by the two dimensions of neuroticism and extraversion. Once a patient has been assessed on these two dimensions, all significant information has been gathered. In effect, if the two-dimensional model of personality disorders is correct, the "structure" of personality disorder symptomatology is shown in Figure 20.1. There is a continuous distribution of patient data along two dimensions that explain the variance in patient symp-

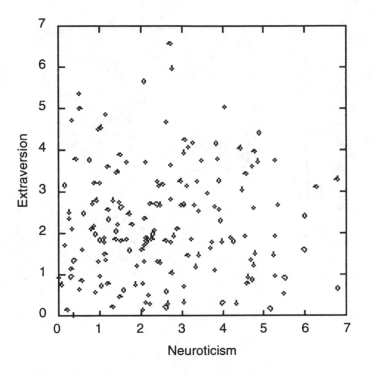

FIGURE 20.1. Results of a test of extraversion (E) and neuroticism (N), consistent with a dimensional model.


toms. In contrast, if a categorical model is correct, the data should be structured as shown in Figure 20.2. The data will form "clusters" of relatively separate but internally homogeneous groups.

An important point to note about categorical and dimensional models, when discussed as structural models, is that these models are consistent with each other; they are not necessarily competing models. A dimensional model is the more basic of the two structural models. A categorical model is a dimensional model with the additional assumption that patient data form descriptive clusters when plotted in the space defined by the dimensions. That is, a categorical structural model assumes that the descriptive data form densities ("clusters"). The categorical model also assumes that there are boundaries between these clusters. A categorical model is a more complex, elaborated version of dimensional model.

The terms "categorical" and "dimensional" can be used to refer not only to structural models, but also to measurement models. As measurement models, "dimensional" and "categorical" relate to how clinical concepts are assessed. Consider the issue of scaling. Typically, measurement scales are

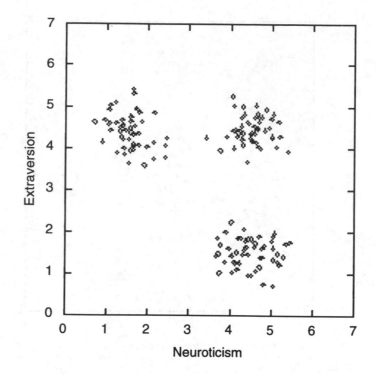

FIGURE 20.2. Results of the same test, consistent with a categorical model.

organized into four levels: "nominal," "ordinal," "interval," or "ratio" (Jacoby, 1991). If a nominal level of measurement is used, then the number associated with a particular value is nothing more than a name. For instance, marital status is a variable with nominal scaling. It does not matter whether marital status is coded single = 1, married = 2, and divorced/widowed = 3, or whether it is coded married = 1, divorced/widowed = 2, and single = 3. In the same way, another nominal variable, gender, can be coded as male = 1 and female = 0 or coded as male = 2 and female = 1. None of these codings is inherently better or worse. The assignment of numbers to a nominal scale is arbitrary. As a result, computing the mean of these numbers is not informative. Variables that have nominal scaling are often called "categorical," because the values of the measurements are organized into categories (e.g., "gender" is subdivided into the categories of "male" and "female").

Another type of scaling involves ratio scales. The numbers associated with ratio scaling are very informative. For instance, consider the measurement of temperature. The difference between 23 °C and 24 °C is of the same magnitude as the difference between 24 °C and 25 °C. Computing the mean of the numbers for temperature is informative; in addition, the value of $0\,°C$ for temperature has a particular meaning. In measurement terms, variables such as temperature are often considered "dimensional," because values for these variables vary continuously along a dimensional scale.

When the terms are used in a measurement context, dimensional variables are associated with higher-level (interval or ratio) scaling than categorical (nominal) variables. This contrasts to the use of these terms in a structural sense, in which categorical models are the more complex and require more assumptions about the descriptive organization of data.

The confusion associated with using the terms "categorical" and "dimensional" in measurement versus structural contexts is important. As an example of this confusion, we will analyze a paper about these models by Frances (1982). He begins by suggesting that, ideally, the categorical model assumes that the disorders in a psychiatric classification represent "classes [that] are defined to be homogeneous, mutually exclusive, and jointly exhaustive. All the criteria for class membership must be met completely by all qualifying members" (p. 517). Notice that in his representation of a categorical model, Frances is referring to "categorical" as a type of structural model. According to this model, the personality disorders should represent relatively discrete "clusters" to which patients can be clearly assigned membership.

Frances argues that the categorical model is not an optimal structural model for the personality disorders. The personality disorders are not mutually exclusive; that is, many patients meet diagnostic criteria for more than one personality disorder. Stated in the language associated with Figure 20.2, the personality disorders do not appear to represent discrete "clusters." Frances suggests that the "dimensional" model may serve as a useful alternative to the categorical model. Dimensional models work best when the data are distributed along a continuous distribution rather than a discrete, binary distribution. Frances uses the concept of color as an example:

> For most purposes, our typology of colors is wonderfully vivid and sufficiently explicit. There may be disagreements and some loss of reliability in distinguishing shades which are quite similar, but the system is nonetheless quite handy when one wants to buy a suit or describe a sunset. If our interest in color is more rigorous, however, the categorical system becomes insufficiently precise. In the study of refraction, a dimensional system measuring wave length is more precise and saves information. (p. 519)

Notice that when making his argument in favor of a dimensional model, Frances has switched to discussing this model within a measurement context. That is, he is talking about "dimensional" as a type of measurement model. His argument is that a "dimensional" approach to assessing color (i.e., a ratio scale assessing wavelengths of light) is more powerful than a "categorical" (i.e., nominal) scaling of color.

Frances then lists four advantages of dimensional systems:

1. Dimensional systems are better in describing border cases—these are described accurately rather than being forced into one or another poorly fitting category.
2. Dimensional systems reduce the halo effect, i.e. the tendency to ignore atypical cases and to see things in stereotyped ways which conform to preconceived categorical definitions.
3. By using a dimensional system, one can manipulate complex data mathematically and include many variables.
4. In reducing dimensions to typologies, information with important predictive value may be lost. (p. 519)

For the last two of these "advantages," Frances is discussing dimensional versus categorical models in a measurement context. For the first advantage, he is arguing that a dimensional structural model is superior when the descriptive data do not conform to a categorical structural model. Advantage 2 refers to neither a structural nor a measurement view of these models, but instead is a psychological argument pertaining to how human beings tend to interpret categorical models (Markman, 1989).

In short, Frances argues for the superiority of a dimensional model over a categorical model. The intent of his argument is to suggest that a dimensional model is superior to a categorical model in a structural context. However, many of his arguments in favor of a dimensional model refer to this model in a measurement context. Also, his argument contrasting these models seems to assume that the field must choose one of these models. Frances does not view these structural models as complementary.

## "HIERARCHY" AND "CLUSTERS"

Two other terms that are often used in confusing and inconsistent ways in discussions of the classification of personality disorders are the concepts of "hierarchy" and "cluster." Consider, for instance, the organization of the 11 DSM-III-R personality disorders into three clusters: Cluster A (the "odd, eccentric" disorders), Cluster B (the "dramatic, erratic" disorders) and Cluster C (the "anxious, fearful" disorders). At a 1991 meeting of the DSM-IV Personality Disorders Work Group, there was an interesting discussion about whether to retain the organization of personality disorders into clusters. The alternative was to list the personality disorders alphabetically. The argument for dropping the clusters was that data on the diagnostic overlap of the personality disorders failed to show that the highest overlap occurred among personality disorders within the same cluster. However, others argued that there were empirical data favoring the clusters. Hyler and others have found that factor-analytic studies of personality disorder data tended to generate factors matching the DSM-III-R three-cluster organization (Hyler & Lyons, 1988; Hyler et al., 1990; Kass, Skodol, Charles, Spitzer, & Williams, 1985).

This interchange concering whether to retain the three clusters of personality disorders involved a confusion about the meaning of the terms "cluster" and "hierarchy" (even though the latter term was not invoked directly). To illuminate this confusion, we new discuss three different meanings of the concept of "hierarchy."

The first meaning of "hierarchy" is associated with a categorical structural model. From this perspective, the hierarchical organization of personality disorders into clusters means that every patient who has an avoidant personality disorder also has a Cluster C personality disorder. This is analogous to biological classification, in which every animal that is a member of the category of house cats (*Felis catus*) is a member of a higher-level category called mammals (*Mammalia*). In terms of this first meaning, a hierarchy is a collection of nested categories.

According to this meaning of "hierarchy," one would expect more diagnostic confusions between categories in the same cluster than between categories in different clusters. That is, it is easier to confuse a jaguar and a cougar than a jaguar and a wolf, because the former belong to the same genus but the latter do not. In the same way, dependent personality disorder should show more diagnostic overlap with obsessive–compulsive personality disorder than it should with borderline personality disorder, because the first two are members of Cluster C, whereas borderline is a Cluster B disorder. Those in the DSM-IV Personality Disorders Work Group who argued for dropping the clusters were referring to this first meaning of "hierarchy." Diagnostic confusions among the personality disorders do not primarily occur within clusters. Diagnostic overlap appears to spread broadly across all personality disorders, regardless of cluster membership (Widiger et al., 1990).

A second possible meaning of hierarchy concerns the nesting of dimensions. For instance, the dimensional concept of IQ can be subdivided on a psychological test such as the Wechsler Adult Intelligence Scale (WAIS) into verbal IQ and nonverbal (performance) IQ. Verbal IQ can be further subdivided into scales on vocabulary, comprehension, and so forth. Thus, the WAIS is organizing its separate subtests into a hierarchy of dimensions. The evidence for the utility of these dimensions comes from factor analyses of WAIS data, which have shown that scales belonging to the same higher-order dimension tend to correlate relatively highly with each other.

When viewed from the perspective of "hierarchy" as referring to nested dimensions, a hierarchical organization of personality disorders into "clusters" suggests that intercorrelation of scores on personality disorders within the same cluster should be higher than the intercorrelations for personality disorders from different clusters. In a series of factor-analytic studies of a self-report inventory to assess the personality disorders, Hyler and his colleagues (Hyler & Lyons, 1988; Hyler et al., 1990) have reported results that support this view. That is, factor analyses of personality disorder scales showed that the antisocial, borderline, histrionic, and narcissistic scales tended to correlate together, forming a higher-order Cluster B dimension.

Notice that the results of Hyler and colleagues support the organization of the personality disorders into three higher-order groups. However, to name these higher order groups as "clusters" is misleading, since, as shown in the earlier discussion of Figures 20.1 and 20.2, the term "cluster" is associated with a categorical structural model. Instead, these higher-order concepts should be renamed Dimension A, Dimension B, and Dimension C.

There is a third way in which the term "hierarchy" has been used when referring to structural models. This third use of the term is what has been described as a "pecking-order" view of hierarchical models (Blashfield, 1990). This model is a variation on a categorical model in which some categories take diagnostic precedence over other categories. For instance, one might argue that diagnosing organic brain syndromes should take precedence over diagnosing mood disorders. There are two reasons for asserting this precedence. First, organic brain syndromes and mood disorders can be confused (e.g., organic delirium of an encephalitis vs. a manic delirium). However, diagnosing an organic delirium takes precedence because rapid intervention is important for the patient's future recovery. Second, organic brain syndromes take diagnostic precedence over nonorganic disorders because the presence of the former may be able to account for many of the symptoms of a nonorganic disorder. For instance, a patient who is experiencing a dementia may hallucinate like a schizophrenic, may have pressured speech like a manic, and may have the autonomic nervous system arousal of someone with an anxiety disorder. On the other hand, a patient with a generalized anxiety disorder should not become disoriented (like a demented patient) or be delusional (like someone with schizophrenia).

This third type of hierarchy is called a "pecking-order" hierarchy because it is analogous to the hierarchical organization of ranks in the military. The rank of colonel takes precedence over the rank of lieutenant in an army. The orders of a colonel will be obeyed over the orders of the lieutenant. Anyone who is a colonel must understand and be responsible for the performance of the lieutenants who are under his or her command. However, there is no membership nesting between these two categories. That is, an individual who is a lieutenant is not also a colonel, nor is a colonel a lieutenant.

The third meaning of "hierarchy" is the meaning that was used by Gunderson and colleagues (Gunderson, 1992; Gunderson et al., 1991) when they proposed that some personality disorders, such as borderline and schizotypal personality disorders, should have diagnostic priority among the personality disorders. This model is consistent with a study by Blashfield and Herkov (1992), which showed that when patients met diagnostic criteria for two or more personality disorders, clinicians tended to make the diagnosis of borderline personality disorder rather than diagnosing all of the comorbid personality disorders.

## FINAL COMMENTS

The confusion about alternative models of psychiatric classification can be exemplified in the use of "borderline personality disorder" as a concept. The name for this disorder, "borderline," stems from early clinical observations of the absence of a no clear boundary between the personality disorders and the psychoses. "Borderlines" were individuals who could appear psychotic, but whose primary psychopathology was that of a personality disorder. Thus, the name of "borderline personality disorder" implied a single severity dimension running from normality to personality disorder to borderline personality disorder to psychosis. However, once the concept of "borderline" was formulated, theorists began to suggest that it referred to a level of personality organization underlying most of the personality disorders. In addition, research suggested that borderline personality disorder was rarely confused with schizophrenia but was much more likely to overlap with major depressive disorder. As a result, the concept of "borderline personality disorder," when used by many contemporary clinicians, refers to a hierarchically dominant (in the pecking-order sense of this term) category among the personality disorders.

## REFERENCES

American Psychiatric Association. (1980). *Diagnostic and statistical manual of mental disorders* (3rd ed.). Washington, DC: Author.

American Psychiatric Association. (1987). *Diagnostic and statistical manual of mental disorders* (3rd ed., rev.). Washington, DC: Author.

American Psychiatric Association. (1994). *Diagnostic and statistical manual of mental disorders* (4th ed.). Washington, DC: Author.

Blashfield, R. K. (1990). Comorbidity and classification. In J. Maser & C. R. Cloninger (Eds.), *Comorbidity in anxiety and mood disorders.* Washington, DC: American Psychiatric Press.

Blashfield, R. K., & Herkov, M. (in press). Investigating clinical adherence to diagnosis by criteria: A replication of Morey and Ochoa. *Journal of Personality Disorders.*

Blashfield, R. K., & McElroy, R. A. (1989). Ontology of personality disorder categories. *Psychiatric Annals, 19,* 126–131.

Clark, L. (1991). *Schedule for normal and abnormal personality.* Dallas, TX: Southern Methodist University.

Eysenck, H. J. (1947). *Dimensions of personality.* London: Kegan Paul.

Eysenck, H. J. (1953). *The structure of human personality.* London: Methuen.

Eysenck, H. J., & Eysenck, S. B. G. (1975). *The Eysenck Personality Questionnarie (EPQ).* London: University of London Press.

Frances, A. (1982). Categorical and dimensional systems of personality diagnosis: A comparison. *Comprehensive Psychiatry, 23,* 516–527.

Grove, W. M., & Tellegen, A. (1991). Problems in the classification of personality disorders. *Journal of Personality Disorders, 5,* 31–41.

Gunderson, J. G. (1992). Diagnostic controversies. *Review of Psychiatry, 11,* 9–24.

Gunderson, J. G., Links, P. S., & Reich, J. H. (1991). Competing models of personality disorders. *Journal of Personality Disorders, 5,* 60–68.

Hyler, S., & Lyons, M. (1988). Factor analsis of the DSM-III personality disorder clusters: A replication. *Comprehensive Psychiatry, 29,* 304–308.

Hyler, S., Lyons, M., Rieder, R., Young, L., Williams, J., & Spitzer, R. (1990). The factor structure of self-report DSM-III Axis II symptoms and their relationship to clinicians' ratings. *American Journal of Psychiatry, 147,* 751–757.

Jacoby, W. G. (1991). *Data theory and dimensional analysis.* Newbury Park, CA: Sage.

Kass, F., Skodol, A., Charles, E., Spitzer, R., & Williams, J. B. W. (1985). Scaled ratings of DSM-III personality disorders. *American Journal of Psychiatry, 147,* 627–630.

Livesley, W. J. (1991). Classifying personality disorders: Ideal types, prototypes, or dimensions? *Journal of Personality Disorders, 5,* 52–59.

Markman, E. M. (1989). *Categorization and naming in children.* Cambridge, MA: MIT Press.

Tellegen, A. (1985). Structure of mood and personality and their relevance to assessing anxiety. In A. H. Tuma & J. D. Maser (Eds.), *Anxiety and the anxiety disorders.* Hillsdale, NJ: Erlbaum.

Watson, D., Clark, L. A., & Tellegen, A. (1988). The Positive and Negative Affect Schedule (PANAS). *Journal of Personality and Social Psychology, 54,* 1063–1070.

Widiger, T., Frances, A., Harris, M., Jacobsberg, L., Fyer, M., & Manning, D. (1991). Comorbidity among Axis II disorders. In J. Oldham (Ed.), *Personality disorders: New perspectives on diagnostic validity.* Washington, DC: American Psychiatric Press.

Wiggins, O. P., & Schwartz, M. A. (1991). Methodological problems with the classification of personality disorders: The significance of existential types. *Journal of Personality Disorders, 5,* 69–81.

# Chapter 21

# Prototypes, Ideal Types, and Personality Disorders: The Return to Classical Phenomenology

Michael A. Schwartz
Osborne P. Wiggins
Michael A. Norko

DSM-III (American Psychiatric Association, 1980) was born from a determination to strengthen the scientific undergirdings of psychiatric diagnoses (Millon, 1986). In this spirit, of firm commitment to scientific rigor, debates have arisen regarding the most effective form of psychiatric classification. Several different forms of classification have been proposed: "polythetic concepts," "dimensions," and "prototypes." These different kinds of classification now compete with one another for the title of "best form of psychiatric classification." In these arguments no one form emerges as the victor, because, as the debates prove, each has its own special usefulness and function. Hence the debates continue unresolved because the proponents of each viewpoint remain able to indicate areas in which their preferred form bears fruitful results.

We suggest that psychiatry, at least at the present point of its development, would profit by retaining the diversity while also achieving an overarching unification in classification. In this chapter we contend that "ideal types," as outlined by Max Weber in sociology and, following Weber, Karl Jaspers in psychiatry, offer an effective way to unify current forms of classification. We explicate the epistemological rationale behind ideal types. In order to draw a contrast with ideal types, we also focus on prototypes. Prototypes in many ways resemble ideal types; it is important, then, to note the similarities and differences. We seek most of all, however, to advocate ideal

An earlier version of this chapter was published in the *Journal of Personality Disorders*, 1989, *3*, 1–9. Copyright 1991 by The Guilford Press. Adapted by permission.

types, not as one competing form of classification among others, but rather as a way of conceptually unifying the other proposed forms—encompassing prototypes, dimensions, and polythetic categories.

By sketching the usefulness of ideal types, we are proposing nothing new. Rather, we are reminding psychiatrists of the old. In the first part of this century, Karl Jaspers advocated the adoption of ideal types in psychiatric classification (Jaspers, 1923), and Karl Schneider fruitfully employed ideal types in the classification of psychopathic personalities (Schneider, 1923a). Because, therefore, of the remarkable similarities between prototypes and ideal types, the recent emergence of prototypes as an important mode of classification signals in a way a return to the classical psychiatry of the early part of this century. Accordingly, in this chapter we contest the view that newer modes of classification constitute a significant advance precisely by rejecting long-standing "classical" forms. Instead, we contend that newer forms of classification, including polythetic concepts and dimensions, constitute a rediscovery of the flexible and versatile modes of classification recognized earlier by Jaspers.

## PROTOTYPES

Prototypes have been thoroughly described by numerous investigators (Rosch & Mervis, 1975; Rosch, 1978; Cantor & Mischel, 1979; Cantor, Smith, French, & Mezzich, 1980; Horowitz, Post, French, Wallis, & Seligman, 1981; Clarkin, Widiger, Frances, Hurt, & Gilmore, 1983; Blashfield, Sprock, Pinkston, & Hodgin, 1985; Livesley, 1985). In psychiatry, prototypes have been most extensively applied in the nosology of personality disorders. This literature usually contrasts prototypes with the "classical" view of categorization. This "classical" view, it is claimed, dominated psychiatric classification until the publication of DSM-III (Cantor et al., 1980; Cantor & Genero, 1986). The "classical" approach to categorization is also called by these authors "monothetic categorization" (Hempel, 1965; Schwartz & Wiggins, 1987). Monothetic categories define a psychiatric disorder by specifying necessary and sufficient conditions for class membership. DSM-III has been praised for moving beyond monothetic classifications to polythetic ones (Kendell, 1983). Polythetic categories provide a list of attributes and then stipulate the number of attributes that an individual must exhibit in order to be included in the category (Beckner, 1959). More recently, investigators have argued that for the classification of psychiatric disorders, prototypes provide an improvement over polythetic concepts (Livesley, 1985).

Prototypes were first developed by cognitive psychologists in studies of "natural categories" (Rosch, 1978; Lakoff, 1987, pp. 12–57). Natural categories are the categories people use in everyday, nonscientific life in the recognition and interpretation of objects in the surrounding world. The cognitive studies showed that these categories are "fuzzy": Boundaries between different categories are difficult to specify; there are numerous borderline cases; members of a class may share very few traits; and class membership falls on a continuum from definite to indefinite. This understanding of natural categories was strongly influenced by Ludwig Wittgenstein's view that the terms of natural language usually express only "family resemblances" among different items (Wittgenstein, 1953, pp. 31–36).

Prototypes initially emerge at the level of sensorimotor or bodily activity. We learn to see things in a certain way because that is the way our human bodies have learned to use them. When I recognize an object as a chair, for instance, I am seeing it as "something to sit on," and I am seeing it as "something to sit on" because that is the way my body has learned to use that particular kind of object (Lakoff, 1987, pp. 46–48). Prototypes thus capture the "interactional properties" of objects: They capture those properties that we humans experience because of the way we interact with things. Accordingly, prototypes do not represent the properties that things possess "in themselves" (i.e., independently of human sensorimotor capacities). Prototypes rather represent objects only as they are mentally processed by us humans— that is, as they exist *relative to us* and to our particular anatomical and neurological makeup (Rosch, 1978; Lakoff, 1987, pp. 50–52). The example of the chair given above should indicate that prototypes are culturally relative, too. Only in certain cultures do people learn to recognize objects with a typical shape as "something to sit on."

Although prototypes initially function at the prelinguistic level of human sensorimotor activity, they can provide a basis for concept formation. Linguistic concepts can be constructed out of prototypes, and these concepts of language then retain many of the features of prelinguistic prototypes (Lakoff, 1987, pp. 58–67). Categories based on prototypes have been fruitfully applied in psychiatric nosology. More specifically, they have been applied in the classification of childhood disorders, depression, functional psychoses, and personality disorders (Blashfield et al., 1985).

Prototypes can be explicitly defined through listing the features of a category. Individuals need not possess all of these features in order to fall into the category; that is to say, the features listed are not "necessary conditions" for class membership. Rather, category membership is a matter of degree (Cantor & Genero, 1986). If the individual possesses more features of the prototype, it is a "better" member of the category. If the individual exhibits fewer features of the prototype, it is a "worse" member. In monothetic categories, on the contrary, membership is never a matter of degree: An individual either is or is not a member of the monothetic class (Hempel, 1965; Blashfield, 1986, p. 367; Livesley, 1986).

Prototypes differ from the polythetic concepts used in DSM-III-R (American Psychiatric Association, 1987). In the polythetic concepts of DSM-III-R, an individual either is or is not a member of the class. Membership is determined by stipulating the *number* of conceptual features the individual must exhibit in order to exemplify the concept (Livesley, 1986). Prototypes, on the other hand, do not specify the number of attributes required for class membership; as noted above, they make class membership a matter of degree.

It should be noted that Rosch (1978) has also shown how prototypes function as "cognitive reference points" in human reasoning. In reasoning about the features, causes, or effects of some entity, we draw inferences based on our knowledge of some "best example" of that entity. Extending this line of thought, Kenneth Schaffner (1986) has demonstrated the fruitfulness of exemplar reasoning in the medicine.

## SCIENTIFIC CONCEPTS AS INVENTIVE CONSTRUCTS

Having outlined the nature of prototypes, we would now like to point to a basic characteristic of scientific conceptualization that must be acknowledged if we are to be able to evaluate the competing forms of classification, including prototypes.

In discussions of classification, writers do not usually recognize the active role of the scientist in *constructing* all forms of categorization. Scientists creatively fashion scientific concepts. Concepts are not simply "read off" objective reality; concepts are actively constructed. Scientific notions are the result of an interaction between the knowing person and the item known. The reality known contributes its part to the concept, but the knowing subject likewise contributes his or her part. Reality contributes data, but scientists must decide which of these data to include and how precisely to connect these data with one another and with unobserved features of reality. The scientist, in other words, is an active *agent* in the production of what comes to be viewed as scientific knowledge.

Any scientist, then, who sets about constructing concepts must make a certain number of decisions, either overtly or covertly (Longino, 1990, pp. 96–102). The scientist must decide to depict reality in certain ways, and must also decide which phenomena to select and how to relate them to one another and to other realities. Other scientists may make other intellectual choices, and thus may depict reality in a different fashion.

The polythetic concepts of DSM-III-R (American Psychiatric Association, 1987) and DSM-IV (American Psychiatric Association, 1994) embody one way to construct scientific classifications. Polythetic concepts thus manifest one set of decisions. Prototypical categories embody an alternative construction and hence a different decision. It is fruitless to ask which of these two forms of classification best represents reality: Each represents reality *from a particular intellectual point of view.* Each was chosen and devised for a particular intellectual purpose (or set of purposes). The form of categorization must be evaluated, then, by reference to how well it serves its particular purpose (or set of purposes). A form of categorization is a means to an end, and that end may not be simply the depiction of reality. Rather, the goal of categorization may consist of facilitating and guiding research, as in the selection of a patient population. The goal may also consist of informing and directing therapy. Concepts are good or bad, depending on how well they serve their appointed goals. Categories are thus not to be judged simply in terms of whether they are true or false reflections of reality, but in terms of how useful or fruitful they are for the various purposes they are designed to serve. They are to be judged in terms of their *heuristic* value in furthering psychiatric work.

Failure to recognize the active role of the knowing subject in the devising of scientific concepts has persisted, we suspect, because of a covert worry that if this active role were admitted, the concepts would appear inescapably "subjective." Thus it has seemed necessary to conceive of the scientific mind as a passive (impartial) receptacle into which reality streams. The mind must do nothing to alter the data directly received from the external world. If the mind should act and thus transform the data, scientific conceptualization would possess no secure foundation in facts (Chalmers, 1982, p. 23). Accordingly, we have long assumed what the philosopher of science Karl Popper has dismissed as "the bucket theory of the mind." Popper (1972) writes:

> According to this view, . . . our mind resembles a container—a kind of bucket—in which perceptions and knowledge accumulate. (Bacon speaks of perceptions as grapes, ripe and in season which have to be gathered, patiently and industriously, and from which, if pressed, the pure wine of knowledge will flow.)
>
> Strict empiricists advise us to interfere as little as possible with this process of accumulating knowledge. True knowledge is pure knowledge, uncontaminated by those prejudices which we are only too prone to add to, and mix with, our perceptions; these alone constitute experience pure and simple. The result of these additions, of our disturbing and interfering with the process of accumulating knowledge, is error. (pp. 341–342)

As a contrast to this traditional view, Popper contrasts his own notion of "the searchlight theory of the mind." Popper emphasizes the fact that even in observing data "we play an intensely active part" (1972, p. 342). Popper focuses on observation in science because it would seem that here, if anywhere in scientific inquiry, the scientist's mind should simply passively receive data coming from outside. But even here Popper claims, "We do not have an observation . . . but we make an observation. [A navigator even works an observation.] An observation is always preceded by a particular interest, a question, or a problem" (1972, p. 342).

According to Popper, then, scientists actively "work" their observations in the service of a particular interest. Indeed, for Popper, the scientist cannot even "have" an observation unless some scientific interest, question, or problem has already been posed, which the observation is then intentionally designed to answer or resolve. Popper's emphasis on the role of "interest" in all scientific work again points to the agency of the scientist in deciding which "questions" to put to reality (Chalmers, 1982, pp. 32–34). This role

of interest need not lead to "subjectivism," however, as long as careful attention is paid to the capacity of evidence to falsify our preconceived designs.

To point to the role of interest in science seems to raise the specter of
subjectivism, because it undeniably discloses the role that "values" play in
science. To have an interest is to be guided by certain values (Fulford, 1989),
and it is also to make choices on the basis of those values. But this is only
to say that scientific concepts are constructed to serve particular purposes
or goals. Concepts that serve one purpose well may serve another only poorly
(Longino, 1990).

What we must notice is that if scientific categories are designed to serve
particular purposes, a single style of categorization, once accepted, may establish a prejudice in favor of its own chosen purpose, to the disregard of
other, equally worthwhile scientific goals. Each form of categorization necessarily remains one-sided; it depicts only certain aspects of reality and dis-
regards others. Consequently, it is essential that one mode of
conceptualization not be deemed the only "truly scientific" one. If this one
form is thought to provide the sole genuinely scientific categories, then those
aspects of reality that can be captured only by developing alternative
categories will be bypassed. It is crucial to recognize that different forms
of conceptualization are needed in order to facilitate different, equally legitimate scientific purposes.

The scientific study of reality requires different forms of categorization
because reality, if stripped of all forms of human conceptualization, consists of an "infinite multiplicity" of data. In order to approach this infinite
multiplicity, we must begin by making some selection. From the unlimited
expanse of data that confronts us, a limited set must be isolated for closer
examination. As Popper says, "An observation is always preceded by a particular interest, a question, or a problem — in short, by something theoretical" (1972, p. 342). Notice that an observation — our direct encounter with
reality — must be *preceded* by an interest, question, or problem. The choice
of the scientific question comes first; then we observe reality. We must first
select which features of reality we wish to study and how we wish to study
them, and then we directly confront those features. Contrary to the bucket
theory of the mind, which would contend that data simply stream in upon
us, Popper writes that "observations are always selective, and . . . they presuppose something like a principle of selection" (1972, p. 343). Again the key
word here is "presuppose": The principle of selection *precedes* the observations. And the principle of selection determines which aspects of reality we
shall observe and which we shall ignore.

This is one point that both Max Weber and Karl Jaspers made with
regard to scientific concepts: In scientific investigations categories must come
first, because observations make sense only when guided and selected by
preconceived categories. This view of Weber and Jaspers evinces their debt
to Immanuel Kant: In the process of scientific inquiry, some categories are
*a priori*. Weber and Jaspers departed from Kant because they believed that

all categories are contingent and subject to revision and redefinition in the light of empirical data. But they nonetheless agreed with him in believing that without concepts observations are blind. In this regard Popper would appear to side with Weber and Jaspers and against the "strict empiricists" (Popper, 1972, pp. 341–361).

## IDEAL TYPES

This view—that scientific inquiry necessarily requires a prior construction of categories, which are then applied to data in order to simplify and organize them—Jaspers took from his friend and mentor, the sociologist Max Weber, and utilized in psychiatric classification. This debt to Weber manifested itself when Jaspers, in *General Psychopathology,* discussed "ideal types" in particular. Weber coined the term "ideal type" (1903–1917, 1956; Schwartz & Wiggins, 1986, 1987). Weber's ideal types, "the Protestant ethic" and "the spirit of capitalism," are well known (Weber, 1904–1905). Jaspers perceived in Weber's methods a way of categorizing those psychiatric disorders that eluded conceptualization as syndromes or disease entities (Jaspers, 1923, p. 611; Schwartz & Wiggins, 1987). For Jaspers, psychiatric diagnoses fell into three groups. Group I included known somatic illnesses with psychic disturbances, such as brain tumors, general paralysis, and endocrinopathies. Group II consisted of the major psychoses, epilepsy, manic–depressive illness, and schizophrenia. Group III encompassed abnormal personalities and neuroses.

Regarding these three groups of disorders (from which, we might note, present-day classifications are derived), Jaspers (1923) wrote:

> *The three main groups of disorders are essentially different from each other.* They have no single unifying and comprehensive viewpoint from which any systematic ordering of these three disease-groups could emerge. With each group we have a different point of view. . . . (p. 610)

Whereas the disorders in Group 1 were "classes of diseases to which a case either does or does not belong" (Jaspers, 1923, p. 611), the disorders in Group III were all conceived as ideal types. Regarding Group II, it is interesting to note that Jaspers believed "we have classes of disease in mind although their definite cause and nature are not known, but in fact one is always confined to types." (Jaspers, 1923, p. 611). And since the original publication of *General Psychopathology,* epilepsy has in fact proven to be a disease with a somatic basis.

Because Jaspers appropriated the notion of ideal types from Weber, we must return to Weber in order to find the most elaborate description of them. From the outset, Weber intended ideal types to be general scientific categories (Weber, 1903–1917). They are thus the products of purposeful intellectual construction. In this regard, they differ from prototypes and Wittgenstein's "family resemblances," which were first described as nonscientific, "natural" devices of categorization. All scientific concepts, Weber thought, are defined in view of the goals those concepts are intended to serve (Weber, 1903–1917). In the case of psychiatry, these goals are the promotion of mental health and the amelioration of mental illness (Schwartz & Wiggins, 1985, 1988). Psychiatric ideal types selectively focus on only those features of human life that are relevant to the goals of psychiatry. For this reason, ideal types are necessarily perspectival or one-sided. The same reality, if approached with different goals in mind, could be conceived from a different perspective or point of view, and this other point of view would yield a different set of concepts.

Weber was always fully aware that ideal types are *human constructs*. They represent human attempts to conceive reality; they do not necessarily represent reality itself. This all-too-human quality of the types becomes especially apparent when one recognizes their one-sided and perspectival character. Because ideal types are from the outset guided by the values we posit, they remain partial and limited and should not be mistaken for absolute truth. As Jaspers was to express this idea in *General Psychopathology*, "[Ideal types] concern perspectives of understanding and not material being" (Jaspers, 1923, p. 434). This does not mean, of course, that ideal types have nothing to do with reality ("material being"). We might better say that ideal types are products of the interaction between the active, knowing mind of the scientist and the data provided by reality.

Weber (1903–1917) described the construction of an ideal type in the following manner:

> An ideal type is formed by the one-sided accentuation of one or more points of view and by the synthesis of a great many diffuse, discrete, more or less present, and occasionally absent concrete individual phenomena, which are arranged according to those one-sidedly emphasized viewpoints into a unified thought-construct. (p. 90)

We focus on reality from the point of view that is dictated by our values. From this point of view, we notice certain features of reality and ignore those features that would become visible only from other points of view. We thus select only certain features of reality as relevant to the point of view we have adopted; we then postulate connections among these selected features. We thus go beyond the data in order to conceive of relationships that underlie them.

Ideal types, moreover, are idealized descriptions of the concrete features of things that are given from this particular point of view. The concrete features of things frequently prove to be difficult to distinguish from one another; their identities may remain fuzzy, fluid, indefinite, and vague. With ideal types, we draw precise and clear conceptual boundaries around these features of things. We conceptually set aside the real indistinctness and ambiguity, and we imagine a "pure" case in which the relevant features are distinct and unambiguous. Furthermore, in actual cases the features may vary so widely that each individual seems unique and incomparable to others. The ideal type, however, specifies manifold features, all of which are not found in each actual case. The features delineated by the ideal type are, as Weber expressed it, "more or less present" and "occasionally absent" in individual cases.

The result is a general category that in all likelihood does not exactly depict any actually existing instance of it. Rather, the category describes a general class that has been deliberately "perfected" and "purified" for intellectual purposes. The scientific mind requires clear, distinct, and precisely defined concepts in order to comprehend reality. And the perfection and purity of the ideal type make it a clear, distinct, and comprehensible concept. The realities themselves are never so clear, distinct, and intelligible; that is why they would remain forever unintelligible if exact concepts were not constructed and applied to them.

Finally, we would like to emphasize the fact that ideal types are very general, comprehensive concepts. Because of their broad generality, more narrowly circumscribed concepts can be subsumed under them. These more specific concepts can then be systematically viewed as subclasses of the more comprehensive class defined by the ideal type. In this way, a unified system of concepts can be developed for the study of some complex phenomenon (e.g., schizophrenia). Weber's ideal type, the Protestant ethic, is very general. It includes within it more specific, explicitly defined notions, such as "inner-worldly asceticism." What Weber in fact developed, then, is an entire battery of useful concepts that all find their comprehensive unity in the overarching category of the Protestant ethic. The result is a detailed and rich system of logically unified concepts. And it stands to reason that any complex reality, such as schizophrenia, may be more fruitfully approached through a unified system of carefully defined concepts rather than through just one notion, such as a single polythetic category.

Ideal types, as a system of interconnected concepts, can then serve as a kind of "theory" for the study of any particular phenomenon. We call this "a kind of 'theory'" because it is not a theory in the usual sense of providing a conceptual representation of reality that will be either true or false. Ideal types, as we have said, are not true or false; they are only helpful or unhelpful in the further investigation of reality. Yet in the further investigation of reality, it would seem to be more helpful to employ a fully defined system of interrelated concepts than to use merely one or two sparsely defined notions.

## SIMILARITIES AND DIFFERENCES
## BETWEEN PROTOTYPES AND IDEAL TYPES

By defining broad general classes, ideal types differ from prototypes. A prototype defines only the "best example" of a class. The best example is, of course, one subclass within the more comprehensive class. The ideal type encompasses, in addition to the best example, all other instances of the class. Prototypes thus fall within the larger domain defined by the ideal type. Similarly, polythetic concepts and dimensions provide more specific way of conceiving of disorders that can be subsumed under the more general ideal type. Thus the definition of the ideal type can provide the larger umbrella under which prototypes, dimensions, and polythetic categories can be unified and systematically related. This systematic organization provided by the overarching ideal type can supply the unity needed to connect the multitude of studies that are to be carried out using prototypes, dimensions, polythetic concepts, and others.

In some respects, however, ideal types resemble prototypes. Both are selective; only selected features of reality are included in the definition of the type. Furthermore, both recognize the fuzziness, indefiniteness, and variability of many of the features found in actual cases. And both overcome the fuzziness and vagueness by defining attributes in a clear and precise way. Moreover, both confront the variability of individual cases by recognizing that different individuals "more or less" conform to the type.

Still, ideal types differ from prototypes in the way in which ideal types deal with this multitude of features. The various features of real things may exhibit no apparent connectedness or unity; as simply phenomenally given, they may appear to be unconnected and disordered. As Weber expressed this idea, the "individual phenomena" may be "diffuse" and "discrete." Nevertheless, in defining ideal types, we try to "synthesize" these features together into a "unified thought-construct" or concept. This means that the scientist imagines connections among the features of reality, although these postulated connections may not be phenomenally apparent. It is here that Jaspers's conception of ideal types again departs significantly from prototypes. A prototype consists of a list of attributes. A list exhibits no conceptual unity; it consists of discrete and separate items. Some of the items on the list may appear to resemble one another, but this resemblance is merely apparent because the list leaves them separate and posits no connection among them. A prototype provides, to borrow Jaspers's words, "a disjointed enumeration" of features (1923, p. 561). For Jaspers, ideal types unify and relate the attributes of the disorder. An ideal type defines a unified whole of which the various attributes are interrelated parts.

Let us indicate how Jaspers himself developed a unified conception of hysterical personality. Jaspers (1923) wrote:

> To characterize the type [of hysterical personality] more precisely we have to fall back on one basic trait. Far from accepting their given dispositions and life opportunities, hysterical personalities crave to appear both to themselves and others as more than they are and to experience more than they are ever capable of. . . . All other traits can be understandably deduced from this. (p. 443)

The various other traits of hysterical personality, such as those listed in prototypes (Livesley, 1986) or in the discussion of histrionic personality disorder in DSM-III-R (American Psychiatric Association, 1987), Jaspers would try
to understand as meaningfully derived from this one. And only such an understanding of the connections of meaning among the manifold traits "uni-
fies" them.

The basic trait, accordingly, does not unify the others by functioning
as some kind of "ultimate cause" or "source" of them. The basic trait is not
an underlying reality that produces the other traits as its effects, but the conceptual whole of which the other traits are parts. The other traits are thus
partial forms of it. There is no real difference between the basic trait and
the others; each of the other traits is the basic trait, but in a particularized
form.

Of course, we may not be able to describe "basic traits" for each of the
personality disorders. We may possess at best only a relatively disjointed list
of traits. But this points to the need to create, test, modify, and refine "unified thought-constructs" as possible basic traits. This is integral to ongoing
scientific work with ideal types in psychiatry. Furthermore, the identification of new types is another aspect of such work. Many of the most important advances in psychiatry have consisted precisely of defining new
personality types that can function as ideal types—for example, Schneider's
psychopathic personalities, Kretschmer's schizothymes and psychothymes,
and Jung's extroverts and introverts.

We wonder, however, whether prototype research as it is currently carried out could generate any new types. Wittgenstein's discussions of natural
language aimed at disclosing how people in their everyday lives use and understand words, such as "game" (Wittgenstein, 1953). Investigations of prototypes aim at disclosing through large-scale surveys of psychiatrists how they
diagnose and understand patients. Just as Wittgenstein did not analyze games,
but rather how people understand the meaning of the word "game," so prototype research cannot further investigate the psychiatric disorders, but
rather what psychiatrists mean by the terms they apply to the disorders. Prototype research, like Wittgensteinian philosophy, is limited to what the
philosopher of science Carl G. Hempel (1970) would call "meaning analysis." Meaning analysis consists of explicating the meaning a word already
has "in use" for some group or community of people. But, as Hempel points
out, meaning analysis is insufficient in empirical science. In addition to it,
the scientist engages in "empirical analysis." Empirical analysts seeks to disclose the properties of the objects to which the words refer. As Hempel (1970)
phrases it, "Empirical analysis is concerned not with linguistic expressions
and their meanings but with empirical phenomena" (p. 658).

Ideal types, however, are not aimed at disclosing how large numbers
of psychiatrists use certain words. They are attempts to study patients and
their disorders. Ideal-type research, then, is far better able to discover new
and better ways of conceptualizing patients and their disorders. This research

is not confined to explicating through meaning analysis how large numbers of people already use certain concepts; new ideal types that improve our understanding of patients can be introduced through empirical analysis. The empirical analysis that Max Weber (1904–1905) undertook created the new ideal types of "the Protestant ethic" and "the spirit of capitalism," ideal types that have proven enormously fruitful for subsequent sociology. Such fruitful concepts could never emerge through a meaning analysis of the ways in which large numbers of early Protestants used the term "ethics."

How, then, do ideal types help us to understand reality better? Weber's "spirit of capitalism" does not aim at describing some underlying spiritual essence of capitalism at work in all capitalist enterprises and countries. His ideal type merely provides a well-defined conceptual tool that may or may not help us make sense of economic activity in a particular country. Ideal types, as we have said, are not either true or false. It does not make sense to ask whether the way in which we have defined the ideal type "histrionic personality" is true or false. Ideal types are only helpful or unhelpful in guiding or orienting further investigations of individual patients. As characterized by both Weber and Jaspers, ideal types are heuristic devices (Schwartz & Wiggins, 1987).

When we apply the ideal type to a particular case, we may find that the case exhibits very few, if any, traits specified by the type. If this is so, then we may conclude that this type cannot help us understand this individual case. Or, if we are still persuaded that the individual case falls within the category, we may be led to ask questions such as "Why is this (typical) trait not present in this case?" If we pose such a question, then we undertake a further inquiry into the particularity of this case, which is still guided by the ideal type.

Suppose, for example, that we detect in a patient, Mr. Herbert, in conformity with the requirements of DSM-III-R, "a pervasive pattern of excessive emotionality and attention-seeking, beginning by early adulthood and present in a variety of contexts" (American Psychiatric Association, 1987, p. 349), including at least four specified DSM-III-R criteria. We may then justifiably diagnose Mr. Herbert as having histrionic personality disorder. Suppose further that Mr. Herbert also seems to exhibit Jaspers's basic trait for hysteria. But imagine that he is not at all "overly concerned with physical attractiveness" (a DSM-III-R criterion for histrionic personality disorder; American Psychiatric Association, 1987, p. 349), and, in addition, that he markedly exhibits "perfectionism that interferes with task completion" (a DSM-III-R criterion for obsessive–compulsive personality disorder; American Psychiatric Association, 1987, p. 356). A psychiatrist who adopts the ideal-type approach might then investigate precisely why the histrionic trait is unexpectedly absent in Mr. Herbert and why the obsessive–compulsive trait is so conspicuously present in him. The ideal type would initially serve in diagnosis, but it would subsequently serve in guiding the ongoing investigations of Mr. Herbert.

Prototypes, unlike ideal types, aim at uncovering the truth about a class of patients. The proponents of prototypes seek to specify in the long run the "correct" definitions of the personality disorders. By contrast, ideal types provide only a (one-sided) point of view from which patients can be further examined. As Jaspers (1923) warned, "Once the study of personality starts to pigeon-hole people into pure types, it comes to grief . . . an individual can never be exhausted by any one type, since this only serves to delineate one aspect of him" (p. 438). And Kurt Schneider (1923b) wrote:

> Psychopathic [i.e., personality] types look like diagnoses but the analogy is a false one. A depressive psychopath is simply a "certain sort of person." People or personalities cannot be labelled diagnostically like illnesses nor like the psychic effects of illness. At most, we are simply emphasizing and indicating a set of individual peculiarities which distinguish these people and in which there is nothing comparable to symptoms of illness. . . . In any detailed portrayal the type is soon lost and other traits not necessarily linked to the special characteristic in question creep in to form a concrete portrait. (pp. 29–31)

This difference between prototypes and ideal types is related to a further one. The proponents of prototypes are trying to define the personality disorders correctly. This aim serves the further goal of uncovering the etiologies of the disorders. If we can reliably delineate separate groups of patients, it is believed, we can study them in order to discover the causes of their disorders. Such reasoning presupposes that the causes will be simple and invariant enough to be captured in this fashion. And, of course, it assumes that there exists some univocal connection between clinical symptomatology and underlying causal mechanisms. These assumptions may prove to be valid. But, at present, we must remain cognizant of the fact that they are mere assumptions that could also prove to be invalid.

The usefulness of ideal types, on the other hand, does not depend upon their ultimate value in uncovering the causal mechanisms of disease. Ideal types can be used by researchers to delineate groups of patients for nomological investigations (Schwartz & Wiggins, 1987). But apart from this, they already serve the clinician in guiding the inquiry into the individual patient.

Some people have complained that DSM-III and DSM-III-R have served the purposes of researchers but not the purposes of clinicians. As long ago as 1874, Hughlings Jackson advocated a dualistic classification system — one system for clinical work and another for research (Stengel, 1963). Since the publication of DSM-III this same idea has been proposed by Zubin (1984) and others (Berner & Katschnig, 1984) for DSM-IV, although it has not been adopted in DSM-IV as published (American Psychiatric Association, 1994). Ideal types, as we envision them, could provide a unified classification scheme that would serve the purposes of both clinicians and researchers.

## CONCLUSION

Ideal types were introduced for the classification of personality disorders by Karl Jaspers. Like so many of Jaspers's timeless insights, his proposed classification scheme has been overlooked in recent years. Present-day discussions of prototypes, however, remind us of the important virtues of ideal types. Because of their similarities to ideal types, prototypes mark a return to some of the classical insights of Jaspers. We maintain that ideal types can help to systematically unify diagnostic categories and the multifarious strands of clinical treatment and empirical research, which, depending on their purposes, may employ polythetic concepts, dimensions, and prototypes.

## REFERENCES

American Psychiatric Association. (1980). *Diagnostic and statistical manual of mental disorders* (3rd ed.). Washington, DC: Author.

American Psychiatric Association. (1987). *Diagnostic and statistical manual of mental disorders* (3rd ed., rev.). Washington, DC: Author.

American Psychiatric Association. (1994). *Diagnostic and statistical manual of mental disorders* (4th ed.). Washington, DC: Author.

Beckner, M. (1959). *The biological way of thought.* New York: Columbia University Press.

Berner, P., & Katschnig, H. (1984). Commentary on R. E. Kendell: "Reflections on psychiatric classification—For the architects of DSM-IV and ICD-10." *Integrative Psychiatry, 2,* 51–52.

Blashfield, R. K. (1986). Structural approaches to classification. In T. Millon & G. L. Klerman (Eds.), *Contemporary directions in psychopathology: Toward the DSM-IV* (pp. 363–360). New York: Guilford Press.

Blashfield, R. K., Sprock, J., Pinkston, K., & Hodgin, J. (1985). Exemplar prototypes of personality disorder diagnoses. *Comprehensive Psychiatry, 26,* 11–21.

Cantor, N., & Genero, N. (1986). Psychiatric diagnosis and natural categorization: A close analogy. In T. Millon & G. L. Klerman (Eds.), *Contemporary directions in psychopathology: Toward the DSM-IV* (pp. 233–256). New York: Guilford Press.

Cantor, N., & Mischel, W. (1979). Prototypes in person perception. In L. Berkowitz (Ed.), *Advances in experimental social psychology* (Vol. 12, pp. 3–52). New York: Academic Press.

Cantor, N., Smith, E., French, R. de S., & Mezzich, J. (1980). Psychiatric diagnosis as prototype categorization. *Journal of Abnormal Psychology, 69,* 181–193.

Chalmers, A. F. (1982). *What is this thing called science?* Brisbane: University of Queensland Press.

Clarkin, J. F., Widiger, T. A., Frances, A., Hurt, S. W., & Gilmore, M. (1983). Prototypic typology and the borderline personality. *Journal of Abnormal Psychology, 90,* 575–585.

Fulford, K. W. M. (1989). *Moral theory and medical practice.* Cambridge, England: Cambridge University Press.

Hempel, C. G. (1965). *Aspects of scientific explanation and other essays in the philosophy of science.* New York: Free Press.

Hempel, C. G. (1970). Fundamentals of concept formation in empirical science. In

G. Neurath, R. Carnap, & C. Morris (Eds.), *Foundations of the unity of science: Towards an international encyclopedia of unified science* (Vol. 2, pp. 651–745). Chicago: University of Chicago Press.

Horowitz, L., Post, D., French, R., Wallis, K., & Seligman, E. (1961). The prototype as a construct in abnormal psychology: 2. Clarifying disagreement in psychiatric judgements. *Journal of Abnormal Psychology, 90,* 575–565.

Jaspers, K. (1923). *General psychopathology* (J. Hoenig & M.W. Hamilton, Trans.). Chicago: University of Chicago Press, 1963.

Kendell, R. E. (1983). DSM-III: A major advance in psychiatric nosology. In R. L. Spitzer, J. B. W. Williams, & A. E. Skodol (Eds.), *International perspectives on DSM-III* (pp. 55–68). Washington, DC: American Psychiatric Press.

Lakoff, G. (1987). *Women, fire, and dangerous things: What categories reveal about the mind.* Chicago: University of Chicago Press.

Livesley, W. J. (1985). The classification of personality disorder: 1. The choice of category concept. *Canadian Journal of Psychiatry, 30,* 353–356.

Livesley, W. J. (1986). Trait and behavioral prototypes of personality disorder. *American Journal of Psychiatry. 143,* 728–732.

Longino, H. E. (1990). *Science as social knowledge: Values and objectivity in scientific inquiry.* Princeton, NJ: Princeton University Press.

Millon, T. (1986). On the past and future of the DSM-III: Personal recollections and projections. In T. Millon & G. L. Klerman (Eds.), *Contemporary directions in psychopathology: Toward the DSM-IV* (pp. 29–70). New York: Guilford Press.

Popper, K. R. (1972). *Objective knowledge: An evolutionary approach.* Oxford: Clarendon Press.

Rosch, E. (1978). Principles of categorization. In E. Rosch & B. L. Lloyd (Eds.), *Cognition and categorization.* Hillsdale, NJ: Erlbaum.

Rosch, E., & Mervis, C. B. (1975). Family resemblances: Studies in the internal structure of categories. *Cognitive Psychology, 7,* 573–605.

Schaffner, K. F. (1986). Exemplar reasoning about biological models and diseases: A relation between the philosophy of medicine and philosophy of science. *Journal of Medicine and Philosophy, 11,* 63–80.

Schneider, K. (1923a). *Psychopathic personalities* (M. W. Hamilton, Trans.). New York: Grune & Stratton, 1958.

Schneider, K. (1923b). *Clinical psychopathology* (M. W. Hamilton, Trans.). New York: Grune & Stratton, 1959.

Schwartz, M. A., & Wiggins, O. P. (1985). Science, humanism, and the nature of medical practice: A phenomenological view. *Perspectives in Biology and Medicine, 26,* 331–361.

Schwartz, M. A., & Wiggins, O. P. (1986). Logical empiricism and psychiatric classification. *Comprehensive Psychiatry, 27,* 101–114.

Schwartz, M. A., & Wiggins, O. P. (1987). Diagnosis and ideal types: A contribution to psychiatric classification. *Comprehensive Psychiatry, 28,* 277–291.

Schwartz, M. A., & Wiggins, O. P. (1988). Scientific and humanistic medicine: A theory of clinical methods. In K. L. White (Ed.), *The task of medicine: Dialogue at Wickenburg* (pp. 137–171). Menlo Park, CA: Henry J. Kaiser Family Foundation.

Stengel, E. (1963). Hughlings Jackson's influence in psychiatry. *British Journal of Psychiatry, 109,* 348–355.

Weber, M. (1903–1917). *The methodology of the social sciences* (E. A. Shils & H. A. Finch, Eds. and Trans.). New York: Free Press, 1949.

Weber, M. (1904–1905). *The Protestant ethic and the spirit of capitalism* (T. Parsons, Trans.). New York: Scribner's, 1958.

Weber, M. (1956). *Economy and society: An outline in interpretive sociology* (E. Fischoff et al., Trans.). Berkeley: University of California Press, 1976.

Wittgenstein, L. (1953). *Philosophical investigations* (G. E. M. Anscombe, Trans.). New York: Macmillan.

Zubin, J. (1984). Commentary on R.E. Kendell: "Reflections on psychiatric classification—For the architects of DSM-IV and ICD-10." *Integrative Psychiatry, 2,* 52–53.

CHAPTER 22

# Toward a Dimensional Model of Personality Disorders

THOMAS A. WIDIGER
CYNTHIA J. SANDERSON

The question of whether mental disorders are optimally classified categorically or dimensionally is a long-standing issue (e.g., Eysenck, 1987; Kendell,
1975; Mezzich, 1979; Presley & Walton, 1973; Tyrer & Alexander, 1979). The
controversy is particularly relevant for the personality disorders, given the
contrasting traditions within personality research and clinical psychiatry.
There have been categorical (typological) models of normal personality traits
and dimensional models of personality dysfunction, but the norm has been
to classify normal personality traits dimensionally and abnormal personality traits categorically (Livesley, 1985; Widiger & Kelso, 1983).

The issue became more salient with the DSM-III placement of the personality disorders on a separate axis (American Psychiatric Association, 1980).
This unique placement was in recognition of the fact that a patient's maladaptive personality traits represent a long-standing mode of functioning that
predates and influences the course, presentation, and treatment of the more
circumscribed mental disorders placed on Axis I (Frances, 1980). "In effect,
the revised multiaxial format requires that symptom states no longer be diagnosed as clinical entities isolated from the broader context of the patient's
lifelong style of relating, coping, behaving, thinking, and feeling—that is,
his or her personality" (Millon, 1981, p. 3).

A personality disorder is not separate or distinct from a patient's personality. It is a description of how the patient characteristically (albeit maladap-
tively) thinks, relates, copes, and behaves, and it is apparent to essentially
all theorists and researchers that personalities do not come in neatly distinct types. The presence of over 2,000 terms in the English language to

433

describe the variety of personality traits is itself a testament to the complexity and diversity of personality (Goldberg, 1982). Nevertheless, DSM-III continued the medical tradition of providing singular, categorical diagnoses to characterize dysfunctional personalities.

Frances (1982) was among the first to discuss this anomaly with respect to DSM-III. His paper was of particular interest because he was an influential member of the DSM-III Advisory Committee on Personality Disorders. The paper has since been cited as opposing the categorical model and advocating the dimensional one, but Frances in fact concluded that the advantages of the categorical model outweighed its disadvantages: "For now, categorical diagnosis is the standard and, with all its problems, it remains the more useful method in everyday clinical psychiatric practice" (1982, p. 524). Millon (1981), another member of the DSM-III Advisory Committee on Personality Disorders, also reviewed this literature and reached the conclusion that "typological models are the preferred schema" (p. 16). Spitzer and Williams (1985) indicated that "even if in the real world a particular personality pattern is distributed on a continuum of severity . . . it may be useful to define a category for that portion of the distribution of the personality pattern that is associated with social or occupational impairment" (p. 592).

Subsequent critiques of the categorical model were provided by Livesley (1985) and by Widiger and Frances (1985) during the time in which DSM-III-R (American Psychiatric Association, 1987) was being prepared. Widiger and Frances (1985), members of the DSM-III-R Advisory Committee on Personality Disorders, recommended the "adoption of a dimensional model of classification" (p. 622). Livesley (1985), however, concluded that "at the present time it is perhaps more appropriate to consider ways to improve current [categorical] classifications, rather than to adopt a dimensional system of unproven relevance" (p. 354). One of the reasons for Livesley's reluctance was the lack of an apparent consensus regarding which dimensional model(s) to include. This concern was acknowledged by Widiger and Frances, but they nonetheless highlighted in particular the interpersonal circumplex (Kiesler, 1986; Wiggins, 1982). They did not advocate replacing Axis II with the interpersonal circumplex, but perhaps they should have been even more circumspect, because their support has since shifted toward the five-factor model (Widiger & Frances, 1994).

The incorporation of a dimensional model into DSM-IV was considered by the DSM-IV Personality Disorders Work Group. A formal review of the relevant empirical literature with recommendations was prepared by Widiger (1991). The purpose of this chapter is in part to provide a summary of this review. However, we also incorporate material that has been published since the appearance of the original review (Widiger, 1992, 1993), discuss the decisions made for DSM-IV by the work group, and make recommendations for future research.

## A CRITIQUE OF THE DSM-III-R CATEGORICAL DISTINCTIONS

Categorical diagnoses would be appropriate if there was a clear distinction between the presence and the absence of a personality disorder. However, no empirical study has ever identified any clear distinction between the presence and absence of a personality disorder, or any clear distinction among near-neighbor personality disorder diagnoses. We found seven studies that explicitly considered these questions, and in each case the authors concluded that the results they obtained were inconsistent with the categorical distinctions. Frances, Clarkin, Gilmore, Hurt, and Brown (1984) obtained personality disorder ratings on 76 psychiatric outpatients and concluded that "the DSM-III criteria for personality disorders do not select out mutually exclusive, categorical diagnostic entities. . . . [The] frequency of multiple diagnoses supports the argument for a dimensional—rather than a categorical—system of personality diagnosis" (p. 1083). Kass, Skodol, Charles, Spitzer, and Williams (1985) obtained personality disorder ratings from a consecutive sample of 609 psychiatric outpatients and concluded that "our data do not lend support to the usefulness of a categorical approach" (p. 628). "Since many more patients had some [maladaptive] personality traits or almost met DSM-III criteria than actually met the full criteria . . . the categorical judgments of DSM-III necessarily resulted in the loss of information" (Kass et al., 1985, p. 630). Zimmerman and Coryell (1990) obtained personality disorder ratings on 808 first-degree relatives of psychiatric patients and never-ill control subjects and concluded that the personality disorder "scores are continuously distributed without points of rarity to indicate where to make the distinction between normality and pathology" (p. 690).

Oldham et al. (1992) administered two semistructured interviews for diagnosing DSM-III-R personality disorders to 100 of 106 consecutive applicants to a long-term inpatient clinic for severe personality disorders. They concluded that "consistent patterns of comorbidity involving narcissistic, avoidant, and histrionic personality disorders suggest that categorical distinctions between them and certain other DSM-III-R personality disorders may be illusory" (p. 213). These authors suggested that the categorical diagnoses be retained only when a patient meets the criteria for just one or two personality disorders (approximately 40% of the cases in their study). "For patients with more than two disorders, a single diagnosis of 'extensive personality disorder' might be made, with a dimensional description of the predominant characteristics" (p. 219). Livesley, Jackson, and Schroeder (1992) administered to 158 patients and 274 community subjects a self-report questionnaire assessing 100 aspects of personality dysfunction. They concluded:

> A class model of personality disorder, such as that apparently underlying the DSM-III-R, implies discontinuities between groups that differ in the presence of personality disorder. Such discontinuities were not apparent in our data. That

continua exist and that a substantial number of persons drawn from the non-clinical population have scores extending into the clinical distribution poses, in our view, great difficulties for the use of a simple class or categorical model. (p. 438)

Nestadt et al. (1990) obtained ratings of histrionic personality disorder symptomatology from a representative sample of a local community ($n$ = 810) and reported that "this personality diagnosis is rather arbitrarily given individuals who extend beyond a cut-off level, yet others less severe but similar in the nature of their dispositional features might have identical symptoms under certain life circumstances" (p. 420). Finally, Nurnberg et al. (1991) obtained systematic assessments of the DSM-III-R personality disorders in 110 outpatients without concurrent major Axis I diagnoses. Their analyses focused on borderline personality disorder, and they concluded that "patients who meet DSM-III-R criteria for borderline personality disorder constitute a very heterogeneous group with unclear boundaries whose overlap with neighboring personality disorder categories is extensive" (p. 1376). They suggested that "a better understanding of personality disorder awaits a paradigmatic shift away from discrete nosologic categories to alternative models" (p. 1376).

There are 93 different ways to meet the DSM-III-R criteria for borderline personality disorder, and 149,495,616 different ways to meet the DSM-III-R criteria for antisocial personality disorder (only 848 possible combinations if one does not count the subcriteria for the conduct disorder and parental irresponsibility items), yet only one diagnostic label is provided in each instance to characterize all of these different cases (i.e., presence of the disorder). One would not need to distinguish among all 149,495,616 different combinations of antisocial criteria to provide a useful description of a patient, but it is evident that not all antisocial individuals are alike with respect to their symptomatology and that many of the differences can be of considerable importance to clinical practice and research (Hare, Hart, & Harpur, 1991). There are 162 different possible combinations of the borderline criteria in persons who would not be given the diagnosis, but all of these cases are simply labeled as not having borderline personality disorder. The inadequacy of diagnosing these and other such patients as simply lacking a particular personality disorder was noted by Skodol (1989) in his overview of DSM-III-R:

Several of my colleagues and I believed that personality traits play such a significant role in determining treatment approach, especially in psychotherapy, that we instituted a scaled system for rating DSM-III personality disorders in the outpatient clinic at the Columbia–Presbyterian Medical Center. . . . Using this system, we found that, in addition to the approximately 50% of clinic patients who meet criteria for a personality disorder, another 35% warrant information descriptive of their personality styles on Axis II. (pp. 385–386)

In the absence of any clear distinction between the presence and the absence of a personality disorder, one might ask on what basis the distinctions were made in DSM-III and DSM-III-R. There was not in fact any empirical support for the thresholds for 9 of the 11 personality disorder diagnoses. They were based simply on the subjective impressions of the Advisory Committee on Personality Disorders (Perry, 1990). The thresholds for the borderline and schizotypal personality disorder diagnoses were based on empirical data (Spitzer, Endicott, & Gibbon, 1979), but this consisted simply of maximizing agreement with a sample of clinical diagnoses. Given that unstructured clinical diagnoses of personality disorders are notoriously inconsistent and unreliable (e.g., Mellsop, Varghese, Joshua, & Hicks, 1982), and that there is no compelling rationale for the point at which a personality becomes disordered (Widiger & Corbitt, 1994), clinical judgments as to the presence versus absence of a personality disorder provide a very questionable and at best circular criterion.

The arbitrary nature of the thresholds and distinctions were evident in a comparison of the DSM-III and DSM-III-R by Morey (1988). The DSM-III-R revisions resulted in "an 800% increase in the rate of schizoid personality disorder and a 350% increase in narcissistic personality disorder" (Morey, 1988, p. 575). Despite the intention of the advisory committee to improve the differentiation among the personality disorders (Widiger, Frances, Spitzer, & Williams, 1988), Morey's data suggested that co-occurrence was in fact increased by the revisions: "Under DSM-III only four personality disorders (narcissistic, histrionic, paranoid, and schizoid) had an overlap of at least 50% with another personality disorder. When DSM-III-R criteria were used, eight of the 11 specific disorders manifested this degree of overlap" (p. 576).

The failure of DSM-III and DSM-III-R to provide clinically meaningful thresholds was evident in a study by McGlashan (1987) concerning the comorbidity of borderline personality disorder and depression. He needed a comparison group of depressives without borderline personality disorder, and therefore obtained depressed persons who did not meet the DSM-III criteria for borderline personality disorder. However, these subjects had on average three of the borderline criteria. "In short, the 'pure' . . . cohort was not pure. . . . The result is that our comparison groups, although defined to be categorically exclusive, may not have been all that different, a fact which, in turn, may account for some of the similarities" (p. 472) between the supposedly pure depressives and the borderlines. The persons who were diagnosed as not having borderline personality disorder did in fact have borderline personality disorder pathology. To characterize these cases as not having borderline personality disorder was misleading (Widiger, Sanderson, & Warner, 1986). McGlashan concluded that the categorical system "emerges as poorly constructed for the study of comorbidity" (1987, p. 473).

The DSM-III-R cutoffs do not identify the point at which personality traits become a personality disorder. This fact provides a considerable handicap for researchers attempting to identify other clinical correlates of the respective disorders. For example, the DSM-III-R threshold for dependent personality disorder does not identify the point at which dependent traits provide a predisposition to depression. Research whose purpose it is to assess the relationship of dependency to depression will then be substantially hindered by the DSM-III-R categorical distinction (Overholser, 1991). Many persons below the threshold for a dependent personality disorder diagnosis will have clinically significant traits of dependency that will be associated with depression, including perhaps those persons with only the single DSM-III-R criterion "feels devastated or helpless when close relationships end" (American Psychiatric Association, 1987, p. 354).

Compelling support for a categorical distinction would be obtained if investigators found that reliability and validity improved with the use of a dichotomous rather than a dimensional rating. A dichotomous variable will show a decreased relation to an external correlate (or at least no change) when it is dimensionalized, whereas a dimensional variable will show a reduced relationship when it is dichotomized (Miller & Thayer, 1989). The former occurs as a result of the inclusion of irrelevant, invalid information. If a more quantitative, dimensional rating simply provided irrelevant, tangential, and/or illusory distinctions, then the additional discrimination required by the dimensional rating would result in a decreased correlation with various external validators. Widiger (1992) summarized the results of 16 personality disorder studies in which the data were analyzed both categorically (i.e., with DSM-III or DSM-III-R diagnoses) and dimensionally (e.g., using the total number of criteria). In all but one instance, the reliability and/or validity data were better with the dimensional analyses, indicating that reliable and valid information is being lost by converting what is either an ordinal, interval, or ratio scale to a nominal scale (Heumann & Morey, 1990).

A dramatic illustration of the fallibility of the categorical distinctions was provided by Pilkonis (1992). Pilkonis assessed the interrater reliability of a DSM-III-R personality disorder diagnosis, using either the Personality Disorder Examination (PDE; Loranger, 1988) or the Structured Interview for DSM-III-R Personality Disorders (SIDP-R; Pfohl, Blum, Zimmerman, & Stangl, 1989) for the assessment. Interrater reliability was low for the categorical decision of any personality disorder present versus no personality disorder present, and much higher when a continuous score was used. More importantly, Pilkonis then selected a single symptom and changed the interviewers' ratings so that they would always agree on this one symptom. Kappa then increased dramatically from .42 to .93 in one group (11 outpatients assessed by five raters) and from .68 to .92 in another group (26 inpatients assessed by two raters) when the PDE was used, and from .61 to .77 and from .51 to .92 in the two groups, respectively, when the SIDP-R was used. Pilkonis also changed the raters' decisions so that they would always disagree with respect to one symptom. Reliability dramatically decreased to .27 and .18 for the inpatient and outpatient groups, respectively, for the PDE, and to

.58 and .35, respectively, for the SIDP-R. These analyses clearly demonstrate the instability of empirical results for categorical diagnoses. Changing the findings for just one symptom from a list of over 100 can produce very dramatic changes in the results. This instability would not occur with the assessment of the reliability for the continuum score.

An application of factor analysis that is relevant to the question of the validity of the categorical model is the comparison of factor solutions across groups that are purportedly distinct with respect to a latent class taxon. Measures that are highly discriminating between such groups should not correlate substantially within the groups, nor should the factor solution of the intercorrelation among such measures be replicated across groups (Eysenck, 1987; Livesley, 1991). Tyrer and Alexander (1979) reported that the factor solutions for the correlations among 24 personality variables assessed by a semistructured interview were replicated across 65 patients with a primary clinical diagnosis of a personality disorder and 65 patients with other diagnoses. Similar findings were reported by Livesley et al. (1992), using a self-report measure of 100 aspects of personality disorder dysfunction, whose intercorrelations were factor-analyzed in a sample of 274 community subjects and 158 patients. Livesley et al. concluded that "the degree of similarity observed between the factor structures across the two samples provides evidence that dimensions of personality disorder are organized in similar ways in the two populations. Personality pathology in a clinical population appears to differ only in quantity rather than quality" (1992, p. 438).

Maximum covariation (MAXCOV) analysis similarly capitalizes on the fact that the covariation between any two signs of a categorical variable will be minimized in groups of subjects who share the class membership and will be maximized in mixed groups, whereas no such variation in covariation will be found across levels of a dimensional variable (Klein & Riso, 1993; Grove & Meehl, 1993; Meehl, 1992). Trull, Widiger, and Guthrie (1990) applied MAXCOV analysis to the DSM-III-R criteria for borderline personality disorder. The charts of 409 patients were systematically coded for symptoms of dysthymia (a presumably dimensional variable), biological sex (a categorical variable), and borderline personality disorder. A clear peak was found for biological sex; the curve was flat for dysthymia; and no peak in the middle of the distribution was found for borderline personality disorder. Trull et al. concluded that "the results are most consistent with the hypothesis that [borderline personality disorder] is optimally conceptualized as a dimensional variable" (1990, p. 47). It should be also be noted, however, that the Trull et al. findings were not unambiguous. The MAXCOV curve for borderline personality disorder did not peak in the center of the distribution, but it did peak at the end of the distribution, which is perhaps inconsistent with both the dimensional and categorical models. Lenzenweger and Korfine (1992) obtained an almost identical finding when they assessed eight indicators of schizotypia in a sample of 1,093 undergraduate college students and suggested that "an upward sweeping right-end peak is consistent with a taxonic [categorical] latent entity that has a low base rate" (p. 570). Lenzenweger and Korfine did not provide a rationale for why taxon with a low base rate would provide a right-end peak. However, it might suggest that the distribution of subjects was approaching an even mix of taxon members and nonmembers as more items were endorsed (e.g., only half of the subjects who endorsed all of the items did in fact have the personality disorder). In any case, future MAXCOV studies need to address this anomaly.

Admixture analysis examines the distribution of canonical coefficient scores derived from a discriminant-function analysis for evidence of bimodality. This technique has suggested the presence of discrete breaks in the distribution of measures of somatoform and psychotic disorders (Cloninger, Martin, Guze, & Clayton, 1985). No published study has yet reported an admixture analysis of personality disorder data. Cloninger (1989) indicated that he applied admixture analysis with personality disorder data and "found that underlying [the] relatively distinct subgroups appeared to be multiple dimensions of personality that were normally distributed" (p. 140). He concluded: "The real take-home message to me is not that we do not have methods to detect relatively discrete groups but that with psychiatric disorders the groups are not totally discrete, and this finding may be consistent with extreme syndromes that develop superimposed on top of underlying dimensional variation" (p. 140).

## ARGUMENTS FAVORING A CATEGORICAL MODEL

The empirical research clearly favors the argument that the DSM-III-R personality disorders do not involve qualitatively distinct disorders. In our opinion, the DSM-III-R personality disorders represent extreme and/or maladaptive variants of personality traits that are present to a varying degree across the entire population. One may then ask why the DSM continues to use a categorical model. Three arguments in favor of the categorical approach have been presented: (1) tradition and familiarity; (2) ease in conceptualization and communication; and (3) consistency with clinical decisions (Davis & Millon, 1993; Frances, 1990, 1993; Gunderson, Links, & Reich, 1991; Millon, 1981, 1991). Each is discussed here in turn.

### Familiarity and Tradition

The categorical system is more familiar than any dimensional model to clinicians. All prior and current diagnoses within the DSM have been categorical, and it would represent a major shift in clinical practice to convert to a dimensional model (Frances, 1990).

It should be noted, however, that no survey has ever documented a preference among practicing clinicians for the categorical format. It may then be presumptive to argue that clinicians prefer the categorical system or would not accept a dimensional classification. Maser, Kaelber, and Wise (1991) surveyed 146 psychologists and psychiatrists in 42 countries with respect to the entire DSM-III-R. "The personality disorders led the list of diagnostic categories with which respondents were dissatisfied" (Maser et al., 1991, p. 275). The personality disorders were considered to be problematic by 56% of the respondents; the second most frequently cited category was that of the mood disorders, cited by only 28%. In response to an optional, write-in question, "35 of 101 respondents (35%) chose to write in personality disorders . . . 'most in need of revision' " (p. 275). Kass et al. (1985) indicated that feedback from staff and trainees during their study on dimensional ratings for the personality disorders suggested that a 4-point severity rating was both feasible and acceptable in routine clinical practice. Similar results were reported in a much earlier study with medical students by Hine and Williams (1975).

Categories are more familiar to, and may at times be preferred by, clinicians. However, this tradition reflects in part a natural inclination toward simplification that fails to appreciate the complexity of personality functioning. Diagnostic categories do provide vivid, clear descriptions (Frances, 1990; Gunderson et al., 1991), but to the extent that most patients do not represent prototypical cases (Clarkin, Widiger, Frances, Hurt, & Gilmore, 1983), these descriptions will be misleading and stereotyping. "There is a tendency, once having categorized, to exaggerate the similarity among nonidentical stimuli by overlooking within-group variability, discounting disconfirming evidence, and focusing on stereotypic examples of the category" (Cantor & Genero, 1986, p. 235). This is most clearly evident in regard to occupational, ethnic, and gender stereotypes, but it can be equally problematic in the diagnosis of mental disorders (Ford & Widiger, 1989; Schacht, 1985). A more quantitative description of the extent to which each personality disorder is evident (or a set of cross-cutting dimensions) would provide a more precise description that would be more informative and less stereotyping. The heterogeneity would then be retained and would inform clinical decisions.

## Ease in Conceptualization and Communication

It has also been argued that even if a dimensional classification of personality functioning is more informative, it would be too difficult and cumbersome in clinical practice (Gunderson et al., 1991; Millon, 1981, 1991). To the extent that a dimensional model retains more information, it requires the acquisition and communication of more information. In practice, however, the personality disorder diagnostic categories of DSM-III-R are more complex and cumbersome than most dimensional models. The DSM-III-R taxonomy includes 104 diagnostic criteria, requiring more than 2 hours for a systematic and comprehensive assessment (e.g., Loranger, 1988; Pfohl et al., 1989). A 2-hour period is substantial, but even this amount of time only allows for an average of 1 minute and 9 seconds to assess each personality disorder criterion. It is then understandable that most clinicians fail to assess the DSM-III-R criteria systematically (Morey & Ochoa, 1989). It is neither practical nor even feasible in routine clinical practice. A rating along five dimensions and relevant facets that did not require the redundant assessments and arbitrary distinctions inherent to the DSM-III-R would probably be easier and simpler.

The DSM-III-R categorical system also results in a variety of confusing multiple diagnoses (Cloninger, 1989; Widiger & Rogers, 1989). Many patients will meet the criteria for as many as five, six, seven, or even more personality disorders, with the average number being approximately three or four (e.g., Skodol, Rosnick, Kellman, Oldham, & Hyler, 1990). Most clinical charts, however, will have just one diagnosis (Gunderson, 1992). The reason why clinicians fail to provide all of the diagnoses that apply is that it is not particularly meaningful to indicate that a patient is suffering from four or five distinct and comorbid personality disorders, each apparently with its own etiology and pathology. It would be simpler and more meaningful to state that the person suffers from one personality disorder characterized by varying degrees of borderline, avoidant, and histrionic traits than to state that the patient is suffering from three different, comorbid personality disorders (Oldham et al., 1992).

## Consistency with Clinical Decisions

The final argument in favor of the categorical model is that clinical decision making tends to be categorical. Treatment decisions are not usually made in shades of grey; many clinicians would therefore convert a dimensional profile to categories in order to facilitate their decisions. The Minnesota Multiphasic Personality Inventory (MMPI), for example, provides the potential for detailed assessments along dimensions, but it is often converted to typological codetypes. There might then be little advantage in increasing the complexity of diagnosis by requiring ratings along a continuum that is ignored in clinical practice.

Consistency with clinical decision making, however, is readily retained in a dimensional model simply by providing recommended cutoff points for various clinical decisions. The reverse option is not possible. Once a categorical diagnosis is provided, the ability to return to a more precise description (e.g., the degree to which the person resembles a prototypical case) cannot be recovered.

It is the case that many clinicians convert an MMPI dimensional profile to a categorical codetype, but it is unlikely that these clinicians would prefer to be given only the codetype and not to be provided with the additional information obtained from the profile description. A dimensional profile also provides the flexibility to use alternative cutting scores for different situations and clinical decisions. It is likely, for example, that some clinical or research situations will require more liberal or more restrictive thresholds than are provided by the DSM-III-R diagnoses. Different cutoff points will be optimal for assessing the need for hospitalization, disability support, or pharmacological intervention, or for determining the predisposition to depression (Finn, 1982; Kendler, 1990). A dimensional profile of the extent to which each personality disorder is present would allow for this flexibility; the categorical diagnoses do not.

# ALTERNATIVE PROPOSALS

A variety of options for addressing the limitations of the categorical model and for incorporating a more dimensional approach were considered by the DSM-IV Personality Disorders Work Group (Task Force on DSM-IV, 1991; Widiger, 1991). These included revising the diagnostic criteria further, implementing hierarchical exclusion rules, providing more specific criteria for a rating of severity, including a table for describing the extent to which each personality disorder is present, and providing an alternative dimensional model in an appendix. These options, and the decisions made regarding each one in DSM-IV as published (American Psychiatric Association, 1994), are discussed here in turn.

## Revision of Diagnostic Criteria

The principal approach of the DSM-IV Personality Disorders Work Group to addressing the limitations of the categorical model has been to revise the diagnostic criteria to improve the differentiation among the categories. It is clearly useful to revise the criteria to improve their clarity and assessment, but this could be an effort to provide a differential diagnosis where there is no meaningful differentiation.

A differential diagnosis assumes that only one diagnosis should be given — for example, that the correct diagnosis is histrionic rather than borderline, or avoidant rather than dependent. However, to the extent that only one diagnosis is given, the description of the patient is likely to be inadequate and misleading. And to the extent that a criteria set describes a distinct personality style, sharing no features or characteristics seen in any other personality disorder, it will probably describe a prototypical case that almost never occurs. Most patients will have a variety of maladaptive personality traits, bearing only a family resemblance to the prototypical case. For instance, patients with avoidant personality disorder will typically possess traits that are seen in patients with the dependent, histrionic, schizoid, and/or borderline personality disorders. A manual that describes prototypical cases will fail to characterize the actual cases, and a manual that describes actual cases will be unable to provide distinct diagnostic categories.

## Hierarchical Classification

A proposal suggested by Gunderson (1992) for addressing the excessive prevalence and co-occurrence of the personality disorders was to include a hierarchical exclusionary algorithm. Hierarchical models have also been
suggested by Morey (1988) and Oldham et al. (1992). DSM-III contained two
such rules within the personality disorders section (American Psychiatric Association, 1980). One could not diagnose schizoid personality disorder if a
patient met the criteria for schizotypal personality disorder, and one could
not diagnose passive–aggressive personality disorder if the patient met the
criteria for any of the other 10 personality disorders. These rules were abandoned in DSM-III-R, because they were virtually ignored by both clinicians
and researchers and because their justification was weak (Widiger et al., 1988).
Clinicians were instead encouraged to provide multiple diagnoses. However,
as Gunderson noted, clinicians have largely ignored this instruction, typically providing only one diagnosis per patient. Gunderson (1992) therefore
suggested that "in practice, there is a hierarchical system that gives precedence to the disorder that is most prototypically evident and that best accounts for the associated symptoms or dysfunction" (p. 19).

There are, however, two fundamental problems with hierarchical exclusionary algorithms. The first is that there is unlikely to be consensus or
clinical acceptance for any particular algorithm. Gunderson (1992) suggested that priority be given "to those diagnoses that are better validated, that
have more functional impairment, or that have primacy for treatment" (p.
19). His own proposal was for the borderline, antisocial, paranoid, and
schizotypal diagnoses to trump the remaining seven DSM-III-R personality
disorders. Given the prevalence of these four diagnoses within clinical settings (Widiger & Rogers, 1989), this would effectively eliminate from future
usage the narcissistic, histrionic, avoidant, dependent, obsessive–compulsive,
schizoid, and passive–aggressive diagnoses. The proposal also did not address the substantial co-occurrence among the borderline, antisocial,
schizotypal, and paranoid diagnoses, failing to specify which among these
four would take precedence when they co-occur.

An alternative to Gunderson's (1992) proposal would be to state that
only the one personality disorder that is most evident or is most important
to treatment should be diagnosed. This would in principle allow any of the
personality disorders to be diagnosed, not constraining the clinician from
giving (for example) a dependent diagnosis in the context of a borderline
diagnosis when the clinician considers the dependent personality disorder
to be more important or useful. This proposal would effectively institute
what probably already occurs in everyday clinical practice. A major limitation, though, is that it might simply encourage the occurrence of idiosyncratic and faddish clinical decisions. The personality disorder of a patient
could change across clinicians, settings, and time as each clinician, setting,
or time suggests a different emphasis. The diagnosis of personality disor-

ders is notoriously unreliable within clinical practice (Mellsop et al., 1982), and this hierarchical rule would simply encourage poor reliability.

The second fundamental problem with a hierarchical rule is that it will not resolve the issue it is trying to address. The empirical fact is that many borderline patients have clinically significant dependent, avoidant, narcissistic, schizotypal, and histrionic traits (Widiger & Frances, 1989). Assigning only the borderline diagnosis to these patients will provide an inadequate and misleading description of their personality disorder pathology. A hierarchical rule eliminates the complexity of personality only by fiat.

The hierarchical rule suggested by Oldham et al. (1992) would be much less problematic than Gunderson's (1992). Oldham et al. suggested that if a patient meets the criteria for only two personality disorders, then both diagnoses should be given. If the patient meets the criteria for three or more, then a diagnosis of "extensive personality disorder" should be given, with "a dimensional description of the predominant characteristics" (p. 219). This proposal would eliminate the conceptual and clinical oddity of diagnosing a patient with three, four, or more purportedly comorbid and distinct personality disorders. One would instead provide just one diagnosis ("extensive"), because the patient is in fact suffering from just one personality disorder characterized by a variety of maladaptive personality traits. Oldham et al.'s proposal failed to address the occurrence of clinically significant traits that are below the threshold for a diagnosis (e.g., clinically significant borderline traits in persons who meet the criteria for an avoidant diagnosis), but it would represent an improvement over the DSM-III-R policy of providing up to 11 personality disorder diagnoses to the same patient.

There are many additional problems and issues with hierarchical exclusionary rules that go beyond the problems peculiar to the personality disorders. Discussions of these issues are presented elsewhere (Blashfield, 1984, 1990; First, Spitzer, & Williams, 1990; Frances, Widiger, & Fyer, 1990; Klein & Riso, 1993). The eventual decision of the Personality Disorders Work Group was not to provide any hierarchical rules in DSM-IV.

## Provision of Explicit Criteria for Severity Rating

In the deliberations of the Personality Disorders Work Group, it was suggested that the DSM-III-R severity rating already provides a dimensional classification. DSM-III-R includes a specification of severity as either mild, moderate, or severe "to indicate the severity of the current disorder . . . at the time of the evaluation when all of the diagnostic criteria are met" (American Psychiatric Association, 1987, p. 24). This rating does recognize that disorders occur in varying degrees of severity, comparable to a "dimensional" proposal considered for DSM-III (Spitzer & Williams, 1985). Spitzer suggested that one could facilitate its usage by providing more explicit criteria. For example, "mild" could be defined as a minimal number of symptoms, resulting in only minor impairment in social or occupational functioning (e.g., reprimands by an employer or arguments with a spouse). "Severe" could be defined as several symptoms in excess of those necessary for the diagnosis, resulting in a marked interference with social and occupational function-ing (e.g., loss of job and divorce).

A severity rating, however, concerns a level of functioning for persons who have a (categorically diagnosed) disorder. It would not be given to per-sons who fail to meet the criteria for a disorder. In addition, the severity rating does not indicate the extent to which a person is (for example) bor-derline or obsessive–compulsive, but rather the degree of dysfunction as-sociated with a person's borderline or obsessive–compulsive personality disorder. A person who is more obsessive–compulsive than borderline could have a higher severity rating for borderline, because a person with just a few borderline symptoms may be more dysfunctional than a person with many obsessive–compulsive symptoms. Finally, it is questionable whether the severity rating could be assessed reliably. Its assessment would require a clinician to determine the specific source of a dysfunction when a patient meets the criteria for more than one personality disorder. For example, a clinician might have to determine whether a marital separation is attribut-able primarily to the borderline, dependent, or paranoid traits. In view of all these objections, the Personality Disorders Work Group eventually decided not to include explicit criteria for a severity rating in DSM-IV.

## Provision of a Table for a More Dimensional Rating

An additional proposal was to provide a table in the introductory text of the section on the personality disorders that would encourage clinicians to consider the extent to which each personality disorder is present (Widiger, 1991). Instead of characterizing each disorder as simply present or absent, the clinician would be encouraged to indicate (for example) whether no traits are present, whether a person represents a subthreshold case, whether the person just barely meets the criteria for the disorder, or whether the patient meets all of the criteria for the disorder. The term "absent" would mean what it implied—an absence of any of the diagnostic criteria. Table 20.1 presents the last version of this proposal.

Six levels are provided in Table 22.1: "absent," "traits," "subthreshold," "threshold," "moderate," and "extreme." The rating in each case was compat-ible with the DSM-III-R format (and could be easily revised for DSM-IV). "Ab-sent" means an absence of any of the specified symptoms. "Traits" means that there are simply one to three symptoms (DSM-III-R recommends that the clinician code personality disorder "traits" on Axis II when the patient meets some of the criteria but not enough to be given the diagnosis; Ameri-can Psychiatric Association, 1987, pp. 16–17). "Subthreshold" means that the person is only one symptom short of having the disorder. "Threshold" means that the person just barely meets the criteria for the disorder. "Moderate"

TABLE 22.1. Proposal for Converting the DSM-III-R Diagnostic Categories
to Dimensional Ratings

| Personality disorder | Number of criteria | | | | | |
|---|---|---|---|---|---|---|
| | Absent | Traits | Subthreshold | Threshold | Moderate | Extreme |
| Paranoid | 0 | 1-2 | 3 | 4 | 5-6 | 7 |
| Schizoid | 0 | 1-2 | 3 | 4 | 5-6 | 7 |
| Schizotypal | 0 | 1-3 | 4 | 5-6 | 7-8 | 9 |
| Antisocial[a] | 0 | 1-2 | 3 | 4-5 | 6-9 | 10 |
| Borderline | 0 | 1-3 | 4 | 5 | 6-7 | 8 |
| Histrionic | 0 | 1-2 | 3 | 4-5 | 6-7 | 8 |
| Narcissistic | 0 | 1-3 | 4 | 5-6 | 7-8 | 9 |
| Avoidant | 0 | 1-2 | 3 | 4 | 5-6 | 7 |
| Dependent | 0 | 1-3 | 4 | 5-6 | 7-8 | 9 |
| Obsessive– compulsive | 0 | 1-3 | 4 | 5-6 | 7-8 | 9 |
| Passive– aggressive | 0 | 1-3 | 4 | 5-6 | 7-8 | 9 |

*Note.* From Widiger (1991, p. 393). Copyright 1991 by The Guilford Press. Reprinted by permission.
[a]Confined to items occurring since the age of 15.

means that the person has more than enough of the criteria, and "extreme" means that all of the diagnostic features are present.

This coding would not be incompatible with the DSM-III-R (or DSM-IV) categorical format, yet would still provide a uniform terminology and method for describing the extent to which a patient has each disorder. The terminology and criteria would facilitate uniform discussion among clinicians and researchers who wish to indicate the extent to which a disorder is present without disrupting the diagnostic system. The table resembles in part a proposal considered for DSM-III (Spitzer & Williams, 1985), but the rating in this case would be based on the extent to which each personality disorder is present, rather than the severity of dysfunction associated with each personality disorder.

There were, however, a few concerns. One was that the table would be too cumbersome for practical use. It seemed unlikely that clinicians would systematically assess all of the criteria for all of the personality disorders and then provide a tabular summary of the extent to which each personality disorder is present. However, the proposal was not to require such a comprehensive rating; the proposal was simply to make the rating available. The table would provide uniform criteria and terminology to be used at times when clinicians or researchers would find it useful to do so. Clinicians would then be given the language and means by which to describe the extent to which each personality disorder is present.

The terminology would be helpful in undermining the characterization of the personality disorders as being simply present or absent. However, this anticipated effect was also a matter of concern. Some felt that it would not be appropriate to apply diagnostic labels (e.g., "subthreshold borderline" or "schizotypal traits") to persons not meeting diagnostic thresholds for the respective disorders. This was already encouraged in DSM-III-R (American Psychiatric Association, 1987, pp. 16–17), but the table would provide additional encouragement. It is our own opinion that persons who fail to meet the DSM-III-R diagnostic thresholds may in fact have maladaptive personality traits (e.g., Skodol, 1989), but the proposal to include the table in DSM-IV was not approved by the Personality Disorders Work Group.

## Inclusion of a Dimensional Model in an Appendix to DSM-IV

The final proposal was to provide an alternative dimensional model in the appendix to DSM-IV for proposed revisions needing further study. The major limitation of this proposal was the absence of a consensus dimensional model. Various dimensional models have been proposed (e.g., Clark, 1990; Cloninger, 1987; Costa & McCrae, 1990; Eysenck, 1987; Harkness, 1992; Kass et al., 1985; Kiesler, 1986; Livesley et al., 1992; Tellegen & Waller, in press), and it was felt that it would not be appropriate at this time for the DSM to favor one particular model over all of the alternatives.

However, the state of controversy, uncertainty, and confusion regarding which personality disorder categories to include in the DSM and how to diagnose them matches or perhaps even surpasses the state of disagreement with respect to the optimal dimensional model. The addition of the avoidant, narcissistic, borderline, and schizotypal diagnoses in DSM-III (American Psychiatric Association, 1980); the addition of the self-defeating and sadistic diagnoses in an appendix to DSM-III-R (American Psychiatric Association, 1987); and the deletion of the self-defeating and sadistic diagnoses, together with the addition of the depressive diagnosis and the reconceptualization of the passive–aggressive (negativistic) diagnosis in an appendix to DSM-IV (American Psychiatric Association, 1994), all suggest considerable disagreement and confusion (Blashfield, Sprock, & Fuller, 1990). There is no basis for estimating how many categorical personality disorders actually exist and which should be included in the manual. As Frances and Widiger (1986) indicated, "it seems likely that an optimal number falls somewhere between the extremes of Fourier's 810 and Hippocrates' four, but it is not clear just where" (p. 247). Each revision of the DSM has resulted in substantial revisions to the diagnostic criteria and the diagnostic thresholds (Morey, 1988). Over 75% of the 104 DSM-III-R personality disorder criteria have been revised in DSM-IV, despite the intention to be conservative (Frances, 1990; Gunderson, 1992).

The authors of the alternative dimensional models, on the other hand, indicate that considerable overlap and convergence exist among their models (e.g., Schroeder, Wormworth, & Livesley, 1992), with disagreements primarily pertaining to the names for and characterization of the dimensions. Nevertheless, the development of a variety of alternative models by leading researchers is interpreted by some as indicating that this perspective is not yet ready for formal recognition within an official nomenclature. "If it is premature to develop a consensus of dimensions and instruments for research purposes, it is certainly premature to suggest that any one system is ready for introduction in a diagnostic manual" (Frances, 1993, p. 110).

There is considerable support for the five-factor model (consisting of the dimensions of neuroticism, introversion vs. extraversion, openness vs. closedness to experience, agreeableness vs. antagonism, and conscientiousness; McCrae & Costa, 1990) for the classification of normal personality functioning (Digman, 1990; Goldberg, 1990; John, 1990; Wiggins & Pincus, 1992). However, this model does not have widespread familiarity and support within psychiatry, and it was argued that because the DSM is a manual for the diagnosis of mental disorders, it should not include normal functioning. On the other hand, to the extent that personality disorders entail extreme and/or maladaptive variants of normal personality traits, it is appropriate and even desirable for a classification of dysfunctional personality to be coordinated with a classification of normal personality traits. There is also substantial empirical support for the ability of the five-factor model to account for and describe the DSM-III-R personality disorders (Clark & Livesley, 1994; Costa & McCrae, 1990; Schroeder et al., 1992; Soldz, Budman, Demby, & Merry, 1993; Trull, 1992; Wiggins & Pincus, 1989). Elsewhere, we and our colleagues (Widiger, Trull, Clarkin, Sanderson, & Costa, 1994) indicate how each of the DSM-III-R and DSM-IV personality disorders would be understood from the perspective of the five-factor model. The five-factor model would provide a description of a patient's entire personality (both normal and abnormal), consistent with the spirit of a comprehensive multiaxial assessment (Costa & McCrae, 1992; Mezzich, 1979).

The inclusion of normal personality functioning would extend the domain of the DSM beyond simply providing a diagnosis of mental disorders. It was therefore suggested that Axis II be confined in DSM-IV to the description of normal personality functioning and that the personality disorders be moved to Axis I. This approach would be useful if the personality disorders were directly related to the normal personality traits (i.e., identified as maladaptive variants of specific dimensions or constellations of dimensions contained on Axis II), but the rationale for this shift was instead to consider the personality disorders as being on a spectrum (continuum) with Axis I mental disorders and distinct from normal personality functioning (Siever & Davis, 1991). In any event, this proposal was rejected.

An initial version of the proposed appendix was to present a compromise model representing the major alternatives (Widiger, 1991). Each of the primary models could be illustrated by providing one or two of its dimensions, indicating in each case how the dimensions from the other models relate to the dimension(s) provided. The advantage of this proposal was that it would represent all of the major formulations in a succinct and balanced fashion, yet would also preserve their distinctive features.

The development of this proposal was comparable to the procedure that was used to develop the criteria for borderline personality disorder. It was evident during the construction of DSM-III that there should be a borderline diagnosis, but there was substantial disagreement regarding its optimal diagnostic criteria (Perry & Klerman, 1978). Spitzer et al. (1979) therefore developed a compromise, consensus model in consultation with leading borderline researchers (Gunderson, Kernberg, Rinsley, Sheehy, and Stone). Disagreement regarding the optimal criteria set still remains (e.g., Zanarini, Gunderson, Frankenburg, Chauncey, & Glutting, 1991), but there was and is agreement that some representation is better than no representation.

The proposal, developed in consultation with Cloninger, Costa, Eysenck, McCrae, Siever, Tellegen, and Wiggins, included seven dimensions: introversion, neuroticism, constraint, antagonism, closedness, reward dependence, and cognitive disorganization. Each dimension was to be defined by one of the alternative models, followed by a description of how dimensions from the other models relate to this dimension. For example, constraint would be defined by the dimensional model of Tellegen and Waller (in press), followed by a brief discussion of how this dimension is similar to and different from psychoticism (Eysenck, 1987), conscientiousness (Costa & McCrae, 1990), novelty seeking (Cloninger, 1987), compulsivity and passive oppositionality (Livesley et al., 1992), and passive–aggressiveness and conventionality/rigidity (Clark, 1990). The major limitation of this proposal was that it would appear to be advocating or giving formal approval to a particular seven-dimensional model. This was not the intention of the proposal because it is unlikely that the optimal dimensional model would consist of these seven dimensions, which simply represented a hybrid compromise among alternative models.

The Personality Disorders Work Group, therefore, recommended that the appendix provide a brief discussion of the advantages and disadvantages of the dimensional approach, along with a brief summary of major alternatives. Table 22.2 presents the summary of the alternative models developed by the coauthors of this chapter and the Personality Disorders Work Group. In the published version of DSM-IV, a similar brief discussion of the topic is provided in the introductory text of the section on the personality disorders (American Psychiatric Association, 1994, pp. 633–634) not in an appendix.


## RECOMMENDATIONS FOR DSM-V


We conclude this chapter with a set of recommendations for research that would facilitate the formal adoption of a dimensional model in DSM-V. We recommend in particular that researchers analyze their personality disorder data dimensionally as well as categorically and consider alternative thresholds for diagnosis; that they include a dimensional model in their data

TABLE 22.2. Draft of Alternative Dimensional Models Statement for an Appendix to DSM-IV

The Personality Disorders Work Group considered presenting a dimensional model in this appendix to DSM-IV, but considered that it was premature to give an official recognition to one particular model. A number of models have been developed and studied across a variety of populations. The number and identity of the dimensions have varied across these studies but the research has also demonstrated substantial convergence and commonality among these alternative models. One approach is to simply use the clusters by which the DSM-IV personality disorder diagnoses are organized (dimensions of odd–eccentric, dramatic–emotional–erratic, and anxious–fearful). Another is to describe more specific areas of dysfunction, including as many as 15 to 40 dimensions (e.g., affective reactivity, social apprehensiveness, cognitive distortion, impulsivity, insincerity, and self-centeredness). An additional approach is to identify the dimensions that may underlie the entire domain of personality functioning. One such model consists of the five dimensions of neuroticism, introversion versus extraversion, closedness versus openness to experience, antagonism versus agreeableness, and conscientiousness, each with a set of facets for a more specific description (e.g., facets of neuroticism may include impulsivity, vulnerability, self-consciousness, angry hostility, anxiety, and depression). Different interpretations have been offered for these five dimensions, and some suggest that there should be two additional dimensions (positive and negative evaluation) whereas others emphasize only three dimensions (e.g., positive emotionality, negative emotionality, and constraint). Additional models emphasize interpersonal trait dimensions (e.g., affiliation and dominance) or neurobiological mechanisms involved in learning and motivation (e.g., reward dependence, harm avoidance, and novelty seeking).

---

collection; that they conduct taxometric studies contrasting the dimensional and categorical models; that they compare alternative dimensional models with respect to external validators; and that they demonstrate the clinical utility of a dimensional model.

## Analyzing Data Dimensionally and Categorically

An initial recommendation is to analyze data with respect to the total number of criteria as well as the categorical diagnoses. It is likely that the results will be much improved with the more quantitative analyses. This should not only facilitate the researchers' testing of the experimental hypotheses; it should also be informative to the authors of DSM-V to demonstrate repeatedly that reliable and valid information is being lost by the categorical distinctions.

It will also be helpful to assess alternative cutoff points with respect to any external validators that are included in a study. Researchers should not be confined to the thresholds provided in DSM-IV, since there is no empirical support for these thresholds. Analyses of alternative cutoff points will be helpful in assessing whether the cutoff points are indeed arbitrary and whether any particular alternative cutoff point will result in more reliable or valid findings.

## Contrasting a Dimensional Model with the DSM-IV Categories

A more demanding suggestion for personality disorder researchers helping to prepare DSM-V is to include at least one alternative dimensional model in their data collection, along with the DSM-IV diagnostic taxonomy. This inclusion would not be particularly expensive, given the availability of self-report inventories for the assessment. Likewise, instead of confining dimensional research to the convergence of a dimensional model with the DSM (e.g., Costa & McCrae, 1990; Trull, 1992; Soldz et al., 1993; Wiggins & Pincus, 1989), future studies should compare the dimensional model and DSM-IV with respect to a validator (e.g., reliability, family history, correlates of personality dysfunction, biological markers, biographic or demographic features, childhood antecedents, or treatment response). Establishing incremental validity over the existing taxonomy would provide particularly compelling data for the dimensional approach.

## Conducting Taxometric Studies

A few studies have used taxometric principles to assess whether the optimal classification of personality disorders would be a dimensional or a categorical model (e.g., Cloninger, 1989; Lenzenweger & Korfine, 1992; Livesley, 1991; Trull et al., 1990; Tyrer & Alexander, 1979). Only one has supported the categorical model (i.e., Lenzenweger & Korfine, 1992). To the extent that the diagnostic taxonomy is to be based upon empirical research, it will be informative to conduct additional taxometric studies that directly assess the validity of the categorical model (Grayson, 1987; Grove & Andreasen, 1989; Grove & Meehl, 1993; Klein & Riso, 1993; Meehl, 1992).

## Comparing Alternative Dimensional Models

A major limitation to the proposal for including a dimensional model in an appendix to DSM-IV was the lack of consensus for a particular model. It is unlikely that there will ever be unanimity, given the commitment of researchers to alternative models (e.g., Clark, 1990; Cloninger, 1987; Livesley et al., 1992; McCrae & Costa, 1990; Siever & Davis, 1991; Tellegen & Waller, in press) and the sociology of scientific debate. It will therefore be important for researchers to compare and contrast their models with one or more alternatives in their future studies. Any one of these models will readily obtain empirical support. It will be more informative to assess empirically the redundant and unique variance provided by a particular model (e.g., Schroeder et al., 1992), as well as whether the model obtains incremental validity when compared directly with a competitor (e.g., Clark, 1993).

## Demonstrating Clinical Utility

A limitation for all of the dimensional models is that their clinical utility is not readily apparent to many clinicians. There are currently no explicit guidelines or recommendations regarding the relevance of particular scores on a scale assessing reward dependence, conscientiousness, or impulsivity to decisions regarding treatment, hospitalization, disability, or other clinical issues. Personality disorder diagnoses such as borderline and antisocial may ultimately prove to be less informative with respect to such decisions than scales assessing the facets of neuroticism, antagonism, and conscientiousness, but at least considerable clinical lore and experience exist in regard to the existing personality disorder diagnoses. In order for a dimensional model to become accepted by clinicians, it will be necessary to indicate how it can be used and applied in everyday clinical practice.

## REFERENCES

American Psychiatric Association. (1980). *Diagnostic and statistical manual of mental disorders* (3rd ed.). Washington, DC: Author.

American Psychiatric Association. (1987). *Diagnostic and statistical manual of mental disorders* (3rd ed., rev.). Washington, DC: Author.

American Psychiatric Association. (1994). *Diagnostic and statistical manual of mental disorders* (4th ed.). Washington, DC: Author.

Blashfield, R. K. (1984). *The classification of psychopathology.* New York: Plenum Press.

Blashfield, R. K. (1990). Comorbidity and classification. In J. D. Maser & C. R. Cloninger (Eds.), *Comorbidity of mood and anxiety disorders* (pp. 61–82). Washington, DC: American Psychiatric Press.

Blashfield, R. K., Sprock, J., & Fuller, A. K. (1990). Suggested guidelines for including/excluding categories in the DSM-IV. *Comprehensive Psychiatry, 31,* 15–19.

Cantor, N., & Genero, N. (1986). Psychiatric diagnosis and natural categorization: A close analogy. In T. Millon & G. L. Klerman (Eds.), *Contemporary directions in psychopathology: Toward the DSM-IV* (pp. 233–256). New York: Guilford Press.

Clark, L. A. (1990). Toward a consensual set of symptom clusters for assessment of personality disorder. In J. Butcher & C. Spielberger (Eds.), *Advances in personality assessment* (Vol. 8, pp. 243–266). Hillsdale, NJ: Erlbaum.

Clark, L. A. (1993). Personality disorder diagnosis: Limitations of the five-factor model. *Psychological Inquiry, 4,* 100–104.

Clark, L. A., & Livesley, W. J. (1994). Two approaches to identifying dimensions of personality disorder: Convergence on the five-factor model. In P. T. Costa & T. A. Widiger (Eds.), *Personality disorders and the five factor model of personality* (pp. 261–277). Washington, DC: American Psychological Association.

Clarkin, J. F., Widiger, T. A., Frances, A. J., Hurt, S. W., & Gilmore, M. (1983). Prototypic typology and the borderline personality disorder. *Journal of Abnormal Psychology, 92,* 263–275.

Cloninger, C. R. (1987). A systematic method for clinical description and classification of personality variants. *Archives of General Psychiatry, 44,* 573–588.

Cloninger, C. R. (1989). Establishment of diagnostic validity in psychiatric illness: Robins and Guze's method revisited. In L. Robins & J. Barrett (Eds.), *The validity of psychiatric diagnosis* (pp. 9–18). New York: Raven Press.

Cloninger, C. R., Martin, R., Guze, S., & Clayton, P. (1985). Diagnosis and prognosis in schizophrenia. *Archives of General Psychiatry, 42,* 15–25.

Costa, P. T., & McCrae, R. R. (1990). Personality disorders and the five-factor model of personality. *Journal of Personality Disorders, 4,* 362–371.

Costa, P. T., & McCrae, R. R. (1992). The five-factor model of personality and its relevance to personality disorders. *Journal of Personality Disorders, 6,* 343–359.

Davis, R. D., & Millon, T. (1993). The five-factor model for personality disorders: Apt or misguided? *Psychological Inquiry, 4,* 104–109.

Digman, J. M. (1990). Personality structure: Emergence of the five-factor model. *Annual Review of Psychology, 41,* 417–440.

Eysenck, H. (1987). The definition of personality disorders and the criteria appropriate for their description. *Journal of Personality Disorders, 1,* 211–219.

Finn, S. E. (1982). Base rates, utilities, and DSM-III: Shortcomings of fixed-rule systems of psychodiagnosis. *Journal of Abnormal Psychology, 91,* 294–302.

First, M. B., Spitzer, R. L., & Williams, J. B. W. (1990). Exclusionary principles and the comorbidity of psychiatric diagnoses: A historical review and implications for the future. In J. D. Maser & C. R. Cloninger (Eds.), *Comorbidity of mood and anxiety disorders* (pp. 83–109). Washington, DC: American Psychiatric Press.

Ford, M., & Widiger, T. (1989). Sex bias in the diagnosis of histrionic and antisocial personality disorders. *Journal of Consulting and Clinical Psychology, 57,* 301–305.

Frances, A. J. (1980). The DSM-III personality disorders section: A commentary. *American Journal of Psychiatry, 137,* 1050–1054.

Frances, A. J. (1982). Categorical and dimensional systems of personality diagnosis: A comparison. *Comprehensive Psychiatry, 23,* 1198–1202.

Frances, A. J. (1990, May). *Conceptual problems of psychiatric classification.* Paper presented at the 143rd Annual Meeting of the American Psychiatric Association, New York.

Frances, A. J. (1993). Dimensional diagnosis of personality—not whether, but when and which. *Psychological Inquiry, 4,* 110–111.

Frances, A. J., Clarkin, J., Gilmore, M., Hurt, S., & Brown, S. (1984). Reliability of criteria for borderline personality disorder: A comparison of DSM-III and the Diagnostic Interview for Borderline Patients. *American Journal of Psychiatry, 42,* 591–596.

Frances, A. J., & Widiger, T. A. (1986). The classification of personality disorders: An overview of problems and solutions. In A. J. Frances & R. E. Hales (Eds.), *Psychiatry update: American Psychiatric Association annual review* (Vol. 5, pp. 240–257). Washington, DC: American Psychiatric Press.

Frances, A. J., Widiger, T. A., & Fyer, M. R. (1990). The influence of classification methods on comorbidity. In J. D. Maser & C. R. Cloninger (Eds.), *Comorbidity of mood and anxiety disorders* (pp. 41–59). Washington, DC: American Psychiatric Press.

Goldberg, L. R. (1982). From ace to zombia: Some explorations in the language of personality. In C. Spielberger & J. Butcher (Eds.), *Advances in personality assessment* (Vol. 1, pp. 203–234). Hillsdale, NJ: Erlbaum.

Goldberg, L. R. (1990). An alternative "description of personality": The Big-Five factor structure. *Journal of Personality and Social Psychology, 59,* 1216–1229.

Grayson, J. (1987). Can categorical and dimensional views of psychiatric illness be distinguished? *British Journal of Psychiatry, 151,* 355–361.

Grove, W. M., & Andreasen, N. (1989). Quantitative and qualitative distinctions between psychiatric disorders. In L. Robins & J. Barrett (Eds.), *The validity of psychiatric diagnosis* (pp. 127–141). New York: Raven Press.

Grove, W. M., & Mechl, P. E. (1993). Simple regression-based procedures for taxometric investigations. *Psychological Reports, 73,* 707–737.

Gunderson, J. G. (1992). Diagnostic controversies. In A. Tasman & M. B. Riba (Eds.), *Review of psychiatry* (Vol. 11, pp. 9–24). Washington, DC: American Psychiatric Press.

Gunderson, J. G., Links, P. S., & Reich, J. H. (1991). Competing models of personality disorders. *Journal of Personality Disorders, 5,* 60–68.

Hare, R. D., Hart, S. D., & Harpur, T. J. (1991). Psychopathy and the DSM-IV criteria for antisocial personality disorder. *Journal of Abnormal Psychology, 100,* 391–398.

Harkness, A. R. (1992). Fundamental topics in the personality disorders: Candidate trait dimensions from lower regions of the hierarchy. *Psychological Assessment, 4,* 251–259.

Heumann, K., & Morey, L. (1990). Reliability and categorical and dimensional judgments of personality disorder. *American Journal of Psychiatry, 147,* 498–500.

Hine, F., & Williams, R. (1975). Dimensional diagnosis and the medical student's grasp of psychiatry. *Archives of General Psychiatry, 32,* 525–528.

John, O. P. (1990). The "Big Five" factor taxonomy: Dimensions of personality in the natural language and in questionnaires. In L. A. Pervin (Ed.), *Handbook of personality: Theory and research* (pp. 66–100). New York: Guilford Press.

Kass, F., Skodol, A., Charles, E., Spitzer, R., & Williams, J. (1985). Scaled ratings of DSM-III personality disorders. *American Journal of Psychiatry, 142,* 627–630.

Kendell, R. (1975). *The role of diagnosis in psychiatry.* Oxford: Blackwell.

Kendler, K. S. (1990). Toward a scientific psychiatric nosology: Strengths and limitations. *Archives of General Psychiatry, 47,* 969–973.

Kiesler, D. J. (1986). The 1982 interpersonal circle: An analysis of DSM-III personality disorders. In T. Millon & G. L. Klerman (Eds.), *Contemporary directions in psychopathology: Toward the DSM-IV* (pp. 571–597). New York: Guilford Press.

Klein, D. N., & Riso, L. P. (1993). Psychiatric disorders: Problems of boundaries and comorbidity. In C. G. Costello (Ed.), *Basic issues in psychopathology* (pp. 19–66). New York: Guilford Press

Lenzenweger, M. F., & Korfine, L. (1992). Confirming the latent structure and base rate of schizotypy: A taxometric analysis. *Journal of Abnormal Psychology, 101,* 567–571.

Livesley, W. J. (1985). The classification of personality disorder: I. The choice of category concept. *Canadian Journal of Psychiatry, 30,* 353–358.

Livesley, W. J. (1991). Classifying personality disorders: Ideal types, prototypes, or dimensions? *Journal of Personality Disorders, 5,* 52–59.

Livesley, W. J., Jackson, D. N., & Schroeder, M. L. (1992). Factorial structure of traits delineating personality disorders in clinical and general population samples. *Journal of Abnormal Psychology, 101,* 432–440.

Loranger, A. (1988). *Personality Disorders Examination (PDE) manual.* Yonkers, NY: DV Communications.

Maser, J. D., Kaelber, C., & Weise, R. E. (1991). International use and attitudes toward DSM-III and DSM-III-R: Growing consensus in psychiatric classification. *Journal of Abnormal Psychology, 100,* 271–279.

McCrae, R. R., & Costa, P. T. (1990). *Personality in adulthood.* New York: Guilford Press.

McGlashan, T. (1987). Borderline personality disorder and unipolar affective disorder: Long-term effects of comorbidity. *Journal of Nervous and Mental Disease, 175,* 467–473.

Meehl, P. (1992). Factors and taxa, traits and types, differences of degree and differences in kind. *Journal of Personality, 60,* 117–174.

Mellsop, G., Varghese, F., Joshua, S., & Hicks, A. (1982). The reliability of Axis II of DSM-III. *American Journal of Psychiatry, 139,* 1360–1361.

Mezzich, J. (1979). Patterns and issues in multiaxial psychiatric diagnosis. *Psychological Medicine, 9,* 125–137.

Miller, M. L., & Thayer, J. F. (1989). On the existence of discrete classes in personality: Is self-monitoring the correct joint to carve? *Journal of Personality and Social Psychology, 57,* 143–155.

Millon, T. (1981). *Disorders of personality: DSM-III, Axis II.* New York: Wiley–Interscience.

Millon, T. (1991). Classification in psychopathology: Rationale, alternatives, and standards. *Journal of Abnormal Psychology, 100,* 245–261.

Morey, L. C. (1988). Personality disorders in DSM-III and DSM-III-R: Convergence, coverage, and internal consistency. *American Journal of Psychiatry, 145,* 573–577.

Morey, L. C., & Ochoa, E. (1989). An investigation of adherence to diagnostic criteria: Clinical diagnosis of the DSM-III personality disorders. *Journal of Personality Disorders, 3,* 180–192.

Nestadt, G., Romanoski, A., Chahal, R., Merchant, A., Folstein, M., Gruenberg, E., & McHugh, P. (1990). An epidemiological study of histrionic personality disorder. *Psychological Medicine, 20,* 413–422.

Nurnberg, H. G., Raskin, M., Levine, P. E., Pollack, S., Siegel, O., & Prince, R. (1991). The comorbidity of borderline personality disorder and other DSM-III-R Axis II personality disorders. *American Journal of Psychiatry, 148,* 1371–1377.

Oldham, J. M., Skodol, A. E., Kellman, H. D., Hyler, S. E., Rosnick, L., & Davies, M. (1992). Diagnosis of DSM-III-R personality disorders by two semistructured interviews: Patterns of comorbidity. *American Journal of Psychiatry, 149,* 213–220.

Overholser, J. C. (1991). Categorical assessment of the dependent personality disorder. *Journal of Personality Disorders, 5,* 243–255.

Perry, J. C. (1990). Challenges in validating personality disorders: Beyond description. *Journal of Personality Disorders, 4,* 273–289.

Perry, J. C., & Klerman, G. L. (1978). The borderline patient: A comparative analysis of four sets of diagnostic criteria. *Archives of General Psychiatry, 35,* 141–150.

Pfohl, B., Blum, N., Zimmerman, M., & Stangl, D. (1989). *Structured Interview for DSM-III-R Personality Disorders (SIDP-R).* Iowa City: University of Iowa, Department of Psychiatry.

Pilkonis, P. (1992, September). *Assessing personality disorders.* Paper presented at New York Hospital–Cornell University Medical Center, Westchester Division, White Plains, NY.

Presley, A. S., & Walton, H. J. (1973). Dimensions of abnormal personality. *British Journal of Psychiatry, 122,* 269–276.

Schacht, T. (1985). DSM-III and the politics of truth. *American Psychologist, 40,* 513–521.

Schroeder, M. L., Wormworth, J. A., & Livesley, W. J. (1992). Dimensions of personality disorder and their relationship to the Big Five dimensions of personality. *Psychological Assessment, 4,* 47–53.

Siever, L. J., & Davis, K. L. (1991). A psychobiological perspective on the personality disorders. *American Journal of Psychiatry, 148,* 1647–1658.

Skodol, A. E. (1989). *Problems in differential diagnosis: From DSM-III to DSM-III-R in clinical practice.* Washington, DC: American Psychiatric Press.

Skodol, A. E., Rosnick, L., Kellman, H. D., Oldham, J. M., & Hyler, S. E. (1990). Development of a procedure for validating structured assessments of Axis II. In J. Oldham (Ed.), *Personality disorders: New perspectives on diagnostic validity* (pp. 47–70). Washington, DC: American Psychiatric Press.

Soldz, S., Budman, S., Demby, A., & Merry, J. (1993). Representation of personality disorders in circumplex and Five-Factor space: Explorations with a clinical sample. *Psychological Assessment, 5,* 41–52.

Spitzer, R., Endicott, J., & Gibbon, M. (1979). Crossing the border into borderline personality and borderline schizophrenia. *Archives of General Psychiatry, 36,* 17–24.

Spitzer, R. L., & Williams, J. B. W. (1985). Classification of mental disorders. In H. L. Kaplan & B. J. Sadock (Eds.), *Comprehensive textbook of psychiatry* (pp. 591–613). Baltimore, MD: Williams & Wilkins.

Task Force on DSM-IV. (1991). *DSM-IV options book: Work in progress.* Washington, DC: American Psychiatric Association.

Tellegen, A., & Waller, N. G. (in press). Exploring personality through test construction: Development of the Multidimensional Personality Questionnaire. In S. R. Briggs & J. M. Cheek (Eds.), *Personality measures: Development and evaluation.* Greenwich, CT: JAI Press.

Trull, T. J. (1992). DSM-III-R personality disorders and the five-factor model of personality: An empirical comparison. *Journal of Abnormal Psychology, 101,* 553–560.

Trull, T. J., Widiger, T. A., & Guthrie, P. (1990). The categorical versus dimensional status of borderline personality disorder. *Journal of Abnormal Psychology, 99,* 40–48.

Tyrer, P., & Alexander, J. (1979). Classification of personality disorder. *British Journal of Psychiatry, 135,* 163–167.

Widiger, T. A. (1991). Personality disorder dimensional models proposed for DSM-IV. *Journal of Personality Disorders, 5,* 386–398.

Widiger, T. A. (1992). Categorical versus dimensional classification: Implications from and for research. *Journal of Personality Disorders, 6,* 287–300.

Widiger, T. A. (1993). The DSM-III-R categorical personality disorder diagnoses: A critique and an alternative. *Psychological Inquiry, 4,* 75–90.

Widiger, T. A., & Corbitt, E. M. (1994). Normal versus abnormal personality from the perspective of the DSM. In S. Strack & M. Lorr (Eds.), *Differentiating normal and abnormal personality* (pp. 158–175). New York: Springer.

Widiger, T. A., & Frances, A. J. (1985). The DSM-III personality disorders: Perspectives from psychology. *Archives of General Psychiatry, 42,* 615–623.

Widiger, T. A., & Frances, A. J. (1989). Epidemiology, diagnosis, and comorbidity of borderline personality disorder. In A. Tasman, R. Hales, & A. Frances (Eds.), *Review of psychiatry* (Vol. 8, pp. 8–24). Washington, DC: American Psychiatric Press.

Widiger, T. A., & Frances, A. J. (1994). Towards a dimensional model for the personality disorders. In P. T. Costa & T. A. Widiger (Eds.), *Personality disorders and the five-factor model of personality* (pp. 19–39). Washington, DC: American Psychological Association.

Widiger, T. A., Frances, A. J., Spitzer, R. L., & Williams, J. B. W. (1988). The DSM-III-R personality disorders: An overview. *American Journal of Psychiatry, 145,* 786–795.

Widiger, T. A., & Kelso, K. (1983). Psychodiagnosis of Axis II. *Clinical Psychology Review, 3,* 491–510.

Widiger, T. A., & Rogers, J. (1989). Prevalence and comorbidity of personality dis-
    orders. *Psychiatric Annals, 19,* 132–136.
Widiger, T. A., Sanderson, C. J., & Warner, L. (1986). The MMPI, prototypal typolo-
    gy, and borderline personality disorder. *Journal of Personality Assessment, 50,*
    540–553.
Widiger, T. A., Trull, T. J., Clarkin, J. F., Sanderson, C. J., & Costa, P. T. (1994). A
    description of the DSM-III-R and DSM-IV personality disorders with the five-
    factor model of personality. In P. T. Costa & T. A. Widiger (Eds.), *Personality dis-
    orders and the five-factor model of personality* (pp. 41–56). Washington, DC: Ameri-
    can Psychological Association.
Wiggins, J. S. (1982). Circumplex models of interpersonal behavior in clinical psy-
    chology. In P. Kendall & J. Butcher (Eds.), *Handbook of research methods in clinical
    psychology* (pp. 183–221). New York: Wiley.
Wiggins, J. S., & Pincus, A. L. (1989). Conceptions of personality disorders and dimen-
    sions of personality. *Psychological Assessment: A Journal of Consulting and Clinical
    Psychology, 1,* 305–316.
Wiggins, J. S., & Pincus, A. L. (1992). Personality: Structure and assessment. *Annual
    Review of Psychology, 43,* 473–504.
Zanarini, M. C., Gunderson, J. G., Frankenburg, F. R., Chauncey, D. L., & Glutting,
    J. H. (1991). The face validity of the DSM-III and DSM-III-R criteria sets for bor-
    derline personality disorder. *American Journal of Psychiatry, 148,* 870–874.
Zimmerman, M., & Coryell, W. (1990). Diagnosing personality disorders in the com-
    munity: A comparison of self-report and interview measures. *Archives of General
    Psychiatry, 47,* 527–531.

# CHAPTER 23

# Possible Contributions from Personality Assessment to the Classification of Personality Disorders

DOUGLAS N. JACKSON
W. JOHN LIVESLEY

A surprising aspect of the process used to develop the different editions of the DSM is the limited use made of developments in disciplines other than psychiatry. This is especially surprising in the case of personality disorders, because other professional groups were represented on the committees responsible for DSM-III (American Psychiatric Association, 1980), DSM-III-R (American Psychiatric Association, 1987), and DSM-IV (American Psychiatric Association, 1994), and because work on personality and personality assessment has obvious relevance for the classification of personality disorders. Psychological assessment is pertinent because psychiatric classifications show several structural and analytic similarities with psychological tests (Blashfield & Livesley, 1991). The most obvious structural parallel is that classification systems consist of diagnostic categories, each defined by a set of diagnostic criteria; these are equivalent to scales and scale items, respectively, of a psychological test. Analytic parallels are seen in the emphasis both place on establishing reliability and validity. Personality research is pertinent because analyses of normal personality functioning may help to define the contents of a classification of personality dysfunction.

Despite these parallels, the architects of the various editions of DSM probably did not consider it necessary to draw upon the systematic body of knowledge on personality assessment or the results of analyses of normal personality structure, because the assumption continues to be made that personality disorders can be classified by means of the same procedures used to classify Axis I disorders. Fundamental to this assumption is the notion that the features of personality disorders are sufficiently self-evident that all that is required to develop a satisfactory system is the consensus of a committee of experts. This approach would be acceptable if the features of personality disorders were distinctive and invariant indicators of different types of pathology. But this is not the case. Instead, diagnostic criteria are samples of the kinds of behaviors shown by patients with personality disorders. Thus, in the development of a classification, the task is to compile criteria sets that are representative of these behaviors and to ensure that the criteria for one disorder are not strongly related to those for other disorders. In this respect, the task of developing a classification of personality disorders resembles that of developing a test to assess multiple dimensions of personality, and it is not one that can readily be accomplished using expert judgment alone.

Personality assessment can contribute to the classification of personality disorders in several ways. First, the conceptual approach underlying structured approaches to test construction (Jackson, 1971), especially construct validation theory (Loevinger, 1957), could provide an overall framework to organize classification research. Second, the procedures developed, and extensively tested, to construct tests could be used to establish and evaluate a classification. Third, the methods used to study personality structure might help to resolve basic issues in the classification of personality disorders that continue to exercise attention, especially the issue of whether a categorical or a dimensional model should be adopted. Finally, the phenotypic structure of normal personality traits resulting from decades of empirical research may help to define the contents of a classification of personality disorders. In this chapter we discuss the first three of these issues; the fourth has been covered by Widiger and Sanderson in Chapter 22 of this volume.

## CONSTRUCT VALIDATION OF A FRAMEWORK FOR CLASSIFICATION RESEARCH

The development and evaluation of a psychiatric classification constitute a lengthy process involving a series of steps, none of which is sufficient but each of which is necessary to establish a satisfactory system. Given the complexity of the process, and the social and scientific significance of the resulting system, it is surprising that so little attention has been paid either to developing a framework within which to organize the process or to defining explicit criteria to guide the selection of diagnostic items and evaluation of the results. This failure is all the more surprising, given the emphasis placed on developing explicit diagnostic criteria for DSM-III. It is as if more stringent standards are applied to the use of a classification than to its compilation.

Psychiatric classifications tend to be compiled and revised in a somewhat informal and arbitrary fashion: A committee of experts is assembled to identify diagnoses, compile diagnostic criteria, and revise earlier classifications. Undoubtedly, the committees deliberating these matters establish

procedural guidelines, and in the case of DSM-IV the literature was carefully reviewed; nevertheless, the approach is not as structured as that used to
construct tests. The closest approximation to a systematic framework is the
understanding that appears to underlie the DSM process: In DSM-III and
DSM-III-R the focus was on establishing diagnostic reliability through the
use of explicit diagnostic criteria, and in DSM-IV the emphasis was placed
on validity. Reliability and validity are treated as if they are distinct issues
that are related only in the sense that reliability is considered to be a necessary precursor of validity (Spitzer & Fleiss, 1974).

In previous articles (Livesley & Jackson, 1990, 1992), we have argued
that the construct validation framework used in psychological test development could provide the conceptual and procedural infrastructure to develop
and evaluate psychiatric classifications. As Skinner (1981) observed, the objective when compiling a classification is to ensure construct validity—that
is, to ensure that the classification covers all relevant diagnoses; that diagnoses are defined and diagnosed using criteria that are representative of
the diagnostic construct, but distinct from criteria proposed for related diagnoses; and that the classification predicts important outcomes. These are,
of course, the goals of psychological assessment (Blashfield & Livesley, 1991).
The construct validation framework originally proposed by Loevinger (1957)
provides the most integrated approach to these issues, and it is surprising
that this approach has not been applied systematically to psychiatric classifications (Skinner, 1981). Loevinger conceptualized construct validation
in terms of three interrelated components: substantive, structural, and external aspects of validity.

The "substantive component" refers to the definition of constructs and
selection of assessment items that together establish a theoretical classification (Skinner, 1981). Central to substantive validity is evidence demonstrating that the classification possesses satisfactory content validity. The DSM-IV
committee has in effect compiled such a theoretical classification, although
we would argue that the process used falls short of the standards expected
in test development. The "structural component" refers to the extent to which
the structural relationships among constructs and items are consistent with
the relationships proposed in the theoretical classification. With a diagnostic classification, this essentially involves demonstrating empirically that
criteria can be assessed reliably and that they cluster into the diagnostic constructs described in the theoretical classification. This component of construct validity complements the substantive component by demonstrating
empirically that criteria that were selected initially because they were considered to conform to the definition of a diagnostic construct are related as
predicted. The substantive and structural components describe the inner
coherence and working of the classification, and hence form the internal
component of validity (Skinner, 1981). A satisfactory diagnostic system must,
however, meet an additional set of criteria: those that establish the external
component of validity.

The "external component" of validity is based on evidence that the classification shows meaningful relationships with relevant external variables. In the case of a psychiatric classification, external validity ultimately rests on evidence that the diagnostic system predicts important clinical outcomes such as prognosis and response to treatment, and that diagnostic constructs are linked to relevant etiological variables. For personality disorders, external validators are difficult to identify. Nevertheless, considerable progress could be made toward a satisfactory system by following procedures that are likely to lead to satisfactory internal validity (Livesley & Jackson, 1992).

It can be seen from this brief overview of Loevinger's analysis of construct validity that it has the potential to provide a comprehensive framework within which to develop and evaluate a psychiatric classification. Contemporary structured approaches to test construction incorporate a set of procedures and criteria designed to ensure the construct validity of the resulting instrument. A further advantage of this approach is that it also provides an integrated framework for conceptualizing and evaluating diagnostic validity. As Loevinger argued, construct validity "is the whole of validity from a scientific point of view" (1957, p. 636), and the three components are "mutually exclusive, exhaustive of the possible lines of evidence for construct validity, and mandatory" (p. 636). Thus validity is considered a unitary concept with multiple facets (Messick, 1988).

It is informative to contrast this approach with psychiatric approaches to validity, which tend either to describe several different forms of validity that are not related in any systematic way or list the kinds of evidence required to validate a diagnostic construct (Robins & Guze, 1970). But perhaps the most important aspect of the application of construct validity to classification is that validity is established incrementally as the classification is constructed and revised. The content validity of the system is established by ensuring that diagnostic criteria are selected to sample all facets of rationally defined diagnoses. Revision of criteria sets on the basis of empirical evaluation establishes structural validity. Only when structural validity is established is it appropriate to pursue external validity. As these steps are completed and the system is modified on the basis of evidence from evaluation studies, it increasingly approximates a valid system.

## ESTABLISHING AND EVALUATING A CLASSIFICATION

Application of test construction methodology to the classification of personality disorders would lead to a very different approach from that used by the DSM committees. An important difference would be the introduction of a more systematic and objective process with explicit procedural rules. This would lead to enhanced content validity, and would reduce the impact of idiosyncratic opinion and the effects of pressure groups and political considerations on the structure and contents of the classification. With DSM-IV the process was more public than it had previously been, and the committee has attempted to communicate the reasons for many decisions, as illustrated by earlier chapters in this volume. Nevertheless, many of the assumptions underlying the exercise are unspecified and hence difficult to evaluate and refute.

## Assumptions

Part of the problem with the formulation of DSM-III, DSM-III-R, and DSM-IV has been the desire to avoid theory and inference. Although initially this restriction was intended to apply only to theories about the etiology of mental disorders, the approach tended to generalize to other theoretical issues. Faust and Miner (1986) have trenchantly challenged the Baconian ideal of identifying "facts" on which to build a diagnostic system in the absence of theory. They point out that complex inferential networks are critical to almost all scientific endeavor; without ideas and concepts, there can be little hope for advances in understanding. Of particular importance for a classification of personality disorders are theoretical assumptions about the way psychopathology is organized. Underlying the DSMs is the neo-Kraepelian assumption that mental disorders are discrete entities (Klerman, 1978; Blashfield, 1984). Unfortunately, this assumption is not stated explicitly, and the precise nature of the discontinuities among disorders on which the classification rests is unclear. This adds to the confusion that Blashfield and McElroy (Chapter 20) note exists about the nature of categorical and dimensional concepts. Yet, as Loevinger demonstrated, the model that underlies any attempt to measure a construct or assess a diagnostic construct has major implications for the way the construct is defined and evaluated (Livesley & Jackson, 1992).

If personality disorders are organized as discrete categories, then the task is not to develop a classification that can differentiate among different degrees of behavior, but rather to differentiate among different types of individuals. Diagnostic items are selected as indicators of a disorder, and they are not necessarily expected to be strongly related to one another. Indeed, there are certain advantages to having items that are relatively unrelated to one another if one's only goal is to predict a criterion (Gulliksen, 1950). If personality disorders represent the extremities of dimensions, however, diagnostic items are summed to provide an estimate of the degree to which the traits defining a disorder are present, and the task in developing the classification is to select items that are correlated with one another to form an internally consistent set. If discontinuities are postulated, several possible bases for the discontinuities exist. For example, a point of rarity could be postulated along a continuous distribution, or distinct clusters of individuals could be hypothesized (see Blashfield & McElroy, Chapter 20).

But the nature of the classificatory model is not the only assumption that needs to be stated explicitly. It is also necessary to state the concept of personality disorders that guides the organization of diagnostic concepts and the selection of criteria. Specific DSM personality disorder diagnoses have diverse origins, including traditional psychoanalytic theory, object relations theory, self psychology, and classical psychopathology. Each of these traditions adopts a somewhat different approach toward understanding and defining personality disorders. Some rely on overt psychodynamic processes and assume differences in personality organization, whereas others are based more on overt behaviors; it is often difficult to unravel the contributions of these diverse traditions. The situation does not lend itself readily to testing hypotheses derived from this implicit set of conceptual systems. Thus the classification system is difficult to confirm or refute in a scientific sense.

## Definitions

Studies on test construction indicate that the validity of any measure is improved if test items are selected on the basis of precise definitions of the construct that is being assessed (Jackson, 1971). In the compilation of a test, the practice is to define the trait construct that the test is intended to measure, subdivide the trait into facets, and select items to assess each facet. This process helps to ensure that items sample all aspects of the behavioral domain addressed by the construct, and it begins to establish the content validity of the test, which is subsequently confirmed using expert judgments. Thus an important aspect of validity is built into the test in the way it is constructed. This is not the way psychiatric classifications are constructed. Instead of defining diagnostic constructs, experts are merely asked to suggest diagnostic items. This means that each expert is forced to rely on a personal and perhaps idiosyncratic understanding of the diagnosis in order to generate items. If an extensive research literature exists on the disorder in question, and there is a consensus regarding an appropriate diagnostic criterion set, this approach works well enough. But without such a literature, the classification runs the risk of becoming little more than a list of the experts' favorite diagnoses and preferred diagnostic criteria.

It could be argued that there is a strong consensus regarding appropriate content for a classification of personality disorders, and that this consensus has been implicit in the development of criteria sets in DSM-III, DSM-III-R, and DSM-IV. When writing and selecting diagnostic criteria for the DSM-III personality disorders, however, the committee generally did so in the absence of empirical data. When some empirical data indicating that some criteria needed to be replaced became available for DSM-III-R and DSM-IV, there were no data or procedures to evaluate the new criteria (Blashfield, Blum, & Pfohl, 1992).

The failure to define diagnoses before selecting diagnostic criteria has contributed to some of the persistent problems with the DSM classification of personality disorders. When classifications are compiled without the benefit of definitions or an extensive empirical literature, there is little as-

surance that the resulting system will possess adequate levels of content validity. Not surprisingly, there is reason to question the content validity of
DSM-III and DSM-III-R (Livesley, Reiffer, Sheldon, & West, 1987; Blashfield
& Breen, 1989), and there is no reason to believe that the situation has improved with DSM-IV (see Hare & Hart's commentary on Chapter 6, this
volume). This is particularly bothersome because, as noted earlier, content
validity is a prerequisite for structural and external validity.

A second problem emanating from this initial failure is that of diagnostic overlap. Most patients with a personality disorder diagnosis meet the
criteria for multiple disorders (Widiger et al., 1990). Although the issue of
"comorbidity" has received considerable attention (see Shea, Chapter 19),
it is far from clear whether this is true concurrence of discrete disorders
or whether it is simply an artifact resulting from the failure to define disorders precisely. Not surprisingly, empirical studies have demonstrated that
other items were frequently more strongly associated with a disorder than
the ones specified in DSM (Bell & Jackson, 1992; Morey, 1988). A further
difficulty is the confusion that occurs because diagnostic criteria differ in
specificity. As Shea points out in Chapter 19, some criteria are relatively
broad trait constructs; others are specific behaviors or symptoms that are
exemplars of a broader trait; and still others are specific historical events.
Given this diversity, it is not surprising that the diagnostic reliability varies
considerably across diagnoses (Mellsop, Varghese, Joshua, & Hicks, 1982; Spitzer, Forman, & Nee, 1979).

A classification of personality disorders should distinguish between
description and definition of the trait constructs defining each diagnosis
and the criteria proposed to diagnose each disorder (Gorton & Akhtar, 1990;
Morey & McNamara, 1987, Livesley, 1987b; Shea, Chapter 19). Delineation
of the trait dimensions underlying the classification of and those associated
with each diagnosis is an essential first step toward establishing a diagnostic
system. In this way, investigators can focus on the concepts to be studied;
can develop definitions of each; and, on the basis of these definitions, can
select behavioral manifestations of these hypothetical constructs that can then
be studied empirically. The search for basic constructs should extend beyond the confines of current classifications to encompass content analyses
of the literature and accumulated clinical wisdom. Elsewhere, we have argued that one approach is to identify the prototypical dimensions and traits
describing personality disorders through a combination of literature review
and expert judgment (Livesley, 1986, 1987; Livesley & Jackson, 1990, 1992).
The important point is that prior to developing criteria sets, it is necessary
to identify and define the characteristics that are likely to be critical and
relevant for classification. The list of characteristics needs to be comprehensive and to have the potential for differentiating between persons with different kinds of personality pathology. Characteristics shared by many different
types of persons, and those that, although differentiating to a degree, are
not prototypical at a conceptual level, are less likely to be useful.

The next step is to select diagnostic items to assess the defined traits. The use of definitions ensures that different item writers have the same understanding of the construct and that items are selected to assess all aspects of the construct. This avoids the problems of poor content validity that arise when items do not represent all aspects of a construct or include items that are more relevant to other constructs. This begins to form the basis for establishing the convergent and discriminant properties of the system. These properties are then enhanced by revisions based on the results of systematic evaluation of the way diagnostic items perform when assessed in samples of patients drawn from different populations.

## Evaluation and Revision

Contemporary classifications tend to be revised in much the same manner as they are developed: A panel of experts is asked to review whatever empirical data are available to identify diagnoses and criteria that do not appear to be performing well, and then to suggest replacements. The experts involved in the revision of DSM-IV have managed this process somewhat better than their predecessors. Attempts were made to develop criteria to evaluate diagnostic items, based on specificity and sensitivity data and on positive and negative predictive power. The problem was that when diagnostic items were replaced because they were lacking in discriminability, there were no data or criteria to guide the selection and evaluation of new items (Blashfield et al., 1992). The item analysis procedures used to evaluate structural validity offer one solution to this problem.

The evidence consistently suggests that dimensional models provide a more satisfactory representation of the features of personality disorder than traditional categorical models do (Livesley, Schroeder, Jackson, & Jang, 1994; Widiger & Sanderson, Chapter 22). This being the case, the diagnostic items for a given disorder should form an internally consistent set and should correlate more with their own diagnosis than with other diagnoses. Items that do not meet this requirement should be deleted and replaced. In this sense, the procedure derived from test construction is not very different from the use of data on sensitivity, specificity, and positive and negative predictive power in DSM-IV. The difference is what happens when replacement items are selected. The procedure used in DSM-IV did not provide any assistance in selecting new items: The committee simply suggested a new item in the hope that it would perform better than the original. When test construction methodology is used, however, in which items are selected for conformity to the definition of the construct being assessed, the performance of other items designed to assess the same construct or facet of a construct can be examined. If these perform satisfactorily, the task is to write a new item to assess this construct. A review of the content and structure of items that perform well will assist this task. On the other hand, if other items assessing the construct or facet also perform badly, either because they do not correlate with the overall diagnostic construct or because they are more strongly related to other diagnoses than to the one for which they were written, the implication is that the construct or facet should be deleted. Similarly, if items assessing all the traits defining a diagnosis do not form an internally consistent set, the implication is that the diagnosis should either be deleted from the classification or extensively redefined. These examples illustrate the major advantages that accrue from the application of test development methodology to the classification of personality disorders. The process of compiling, evaluating, and revising the system becomes orderly, and the classification is modified in a rational way on the basis of evaluation data.

## EMPIRICAL ANALYSIS OF PROBLEMS IN CLASSIFICATION

The techniques and procedures used in test construction offer a means to investigate and perhaps resolve some of the basic problems facing the classification of personality disorders. We want to mention two such issues: (1) whether the manifest features of personality disorders are organized into the diagnostic categories proposed by DSM-IV, or whether there is a more optimal way to represent the phenotypic structure of personality disorders; and (2) whether distinct types of personality disorders can be identified.

The methods and techniques in widespread use in personality assessment and test development offer, according to Blashfield (1984, p. 259), an alternative to the political posturing, "obsessive thinking and armchair philosophizing" that has characterized many discussions of the classification of psychopathology. We share with Blashfield the belief that empirical methods offer the promise of confronting the rather staggering array of unsolved problems facing the classification of personality disorders. Resolution of these problems through the quantitative methods of personality assessment has not yet occurred, although some progress is being made. Effective application of the methods of personality assessment research to both of these issues requires that certain preconditions by met—namely, that the initial classification is carefully defined, and that valid measurement instruments are developed. The issue of definition has been addressed extensively above. The only point that we emphasize here is that the constructs used to define diagnoses should cover the overall domain of personality disorders. Only then will it be possible to investigate alternative clusterings of these features to the one proposed in DSM-IV. Unfortunately, steps were not taken to ensure that this occurred in DSM-III, DSM-III-R, or DSM-IV. Consequently, future studies of DSM-IV criteria sets will convey only limited information.

Definitions are also required to establish (Widiger et al., 1990) valid measures for classification research. The high level of comorbidity found among disorders, the empirical confusion between and among purportedly distinct disorders, and the confusing lack of an explicit rationale for including or excluding criteria do not provide a firm foundation for simple one-to-one translations of criteria sets into assessment instruments. In the absence of such measures, empirical studies will not yield useful or interpretable results. Yet surprisingly little attention has been paid to the validity of measures currently used in personality disorder research or to the way the classification should be formulated to facilitate the development of measurement instruments. Regardless of whether measures are designed as psychometric instruments or as clinical interviews, they must nevertheless show certain psychometric properties if they are to provide useful data. For example, measures that contain a great deal of method variance, item overlap, and excessive interscale correlations are unlikely to provide a valid basis for classification research. Nor are scales lacking evidence for reliability and for convergent and discriminant validity. This kind of failure is perhaps the primary reason why otherwise well-designed studies, such as those based on the Millon Clinical Multiaxial Inventory-II (Lorr & Strack, 1990) and the Minnesota Multiphasic Personality Inventory (MMPI; Nerviano & Gross, 1983), did not yield a higher level of differentiation than might have been expected.

## Phenotypic Structure of Personality Disorders

A fundamental question pertaining to the classification of personality disorders is whether the 10 diagnoses listed in DSM-IV are the most optimal way to represent personality disorders — that is, whether the features defining personality disorders are organized into the diagnostic constructs listed in DSM-IV. The development of a preliminary classification using test construction methodology would provide the requirements to evaluate this aspect of diagnostic validity. As Torgersen notes in his commentary on Chapters 3–5 of this volume, factor-analytic procedures provide the most convenient way to investigate this issue. Viewed from a personality assessment and test construction perspective, this issue is similar to a consideration of the evidence required to support of the contention that a given test is composed of several scales and subscales.

Several factor analyses of the descriptive features of personality disorders have been reported. Kass, Skodol, Charles, Spitzer, and Williams (1985), for example, reported a factor analysis of DSM-III criteria rated in a sample of patients. Although 11 factors were extracted as predicted by DSM-III, individual factor content showed limited correspondence with DSM-III diagnoses. Similar results were reported by Clark (1990) and Harkness (1992) in separate studies, in which clinical judgment data rather than patient observations were analyzed. Clark asked clinical judges to sort DSM-III Axis II and relevant Axis I criteria according to likely co-occurrence. Harkness used a similar procedure limited to DSM-III-R Axis II criteria. Although the number of factors extracted differed substantially in the two studies, largely because Clark used a more conservative criterion for extracting additional factors than Harkness did, the results were consistent in the sense that little correspondence with DSM-III or DSM-III-R diagnoses were observed.

Our studies have yielded similar results, although we used a different approach. In order to ensure that the initial set of constructs that were the basis for factor analysis were not confined to DSM-III-R criteria but were representative of the overall domain, the clinical literature on personality disorders was content-analyzed, and clinical judges were asked to identify the most prototypical features (Livesley, 1986, 1987a). This procedure resulted in approximately 100 traits. A self-report instrument was then developed to assess each trait and was administered to several groups of subjects. Factor analysis of each of these data sets yielded a 15-factor structure that was stable across the different samples (Livesley, Jackson, & Schroeder, 1989, 1992). These factors were used to define 18 basic personality disorder dimensions, which are discussed later in this chapter. This structure provides little support for the DSM-IV model; most factors showed little resemblance to DSM-III-R diagnoses.

The significance of the failure of factor-analytic studies to support the DSM-III-R position is enhanced by the fact that they are consistent across investigators and types of data. As Harkness (1992) pointed out, although the number of factors extracted differed considerably across studies (with Clark extracting 22 factors, Harkness extracting 39, and ourselves extracting 15) examination of factor content reveals considerable similarity. Differences are largely due to a single factor in one study's being partitioned into several factors in another study (Clark & Livesley, 1994).

Although these studies provide little support for either the simple categorical model used in DSM-IV or the actual contents of many diagnostic categories, multivariate studies do support the hierarchical model used in DSM, in which diagnoses are organized into three higher-order structures. Higher-order analyses of the 18 basic dimensions yielded four or five factors, according to whether clinical or general population data were examined. We have tentatively labeled these factors Lability, Antagonism, Social Unresponsiveness, Compulsivity, and Impulsive Stimulus Seeking (see also Livesley, 1991; Schroeder, Wormworth, & Livesley, 1992, 1994).

Multivariate studies can contribute not only to establishing the contents of a valid classification of personality disorders, but also to evaluating the question of whether personality disorders are best classified using a categorical or dimensional model. The idea that personality disorders can be described, as in DSM-IV, in terms of a set of discrete categories or a series of "fuzzy sets" or prototypes (Cantor, Smith, French, & Mezzich, 1980; Livesley, 1985), in which diagnostic categories can be represented by ideal types to which a particular patient is more or less related, is a central assumption underlying categorical diagnosis. In principle, such an assumption is testable; nevertheless, much of the debate on the issue is theoretical and rational.

The categorical model for classifying phenotypic traits has measurement implications that can be tested empirically. As Eysenck (1987) has pointed out, the model predicts that the intercorrelations among traits delineating personality disorders should differ in samples that vary with regard to the presence of personality disorders. For example, if a category of borderline personality disorder is postulated, defined by traits such as affective lability, impulsivity, and identity disturbance, then the expectation is that the correlation among these features observed in a sample of patients with the disorder will differ from that observed in a general-population sample. If, on the other hand, borderline is considered to be an extreme position on a dimension that is also present in the general population, then the expectation is that the intercorrelations will be the same in the two samples; the only difference will be in the magnitude of the scores. The different levels of intercorrelation can be compared by investigating the factorial structure of the features of the personality disorder in a personality-disordered sample and a non-personality-disordered sample.

Tyrer and Alexander (1979) found a similar factorial structure underlying personality traits in two samples of patients, one sample with a personality disorder diagnosis and the other with other psychiatric disorders. We (Livesley et al., 1992) compared the structure underlying 100 scales designed to assess traits delineating personality disorders in two samples: a clinical sample of 158 patients with a primary personality disorder diagnosis, and a sample of 274 general-population subjects. Separate factor analyses revealed similar structures in the two samples. In other studies, Livesley and Schroeder (1990, 1991) obtained similar results when DSM-III-R diagnoses were examined separately.

These results suggest that the differences between personality-disorderd and non-personality-disordered samples are quantitative rather than qualitative. If the iterative approach of personality assessment were to be applied systematically to the classification of personality disorders, these results, if replicated, could be used to modify the contents (diagnostic constructs and diagnostic items) of the initial theoretical classification, and the structure of the system could be changed to incorporate a dimensional model with dimensions organized hierarchically.

## Typal Structure of Personality Disorders

The conclusion that the traits describing personality disorders appear to be continuously distributed is not inconsistent with the simple categorical model of DSM-IV. As Blashfield and McElory (Chapter 20) point out, however, dimensional assessment could be used to identify clusters of individuals who are relatively distinct from one another. What would be more reasonable than to test the DSM-IV assumption of discrete categories by subjecting a set of measures to the methods of numerical taxonomy or cluster analysis (Aldenderfer & Blashfield, 1984; Anderberg, 1973; Milligan & Cooper, 1987; Sneath & Sokal, 1973) to resolve the issue once and for all?

## Considerations Pertaining to Clustering Algorithms

The kind of clustering undertaken depends intimately on the underlying models of psychopathology to be tested (see Blashfield & McElroy, Chapter 20). Again, it is important that future editions of DSM specify in detail the model that underlies the system. For example, the idea that personality disorder diagnoses can be represented by differently shaped profiles of underlying traits is a different conception from one in which personality disorder diagnoses are determined by the presence or absence of discrete signs or categorical items.

In addition to choosing the dimensions and corresponding measures that contain the information necessary to initiate a classification study, a number of critical decisions must be made regarding the numerical procedures. These decisions bear intimately on the nature of the classification likely to be obtained. Because there are literally hundreds of variations of clustering methods, and because the statistical and formal foundations have often not been delineated, there is clearly an important art to integrating the substantive nature of the domain and the method employed. It is particularly the case with personality pathology that an investigator's formal conception of pathology must be integrated with decisions at each step. Milligan and Cooper (1987) outline five important decisions to be made, after the investigator has decided on the entities to be clustered and the variables to be used: (1) deciding whether or not to standardize the data, and, if so, how to do it; (2) deciding on a dissimilarity measure and thinking through the implications of this decision; (3) choosing a clustering method and determining whether or not the choice is congruent with the investigator's concept of a diagnostic cluster; (4) deciding on a rule for the number of clusters; and (5) interpreting, testing, and validating the obtained array of clusters. This yields a Euclidian space within a dimensional framework, with the patients represented as points in the space. The investigator is required to decide not only how many dimensions to retain, but what constitutes a cluster and how to interpret it. Finally, the investigator faces the questions of whether or not the cluster will be replicated in a new sample and how the external behavior of individuals comprising a given cluster differs from that of individuals in a different cluster. This question is unfortunately complicated by the fact that software packages typically do not permit easy crossreplication of clustering results.

It is clear that these many questions (and others) will not be addressed in the same manner by different investigators. Accordingly, there will be less than perfect agreement regarding clustering results. But clustering methods nevertheless provide the most rational alternative to the indecisive political lobbying and "armchair philosophizing" to which Blashfield (1984) referred. They offer a means to identify clusters of individuals on the basis of their profile on a series of dimensions.

As an example of the problems that might arise in a particular study,

suppose that an investigator has administered a profile measure of personality disorder dimensions to a substantial number of patients. Should the
variables be standardized? Standardizing variables tends to give each variable equal weight in the sample—but perhaps variables with greater variance
are more important and should remain unstandardized. If the profiles are
elevated because the patients are generally expected to be high on the variables, or if the patients do not constitute a representative sample of patients,
perhaps profiles should be standardized in terms of the general population,
not their own groups; however, this might reduce the dissimilarities among
their profiles. Should the profiles be double-standardized—that is, standardized in terms of both scale scores and people? This has the effect of
eliminating variations in scatter between people, which could be diagnostically important. What kind of dissimilarity measure should be used? If the
complement of the correlation coefficient is used, information about profile elevation is lost, which might bear on the severity of symptoms. Suppose an ordination clustering algorithm is chosen, based on transposed
components or factor analysis?

Despite these problems, there are many advantages to such an approach.
First, this approach begins by correlating profiles and identifying profiles
that are similar and dissimilar. Because the correlation coefficient ignores
differences in the elevation of the profile (Skinner, 1978), one can identify
clusters of profiles that are similar in shape without the interference of differences in elevation, which are sometimes attributable to response biases or
differences in general psychopathology. A second advantage of this procedure from a statistical viewpoint is that it takes into account the entire profile rather than focusing on a few high points, as has traditionally been done
with MMPI profiles.

A third advantage is that it is possible to treat the basis for the differences in terms of a set of dimensions. Persons clustering together with high
or low scores on a particular dimension share key characteristics that are
potentially interpretable and diagnostically relevant. In another domain, that
of vocational interest profiles for different occupational groups, Jackson and
Williams (1975) reported that more than two dozen meaningful occupational
clusters could be identified. They found, for example, that more than a dozen
groups of physicians in different medical specialties (e.g., psychiatry, internal medicine, and pathology) were all associated in a single cluster that could
be differentiated from other occupational groups. Fourth, it is possible to
cross-validate clusters analytically by comparing clusters obtained from the
same or different populations (Skinner, Read, & Jackson, 1976). Fifth, modal
profile analysis provides a quantitative basis for classifying personality in
using computer-based actuarial taxonomies that are more parsimonious than
those based on clinical experience (Skinner & Jackson, 1978). Finally, weights
obtained for profile types using such a clustering algorithm can be obtained
and applied to new algorithms that seek to classify individuals in terms of
their probability of falling within a cluster or diagnostic classification.

Modal profile analysis combines a dimensional framework with a clustering approach, so that one obtains typal dimensions based on profile patterns (see also Blashfield & McElroy, Chapter 20). In the future, individuals showing a similarity to one of these identified types may be assumed to have similar characteristics when compared with others defining the type. We submit that such a classification will be more stable than one in which diagnoses and diagnostic criteria are based on a consensus of expert clinical judgment, where small changes have been shown to have substantial and unanticipated effects (Blashfield et al., 1992). Furthermore, such a classification system is more consistent with modern thinking regarding the dimensional nature of personality disorders (Schroeder et al., 1994; Widiger & Sanderson, Chapter 22; Widiger & Frances, 1994).

## Modal Profile Analysis of Clinical and General-Population Samples

To illustrate this approach, we applied modal profile analysis to two groups: 158 patients diagnosed as having a personality disorder, and 274 individuals drawn from the general population (Livesley et al., 1992). Both groups completed a questionnaire comprised of 100 personality scales. These scales were reduced via principal-components factor analysis to 18 dimensions and assessed via the Dimensional Assessment of Personality Problems (DAPP; Livesley & Jackson, in press). These dimensions are listed below in Figure 23.1–23.3. As noted previously, a remarkable feature of the factor-analytic results is that the factor structures present in the clinical and general-population samples were highly similar. Accordingly, it was possible to identify factor scores for each individual in both clinical and general-population groups for each of the 18 personality pathology dimensions, based on the weights for the 100 scale scores obtained by each individual. But there was a complication in this analysis—namely, that patients generally obtained higher factor scores than persons in the general population. Thus, if we generated modal profiles characterizing each cluster for the patient group and the general-population group separately, the patient clusters would be compared with the set of patients, and clusters from the general population would be compared with persons drawn from the general population. This would render the two sets of profiles incomparable. Thus, a patient cluster showing a score at the 50th percentile on affective lability might score at the 85th percentile if compared with the nonpatients. Accordingly, we decided to standardize the patient group using the mean and standard deviation from the general-population group. Thus, a score falling at the 75th percentile in one group would be directly comparable with a score falling at the 75th percentile in the second group.

Having standardized both sets of individual factor scores in terms of the general-population summary statistics, we sought to cluster these using modal profile analysis. Because the groups were relatively large and would have resulted in very large correlation matrices if one individual's profiles were correlated with all of the other individuals' profiles, we employed singular value decomposition—a statistical technique that essentially allows one to proceed directly from the data matrix to the underlying principal components representing the dimensions along which people are clustered, without the necessity of computing correlations.

We obtained 17 dimensions in both the clinical and general-population groups. If an individual's profile correlated with an absolute value of above .50 with the profile represented by the positive or negative pole of one of the 17 dimensions, we classified that individual as falling within the cluster. Using that criterion for classification, we found that 84.8% of the clinical sample and 83.2% of the general-population sample could be classified.

These findings have three important implications:

1. Individuals in the general population and clinically diagnosed patients show variations in patterns of personality pathology. The clusters that emerged in the two groups were in many cases similar, although not identical. In general, clinical clusters showed stronger definition in the sense that there were more extremely high and low scores, although many of the clusters for the general population were also well defined.

2. The high classification rates for both groups support a dimensional formulation for personality disorders. General population respondents showed variations in patterns of personality pathology, as did patients.

3. The findings regarding 17 bimodal dimensions, which reflect 34 distinct types, suggest that diagnostic systems such as DSM-III-R and DSM-IV (which contain 11 and 10 diagnostic categories, respectively) may not reflect the complexity of personality disorders as this is revealed in empirical findings. Certainly evidence for the complexity of personality disorders based on our findings is not sufficiently revealed in the five-factor or "Big Five" model of personality (Costa & Widiger, 1994).

An illustration of the distinct variations in personality pathology might be in order. Corbitt (1993) has analyzed a clinical case of narcissistic personality disorder, "Patricia," in terms of the five-factor model. Thus, Corbitt has implicitly suggested that this person's profile on the five factors and each of their facets is prototypical of narcissistic personality disorder. Corbitt notes that "Patricia" has high scores on neuroticism and conscientiousness, a low score on agreeableness, and scores in the more neutral range on extraversion and openness.

Although Corbitt's discussion of this case, integrating the Big Five factors with facets of each factor, is sensitive and of considerable interest to clinicians, the suggestion (based presumably on DSM-III-R and DSM-IV) that there is only one type of narcissism and that narcissistic personality disorder is adequately reflected in a single profile—whether of the Big Five personality dimensions or of facets comprising these—is not consistent with our data. Our data indicate more than one cluster of individuals who have nar-

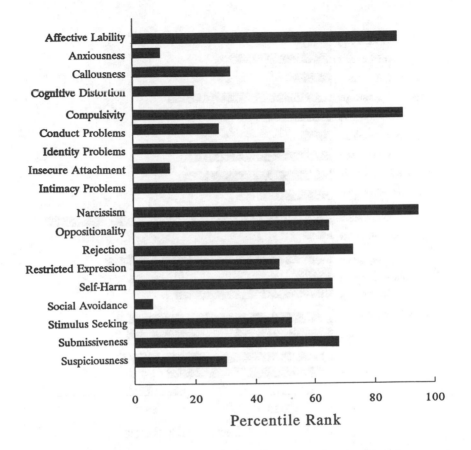

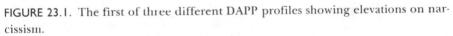

FIGURE 23.1. The first of three different DAPP profiles showing elevations on narcissism.

cissism as a prominent feature. In some sense, each cluster could be described as narcissistic, but the clinical syndromes are quite distinct from one another. Compare Figures 23.1, 23.2, and 23.3. Of a total of 158 patients, there were 4 who were classifiable in the cluster characterized by the DAPP profile depicted in Figure 23.1, four in the cluster presented in Figure 23.2, and four in the cluster represented in Figure 23.3. (Although there were just 4 patients classifiable into each of these clusters, the modal profile analysis employed the data from all 158 patients to define the modal profiles.) Each of these clusters shows an elevation for narcissism above the 90th percentile, but otherwise the profiles are quite distinct.

The profile represented in Figure 23.1 is characterized by high scores, in addition to narcissism, on compulsivity, affective lability, and rejection, with notably low scores on social avoidance and anxiousness. The profile represented in Figure 23.2 is quite different. In addition to a high narcis-

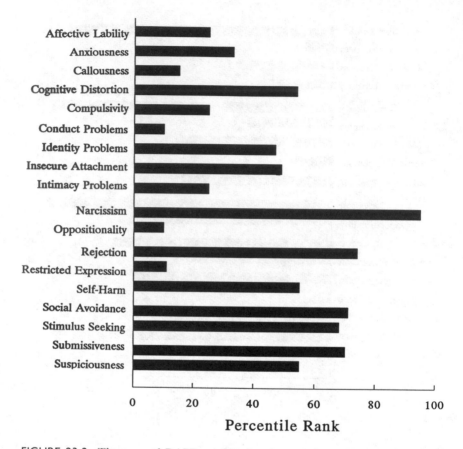

FIGURE 23.2. The second DAPP profile showing an elevation on narcissism.

sism score, there are distinct elevations for social avoidance, stimulus seeking, and suspiciousness. Neither of the profiles in Figures 23.1 and 23.2 shows
an elevation on intimacy problems or callousness, as shown in the profile
represented by Figure 23.3. Here we have elevations, in addition to narcissism, for scales measuring callousness, intimacy problems, and suspiciousness, with notably low scores on rejection and stimulus seeking. These results
help to explain the high overlap noted between narcissistic and other personality disorders (see Gunderson, Ronningstam, & Smith, Chapter 9). Experienced clinicians will recognize these different "types" of narcissistic
individuals. Indeed, the association of narcissistic features with the features
of antisocial personality disorder has been noted by Widiger and Corbitt
in Chapter 6 (see also Livesley & Schroeder, 1991). If these "types" were to
be lumped together into one category of "narcissistic personality disorder,"
very disparate personalities would be represented in a single category—one

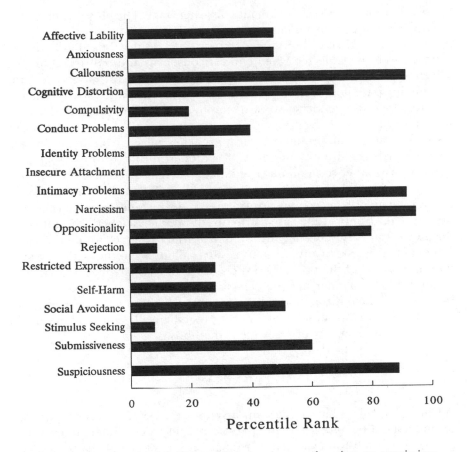

FIGURE 23.3. The third DAPP profile showing an elevation on narcissism.

that would do little justice to their uniqueness. The result of such undifferentiated classification would be confusion on the part of the inexperienced clinician who had not yet developed skepticism about the rigorousness of personality disorder diagnosis. With little more clinical experience, such a novice clinician might reasonably conclude that patients with the same diagnosis of "narcissistic personality disorder" are almost as distinct from one another as are patients falling in different diagnostic groups.

Our findings that personality-disordered patients can be clustered analytically into as many as 34 groups has implications that in some ways are perplexing. Clearly, the findings from our modal profile analysis show that personality disorders are much more complex than can be represented in the prevailing set of diagnostic categories. In fact, this complexity might even challenge the clinician's cognitive intuitive capacity to represent these disorders. But, as we have indicated, experienced clinicians will not be surprised

at the different forms that personality disorders take. The illustration of narcissistic pathology is by no means exceptional; we could easily have reported on several other differentiated types. Our results thus highlight the
differences to be expected when clinical consensus and political lobbying
are employed as the primary basis for a diagnostic classification system for
personality pathology, as compared with data-based analytical approaches.
Whereas there is a tendency toward simplicity in human judgment, involving an inevitable leveling of distinctions traceable to the frailties and vagar-
ies of human cognition, analytical approaches permit complexity where
complexity is required by the data. It is a question for future research to
determine whether computer-assisted diagnosis (e.g., in combining features
and dimensional configurations quantitatively) will contribute to improved
accuracy in identifying complexity where complexity is present. Alternatively,
perhaps more empirically based structured interviews aimed at identifying
diagnostic categories that are anchored in a firmer research foundation may
be equal to the task. In any case, our results call for a careful, critical examination not only of the present DSM classification of personality disorders,
but indeed the manner in which classifications are determined. Our findings support the position that a diagnostic classification scheme be supported not only by clinical judgment, but by systematically collected empirical
data based on a variety of assessment methods.

## OVERVIEW

We have argued, as have others, for a systematic, research-based approach
to understanding and classifying personality disorders. Such an approach
leans substantially on experience from general personality assessment and
research, but not on the blind empiricism that has historically characterized
some of the personality assessment literature. Rather, we are arguing for the
use of personality constructs that are based in theory, consistent with what
is known clinically about personality pathology, and validated empirically
by seeking a triangulation of methods (e.g., using clinical judgments and other
empirical methods to validate the scores obtained by patients on clinically
significant questionnaire dimensions of personality pathology). Furthermore,
we are concerned with obtaining empirical evidence for clusters of personality pathology, with identifying the bases on which we can distinguish the
degree and quality of pathology, and with determining how we can distinguish normality from disordered personality. We submit, as have others that
normality and personality pathology represent a continuum. This viewpoint
conceptualizes the large majority of persons as being to some extent classifiable in terms of some degree of personality pathology. The critical
research question is the determination of which constellations and what
degree of deviation represent a level of pathology that is appropriately diagnosed. We hope and expect that increased understanding of the com-

plex phenomena of personality pathology will be better achieved through the use of systematic cumulative knowledge regarding conceptions of diagnostic categories, the personality dimensions that characterize persons falling into these categories, methods for their evaluation, and empirical research seeking to validate a variety of methods (including, but not limited to, clinical judgment).

## REFERENCES

Aldenderfer, M. S., & Blashfield, R. K. (1984). *Cluster analysis.* Beverly Hills, CA: Sage.

American Psychiatric Association. (1980). *Diagnostic and statistical manual of mental disorders* (3rd ed.). Washington, DC: Author.

American Psychiatric Association. (1987). *Diagnostic and statistical manual of mental disorders* (3rd ed., rev.). Washington, DC: Author.

American Psychiatric Association. (1994). *Diagnostic and statistical manual of mental disorders* (4th ed.). Washington, DC: Author.

Anderberg, M. R. (1973). *Cluster analysis for applications.* New York: Academic Press.

Bell, R. C., & Jackson, D. N. (1992). The structure of personality disorders in DSM-III. *Acta Psychiatrica Scandinavica, 85,* 279–287.

Blashfield, R. K. (1984). *The classification of psychopathology.* New York: Plenum Press.

Blashfield, R. K., Blum, N., & Pfohl, B. (1992). The effects of changing Axis II diagnostic criteria. *Comprehensive Psychiatry, 33,* 245–252.

Blashfield, R. K., & Breen, M. J. (1989). Face validity of the DSM-III-R personality disorders. *American Journal of Psychiatry, 146,* 1575–1579.

Blashfield, R. K., & Livesley, W. J. (1991). Metaphorical analysis of psychiatric classification as a psychological test. *Journal of Abnormal Psychology, 100,* 262–270.

Cantor, N., Smith, E. E., French, R., & Mezzich, J. (1980). Psychiatric diagnosis as prototype categorization. *Journal of Abnormal Psychology, 89,* 181–193.

Clark, L. A. (1990). Toward a consensual set of symptom clusters for assessment of personality disorder. In J. Butcher & C. Spielberger (Eds.), *Advances in personality assessment* (Vol. 8, pp. 243–266). Hillsdale, NJ: Erlbaum.

Clark, L. A., & Livesley, W. J. (1994). Two approaches to identifying the dimensions of personality disorder: Convergence on the five-factor model. In P. T. Costa & T. A. Widiger (Eds.), *Personality disorders and the five-factor model of personality* (pp. 261–277). Washington, DC: American Psychological Association.

Corbitt, E. M. (1994). Narcissism from the perspective of the five-factor model. In P. T. Costa & T. A. Widiger (Eds.), *Personality disorders and the five-factor model of personality* (pp. 199–203). Washington, DC: American Psychological Association.

Costa, P. T., & Widiger, T. A. (Eds.). (1994). *Personality disorders and the five-factor model of personality.* Washington, DC: American Psychological Association.

Eysenck, H. J. (1987). The definition of personality disorders and the criteria appropriate to their definition. *Journal of Personality Disorders, 1,* 211–219.

Faust, D., & Miner, R. A. (1986). The empiricist and his new clothes: DSM-III in perspective. *American Journal of Psychiatry, 143,* 962–966.

Gorton, G., & Akhtar, S. (1990). The literature on personality disorders 1985–1988: Trends, issues, and controversies. *Hospital and Community Psychiatry, 41,* 39–51.

Gulliksen, H. (1950). *Theory of mental tests.* New York: Wiley.

Harkness, A. R. (1992). Fundamental topics in the personality disorders: Candidate trait dimensions from lower regions of the hierarchy. *Psychological Assessment: A Journal of Consulting and Clinical Psychology, 4,* 251–259.

Jackson, D. N. (1971). The dynamics of structured personality tests. *Psychological Review, 78,* 229–248.

Jackson, D. N., & Williams, D. R. (1975). Occupational classification in terms of interest patterns. *Journal of Vocational Behavior, 6,* 269–280.

Kass, F., Skodol, A. E., Charles, E., Spitzer, R. L., & Williams, J. B. W. (1985). Scaled ratings of DSM-III personality disorders. *American Journal of Psychiatry, 142,* 627–630.

Klerman, G. L. (1978). The evolution of a scientific nosology. In J. C. Shershow (Ed.), *Schizophrenia: Science and practice* (pp. 99–121). Cambridge, MA: Harvard University Press.

Livesley, W. J. (1985). The classification of personality disorder: I. The choice of category concept. *Canadian Journal of Psychiatry, 30,* 353–358.

Livesley, W. J. (1986). Trait and behavioral prototypes of personality disorder. *American Journal of Psychiatry, 143,* 728–732.

Livesley, W. J. (1987a). A systematic approach to the delineation of personality disorder. *American Journal of Psychiatry, 144,* 772–777.

Livesley, W. J. (1987b). Theoretical and empirical issues in the selection of criteria to diagnose personality disorders. *Journal of Personality Disorders, 1,* 88–94.

Livesley, W. J. (1991). Classifying personality disorders: Ideal types, prototypes, or dimensions? *Journal of Personality Disorders, 5,* 52–59.

Livesley, W. J., & Jackson, D. N. (1990). Construct validity and the classification of personality disorders. In J. Oldham (Ed.), *Personality disorders: New perspectives on diagnostic validity* (pp. 3–22). Washington, DC: American Psychiatric Association.

Livesley, W. J., & Jackson, D. N. (1992). Guidelines for developing, evaluating, and revising the classification of personality disorders. *Journal of Nervous and Mental Disease, 180,* 609–618.

Livesley, W. J., & Jackson, D. N. (in press). *Dimensional assessment of personality problems (DAPP).* Port Huron, MI: Sigma Assessment Systems, Inc.

Livesley, W. J., Jackson, D. N., & Schroeder, M. L. (1989). A study of the factorial structure of personality pathology. *Journal of Personality Disorders, 3,* 298–306.

Livesley, W. J., Jackson, D. N., & Schroeder, M. L. (1992). Factorial structure of traits delineating personality disorders in clinical and general population samples. *Journal of Abnormal Psychology, 101,* 432–440.

Livesley, W. J., Reiffer, L. I., Sheldon, A. E. R., & West, M. (1987). Prototypicality of DSM-III personality criteria. *Journal of Nervous and Mental Disease, 175,* 395–401.

Livesley, W. J., & Schroeder, M. L. (1990). Dimensions of personality disorder: The DSM-III-R Cluster A diagnoses. *Journal of Nervous and Mental Disease, 178,* 627–635.

Livesley, W. J., & Schroeder, M. L. (1991). Dimensions of personality disorder: The DSM-III-R Cluster B diagnoses. *Journal of Nervous and Mental Disease, 179,* 320–328.

Livesley, W. J., Schroeder, M. L., Jackson, D. N., & Jang, K. L. (1994). Categorical distinctions in the study of personality disorder: Implications for classification. *Journal of Abnormal Psychology, 103,* 6–17.

Loevinger, J. (1957). Objective tests as instruments of psychological theory. *Psychological Reports, 3,* 635–694.

Lorr, M., & Strack, S. (1990). Profile clusters of the MCMI-II personality disorder scales. *Journal of Clinical Psychology, 46,* 606–612.

Mellsop, G., Varghese, F., Joshua, S., & Hicks, A. (1982). The reliability of Axis II of DSM-III. *American Journal of Psychiatry, 139,* 1360–1361.

Messick, S. (1988). Validity. In R. L. Linn (Ed.), *Educational measurement* (3rd ed., pp. 13–103). New York: Macmillan.

Milligan, G. W., & Cooper, M. C. (1987). Methodology review: Clustering methods. *Applied Psychological Measurement, 11*(4), 329–354.

Morey, L. C. (1988). A psychometric analysis of the DSM-III-R personality disorder criteria. *Journal of Personality Disorders, 2,* 109–124.

Morey, L. C., & McNamara, T. P. (1987). On definitions, diagnosis, and DSM-III. *Journal of Abnormal Psychology, 96,* 283–285.

Nerviano, V. J., & Gross, H. W.. (1983). Personality types of alcoholics on objective inventories: A review. *Journal of Studies on Alcohol, 44,* 837–851.

Robins, E., & Guze, S. B. (1970). Establishment of diagnostic validity in psychiatric illness: Its application to schizophrenia. *American Journal of Psychiatry, 126,* 983–987.

Schroeder, M. L., Wormworth, J. A., & Livesley, W. J. (1992). Dimensions of personality disorder and their relationships to the Big Five dimensions of personality. *Psychological Assessment: A Journal of Consulting and Clinical Psychology, 4,* 47–53.

Schroeder, M. L., Wormworth, J. A., & Livesley, W. J. (1994). Dimensions of personality disorder and the five-factor model of personality. In P. T. Costa & T. A. Widiger (Eds.), *Personality disorders and the five-factor model of personality* (pp. 117–127). Washington, DC: American Psychological Association.

Skinner, H. A. (1978). Differentiating the contribution of elevation, scatter and shape in profile similarity. *Educational and Psychological Measurement, 38,* 297–308.

Skinner, H. A. (1981). Toward the integration of classification theory and methods. *Journal of Abnormal Psychology, 90,* 68–87.

Skinner, H. A., & Jackson, D. N. (1978). A model of psychopathology based on an integration of MMPI actuarial systems. *Journal of Consulting and Clinical Psychology, 46,* 231–238.

Skinner, H. A., Reed, P. L., & Jackson, D. N. (1976). Toward the objective diagnosis of psychopathology: Generalizability of modal personality profiles. *Journal of Consulting and Clinical Psychology, 44,* 111–117.

Sneath, P. H. A., & Sokal, R. R. (1973). *Numerical taxonomy.* San Francisco: W. H. Freeman.

Spitzer, R. L., & Fleiss, J. L. (1974). Re-analysis of the reliability of psychiatric diagnosis. *British Journal of Psychiatry, 125,* 341

Spitzer, R. L., Forman, J., & Nee, J. (1979). DSM-III field trials: I. Initial inter-rater diagnostic reliability. *American Journal of Psychiatry, 136,* 815–817.

Tyrer, P., & Alexander, M. S. (1979). Classification of personality disorder. *British Journal of Psychiatry, 135,* 163-167.

Widiger, T. A., Frances, A. J., Harris, M., Jacobsberg, L., Fyer, M., & Manning, D. (1990). Comorbidity among Axis II disorders. In J. Oldham (Ed.), *Personality disorders: New perspectives on diagnostic validity* (pp. 163–194). Washington, DC: American Psychiatric Press.

Widiger, T. A., & Frances, A. J. (1994). Toward a dimensional model for the personality disorders. In P. T. Costa & T. A. Widiger (Eds.). *Personality disorders and the five-factor model of personality* (pp. 19–39). Washington, DC: American Psychological Association.

# CHAPTER 24

# The Challenge of Alternative Perspectives in Classification: A Discussion of Basic Issues

LEE ANNA CLARK

The chapters in this section each address classification in the domain of personality disorder from perspectives other than that of the currently prevailing taxonomy, and yet every one of them considers issues that are fundamental to the development of scientific knowledge—issues regarding the role of theory and its relations to empirical data. It is no secret that the official classification of personality disorders (and indeed of all mental disorders) embodied in the DSMs represents a compromise among the often competing interests of clinicians, researchers, educators, and statisticians with various training backgrounds and diverse orientations (Frances, Pincus, Widiger, Davis, & First, 1990). This fact tends to be forgotten, however, in the day-to-day usage of the classification system. Despite the explicit statement in DSM-III-R that "the diagnostic criteria are based on clinical judgment, and have not been fully validated" (American Psychiatric Association, 1987, p. xxiv), there is widespread acceptance of the DSM criteria as definitive. To be sure, we can hardly expect otherwise of such users as third-party payers, who appropriately turn to external authority as the initial basis for their decisions (we would certainly not wish them to develop their own classification system). And, on the other end of the continuum, let us dismiss out of hand those who reject the DSM for scientifically ill-founded reasons (e.g., "I don't believe in labeling people," "Diagnosis doesn't matter; it's the clinical formulation that counts," "The DSM pathologizes and I like to focus on strengths," etc.)

What is disturbing is that, aside from a handful of those who are interested in classification per se, researchers who submit either manuscripts for publication or grant applications for funding typically use the DSM to diagnose their subjects without devoting much (if any) thought to the committee-based nature of, and the relative lack of empirical bases for, its diagnostic criteria. Much attention may be paid to obtaining reliable diagnoses through the use of structured or semistructured interviews administered by carefully trained research assistants, but the operating assumption is that if these procedures are followed, the resulting patient groups *ipso facto* represent valid diagnostic categories. Again with the exception of those relatively few researchers who concern themselves directly with such issues, inconsistent or unexpected findings are rarely attributed to problems in the diagnostic system; rather, they are thought to stem from such things as measurement error, comorbidity, or sampling error attributable to different settings or small samples. Of equal concern is the fact that these attitudes are also typically held by those who evaluate research submissions: A work is in danger of serious criticism if the DSM was *not* used in diagnosis.

In this context, it is refreshing to be confronted by a series of chapters that all address very basic issues in the formulation of diagnostic taxonomies. Although it is important that some researchers investigate such details as the effect of lengthening a symptom duration requirement for diagnosis from 1 month to 6 months, it is also crucial that others reconsider the fundamental assumptions underlying the very process of taxonomic development. The writers in this section address questions of epistemology, natural versus artificial classification, operational definitions versus open concepts, structural versus measurement models, incremental validity of dimensional over categorical systems, and "ideal types" versus "prototypes," to mention but a few of the topics discussed. Although each chapter offers a different perspective and advocates a different approach, the authors share a basic concern for the process of science, a balanced appreciation for the breadth and complexity of their subject and the importance of discerning order in that complexity, a respect for precision in both terminology and procedures, and a consideration of the difference between values and truth. In this chapter, I discuss common themes that emerge across the chapters as well as in others' writings, challenge inconsistencies or illogic, and attempt to reconcile at least some of the apparent differences and discrepancies.

## MODELS OF PERSONALITY DISORDER: TERMINOLOGICAL ISSUES

A recurrent concern is that the terminology used to discuss the classification of personality disorder is often ambiguous, confusing, or inconsistent. Indeed, even within these chapters, similar issues are discussed using different terminology, or the same terms are applied in somewhat different ways. For example, the chapters by Blashfield and McElroy (Chapter 20), Jackson and Livesley (Chapter 23), and Shea (Chapter 19) each consider how relations among traits or symptoms account for or define the psychopathology: Distinctive configurations of features or traits suggest that personality disorders may be categorical, whereas the failure to find such clusters favors a dimensional view of personality disorders. Blashfield and McElroy specifically refer to these two types of feature/trait organizations as "structural" models, whereas in Jackson and Livesley's discussion, which is based on Loevinger's (1957) construct validation approach, the "structural component" refers to the extent to which the observed relations are consistent with the theoretical model. Thus, it has both empirical and theoretical aspects. This seems to go beyond Blashfield and McElroy's notion of structural models. In this more elaborated view (which is discussed in more detail later), the substantive component defines the diagnostic features or traits, whereas the structural component delineates their interrelations and how each feature is diagnosed. Thus, the term "structural" is used in these two chapters in both overlapping and distinctive ways. It is used to make the common point that the organization of psychopathological features may be either categorical or dimensional; yet it is further elaborated in different ways.

Blashfield and McElroy further state that what differentiates categorical from dimensional structural models is not whether they posit the existence or nonexistence of dimensions per se, but whether or not there are supposed discontinuities or points of rarity along these dimensions. Shea also notes that it may be *combinations* of dimensions that are categorical. In this view, categorical and dimensional structural models are not mutually exclusive; rather, the former may represent a subset of the latter. Interestingly, Blashfield and McElroy neither rule out nor discuss nondimensional categorical structural models; perhaps they ignore them because, although they represent an interesting theoretical possibility, there are few if any empirical data on personality disorders to support them. Jackson and Livesley also mention them only briefly (without using this terminology); however, the ideal types described by Schwartz, Wiggins, and Norko in Chapter 21 (discussed later) may fall under this rubric.

Moreover, Blashfield and McElroy explicitly distinguish structural models from measurement models. Specifically, their discussion of measurement models focuses on whether personality disorders themselves are represented as simple nominal scales (categorical model) or based on variables with interval or ratio scaling (dimensional model). Thus, according to these writers, measurement and structural models are independent: For example, a dimensional measurement model may be consistent with a categorical structural model, given one or more points of rarity on the relevant dimension(s). Although measurement is clearly a core issue in the structural component discussed by Jackson and Livesley, this separate terminology is not used. Moreover, these writers imply that the measurement and theoretical models should be consistent (e.g., the theoretical and measurement models should both be categorical). Shea, in turn, notes the lack of clarity regarding the relation between conceptualization (model) and criteria (i.e., measurement) for the DSM personality disorders.

At first glance, therefore, it appears that these chapters, each attempting to clarify the debate about categorical and dimensional models of personality disorder, present only partially overlapping views. However, the more one delves into them, the more it appears that they are actually in close agreement and that they are separated only by differences in terminology.

Yet another terminological inconsistency creates additional confusion: Specifically, the term "dimensional" is used with two widely different meanings. One view of dimensions considers the question of whether each diagnosis represents a pathological entity distinct from normality and from other personality disorders (categorical model) or represents the extreme end of a continuously distributed latent factor (I term this view a "latent-entity dimensional model"). In this latter view, the latent factors presumably shade into normality at lower ends of the continuum. There also is no apparent assumption that the latent factors representing the different personality disorders are independent; rather, they may be correlated among themselves.

By contrast, the term "dimensional" is also used in reference to personality traits (I term this view a "trait dimensional model"). In discussions of categorical versus dimensional models, this view of dimensions considers the question of whether or not individuals' standings along a set of personality trait dimensions are patterned in such a way that discernible clusters are formed. Unlike a latent-entity dimensional model, which hypothesizes the existence of a latent dimension corresponding to each personality disorder, a trait dimensional model makes no statement whatsoever about the existence of personality disorder per se. Rather, it offers a trait structure with which to describe observed manifestations of personality, both adaptive and maladaptive. Trait dimensional models themselves are indifferent to whether or not these form replicable patterns (i.e., categories) within either the normal or abnormal range (i.e., personality types or disorders, respectively).

The admixture of these two types of dimensional models has obscured debate regarding categorical versus dimensional models of personality disorder. For example, in their critique (in Chapter 22) of the DSM-III-R categorical distinctions, Widiger and Sanderson's discussion of the superiority of dimensional over categorical approaches almost invariably references latent-entity models. It is not until late in their chapter that Widiger and Sanderson introduce their favored approach, a trait dimensional model (the five-factor model), as an alternative to the DSM. However, it is not at all clear that the data favoring a latent-entity dimensional approach can be applied to support trait dimensional approaches. The cited studies typically compared DSM-III-R categorical ratings (presence vs. absence) to latent-entity dimensional scores that used an $X$-point rating scale or simply the number of criteria met. It is noteworthy that these two types of ratings share the presumption of the existence of the specific disorders being assessed. Thus, what is being compared in these studies is two different measurement (à la Blashfield and McElroy) models for the same set of personality disorders.

In this context, the similarity of the latent-entity dimensional model to the prototype model of diagnosis discussed by Schwartz et al. in their chapter is also noteworthy. In both models, a given set of disorders (e.g., the current DSM diagnoses) is accepted as defining, respectively, the target latent entities or prototypes, and pathology is assessed by degree rather than dichotomously. Where these approaches appear to differ is that advocates of a prototype approach emphasize the constructed nature of the target entities, whereas those who favour the latent-entity dimensional model are more likely to view them as reality-based. I return to this point in a later section.

As stated earlier, in contrast to prototype and latent-entity dimensional models, trait dimensional models of personality disorder make no assumptions about the existence of any particular type of psychopathology, although they build upon the DSM definition of personality disorders as inflexible and maladaptive personality traits. Trait dimensional models maintain that the fundamental dimensions underlying this domain are not the personality disorders themselves, but sets of dysfunctional traits used to describe personality disorder. This is the type of dimensional model referred to by Shea and, for the most part, by Jackson and Livesley.

With this concept of dimensions, the outcome of the assessment process is not ratings on a set of diagnoses but a profile of personality traits (Clark, in press; Widiger & Frances, 1994). At this stage, therefore, trait dimensional models are descriptive rather than classificatory models. Whether and how the results of a trait dimensional assessment can be used to classify individuals are further questions. Thus, implementation of a trait dimensional model for assessing personality disorder would represent a far more radical departure from the DSM taxonomy than would adopting a latent-entity dimensional approach based on the current system.

The application of trait dimensional approaches to personality disorder is promising, but still relatively untested. As noted by Shea, given its conservative mandate, rejection of this model by the DSM-IV Personality Disorders Work Group is not surprising. However, given the robust finding that increased reliability and validity are obtained with the use of interval and ratio scales compared to nominal scales (Widiger, 1992), and the fact that latent-entity dimension models also retain more clinically relevant information than categorical models (Clark, in press), the lack of endorsement of a latent-entity dimensional model in the DSM-IV clearly suggests that additional factors are needed to explain the persistent endorsement of the categorical approach by the work group.

When Widiger and Sanderson state the arguments favoring categorical models, they mention a set of issues largely unrelated to questions of science, raising instead concerns that are educational (tradition/familiarity), professional (ease in conceptualization/communication), and practical (clinical decision making) in nature. One way in which these issues can be addressed is by using cutoffs with a latent-entity dimensional model to convert interval measurements into categorical diagnoses—an option that Widiger and Sanderson note was considered by the Personality Disorders Work Group. Such an approach could reconcile the scientific desire for an empirically based theoretical/structural and measurement model with the perceived need for a user-friendly classification system. However, this possibility was rejected as a solution to the large gap between data and officialdom, in part because it was perceived as "too cumbersome for practical use" (Widiger & Sanderson, Chapter 22, p. 447).

It is possible that latent-entity dimensional approaches were rejected because the work group recognized that they do not represent a radical conceptual departure from the current system, and therefore felt that the disruption caused by adopting a different measurement model for the same set of diagnoses could not be justified. That is, the ultimate validity of the latent-entity dimensional approach depends in turn upon the validity of the personality disorders on which the latent factors are based. Adopting a different measurement model does not address the validity of the disorders themselves, which has been the subject of as much (or more) criticism as the categorical measurement model. Moreover, treating disorders as continua (or as prototypes) rather than as dichotomous categories would not resolve the often-cited problem of within-diagnosis symptom heterogeneity. Latent-entity dimensional and prototype models are not as theoretically inconsistent with heterogeneity as are classical categorical models, but the criticisms have been leveled largely at the clinical difficulties of dealing with within-group heterogeneity, not at inconsistency with the underlying theoretical model.

Finally, latent-entity dimensional and prototype models neither solve nor provide a theoretical basis for understanding the problem posed by the high levels of mixed personality pathology that are observed routinely in clinical settings. Thus, despite that fact that these alternative models provide a better fit with the empirical data, they do not offer solutions to some of the more difficult and persistent practical and theoretical problems in the assessment of personality disorder. Nevertheless, it seems likely that all of these reasons for rejecting latent-entity dimensional and prototype models are still insufficient to explain the persistence of the categorical approach, and that other, more psychological or political factors also may be involved.

## EMPIRICISM, POSITIVISM, CONSTRUCTIONISM, RELATIVISM, PRAGMATISM, AND REALISM

The terminological and related issues just discussed provide a language and a framework for consideration of fundamental concerns in the study of personality disorder that are also addressed in this set of chapters. One recurring theme is that blind or naive empiricism is unlikely to advance our understanding of personality disorder very far beyond our current state of knowledge. For example, Schwartz et al. argue that without guiding concepts, empirical observations are uninterpretable, or at best will be organized at the very basic level of sensorimotor activity. Similarly, Davis and Millon state in Chapter 18 that the purely empirical approach can encompass reliability, but cannot address questions of validity. Moreover, they argue that whether or not a theory is explicit and well articulated, there are no theory-free observations. Thus, naive empiricists deceive themselves by believing that they are observing nature directly. Furthermore, pure empiricism is limited to the compilation of observational "facts" and the refinement of others' constructs. It points in no direction for the generation of new realms of observation.

To illustrate this point with an example from a different field, Weinberg (1992) tells a story of two physicists who, unbeknownst to each other and nearly at the same time in different countries, performed the same experiment with the same result. One of them, J. J. Thomson, hypothesized that his observations suggested the existence of a theoretical entity—which he named the "electron"—whereas the other, Walter Kaufmann, was a positivist and would not name a thing that he could not observe. As a result of their respective conclusions, only Thomson continued his experimentation and, after obtaining many more observations that supported his hypothesis, became known as the discoverer of the electron. The point of this story with regard to personality disorder is not that we should reify our diagnostic categories, but rather that a philosophical stance can influence how investigators proceed to explore and to explain their data, with the result that entirely new fields of knowledge may or may not be generated.

There are obvious parallels between theoretical approaches to personality disorder classification and the process of construct validation. The writings of such theoretical psychometricians as Cronbach, Meehl, and Loevinger thus provide a foundation for many of the points articulated in the present set of chapters. For example, one clear strength of a theoretical approach is its ability to synthesize diverse types of information into a coherent whole, in contrast to the "operational definition'" approach, which views each type of data as a thing unto itself and "involves the acceptance of a set of operations as an adequate definition of whatever is to be measured" (Bechtoldt, cited in Cronbach & Meehl, 1955, p. 282). The construct validation approach was developed in response to an overemphasis on criterion-related validity, which insisted on a rigorously empirical but atomistic one-construct/one-criterion approach. As Cronbach and Meehl (1955) note, "Construct validity must be investigated whenever no criterion or universe of content is accepted as entirely adequate to define the quality to be measured" (p. 282). Personality disorders easily meet this definition.

On the other hand, one difficulty with embracing a theoretical approach, with its emphasis on abstract and inferential entities, is that it is possible for theoretical formulations to be related to observables so indirectly that empirical tests of their validity become impossible. Such "open concepts,"as Davis and Millon call them in their chapter, "may become so circuitous in their references that they become tautological and completely decoupled from the empirical realm" (Chapter 18, p. 380). Cronbach and Meehl (1955), however, deal firmly with this concern: *The answer is that unless the network makes contact with observables, and exhibits explicit, public steps of inference, construct validation cannot be claimed"* (p. 291; emphasis in original).

Similarly, Jackson and Livesley address this issue from the outset by outlining a procedure for the development of a scientifically valid classification system for personality disorders. Their general approach is firmly theoretical (e.g., "the objective when compiling a classification is to ensure construct validity"—Chapter 23, p. 461); yet they emphasize that the theoretical concepts and their interrelations that define the classification system must be clearly articulated and empirically tested. Thus, the contrast made both in these chapters and in the classic writings on construct validity is not simply between empiricism and theory, which complement and are dependent on each other, but between blind empiricism unguided by any explicit theory and abstract theory untied to any observables. Although it is easy to grasp that both extremes should be shunned, it is also important to recognize that there are clear philosophical differences even among researchers who do reject both extremes, in terms of the emphasis they place on the importance of empiricism versus theory. Writers of both persuasions often argue for their position by rejecting the straw target of the opposite extreme (and, regrettably, it would not be hard to find examples in the published literature that approximate each extreme). However, these arguments should not be taken as seriously as those of writers who contrast their position with that of a moderate view on the opposing side.

A second recurring theme is whether the entities we seek to describe are in some sense real or whether they represent conceptual constructions that have utility but not truth value. It is important not to draw this distinction too firmly, for there are respects in which these two viewpoints converge. For example, Schwartz et al. (who argue strongly for the constructionist viewpoint) state that ideal types provide a unified view of a disorder through definition of the interrelations of its attributes, whereas Davis and Millon (who advocate scientific realism) state that theories provide coherence by integrating components in a logical, consistent, and intelligible manner. Clearly, these views have much in common. Moreover, all but the most ardent constructionists acknowledge that their concepts have some basis in reality, while only the most arrogant of scientific realists would suggest that we can ever be certain that there is an objective reality that we can know. Nevertheless, the philosophical differences between constructionism and realism reflect rather different attitudes regarding the relation between theory and empirical reality.

For example, as constructionists, Schwartz et al. argue that it is fruitless to ask whether the particular classification model one adopts "represents reality" (Chapter 21, p. 420); rather, they state that a system must be judged on the basis of its utility, which may vary for different purposes. These authors emphasize that this is not an endorsement of subjectivism, because it is also important for constructs to be open to modification based on empirical observation. Nevertheless, they stress the active and creative role of the scientist in selecting the data (from which concepts are constructed) to be observed.

On the other hand, speaking as scientific realists, Davis and Millon state that the dream is to be freed from "representational blinders" and to know "the inner essences of reality" (Chapter 18, p. 378), which in the case of personality disorder is "the substantive structural and functional variables which comprise personology and its nexus with psychopathology" (Chapter 18, p. 378). To be sure, it is acknowledged that constructs have their "origins in the mind of a reflective scientist" (Chapter 18, p. 381). Moreover, there is the recognition that all such human constructions may fall short of an ideal taxonomy that represents nature as it is. Yet it is also clear that the goal is nonetheless a classification system that captures the "true" state of nature.

Schwartz et al. thus appear to endorse a scientific relativism or pragmatism, whereas Davis and Millon seek to know an absolute truth. The essential difference between these two positions is well captured by Schwartz et al.'s statement that "A form of categorization is a means to an end, and that end may not be simply the depiction of reality" (Chapter 21, p. 420). In response, Davis and Millon might well reply that "only just such a taxonomy [i.e., with true validity] will prove ultimately scientifically satisfying . . . to the researchers and clinicians who must work inside it" (Chapter 18, p. 379).

Given that both the constructionists' and realists' stances are rather abstract, perhaps even esoteric, it is worth pondering what effect (if any) such philosophical differences would have on the way in which personality disorder researchers conduct their work. Consider, for example, Schwartz et al.'s statement that ideal types serve only as "a kind of 'theory' " (Chapter 21, p. 425) because they do not provide a conceptual representation of reality that is either true or false, but only one that is helpful or unhelpful in further investigations. In their view, different forms of categorization are actually required, because reality consists of an "infinite multiplicity" of data, from which scientists select a limited set on which to focus (Chapter 21, p. 422). By contrast, Davis and Millon advocate an approach in which one of the fundamental questions is "Why these categories rather than others?" (Chapter 18, p. 391). That is, the theory itself must include an intrinsic justification for the very selection of categories or types that it seeks to explain. According to Davis and Millon, anything else is a "pseudoscience that provides a service to the larger society, establishing diagnostic standards according to extrinsic standards" (Chapter 18, p. 392).

It is easy to imagine that researchers who hold the former view would be more content working to improve the external validity of an established nosological framework, whereas those espousing the latter would be more likely to pursue their own theoretical vision. Moreover, in conducting empirical studies to test current categories, constructionist researchers would probably argue (e.g., as does Kendler, 1990) that validity itself is pluralistic rather than a monolithic entity. For example, suppose that one type of validator (e.g., clinical course) supports a certain conceptualization of a disorder, while another type (e.g., genetic similarity data) supports a different conceptualization of the same disorder. Scientific constructionists might not feel compelled to choose between these apparently conflicting data, but could argue that each conceptualization "represents reality *from a particular intellectual point of view*" (Schwartz et al., Chapter 21, p. 420; emphasis in original). By contrast, to researchers espousing a scientific realist approach, these data present a conceptual challenge. Because neither conceptualization can account fully for the data produced by the two types of validators, the theory itself must be changed through the generation of new constructs and the elimination or modification of others.

## SCIENTIFIC CLASSIFICATION AND PSYCHOMETRIC THEORY

As mentioned earlier, the parallels between taxonomic development and construct validation are compelling, and Jackson and Livesley explicitly embrace Loevinger's (1957) construct validation approach in their discussion. Again, as intimated earlier, the essence of this approach is that there are three essential components to the delineation, measurement, and validation of any complex construct: substantive, structural, and external. Loevinger argues that the division of validity into four types (content, concurrent, predictive, and construct) carries the disturbing implication that each stands on its own, rather than that they exist in some logical relation to one another. Moreover, each type of validity has tended to become attached to different types of constructs. For example, measures of achievement emphasize content validity, whereas constructs of specific aptitudes may focus on criterion validity. In contrast, Loevinger insists that all types of validity are subordinate to construct validity and that each must be considered in the validation of a construct.

Beginning with the substantive component, Loevinger places considerable emphasis on content validity. Quite reasonably, she notes that it is far easier to cull features that are shown empirically to be unrelated to a construct than it is to evaluate at some later point whether there are essential features that are missing. Thus, one of her major points is that the initial conceptualization of a construct should be sufficiently broad as to encompass all reasonable possibilities, and that the set of exemplars developed to represent the construct should reflect this breadth.

This concern is echoed both by Jackson and Livesley and by Shea, who also emphasize the importance of developing adequate criterion sets based on clearly defined constructs for personality disorders. Interestingly, whereas in earlier writings Livesley and Jackson (1992) have advocated reliance on aggregated expert opinion for the formulation of diagnostic content, in Chapter 23 they seem to argue for a more strongly data-based approach. Specifically, they question whether the set of DSM diagnoses organize the features of personality disorders optimally, whereas previously they were willing to rely on "systematic samples of experts . . . to identify the diagnostic construct that they consider important" (Livesley & Jackson, 1992, p. 613). Their earlier approach seems more similar to Schwartz et al.'s constructionist model, whereas the stance of their current chapter shares the view espoused by Davis and Millon that "one cannot merely accept any list of kinds or dimensions as given, even if it has been arrived at by committee consensus" (Chapter 18, p. 391).

What guiding principles, then, should be used to formulate the particular set of personality disorders to be studied further? Jackson and Livesley note that the current situation—in which the disorders have different theoretical origins—is difficult to test scientifically. Yet no fully articulated theoretical model exists, so a more completely theoretical approach (as Davis and Millon appear to advocate), in which the criterion sets are derived from prior postulated dimensions, seems premature. It is noteworthy that in the more theoretical sections of their chapter Jackson and Livesley express ideas quite close to Davis and Millon's ideal (in particular regarding the structural component of a classification system for personality disorders), but their empirical explorations are less abstract and more closely tied to what Davis and Millon term "sense-near representations." This blend of theory and data seems in harmony with the spirit of construct validity.

In this context, it is relevant to note Blashfield and McElroy's description of the three ways that the term "hierarchy" has been used in personality disorder research. Although they do not use this terminology in their chapters (cf. Livesley & Jackson, 1992), both Jackson and Livesley and Shea support a view of personality disorders consistent with the second meaning described in the Blashfield and McElroy chapter—that is, hierarchy as "nested dimensions." In this view, trait exemplars form the lowest level of the hierarchy; together they define a trait dimension at the next higher level. Typically, the trait dimensions will be identified on the basis of the covariation of their exemplars (Watson, Clark, & Harkness, 1994). Trait dimensions, in turn, may jointly define the next hierarchical level of diagnostic constructs. Blashfield and McElroy note that if this higher hierarchical level is also identified on the basis of trait covariation, then the emergent constructs should be labeled as dimensions rather than categories.

It is important to note, however, that nested hierarchical models are not necessarily dimensional, as the example of hysterical/histrionic personality offered by Schwartz et al. illustrates. In their view, a diagnosis may consist essentially of a single core trait at the highest level of the hierarchy that provides the unified concept for the diagnosis. What appear to be other, phenotypically distinct characteristics of the disorder are then viewed as lower-order manifestations of the core trait.

An advantage of the trait dimensional hierarchical model, in which the different traits composing each diagnosis are defined and assessed separately, is that it is open to empirical testing and to the possibility of revision of the underlying constructs based on data. The existence of discrete personality disorders may be confirmed or disconfirmed using a trait dimensional approach. Thus, a categorical model of personality disorders is compatible with, but neither dictated nor rejected by, trait dimensional models.

In Davis and Millon's terminology, trait dimensional models represent descriptive empirical approaches with more emphasis on "sense-near representation" than more theoretical models. Although Davis and Millon eschew descriptive approaches as typically not engaging theoretical reflection (and it must be admitted that trait dimensional models have no *a priori* explanatory value in the sense of being able to answer Davis and Millon's question "Why these categories rather than others?"), rejection of theory is not a necessary aspect of a trait dimensional approach. For example, Tellegen and Waller (in press) describe a comprehensive approach to personality test construction, in which there is continual interplay between theory and data. Moreover, Tellegen (1993) — himself a long-time researcher of trait dimensions — has raised the question of whether the dimensions of the five-factor model are "real" in the way that the scientific realist uses the terms, or have only heuristic value in the constructionist sense of constructs.

Given the concern that we are still quite ignorant with regard to the structure of personality disorders, adopting an approach that is somewhat closer to behavioral observation — but still is capable of offering a low-level theoretical framework on which to base the development of more complex taxonomies — would appear to strike a reasonable balance between mindless empiricism and abstract theory, while still providing input for those who would proceed to the diagnostic level via clinical consensus. This seems to be the thrust of Jackson and Livesley's modal profile analysis, as well as of Shea's general approach.

In this context, it is interesting to consider the five-factor dimensional model advocated by Widiger and Sanderson. This model, described by Davis and Millon as a "descriptive polytaxonic empirical approach" (Chapter 18, p. 387), has an interesting measurement history. It first emerged from attempts to systematize the trait terms in the English language — an approach that can be termed "bottom up," as the original data of common-language terms are low on the structural hierarchy of personality constructs (Watson et al., 1994). As the model gained in prominence, assessment measures were developed directly on the basis of broad, general conceptualizations of the factors (e.g., Costa & McCrae, 1985), with the subsequent application of a "top-down" approach by the elaboration of the lower, "facet" level of the trait domains (Costa & McCrae, 1992).

It is interesting to speculate as to how much this latter step was initiated because of data indicating that the highest level of the hierarchy (i.e., the five factors themselves) had less explanatory power with regard to such phenomena as personality disorders than did the lower-order, facet level (or other instruments directly assessing lower-order, primary traits). That is, Loevinger's third component of construct validity — the external component—may have played a role in this development. Many of the traditional methods of validation (e.g., hypothesized group mean differences, convergent and discriminant validity with other measure of the diagnostic construct, concurrent validity correlations with relevant variables, and predictive validity in terms of course and outcome) are incorporated in the external component. Establishing the external component of construct validity involves elaboration of the broader network in which the diagnostic construct is embedded. It is interesting that there is little argument about the relevance and importance of this aspect of validity. As mentioned earlier, researchers with different philosophical positions regarding the reality of diagnostic constructs would take rather different stances in response to the emergence of conflicting data, but no one argues that inconsistencies can be ignored.

## TOWARD A SCIENTIFIC CLASSIFICATION OF PERSONALITY DISORDER

The chapters in this section discuss a range of philosophical issues relevant to future developments in the classification of personality disorder. Moreover, although different approaches have been advocated, there is general agreement that the development of a theoretical basis for personality disorders is important to advance the field; it is further agreed that this theory should be consistent with our knowledge base and sufficiently explicit as to be empirically testable. In contrast, the DSM-IV is touted as more empirically based than its predecessors—utilizing research findings through a three-part process of literature reviews, data reanalyses, and focused field trials—but there is little or no mention of theory in the development of the DSM-IV.

Although it is to be hoped that the revisions incorporated into DSM-IV process will increase the validity of some criteria sets and document more clearly the existing validity of others, the overall impact of these revisions is as yet unclear, especially in the absence of a theoretical framework within which to consider the available data. The fact remains that a relatively small proportion of the reviewed literature has evaluated the diagnostic criteria in relation to any alternatives (Frances et al., 1990). Without consideration of alternative criteria, validity can be enhanced only by eliminating poor criteria, not by adding valuable new ones. Moreover, most of the reviewed research has addressed issues only of convergent and not also of discriminant validity; that is, relatively few studies considered a diagnosis in the context of the entire domain of personality disorders, in order to determine whether the phenomenon of interest was specific to the target diagnosis or shared across multiple diagnoses. The potential improvement in the DSM-IV diagnostic criteria based on the accumulated research is limited by these research biases. The data reanalyses and especially the field trials are less subject to these biases, but they represent a small subset of the full panoply of diagnoses; for example, from Axis II, only antisocial personality disorder was included in the field trials.

It is heartening that—despite continued recognition of the multiple uses to which the DSMs are put—the emphasis in DSM-IV is "on explicit documentation and review of evidence" (Frances et al., 1990, p. 1440). Nevertheless, we must guard against the possibility that this emphasis "will degenerate into pseudoscience, in which we pretend to be 'objective' and 'empirical' when, in reality, we are making informed value judgments" (Kendler, 1990, p. 972). In the language of the current set of chapters, we must be concerned that the DSM-IV process may be largely one of naive empiricism, which believes that "what you see is what you get" (Davis & Millon, Chapter 18, p. 382). It is likely that this increased emphasis on empirical data will impart to the new manual a greater degree of scientific respectability. Let us hope that it does not simultaneously foster further mindless acceptance of the diagnoses and their criteria, but that the ideas set forth in this section will gain an audience interested in pursuing more basic taxonomic questions that are grounded in theory, as well as in improving diagnoses through micromanagement at the criterial level.

## REFERENCES

American Psychiatric Association. (1987). *Diagnostic and statistical manual of mental disorders* (3rd ed., rev.). Washington, DC: Author.

American Psychiatric Association. (1994). *Diagnostic and statistical manual of mental disorders* (4th ed.). Washington, DC: Author.

Clark, L. A. (in press). Dimensional approaches to personality disorder assessment and diagnosis. In C. R. Cloninger (Ed.), *Personality and psychopathology*. Washington, DC: American Psychiatric Press.

Costa, P. T. Jr., & McCrae, R. R. (1985). *The NEO Personality Inventory manual*. Odessa, FL: Psychological Assessment Resources.

Costa, P. T. Jr., & McCrae, R. R. (1992). *Revised NEO Personality Inventory (NEO-PI-R) and NEO Five-Factor Inventory (NEO-FFI) professional manual*. Odessa, FL: Psychological Assessment Resources.

Cronbach, L. J., & Meehl, P. E. (1955). Construct validity in psychological tests. *Psychological Bulletin, 52*, 281–302.

Frances, A. J., Pincus, H. A., Widiger, T. A., Davis, W. W., & First, M. B. (1990). DSM-IV: Work in progress. *American Journal of Psychiatry, 147*, 1439–1448.

Kendler, K. S. (1990). Toward a scientific psychiatric nosology: Strengths and limitations. *Archives of General Psychiatry, 47*, 969–973.

Livesley, W. J., & Jackson, D. N. (1992). Guidelines for developing, evaluating, and revising the classification of personality disorders. *Journal of Nervous and Mental Disease, 180*, 609–618.

Loevinger, J. (1957). Objective tests as instruments of psychological theory. *Psychological Reports, 3*, 635–694.

Tellegen, A. (1993). Folk concepts and psychological concepts of personality and personality disorder. *Psychological Inquiry, 4*, 122–130.

Tellegen, A., & Waller, N. (in press). Exploring personality through test construction: Development of the Multidimensional Personality Questionnaire. In S. R. Briggs & J. M. Cheek (Eds.), *Personality measures: Development and evaluation* (Vol. 1). Greenwich, CT: JAI Press.

Watson, D., Clark, L. A., & Harkness, A. (1994). Structures of personality and their relevance to the study of psychopathology. *Journal of Abnormal Psychology, 103,* 18–31.

Weinberg, S. (1992). *Dreams of a final theory.* New York: Pantheon.

Widiger, T. A. (1992). Categorical versus dimensional classification: Implications from and for research. *Journal of Personality Disorders, 6,* 287–300.

Widiger, T. A., & Frances, A. J. (1994). Towards a dimensional model of personality disorders. In P. T. Costa Jr. & T. A. Widiger (Eds.). *Personality disorders and the five-factor model of personality* (pp. 19–39). Washington, DC: American Psychological Association.

# CHAPTER 25

# Past Achievements
# and Future Directions

W. JOHN LIVESLEY

When we look back at the progress that has occurred in the study of personality disorder since DSM-III was published (American Psychiatric Association, 1980), it is apparent that the field has in a sense come of age. In the late 1970s, when DSM-III was under development, it was rare to open a major journal to find an empirical paper on the subject. Although psychiatrists had long recognized the clinical importance of personality disorders, this recognition was rarely translated into empirical inquiry. Now such articles are commonplace, and it will not have escaped the reader's attention that most of the empirical work cited in this volume was conducted in the 1980s and 1990s. Much of the credit for this change belongs to DSM-III. The decision to place personality diagnoses on a separate axis forced the recognition that these are important clinical conditions that are frequently encountered in everyday practice. At the same time, the decision to develop explicit diagnostic criteria as for other mental disorders encouraged empirical research. The main innovation of DSM-III-R (American Psychiatric Association, 1987) was the introduction of more specific behavioral criteria. DSM-IV (American Psychiatric Association, 1994) has consolidated these advances and introduced important changes into the revision process.

## ACHIEVEMENTS AND ADVANCES OF DSM-IV

The initial decision that revisions introduced in DSM-IV would be conservative left little room for radical changes or for the introduction of alternative taxonomic principles. Only minor changes in criteria sets and the addition or elimination of the occasional diagnosis were possible. The result is that the DSM-IV system differs little from its predecessor and contains little that is new or innovative, so that those looking for more fundamental changes will be disappointed with the results of the Personality Disorders Work Group's deliberations. It could be argued, however, that the current state of knowledge does not justify more fundamental change, and that all that was appropriate was some fine-tuning of the system. If this is the case, DSM-IV has certainly attained its objectives. Diagnoses are more clearly defined, criteria are more precise, and some ambiguities have been resolved.

But DSM-IV has also introduced some important changes, the most significant being the extensive use of systematic reviews of the literature and reanalyses of empirical data. The work group's insistence that changes be based on empirical data, although an obvious requirement, was an important affirmation of the importance of information gained through the routine application of scientific methodology. This consolidates the advance that DSM-III made in moving the study of personality disorders from the intuitive domain to that of explicit criteria sets and systematic empirical analysis. Although the impact on DSM-IV has not been extensive, this requirement sets the stage for a data-based classification in the future. In retrospect, this may well be seen to be the most important contribution of DSM-IV to the classification of personality disorders.

The use of systematic reviews of the empirical literature is also important because it has begun the process of depoliticizing the classification of mental disorders. All too often in the past, the structure and contents of psychiatric classifications have involved compromise among the requirements and demands of different influence groups. Although compromise is perhaps necessary at some stages in the evolution of classifications that seek to gain widespread acceptance, this is obviously not the way to develop a scientific system. Insistence that revisions and changes be justified on the basis of empirical data reduces the impact of lobby groups and personal opinion on the nature and contents of a classification. Again, this bodes well for the future of classification and classification research.

Because the DSM-IV classification differs so little from DSM-III-R, it possesses the same strengths and suffers from the same limitations. As many of the authors in this volume note, the classification of personality disorders is far from resolved, and there are some formidable taxonomic challenges to overcome before we have a valid system. It may be useful to remind ourselves of some of these problems, because they will set the agenda for DSM-V.

## LIMITATIONS OF DSM-IV

### Descriptive Limitations

A shortcoming of DSM-IV—and perhaps the greatest obstacle to progress in the study of personality disorders—is the failure to provide an agreed-upon nomenclature to describe the basic traits that constitute personality disorders (see Shea, Chapter 19). What is needed is a personality disorder equivalent to the lexicons available to describe the phenomenology of mental state disorders, such as the glossary to DSM or the lexicon for use with the Present State Examination (Wing, Cooper, & Sartorius, 1974). In general, the importance of description has not been recognized in the study of personality disorders. Whereas classical texts on psychopathology contain detailed definitions and descriptions of the phenomenology of mental state disorders, the literature on personality disorders relies on everyday language. The availability of a wide variety of descriptive terms in natural language seems to have created the impression that a systematic nomenclature is unnecessary. Consequently, the basic features of personality disorders remain undefined, causing confusion about the meaning of terms such as "identity disturbance" and "impulsivity" that reduces diagnostic reliability. Description, however, is fundamental to classification (Livesley, 1991), and implementation of Shea's recommendation that the basic constructs underlying personality disorders be specified and defined would provide a more solid basis for empirical research and theory development.

Linked to the need for a standard nomenclature is the problem of content validity. Content validity was a problem with both DSM-III and DSM-III-R (Blashfield & Breen, 1989; Blashfield & Haymaker, 1990; Livesley, Reiffer, Sheldon, & West, 1987); the use of similar methods to develop DSM-IV, and the failure to adopt standard procedures to evaluate content validity, do not instill confidence that the problem has been addressed. Indeed, commentators in this volume question the content validity of specific diagnoses (see, e.g., Hare & Hart's commentary on Chapter 6). But the limitations of DSM-IV as a descriptive system are not confined to poor content validity. The diagnoses and criteria listed on Axis II are too heterogeneous in content, too variable in breadth of content, too poorly defined, and overlap too much to meet the requirements of measurement and theory construction.

## Categorical Model

A fundamental problem with DSM-IV noted in most of the commentaries on specific diagnoses is the continued use of a categorical model. This, more than anything else, limits the value of DSM-IV for research purposes. It also creates pseudoproblems such as diagnostic overlap that continue to exercise investigators' attention. As Blashfield and McElroy point out in Chapter 20, the problem of whether personality disorders should be classified according to a dimensional or a categorical model is more complex than most discussions acknowledge. Nevertheless, the simple categorical model adopted by DSM-IV is not supported by empirical research. The results of all relevant studies consistently support a dimensional model of phenotypic traits of personality disorders (Livesley, Schroeder, Jackson, & Jang, 1994). Ultimately, the DSM system will have to incorporate these empirical data.

## Problems of Political Influence and Philosophical Bias

In many ways, the DSM-IV classification of personality disorders is more like a political or philosophical statement than a scientific classification. Reliance on the consensus of experts as revealed during committee deliberations is not in itself a problem, although (as Widiger and Sanderson note in Chapter 22) this approach only works well when the phenomena of a disorder are easily identified and an extensive body of empirical information exists. Rather, problems arise because the basic assumptions on which the system depends are not stated explicitly in the ways expected of a scientific system, and because all too often philosophical and political positions rather than empirical data determine the decisions about diagnoses and criteria.

Although an attempt was made to remedy some of these problems when compiling DSM-IV by attempting to ensure that decisions were based as far as possible on empirical data, the decision to be conservative and to rely largely on committee processes compromised the advances that could have been made. The impact of prior assumptions on specific diagnoses is clearly illustrated in regard to antisocial personality disorder by Hare and Hart's commentary on Chapter 6. Preliminary decisions about the conceptualization of the disorder led to studies that served to perpetuate the earlier concept rather than to explore alternative conceptualizations.

At a more fundamental level philosophical positions about the nature of mental disorders—especially the neo-Kraepelinian position that mental disorders are discrete entities—imposed a rigid structure on the classification. This preconception reduced the impact of empirical findings, especially those relating to the issue of dimensional versus categorical models, and minimized the extent to which the committee drew upon the results of decades of research on normal personality structure. Indeed, in instances where empirical data conflict with implicit philosophical assumptions, it is difficult to escape the conclusion that unstated presuppositions determined the outcome. Perhaps this was and is inevitable with a system that has to meet diverse needs and satisfy diverse groups, but nevertheless it has reduced the DSM-IV classification's scientific value and resulted in a system that is more severely flawed than necessary, given the current state of knowledge.

## Reliance on Arbitrary or Semantic Rather than Behavioral Distinctions

A consequence of the assumption of discrete disorders is that DSM-IV has been forced to make arbitrary decisions that are inconsistent with the data, or subtle semantic distinctions, in order to differentiate between disorders. The arbitrary nature of some decisions is seen in the way the final criteria set for antisocial personality disorder was determined. Widiger and Corbitt (Chapter 6) have reported:

Two of the items with content unique to the PCL-R ("lacks empathy" and "inflated and arrogant self-appraisal") were significantly associated with the DSM-III-R antisocial personality disorder diagnosis and with the external validators of antisocial personality disorder (e.g., clinicians' and interviewers' impressions and the self-report measures of antisocial personality disorder/psychopathy), but these items are included within the DSM-III-R criteria for narcissistic personality disorder. The field trial suggested that their inclusion within the DSM-IV antisocial personality disorder criteria set would increase the overlap of the antisocial and narcissistic personality disorders and complicate their differentiation." (p. 119)

Empirical data consistently show that some "narcissistic" features are associated with antisocial personality disorder. To ignore this empirical fact leads to a system that differentiates among diagnoses on paper but not in practice. The result is a classification with boundaries between disorders that are largely artificial.

## FUTURE DIRECTIONS

### Conceptual Analysis

It is probable that the most important contributions to the study of personality disorders in the immediate future will be conceptual and theoretical in nature. Although the progress made in establishing empirical research during the last two decades has provided a refreshing counterbalance to the earlier emphasis on clinical report, there has been a tendency to rely on "blind" empiricism to an untoward degree. The use of systematic reviews of the empirical literature for DSM-IV was a positive advance that needs to be buttressed in DSM-V with conceptual and theoretical analysis.

To this point, conceptual research and empirical studies guided by theoretical considerations have been rare. Yet the problems that confront classification studies are largely conceptual in nature. The decision to include depressive personality disorder in the appended diagnoses highlights many of these conceptual problems by raising multiple questions about the definition of personality disorders, the relationship between personality disorders and other mental disorders, the grounds for differentiating between axes, and the relationship of personality disorders to fundamental dimensions of personality such as neuroticism. These issues are not unique to depressive personality disorder, and it is unlikely that much further progress will be made toward developing a valid classification until they have been addressed more successfully. Unfortunately, however, conceptual analysis of the depth required is not popular. It is difficult to fund, and it does not generate information that is readily published. A further difficulty is that the DSM process for formulating the classification is not structured in a way that encourages a detailed analysis of fundamental problems.

Nevertheless, these problems are inescapable, and the direction that empirical research is likely to take over the next decade will undoubtedly bring them to the fore. The increasing use of data-based dimensional models in clinical research and routine clinical evaluation, for example, will force a reappraisal of the distinctions among personality disorder, normal personality, and other mental disorders. If the features of personality disorder are described as a profile of scores on a series of quantitatively variable dimensions, such questions as what constitutes a personality disorder, how normal and disordered personalities differ, and the distinction between personality disorders and other mental disorders become inescapable.

## Distinction between Axis I and Axis II

The fundamental distinction that the DSM system makes between personality disorders and Axis I disorders is one conceptual issue that is likely to receive increasing scrutiny. DSM-III did not provide a convincing rationale for the distinction. It was justified initially on the pragmatic grounds that it was necessary to emphasize personality disorders because they were likely to be overlooked in the presence of more florid Axis I disorders. Possible reasons for asserting that there are fundamental differences between personality disorders and other mental disorders include etiology, form and nature of psychopathology, and temporal stability. Recent empirical studies raise doubts about the validity of these ideas (Livesley et al., 1994).

Twin studies indicating a large genetic component in the traits of personality disorders (Kendler & Hewitt, 1992; Livesley, Jang, Jackson, & Vernon, 1993) and other studies have identified substantial neurochemical and physiological correlates (Siever & Davis, 1991). Thus there is currently no reason to believe that the etiology of personality disorders differs in any fundamental way from that of other mental disorders. Similarly, there do not appear to be fundamental differences in phenomenology or temporal stability between the two groups of disorders.

For these reasons, it will be necessary to reconsider the distinction between Axis I and Axis II. One possible reconceptualization that warrants attention would involve the inclusion of personality disorders on Axis I along with other mental disorders, and retention of Axis II to code personality traits (Livesley et al, 1994).

## Alternative Models

As noted several times in this volume, alternative ways to represent personality disorders are only just beginning to be explored in detail. Disenchantment with the categorical model of DSM has led to increased interest in dimensional models. As Clark has noted in Chapter 24, simply converting DSM diagnoses into dimensions is unlikely to meet the mounting criticism of the categorical approach. The problem is not only that a categorical model is not consistent with the data, but also that the features of personality disorders do not appear to be organized into the patterns suggested by DSM. For this reason, models based on a well-established structural representation of normal personality traits (e.g., the five-factor model), or derived specifically from analyses of the traits describing the personality disorder domain, are more promising. Given the empirical evidence to date, there appears little doubt that future classifications will incorporate some type of dimensional system. It may not, however, be a purely dimensional model, because as Blashfield and McElroy have noted (Chapter 20), dimensional and categorical models are not incompatible.

Prior to compilation of DSM-V, it would be extremely useful if information were available from studies comparing the goodness of fit of different models across different measures and samples, so that an informed decision about the type of system to adopt could be made on the basis of empirical data. Comparisons need to be made among categorical, dimensional, and mixed models. Each of these types of model has measurement implications that can be evaluated empirically. Thus far evaluations of different models have been limited and largely confined to comparisons between simple dimensional and simple categorical structures. More complex models that attempt to identify dimensional types based on a profile of trait dimensions have only recently begun to receive attention. These approaches are especially interesting because they retain the practical advantages of categories or types within a dimensional framework that offers a better representation of the basic data. Investigations of this type depend upon reliable and valid instruments to assess the basic constructs or dimensions associated with personality disorder. Structured interviews that assess DSM-IV criteria sets will need to be supplemented with broader-based instruments with superior psychometric properties.

## Functional Analysis of Personality Disorders

The major focus of empirical evaluation of personality disorders has been descriptive and taxonomic. Attention has been focused on the structural aspects of Axis II in order to establish reliable and efficient diagnostic criteria. Classification, however, has much to gain from an analysis of the dysfunction associated with a diagnosis of personality disorder. Although DSM defines personality disorders in terms of inflexible and maladaptive traits that result in impaired social or occupational functioning, relatively little attention has been paid to systematic analysis of this impairment. The concept of personality disorders implies that impairment is stable across a wide variety of situations and over substantial periods of time, but we know little about the stability of these behaviors or about the ways they are influenced by circumstances. This type of information will be central to establishing a satisfactory definition of personality disorders and to the establishment of diagnostic validity. A start has been made with work on the cognitions associated with personality disorder diagnoses (Beck, Freeman, & Associates, 1990), and this promises to be a fruitful line of inquiry with clinical and taxonomic implications.

## CONCLUSIONS

When one reviews the substantial changes in the field since DSM-III was published, any sense of achievement is tempered by disappointment with what has actually been achieved. The increase in scientific knowledge has been limited, and, as the chapters and commentaries in this volume amply demonstrate, minimal progress has been made toward resolving the basic problems that confronted the field when DSM-III was first compiled. Curiously, DSM itself seems to have contributed to these limited accomplishments. The powerful impact of DSM-III not only stimulated empirical research but also shaped the research agenda. Research has concentrated on the contents of the DSM system, particularly evaluation of criteria sets. Rarely have more fundamental issues been addressed or has research been conducted using alternative approaches and concepts. The well-deserved status of DSM has led to uncritical acceptance of Axis II diagnoses and criteria sets, which have achieved a degree of credibility that is not warranted by the somewhat arbitrary manner in which Axis II was compiled. When investigators have been critical, they still have tended to operate within the system; investigations of alternative approaches are uncommon.

The danger is that DSM-IV will ossify the classification of personality disorders at a premature stage. It is perhaps paradoxical that the force that led to growth in interest in personality disorders now threatens to become an impediment to the evolution of the field. The decision to adopt a conservative approach when considering the changes to introduce in DSM-IV may well intensify the problem. The minor revisions will mean that the results of research conducted on the basis of DSM-III-R criteria sets will probably not generalize to diagnoses based on DSM-IV criteria sets, and this is likely to encourage replication of earlier studies using the new criteria, with minimal benefits.

The classification, and hence the study, of personality disorders are at something of a crossroads. The DSM approach (and that of the *International Classification of Diseases* as well), based on discrete diagnoses and committee-generated diagnostic criteria, has probably been taken to its limits. Indeed, it could be argued that all the advantages that accrue from this approach were probably realized with DSM-III-R and that DSM-IV's main contribution is procedural. If one can predict anything with any confidence, it is that future classifications—especially those used for research purposes—will look very different. Already empirical research has begun to leapfrog DSM-IV, with the increasing use of dimensional models based on constructs that are very different from DSM diagnoses. Categorical models, if retained, will differ from the simple polythetic model of DSM-IV. More complex models (such as typal models based on trait dimensions) have been discussed for some time, and they are just beginning to find their way into empirical studies. These developments promise to be more in accord with empirical data and to provide a more satisfactory representation of the complexity of personality phenomena. They also hold the hope of integrating empirical observation and theory development. These developments are encouraging; the study of personality disorders is in a healthy state, and the field is growing rapidly. Although it is likely that DSM-IV will be left behind, it is important to recall that DSM-III, DSM-III-R, and DSM-IV were what provided the stimulus for the empirical research that will lead to their successor. This is a fine achievement—indeed, all that can be expected from a classification.

## REFERENCES

American Psychiatric Association. (1980). *Diagnostic and statistical manual of mental disorders* (3rd ed.). Washington, DC: Author.

American Psychiatric Association. (1987). *Diagnostic and statistical manual of mental disorders* (3rd ed., rev.). Washington, DC: Author.

American Psychiatric Association. (1994). *Diagnostic and statistical manual of mental disorders* (4th ed.). Washington, DC: Author.

Blashfield, R. K., & Breen, M. (1989). Face validity of the DSM-III-R personality disorders. *American Journal of Psychiatry, 146,* 1575–1579.

Blashfield, R. K., & Haymaker, D. (1990). A prototype analysis of the diagnostic criteria for DSM-III-R personality disorders. *Journal of Personality Disorders, 2,* 272–280.

Beck, A. T., Freeman, A., & Associates. (1990). *Cognitive therapy of personality disorders.* New York: Guilford Press.

Kendler, K. S., & Hewitt, J. (1992). The structure of self-report schizotypy in twins. *Journal of Personality Disorders, 6,* 1–17.

Livesley, W. J. (1991). Classifying personality disorders: Ideal types, prototypes, or dimensions? *Journal of Personality Disorders, 5,* 52–59.

Livesley, W. J., Jang, K. L., Jackson, D. N., & Vernon, P. A. (1993). Genetic and environmental contributions of dimensions of personality disorder. *American Journal of Psychiatry, 150,* 1826–1831.

Livesley, W. J., Reiffer, L. I., Sheldon, A. E. R., & West, M. (1987). Prototypicality ratings of DSM-III criteria for personality disorders. *Journal of Nervous and Mental Disease, 175,* 395–401.

Livesley, W. J., Schroeder, M. L., Jackson, D. N., & Jang, K. L. (1994). Categorical distinctions in the study of personality disorder: Implications for classification. *Journal of Abnormal Psychology, 103,* 6–17.

Siever, L. J., & Davis, K. L. (1991). A psychobiological perspective on personality disorders. *American Journal of Psychiatry, 148,* 1647–1658.

Wing, J. K., Cooper, J. E., & Sartorius, N. (1974). *The description and classification of psychiatric symptoms: An instruction manual for the PSE and Catego system.* London: Cambridge University Press.

# Index